# Student Quick Tips

Use this Student Quick Tips guide for a quick and easy start with McGraw-Hill Connect. You'll get valuable tips on registering, doing assignments, and accessing resources, as well as information about the support center hours.

## Getting Started

**TIP:** To get started in Connect, you will need the following:

* Your instructor's Connect Web Address

  Sample of Connect Web Address:

  http://www.mcgrawhillconnect.com/class/instructorname_section_name

* Connect Access Code

**TIP:** If you do not have an access code or have not yet secured your tuition funds, you can click "Free Trial" during registration. This trial will provide temporary Connect access (typically three weeks) and will remind you to purchase online access before the end of your trial.

## Registration and Sign In

1. Go to the Connect Web Address provided by your instructor
2. Click on **Register Now**
3. Enter your email address

**TIP:** If you already have a McGraw-Hill account, you will be asked for your password and will not be required to create a new account.

4. Enter a registration code or choose **Buy Online** to purchase access online

5. Follow the on-screen directions

**TIP:** Please choose your Security Question and Answer carefully. We will ask you for this information if you forget your password.

6. When registration is complete, click on **Go to Connect Now**

7. You are now ready to use **Connect**

## Trouble Logging In?

- Ensure you are using the same email address you used during registration

- If you have forgotten your password, click on the "Forgot Password?" link at your Instructor's Connect Course Web Address

- When logged into Connect, you can update your account information (e.g. email address, password, and security question/answer) by clicking on the *"My Account"* link located at the top-right corner

## Home (Assignments)

**TIP:** If you are unable to begin an assignment, verify the following:

- The assignment is available (start and due dates)

- That you have not exceeded the maximum number of attempts

- That you have not achieved a score of 100%

- If your assignment contains questions that require manual grading, you will not be able to begin your next attempt until your instructor has graded those questions

**TIP:** Based on the assignment policy settings established by your Instructor, you may encounter the following limitations when working on your assignment(s):

* Ability to Print Assignment

* Timed assignments – once you begin a "*timed assignment*," the timer will not stop by design

**TIP:** "*Save & Exit*" vs. "*Submit*" button

* If you are unable to complete your assignment in one sitting, utilize the "*Save & Exit*" button to save your work and complete it at a later time

* Once you have completed your assignment, utilize the "*Submit*" button in order for your assignment to be graded

## Library

**TIP:** The *Library* section of your Connect account provides shortcuts to various resources.

* If you purchased ConnectPlus, you will see an *eBook* link, which can also be accessed from the section information widget of the *Home* tab

* *Recorded Lectures* can be accessed if your instructor is using *Tegrity Campus* to capture lectures. You may also access recorded lectures when taking an assignment by clicking on the projector icon in the navigation bar

* Many McGraw-Hill textbooks offer additional resources such as narrated slides and additional problems, which are accessible through the *Student Resources* link

## Reports

**TIP:** Once you submit your assignment, you can view your available results in the *Reports* tab.

- If you see a dash (-) as your score, your instructor has either delayed or restricted your ability to see the assignment feedback

- Your instructor has the ability to limit the amount of information (e.g. questions, answers, scores) you can view for each submitted assignment

## Need More Help?

**CONTACT US ONLINE**

Visit us at:

www.mcgrawhillconnect.com/support

Browse our support materials including tutorial videos and our searchable Connect knowledge base. If you cannot find an answer to your question, click on "Contact Us" button to send us an email.

**GIVE US A CALL**

Call us at:

1-800-331-5094

Our live support is available:

Mon-Thurs:  8 am – 11 pm CT
Friday:     8 am – 6  pm CT
Sunday:     6 pm – 11 pm CT

The School of Applied Physiology at Georgia Tech evolved from the Department of Health and Performance Sciences which was established in 1990. This evolution led to the expansion of a one-laboratory department conducting research primarily in exercise physiology into a multi-laboratory school devoted to the study of all levels of physiological systems as they relate to both basic and applied movement control. In addition, the school now offers two graduate programs, a Master's in Prosthetics and Orthotics as well as a PhD in Applied Physiology.

As we've transitioned, we have managed to keep our dedication to undergraduate students via the Health Concepts and Strategies course as well as through electives offered as part of an undergraduate Certificate in Applied Physiology. These electives include exercise physiology, anatomy and physiology, nutrition and biomechanics.

Though the School of Applied Physiology has grown and now serves multiple roles within the institute, it is still our mission to impress upon undergraduate students the value of positive health behaviors and to arm them with the information and tools to make good choices and implement change to preserve or improve their health. We promote the multidimensional model of health that acknowledges the balance of many areas of one's life, and give students the opportunity to identify the application of this model in their lives. It is our hope that Georgia Tech students will flourish here, that they will accept the responsibility to look after their own health and that they will avail themselves of the numerous campus resources that can support them in this effort.

In Health,

The Faculty of the School of Applied Physiology

Select Chapters from

# iHealth
## AN INTERACTIVE FRAMEWORK

**SECOND EDITION**

### PHILLIP B. SPARLING
Georgia Institute of Technology

### KERRY J. REDICAN
Virginia Polytechnic Institute and State University

With Select Chapters from

# Core Concepts
# in Health

**TWELFTH EDITION**

### PAUL M. INSEL
Stanford University

### WALTON T. ROTH
Stanford University

Custom Edition for Georgia Institute of Technology

 **Learning Solutions**

Boston   Burr Ridge, IL   Dubuque, IA   New York   San Francisco   St. Louis
Bangkok   Bogotá   Caracas   Lisbon   London   Madrid
Mexico City   Milan   New Delhi   Seoul   Singapore   Sydney   Taipei   Toronto

The McGraw·Hill Companies

Select Chapters from
*iHealth: An Interactive Framework*, Second Edition
With Select Chapters from
*Core Concepts in Health*, Twelfth Edition
Custom Edition for Georgia Institute of Technology

This book is a McGraw-Hill Learning Solutions textbook and contains select material from:
*iHealth: An Interactive Framework*, Second Edition by Phillip B. Sparling and Kerry J.
Redican. Copyright © 2013, 2011 by The McGraw-Hill Companies, Inc.
*Core Concepts in Health*, Twelfth Edition by Paul M. Insel and Walton T. Roth.
Copyright © 2012, 2010, 2008, 2006, 2004, 2002, 2000, 1998, 1996, 1994, 1991,
1988, 1985, 1982, 1979, and 1976 by The McGraw-Hill Companies, Inc.
Both reprinted with permission of the publisher. Many custom published texts are
modified versions or adaptations of our best-selling textbooks. Some adaptations are
printed in black and white to keep prices at a minimum, while others are in color.

1 2 3 4 5 6 7 8 9 0 QDB QDB 14 13 12

ISBN-13: 978-0-07-770121-5
ISBN-10: 0-07-770121-6
Part of
ISBN-13: 978-0-07-770122-2
ISBN-10: 0-07-770122-4

*Learning Solutions Consultant: Judson Harper*
*Production Editor: Constance Kuhl*
*Printer/Binder: Quad/Graphics*

contents in brief

# contents in detail

contents in detail

Part III

# contents in detail

# iHealth

## An Interactive Framework

## The *iHealth* Story

iHealth started with instructors like you. Through extensive research, ranging from online surveys to multiday symposia, McGraw-Hill learned that personal health instructors were looking for a new kind of teaching tool—one that provides a framework for efficiently covering key topics in a limited period of time, that offers the flexibility to meet personal instructional goals and student needs, and that effectively engages their students. Phillip Sparling and Kerry Redican, themselves participants in this research, were so enthusiastic about this new type of tool that they decided to build it themselves. The result is iHealth, an integrated print–digital learning system that is engaging, flexible, and innovative so as to meet the needs of today's students and educators.

## You Made *iHealth* Even Better . . .

iHealth improved because of instructors like you. The new edition of iHealth is better because we watched how you use iHealth and listened to what you said about it.

- The **LearnSmart** adaptive assessment program creates personalized study plans for your students, giving them a tool that is shown to improve grades. The new iHealth test bank is aligned with the LearnSmart objectives, improving the way in which you can assess your students' mastery of the concepts.

- New and updated online articles and health assessments are easier to assign and grade. New documentary-style videos called **College Health Reports** provide a relevant, balanced look at issues facing today's college students, such as tattooing and tanning salons.

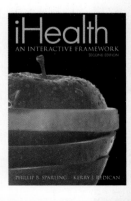

- The **Connect** platform now offers full integration with Blackboard, and through McGraw-Hill Campus, quick and easy integration with *any* course management system. New Connect enhancements also include easy uploading of your own course or assignment-level files, new social networking tools, and improved online performance.

# Why *iHealth* Works

*iHealth* is used by hundreds of instructors and thousands of students because it provides a foundation for building solid research skills, critical thinking skills, and behavior change skills that will enable students to make good decisions and live a more fulfilling life.

## *iHealth* Gives Students What They Want

McGraw-Hill listened to students, who said they want:

- **A concise, accessible book.** iHealth presents essential health concepts in a clear, concise, portable text that is available in print and eBook formats. iHealth is a handbook for a lifetime of health and wellness.
- **Relevant multimedia content.** New videos on tattoing, tanning salons, drinking and driving, and stress explore health-related issues relevant to today's college students. Updated online articles and health risk assessments put concepts in a real-world context, motivating students to think critically, build research skills, and apply what they learn to their own lives.
- **Dynamic personalized learning plans.** LearnSmart for iHealth, an unparalleled adaptive diagnostic tool, makes students aware of their knowledge of a particular subject area and builds an individualized learning plan to help them gain mastery of the material. With LearnSmart, students are able to study more efficiently and effectively, be more informed participants in class discussions, and perform better on quizzes and exams.

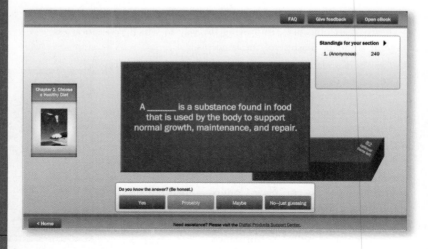

# *iHealth* Gives Instructors What They Need

McGraw-Hill listened to instructors, who said they want:

- **More time.** iHealth's concise 13-chapter framework and auto-graded assignments enable instructors to maximize limited class hours while also providing the flexibility to cover additional topics and themes to fit the needs of their course.

- **Tools to build critical thinking and research skills.** iHealth's rich library of interactive assignments—including online articles, video activities, and health risk assessments—are designed to give instructors the resources to teach their students research skills, critical thinking skills, and behavior change skills that will last a lifetime.

- **Flexibility.** The online components that accompany iHealth, powered by the Connect platform, allow instructors the flexibility to design the course that they want and that best suits their students' needs. Using

Connect, instructors can now upload and create an assignment around any article, video, or podcast of their choice, further enhancing the flexibility of iHealth and providing more opportunities for customization.

■ **Seamless integration with Blackboard.** Through a partnership between McGraw-Hill and Blackboard, the iHealth online components can now be easily and seamlessly integrated with the Blackboard course management system. Among other things, this integration enables Connect activities, assessments, grades, and other content to appear within your university's Blackboard system. Setup is fast, easy, and flexible, and students can access Connect using their university logins.

■ **McGraw-Hill Campus.** Regardless of what course management system your school uses, McGraw-Hill now makes it quick and easy for *all* faculty to find just the right online and digital resources, at no additional cost. McGraw-Hill Campus will provide all faculty and students streamlined access to unlimited digital resources at no additional costs and will enable quick, simple connections between McGraw-Hill Connect and multiple learning management systems.

# Author Acknowledgments

Many people at McGraw-Hill made iHealth possible. A few folks deserve special mention:

Nick Barrett, who shared our vision and began the project in 2004, Chris Johnson who shepherded the project from infancy to graduation, and development editors Erin Strathmann and Emily Pecora who showed finesse and patience from start to finish.

We also gratefully acknowledge Lydia Kim, Briana Porco, Kate Engelberg, Rhona Robbin, Margaret Young, Melanie Field, Jennifer Gordon, Bill Glass, Julie Bickar, Mike Ryan, and Steve Debow. Each helped in different ways, at different points—but all as a team toward our shared goal of seeing iHealth become a reality. Many others unnamed also contributed. Our thanks to all.

Lastly, it's our pleasure to thank a number of our fellow college teachers from across the nation (cited below) for their feedback and insights during the development and production of iHealth. Your contributions are sincerely appreciated.

Phillip B. Sparling
Kerry J. Redican

## Academic Reviewers

Michael Aboussleman
*Kingsborough Community College*

Allen Adeimy
*Glenville State College*

Al Bacchus
*Washington Adventist University*

Camilla Bantum
*Butte Community College*

Jeremy Barnes
*Southeast Missouri State University*

Elizabeth Belzer
*Chabot College*

Francis Bolden
*Washington Adventist University*

Christine Bouffard
*Waubonsee Community College*

Brian Brabham
*University of Mary Hardin–Baylor*

Toby Brooks
*Rend Lake College*

Brenda Bruner
*Nipissing University*

Ni Bueno
*Cerritos College*

Karen Ann V. Cameron
*Alvernia University*

Annette Carrington
*North Carolina Central University*

Claudia Dempsey
*Liberty University*

Char DeSmith Foth
*Hutchinson Community College*

Amber Dills
*Beaufort Community College*

Vickie Dugan
*Porterville College*

Rachelle Duncan
*Oklahoma State University, Institute of Technology*

Paul Finnicum
*Arkansas State University*

Kathleen Flynn
*University of the Cumberlands*

Joseph D. Gar
*West Kentucky Community and Technical College*

Todd Garner
*University of Arkansas–Pine Bluff*

Jessica Gillette
*Central Christian College*

Ronald Glahn
*Porterville College*

Leslie Gollop
*Tallahassee Community College*

Melissa Grim
*Radford University*

Steve Hartman
*Citrus College*

Dina Hayduk
*Kutztown University*

Sharrie Herbold
*Lane Community College*

Sherika Highman
*Tallahassee Community College*

Harold Horn
*Lincoln Land Community College*

Rose Jean-Baptiste
*William Paterson University*

Belinda L. Jones
*North Carolina Central University*

William D. Kernan
*William Paterson University*

Brianne Kilbourne
*Liberty University*

Denise Kreski
*University of Nebraska–Omaha*

Aisha Kudura
*New Mexico State University*

Garry Ladd
*Southwestern Illinois College*

Deneen Long-White
*Howard University*

Greg Lonning
*Luther College*

Deanna Lowe
*Butte Community College*

Elaine Lucas
*Spoon River College*

Shannon Lugaila
*University of Pittsburgh*

Pamela N. Lusk
*Genesee Community College*

Vincent Lyons
*Ohio State University*

Nancy Mankin
*Oral Roberts University*

Darlene Martin
*Liberty University*

Michara Mayes
*Texas Southern University*

Eugene A. McAdoo
*Kaskaskia College*

Dean Mcgovern
*University of Montana*

Jesus Medina
*Gaston College*

Paul Miller
*Bethany University*

Paul Miller
*Kean University*

Gloria C. Moore
*Kingsborough Community College*

Richard Morris
*Rollins College–Winter Park*

Tim Mosby
*St. Louis Community College*

Holly Turner Moses
*University of Florida–Gainesville*

Michelle Ness
*Cecil College*

Craig Newton
*Middle Georgia College*

Brad Odum
*Kaskaskia College*

Kay Perrin
*University of South Florida–Tampa*

Jason Porter
*Liberty University*

M. La Verne Reid
*North Carolina Central University*

Lindsey Reider
*Onondaga Community College*

Daniel Roman
*Washington Adventist University*

Cindy Schendel
*Shenandoah University*

Donald Schultz
*Liberty University*

Kim Seddon
*Niagara County Community College*

Robin Shepherd
*Danville Community College,*
*Rappahannock Community College*

Agneta Sibrava
*Arkansas State University*

Tamara Knott Silva
*Pasadena City College*

Jacob M. Silvestri
*Hudson Valley Community College*

Amy H. Smith
*Virginia Tech*

Mona Smith
*Georgia Gwinnett College*

Teresa Snow
*Georgia Institute of Technology*

John Strong
*Niagara County Community*
*College*

Phillip Taugher
*University of Wisconsin–Milwaukee*

Kristen Tice
*University of South Carolina*

Gilian Tyndall
*Carteret Community College*

Lesley Wasilko
*Montgomery College–Rockville*

Ronald Webb
*Tallahassee Community College*

Kathy Werheim
*William Paterson University*

Tim Wills
*Rend Lake College*

Elizabeth Zicha
*Muskingum University*

## Symposia Attendees

Daniel Adame
*Emory University*

Becky Allen
*Reedley College*

Vikki Armstrong
*Fayetteville State University*

Tami Ashford-Carroll
*Benedict College*

Donna Bacon
*Nassau Community College*

Brian Barthel
*Utah Valley State College*

Tia Bennett
*Northeastern State University*

Deborah Blair
*Sacramento City College*

Dede Bodnar
*San Diego City College*

Christine Bouffard
*Waubonsee Community College*

Jodi Brookins-Fisher
*Central Michigan University*

Charlene Brown
*Western Michigan University*

Curtiss Brown
*Solano Community College*

Larry Bryant
*Georgia Southern University*

Karen Camarata
*Eastern Kentucky University*

Annette Carrington
*North Carolina Central University*

Steve Chandler
*Florida A&M University*

Kim Clark
*California State University–
San Bernardino*

Cindy Corn
*Rend Lake College*

Marianne Crocker
*Ozarks Technical Community College*

Brent Damron
*Bakersfield College*

Kathi Deresinski
*Triton College*

Steve Dion
*Salem State College*

Shae Donham-Foutch
*Northeastern State University*

Eva Doyle
*Baylor University*

Lynne Edmondson
*Alabama A&M University*

Carrie Edwards
*Southeastern Louisiana University*

Kelly Falcone
*Palomar College*

Jennifer Fay
*Arizona State University*

Gabrielle Floyd
*Texas Southern University*

Rachelle Franz
*University of Central Oklahoma*

Kathi Fuller
*Western Michigan University*

Kathleen Gilbert
*Indiana University*

Christine Harrison
*Montgomery College–Rockville*

Del Helms
*Mt. San Jacinto College–Menifee*

Tonya Huff
*Riverside City College*

Jerolyn Hughes-Golightly
*Alabama A&M University*

Kim Hyatt
*Weber State University*

Emina Ibragic-Burak
*University of Vermont*

Allen Jackson
*Chadron State College*

Kris Jankovitz
*California Polytechnic State University–
San Luis Obispo*

David Jolly
*North Carolina Central University*

Chester Jones
*University of Arkansas–Fayetteville*

Walter Justice
*Southwestern College*

William Kernan
*William Paterson University*

Mark Kittleson
*Southern Illinois University, Carbondale*

Raeann Koerner
*Ventura College*

John Kowalczyk
*University of Minnesota–Duluth*

Jennifer Langeland
*Western Michigan University*

Grace Lartey
*Western Kentucky University*

Randy Maday
*Butte Community College*

Lori Mallory
*Johnson County Community College*

Brian McFarlin
*University of Houston*

Marshall Meyer
*Portland Community College–Sylvania*

Craig Newton
*Middle Georgia College*

Alison Oberne
*University of South Florida–Tampa*

Kay Perrin
*University of South Florida*

Grover Pippin
*Baylor Univeristy*

Elaine Popp
*Humber Institute of Technology
and Advanced Learning*

Linda Rankin
*Idaho State University*

Dollie Richards
*Salt Lake Community College*

Thurman Robins
*Texas Southern University*

Karla Rues
*Ozarks Technical Community College*

Linda Schaffer
*Mira Coasta College*

Shawna Shane
*Emporia State University*

Cindy Shelton
*University of Central Arkansas*

Jacob Silvestri
*Hudson Valley Community College*

Carol Smith
*Elon University*

John Smith
*Springfield College*

Cynthia Smith
*Central Piedmont Community
College*

Bernard Smolen
*Prince George's Community College*

Jiri Stelzer
*Valdosta State University*

Bridgette Stewart
*University of West Georgia*

Debra Sutton
*James Madison University*

Michele Sweeney
*Salem State University*

Laura Sweet
*Eastern Michigan University*

Gayle Truitt-Bean
*Clarion University*

Steve Trujillo
*University of Western Ontario*

Holly Turner
*University of Florida–Gainesville*

Karen Vail-Smith
*East Carolina University*

Danielle Wadsworth
*Auburn University–Auburn*

Resa Walch
*Elon University*

David Wassmer
*Harrisburg Area Community College*

Cecilia Watkins
*Western Kentucky University*

Jae Westfall
*The Ohio State University*

Virginia White
*Riverside City College*

Wayne Wylie
*Texas A&M University*

Cathy Dooly
*Lander University*

Max Faquir
*Palm Beach Community College–Boca Raton*

Jennifer Han
*University of Oklahoma*

Jody Hart
*John A. Logan College*

Dina Hayduk
*Kutztown University*

Allen Jackson
*Chadron State College*

Mark Kittleson
*Southern Illinois University–Carbondale*

Garry Ladd
*Southwestern Illinois College*

Grace Lartey
*Western Kentucky University*

Barbara Long
*Bridgewater College*

Susan Lyman
*University of Louisiana–Lafayette*

Calvin Maginel
*Southeast Missouri State University*

Patty Marcum
*University of Southern Indiana*

Catherine McKay
*Bridgewater College*

Bridget Melton
*Georgia Southern University*

Tomas Mendez
*College of Charleston*

Julie Merten
*University of North Florida*

Juli Miller
*Ohio University*

Peggy Oberstaller
*Lane Community College*

Ramani Rangavajhula
*San Jose State University*

Raymond Reinertsen
*University of Wisconsin–Superior*

Lisa Fender Scarr
*University of Akron*

Karen Vail-Smith
*East Carolina University*

Scott Wolf
*Southwestern Illinois College*

Ottely Wright
*Chadron State College*

Connie Zuercher
*Sacramento City College*

# Beta Edition Reviewers

Kathleen Allison
*Lock Haven University*

Paul Ankomah
*North Carolina A&T State University*

Martha Beagle
*Berea College*

Christine Bouffard
*Waubonsee Community College*

Dwalah Fisher
*Texas Southern University*

Mark Kittleson
*Southern Illinois University*

Jon Kreissig
*Montgomery College*

Laura Massey
*University of Arkansas Community College–Hope*

Eric Nehl
*Emory University*

Kristen Olmos
*Lane Community College*

Linda Romaine
*Raritan Valley Community College*

Brenda Simonson
*Niagara County Community College*

## Academic Roundtable Participants

Daniel Adame
*Emory University*

Elaine Bryan
*Georgia Perimeter College*

Valerie Burge-Hall
*Hampton University*

Tiffany Fuller
*North Carolina A&T State University*

Ping Johnson
*Kennesaw State University*

Jennifer Koch
*University of West Georgia*

Eric Nehl
*Emory University*

Steve Owens
*Tallahassee Community College*

Teresa Peeples
*College of Coastal Georgia*

Serena Reese
*Virginia State University*

Linda Rosskopf
*Georgia Institute of Technology*

Teresa Snow
*Georgia Institute of Technology*

Debra Sutton
*James Madison University*

Stephen Vaughan
*Virginia State University*

LaShawn Wordlaw-Stinson
*North Carolina Central University*

Bonnie Young
*Georgia Perimeter College*

## College Health Report Video Series

Karen Vail Smith, Producer and Writer
*East Carolina University*

Charles Baldwin, Producer
*East Carolina University*

Kristen Hunter, Reporter
*East Carolina University*

Learning is like rowing
upstream. Not to
advance is to fall
backward.

— CHINESE PROVERB

# Chapter 1

FOUNDATIONS OF PERSONAL HEALTH

In Chapter 1, we provide a framework for understanding
fundamental health topics, from health behaviors and medical
conditions to health care considerations. This orientation can
guide you in optimizing your health. We review the modern
concept of health followed by the crosscutting themes of
health literacy, health risk, impact of health advances, and
health behavior change.

**LIFE EXPECTANCY** rose dramatically in the United States during the 20th century. Life expectancy for Americans born in 1900 was 47 years, whereas for those born in 2010, life expectancy is 78 years. Thirty-one years is a phenomenal gain in average lifespan. Yet, researchers who study the biology of human aging believe that most of us are still dying prematurely. They contend that with prudent lifestyles, young people in America today can expect to live to an average age of 90 years.

The trends are evident. In the year 2010, over 11 million Americans were 80 years or older, and nearly 80,000 were centenarians—100 years or older. Lizzie Brown of Fayetteville, Georgia, took everything in stride and lived to 111. At 110 she was still tending her garden at the house in which she had lived for the past 62 years. Among long-lived celebrities, Bob Hope reached 100 and was still performing in his mid-90s, UCLA basketball coach John Wooden lived to 99 and remained active giving talks until his last year, and Les Paul, inventor of the steel guitar, gave a concert the week before his death—at age 94! Yet, we all also know of older folks in assisted care homes or convalescent centers who are only in their 70s. Many will reside in these facilities for years or even decades. This thought gives us pause.

Undeniably, a full life is what we long for, and it is much more than merely being alive. How does this relate to being healthy? How do we go about making smart decisions and establishing healthy behaviors? If we invest the time and effort to truly improve our health status, are there immediate paybacks, or are the benefits only to be gained in the years and decades ahead? How much control do we actually have in living a long and full life? Our aim in writing *iHealth: An Interactive Framework* is to address these fundamental questions.

Article 1.1

## ➤ Modern Concept of Health

**Health** is a universal term used widely in everyday language. We all have a general sense about what the term means but are unsure about specific definitions. Has the definition of *health* changed over time? How should the term *health* be used today? Let's take a closer look. We'll begin by defining health and then discuss its dimensions and how the meaning of health is influenced by social and cultural factors.

> **Health** is a dynamic human condition with multiple but intertwined dimensions—physical, emotional, social, intellectual, spiritual, and environmental. Health can be viewed as a continuum with positive and negative poles. Positive health is associated with a capacity to enjoy life and to withstand challenges. Negative health is associated with illness and disease and, in the extreme, with premature death.

For over 50 years, the World Health Organization (WHO) has defined health as a state of complete physical, mental, and social well-being and not merely the absence of disease or infirmity. Yet, for most of us, the importance of health becomes clear only when we are sick or injured. Consequently, our reflexive perspective on the meaning of health is to dichotomize it. One is either healthy or unhealthy, with a continuum existing only on the unhealthy side depending on the severity of the illness. This lopsided and mistaken view has a serious unintended consequence—it limits human development and potential. This narrow view overlooks the existence of the broad continuum on the positive side of health. With little conscious intention, most young adults simply drift along on the positive side of the continuum. The good news is that by becoming more aware of what it means to be healthy, we can take steps to improve our own health.

Quality of life is an important related concept. Most succinctly, the phrase *quality of life* refers to our overall sense of well-being. **Quality of life** is a subjective rating of the difference between our hopes and expectations and our present experience. Health professionals sometimes have patients rate their quality of life to measure the effects of disorders and disabilities as well as medical treatments. These ratings can then be used to help guide medical decisions. Some treatments can seriously impair a person's ability to enjoy normal life activities without providing appreciable benefit, while others can greatly enhance quality of life. For most young adults, quality of life is synonymous with overall enjoyment of life and highly dependent on their current and expected health.

The relationship between quality of life and longevity is illustrated in Figure 1.1. From adolescence into young adulthood, we have increasing control over lifestyle choices and set the trajectory for our quality of life. The lower curve and the upper curve represent two hypothetical boundaries within which individual lifespan curves can be drawn. The upper curve reflects an individual who maximizes lifestyle choices and healthy behaviors. This leads to *both* a full life and a long life, reaching the 90-year potential and perhaps beyond. Ideally, the end of life is preceded by a sharp decline of short duration, with only a few weeks or months of deteriorating function and loss of independence, as in the case of Lizzie Brown.

> **Quality of life** is one's overall sense of well-being or enjoyment of life. It's a subjective rating of the difference between a person's hopes and expectations and his or her present experience, and it is sometimes used in medical settings to help assess the effects of disease, disability, and treatments.

**FIGURE 1.1    ALTERNATE PATHS OF WELL-BEING**

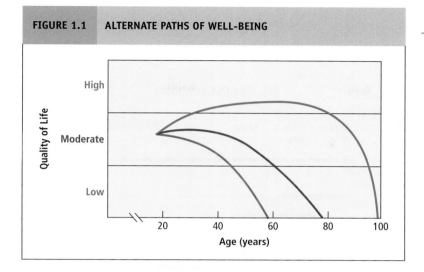

In contrast, the lower curve represents a person who is unaware of or uninterested in a healthy life and adopts unhealthy behaviors. This compromises quality of life and substantially shortens a normal biological lifespan. Death at 60 rather than 90 is life truly cut short, yet sadly we all have firsthand knowledge of premature deaths and incomplete lives. Moreover, in this scenario, many years of low quality of life may precede the person's early death.

The middle curve depicts the path of many Americans who are aware of key health issues but unsuccessful in effectively translating their knowledge into healthier lifestyle behaviors. Note that the area between the lower and upper curves is large—it is high (along the Quality of Life axis) and wide (along the Age, or longevity, axis). Within these broad bounds, we can have enormous control on setting our own course. This is the potential area for growth available to us.

As in the WHO definition, health is often referred to as a state of optimal functioning, which implies the highest achievable level physically, mentally, and socially. In contrast, a contemporary perspective views health not as a state of being but as a goal that people continually work toward throughout their life. In Figure 1.2, health is depicted as a continuum extending from critical illness to optimal health. The traditional "treatment model" focuses on the left side of the continuum, and its emphasis is on freedom from sickness and disease. The proactive "optimal health model" focuses more on the right side of the continuum and the challenge of maximizing potential and quality of life.

Humans are goal-oriented creatures. We like to set goals and then work to achieve them. The goal of better health is no exception. To craft

**FIGURE 1.2    TWO VIEWS OF HEALTH**

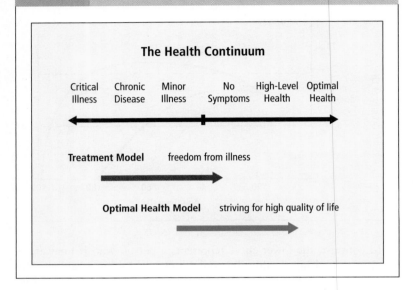

The Health Continuum

Critical Illness — Chronic Disease — Minor Illness — No Symptoms — High-Level Health — Optimal Health

Treatment Model    freedom from illness

Optimal Health Model    striving for high quality of life

a plan, we need to know what factors influence movement along the health continuum, especially those we can control or modify. As it turns out, the most important factors are those associated with lifestyle—for example, factors related to eating, exercising, sleeping, drug use (including alcohol and tobacco), and stress. To a great extent, we are in charge on these matters. By choosing which behaviors to develop and which to avoid, each of us sets the course for moving forward (or falling back) along the health continuum.

Uncontrollable (or nonmodifiable) factors can also influence our health. These include heredity, age, gender, and race. Occasionally unfavorable genetic combinations result in hereditary diseases such as cystic fibrosis, sickle cell anemia, and type 1 (juvenile) diabetes. Fortunately, today most inherited diseases can be effectively treated or managed. The uncontrollable factors of age, gender, and race—in addition to being essential parts of who we are—are useful categories for researchers studying diseases in populations. Yet, for us as individuals, our gender and race have no inherent positive or negative qualities that limit our movement along the health continuum across the broad span of our adult years.

Throughout *iHealth* an emphasis is placed on understanding modifiable factors and how to maximize lifestyle behaviors for a full and long life. Admittedly, there are no guarantees, because life is unpredictable.

Every day, unexpected accidents and deaths occur that are beyond people's control. This serves to remind us that good health is about having the best quality of life possible for whatever conditions we face or however many years we may have. In short though, a healthy lifestyle dramatically improves the odds for a full life, both today and in the future. Men and women of all races can be proactive about their health and reap the benefits today as well as tomorrow.

## DIMENSIONS OF HEALTH

The modern view is that health is multidimensional. Scholars point out that the characteristic of multidimensionality is of fundamental importance to truly understanding health. This view counters the popular notion that health is simply physical well-being. Expanding upon the three dimensions (physical, mental, social) cited in the WHO definition, the contemporary view typically encompasses six dimensions of health: physical, emotional, social, intellectual, spiritual, and environmental. A brief description of each dimension follows.

### *Physical Dimension of Health*

The physical dimension of health encompasses the functional operation and soundness of the body. How well are you able to perform activities of daily living such as dressing, cooking, walking, and driving? Can you perform routine tasks efficiently without becoming overly fatigued? Do you get regular medical checkups? Do you follow preventive health practices known to optimize physical health—namely, eating prudently, exercising regularly, avoiding substance abuse, wearing seat belts, minimizing sun exposure, and getting immunizations? For centuries, health was equated only with physical health. Today, physical health, although the predominant dimension at times, is recognized as only one of six dimensions that underlie our health.

Self Assessment 1.1

### *Emotional Dimension of Health*

The emotional dimension is associated with the ability to deal with personal feelings in a positive and constructive manner, to cope with stress, and to live independently. How is your outlook on life? Could your outlook be improved? Positive approaches to our emotions characterized by flexibility, balance, and resiliency help us deal effectively with feelings such as anger, happiness, fear, guilt, and love. A strong emotional dimension is a key to greater life satisfaction.

### *Social Dimension of Health*

Closely tied to emotional health, the social dimension is the ability to interact effectively with other people, to develop satisfying interpersonal relationships, and to fulfill social roles. Do you have friends in whom you can confide? Do you have friends who feel comfortable confiding in you? Do you get along well with others and show respect regardless of your differences? Hallmarks of social health are the capacity for intimacy, meaningful relationships with family and friends, and participation in community activities. Young adulthood is a particularly important time for developing and broadening social skills.

### Intellectual Dimension of Health

The intellectual dimension is reflected in our ability to question and evaluate information, to think and learn from a variety of experiences, and to be open to new ideas. Do you enjoy solving problems, learning new skills, and exploring new ideas? The academic challenges of college emphasize the development of intellectual health. Make the most of these opportunities. Critical thinking and problem solving are fundamental lifelong pursuits that enable us to continue learning new material and master new skills.

### Spiritual Dimension of Health

Being spiritual doesn't mean belonging to a formal religion, although religion is part of this dimension for many people. The essential component of spiritual health is a commitment to a set of values or principles that guide our actions. This commitment is usually but not always based on a belief in a greater force. This greater force may be a god or simply an acknowledgment of a higher power or order in the universe. Atheists can have sacred sets of values to live by just as Christians, Muslims, and Jews have divine beliefs to guide them. Spiritual health often involves a dedication to nurture all living beings out of respect for the interrelatedness of all life. The basis for leading a moral and ethical life is rooted in spiritual health.

### Environmental Dimension of Health

The importance of the environmental dimension of health is highlighted by the immense growth in the field of ecology (interactions between organisms and their environment) and, in particular, knowledge about environmental risks to human (and animal) health. This dimension focuses on the state of the environment and the conditions in which we live. Primary environmental concerns include air and water quality and management of wastes and harmful substances, as well as our unsustainable use of natural resources and the steady rise in human population. Our health is dependent on understanding that we are part of the natural world, not separate from it. In turn, our responsibility is to be good stewards of the earth and to find solutions that are ecologically sound.

The dimensions of health do not exist as separate elements. Rather, each dimension relates to all others. As one dimension is affected, so too are the others. Just as individual threads are braided together to form a single cord, so too are the dimensions of health. Each thread or dimension contributes to the overall balance, quality, and strength of the whole.

## DIVERSITY AND HEALTH

Over the past decade, the issue of diversity has come to the forefront. The changing demographics of the United States are illustrated with the following examples from the U.S. Census of 2010:

- Just over one-third of the population reported their race/ethnicity as other than non-Hispanic White (i.e., "minority"), representing a growth of 29 percent over the decade.
- The Hispanic, African American, and Asian populations now comprise 16, 13, and 5 percent respectively of the total population.
- Texas joined California, the District of Columbia, Hawaii, and New Mexico in having a "majority–minority" population, where more than 50 percent of the population is a minority group.
- Fifty-seven percent of college students are women, and over 60 percent of adult women are in the workforce.
- Family structures continue to change. As an example, the proportion of young adults (ages 25–34) never married (46%) is now higher than the proportion married (45%).
- Immigration to the United States over the past decade was at an all-time high, averaging over 1 million per year.

We see diversity in ordinary encounters with individuals and groups who may differ widely in attitudes, values, and beliefs—cumulatively referred to as *culture*. Diversity is sometimes criticized as a form of political correctness, but that is an unfortunate and shortsighted view. The following quote from Sara Corbett's *New York Times* article "The Long Road from Sudan to America" introduces us to three young refugees from Sudan:

> One evening in late January, Peter Dut, 21, leads his two teenage brothers through the brightly lit corridors of the Minneapolis airport, trying to mask his confusion. Two days earlier, the brothers, refugees from Africa, had encountered their first light switch and their first set of stairs. An aid worker in Nairobi had demonstrated the flush toilet to them—also the seat belt, the shoelace, the fork. And now they find themselves alone in Minneapolis, three bone-thin African boys confronted by a swirling river of white faces and rolling suitcases.

This description sets a sharp contrast between the lives of these African refugees and those of the Americans who walked by them in the airport. What is ordinary and routine for many may indeed be novel and wondrous for others. Most of us can hardly imagine the environment

Colleges and universities are among the most ethnically diverse places in America.

and circumstances from which these three brothers escaped. Should it be surprising that cultural background and life experiences invariably shape how we perceive one another and the world in which we live?

Of all the places in America, colleges and universities are among the most diverse. A large lecture class may have students who are urban and rural, wealthy and poor, and religious and nonreligious. Students may include devout Christians, Jews, and Muslims alongside agnostics and atheists. Students representing many nationalities from both developed and developing countries and various ethnic groups may be present. Many may speak English as a second language. Students may differ in sexual orientation, and some may be part of a nontraditional family structure. With this medley in mind, it's easier to understand why perceptions and knowledge of health concepts and issues vary so widely.

Discussing diversity is important because many health topics such as stress, mental health, nutrition, drug use, chronic diseases, and infectious diseases are strongly related to culture. Examples include social stressors (prejudice, economic oppression), mental health disorders (depression, suicidal behavior), food choices (ethnic diets), and drug use patterns (tobacco, alcohol, other drugs). Gaining insight into how the concept of health varies among different religious, ethnic, and cultural groups helps each of us better define the meaning of health in our own lives. This theme will be followed throughout *iHealth* and highlighted in selected readings.

The diversity of the American population is a great asset. It is also one of our nation's greatest challenges because profound health disparities exist between the mainstream population and various subpopulations such as African Americans, Hispanics, American Indians, and residents of Appalachia. Health disparities are a reality faced daily by employers, educators, and health professionals. A primary goal of public health is to reduce health disparities through research, education, and improved access to heath care. In the wealthiest and most technologically advanced country in the world, affordable and equitable health care should be available to everyone.

✓ **NEED TO KNOW**

The concept of health is much more than simply not being sick. Health is multidimensional, dynamic, and influenced by social and cultural norms. Our overall health status and the associated quality of life are largely determined by our lifestyle choices and behaviors.

## ➤ Health Literacy

**Health literacy** can be defined as the degree to which individuals have the capacity to obtain, process, and understand basic health information and services needed to make appropriate health decisions. Health literacy programs are traditionally targeted to the poor, the elderly, and those with little education. Yet, health literacy is not solely a matter of formal education or access to health information. The Institute of Medicine estimates that nearly half of all American adults have difficulty understanding and using health information. The challenge of becoming health literate becomes clearer when considered within the context of our consumer-driven society. More than ever before, consumption defines who we are and what we do.

We are immersed in advertising throughout our waking hours. American children and adolescents watch an average of three to four hours of television a day. Young children recall Ronald McDonald, Tony the Tiger, and the Budweiser Frogs as easily as Santa Claus, Mickey Mouse, and Bugs Bunny. Beyond the screen, advertising in other forms from signage to apparel is increasingly found throughout schools. The American Academy of Pediatrics is one of many professional groups to point out that excessive or uncontrolled exposure to television, movies, music, video games and the Internet is associated with increased risk for an array of health problems from obesity and eating disorders to substance abuse, promiscuity, and aggressive behaviors.

Advertisers shape our consumer desires and create values in products by portraying them as having the power to change us into "more desirable" people. Commercials feature adults who are attractive, happy, energetic, and often hip or sensuous too. The underlying message is we can be like them if we use those products. Mega shopping malls have become a cultural primer for telling us how we should dress, furnish our homes, and spend leisure time. Luxuries have become necessities and

Article
1.2

**Health literacy** is the ability to obtain, process, and understand basic health information and services needed to make appropriate health decisions.

Advertising, a major industry in itself, is adept at creating messages to sell products. In the 1940s, the nonprofit Ad Council created a new type of advertising known as public service announcements (PSAs) to bring about positive social change, including better health. The Ad Council remains active today but its resources are limited **(www.adcouncil.org).**

Another approach to communicating healthy messages is to dispel the illusion of advertising with spoof ads. Cigarette and alcohol ads are especially ripe targets. Adbusters, a Canadian advocacy advertising agency and publisher of *Adbusters* magazine, has produced several memorable ones. Their "Absolute on Ice" parody ad evokes a stark contrast to the original ad and makes one think twice about the downsides of excessive drinking. (The product being parodied is Absolut, a vodka.) See other spoof ads such as Joe Chemo, a takeoff on Joe Camel, at **http://adbusters.org/spoofads.**

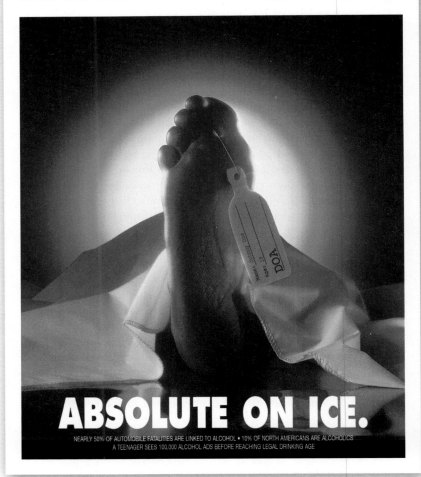

lifestyles can be purchased. As an interesting side note, Barry Schwartz, Ph.D., a professor of psychology at Swarthmore College, suggests that our nearly unlimited choices have resulted in additional stress for the modern consumer—the paradox of choice.

In the health marketplace, frauds and hoaxes remain commonplace. For any ailment or disease, there exist literally hundreds of products, most of which are bogus. Regardless of the source—the Internet, newspapers, magazines, radio, television, neighbors, colleagues—the best advice remains "buyer beware." It is tempting to assume that being college educated ensures the ability to sort out the confounding influences and misleading claims from science-based information. But this is true only if we remain health literate. Health literacy is dependent upon self-directed learning, effective communication, and critical thinking.

## SELF-DIRECTED LEARNING

Self-directed learning is a process in which the individual controls both the learning objectives and the means of learning, with or without the help of others. You are in charge—you determine what should be learned, what resources and methods should be used, and how the success of the effort should be measured. This is in contrast to most college courses and workplace training classes, in which the learning objectives, methods, and evaluation are set by the teacher or employer.

To a large degree, most adult learning is self-directed. A person's objective may be to improve family life, enjoy the arts, participate in a hobby, or to research a medical question. For many people, however, the extent of self-directed learning is quite limited. They may not engage in self-directed learning because they lack the confidence, resources, independence, or some combination of the three. Thankfully, these barriers can be overcome with motivation and guidance.

First and foremost, the Internet is a rich resource for the self-directed learner. To become a savvy health consumer, it's essential to learn the basic skills of using the Internet. This will allow you to expand on and update material presented in *iHealth*. The first step is to recognize that you need to carefully and critically evaluate information on the Internet because anyone can post information. For instance, you and your friends may have your own websites. Unlike reference books and refereed journal articles, a rigorous review and evaluation by experts prior to posting or "publishing" on the Internet is not required.

As an initial screening procedure, note that certain web addresses (or URLs)—namely, those with the ".org" (nonprofit organization), ".gov" (federal government), and ".edu" (college/university) extensions—are more likely than the ".com" (commercial business) websites to lead to authoritative information. As health decision makers, our primary aim

*The HON Code Icon indicates a website is certified as a trustworthy health resource based on the following principles:*

1. **Authoritative:** Any medical or health advice provided or hosted on the site comes from medically trained and qualified professionals. In the event a piece of advice comes from a nonmedically qualified source or organization, that is also made clear.

2. **Complementarity:** Information provided supports, but does not replace, the doctor-patient relationship.

3. **Privacy:** Data regarding individual patients or visitors to the health-related website remain confidential.

4. **Attribution:** When appropriate, the site contains clear references to source data and, where possible, specific HTML links to that data. The date when a clinical page was last modified is clearly displayed.

5. **Justifiability:** Any claims related to benefits or performance of a specific treatment, product, or service is supported by appropriately balanced evidence in the manner outlined above in Principle 4.

6. **Transparency:** The site designers seek to provide information in the clearest possible manner and provide contact addresses for visitors who seek further information or support. The Webmaster displays his/her email clearly throughout the site.

7. **Financial Disclosure:** The site identifies its funding sources clearly.

8. **Advertising Policy:** The site clearly distinguishes editorial content from advertising.

Source: Reprinted by permission of HON, Health on the Net Foundation.

is to find credible and reliable information—not to buy a product! We should look for information that is factual, current, written in everyday language, and sponsored by a reputable group.

The following websites are excellent resources for health information and all abide by the Health on the Net (HON) Foundation Code of Conduct, a set of ethical principles to guide the presentation of health and medical information (Figure 1.3). Created in 1995 to cope with the unprecedented volume of health care information available, HON—a nonprofit, non-governmental organization—reviews and certifies websites to protect consumers from misleading health information. Look for the HON icon on the opening page of a health or medical website as a sign of credibility and trustworthiness. Among those listed below, WebMD is the most popular. The other sites listed are included in the Medical Library Association's top 10 most useful websites. It should be noted that even with reputable sites, it's a good practice to read your desired topic at more than one source and to cross-check information:

1. WebMD **www.webmd.com** A leading, for-profit provider of health information, recognized for timely and accurate medical journalism and effective health communication
2. MayoClinic **www.mayoclinic.com** Sponsored by the renowned Mayo Clinic, the world's first and largest not-for-profit medical practice
3. MedlinePlus **http://medlineplus.gov** Sponsored by the National Library of Medicine and National Institutes of Health (NIH)
4. Healthfinder.gov **www.healthfinder.gov** Sponsored by the Office of Disease Prevention and Health Promotion, U.S. Department of Health and Human Services (HHS)
5. Centers for Disease Control and Prevention (CDC) **www.cdc.gov** Leading federal agency for preventing and controlling disease, injury, and disability
6. FamilyDoctor.org **www.familydoctor.org** Sponsored by the American Academy of Family Physicians, the nation's largest association of family doctors

A few carefully selected websites will be presented in each chapter. Since web addresses sometimes change, occasionally there may be a link that no longer works. If that happens, refer to the *iHealth* web page for updates.

## EFFECTIVE COMMUNICATION

The importance of developing written and oral communication skills cannot be overstated, especially in today's world of smart phones and social media. Every day we communicate with different people in many ways and settings. Yet, good communication skills are not routinely learned in school so it's left to each of us to master them as self-directed learners. Regular investments of time and effort to improve communication skills will yield great returns. The likelihood for miscommunication when dealing with medical or health issues is enormous. Let's consider three different scenarios.

### Scenario One

You are waiting in the exam room to see a physician. You have been told to take off your clothes and put on an exam gown. You have an odd illness you have never experienced before. Or you may have a hunch about what's going on but hope it's not true. You know your time with the doctor will be short, perhaps 5 to 10 minutes. And on top of that, you are feeling really lousy—that's why you've come to the doctor in the first place! This situation is predictably stressful and not conducive to good communication. Common barriers are intimidation, embarrassment, and fear. Many people are intimidated by the medical setting, being half-clothed, and the status of the doctor. They may be embarrassed due to the personal nature of the condition they need to reveal. Some are fearful they may have a serious condition. It's no wonder we often cannot recall exactly what the doctor said or we forget to ask a question. How to prepare for a doctor's appointment and how to get your questions answered are discussed in Chapter 13.

### Scenario Two

Your elderly neighbor has asked you to drive her to her doctor's appointment. As you take her home, she tells you that she has diabetes. But she is confused. She relates, "I think some of the words . . . [during the office visit and in brochures], they ought to explain in simple English. Everybody hasn't graduated from high school or college. They should just speak or put them down in plain English." Like millions of

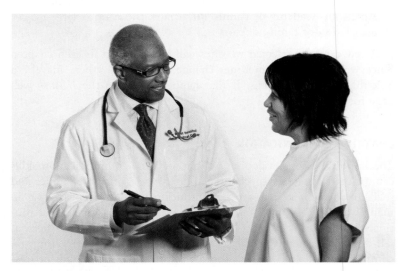

Many people struggle to communicate effectively with physicians due to embarrassment, fear, or time constraints.

Americans, she is struggling with "medspeak," the specialized language of health professionals. The overuse of medical jargon has created a communication barrier for the public. As health professionals work to minimize their use of medspeak with patients, we as health consumers should increase our understanding of basic health and medical terms.

### Scenario Three

You are in the pharmacy line at the drugstore and hear a disjointed conversation between the pharmacist and a Hispanic man in front of you. Although he has a heavy accent, his English is understandable. But it is unclear if he completely comprehends the pharmacist's instructions about how the medication should be taken. Communication problems are not limited to obvious language differences between patients and health care providers. They may also exist between people who come from different regions of the country or who have different values or expectations about health care. It is important to remember that one's customs and beliefs should be considered when communicating health messages.

## CRITICAL THINKING

The term *critical thinking* is widely used but not well understood. Most would say it has something to do with logic or analysis, but these terms provide only a partial description. Essentially, critical thinking is careful and deliberate determination of whether to accept, reject, or suspend judgment. These are often the *why* questions. Critical thinking has two components: first, a set of skills to process and generate information and beliefs, and second, the habit—based on intellectual commitment—of using those skills to guide behavior. This is in contrast to the mere acquisition of information, the simple possession of skills, or the use of those skills as an exercise without giving any thought to their results.

Critical thinking is driven by asking the *right* questions. Critical thinking is *not* involved when teachers feed students endless facts for simple recall or when students sit in silence except for superficial or ill-informed questions. Both examples are dead ends. In contrast, good teaching and good questions lead to more questions and eventually to true learning. Overcome lifeless classrooms by asking thought-provoking questions. Learn the skills and establish the habit of critical thinking. From time to time, we are all subject to undisciplined and irrational thought. But is it the norm or the exception? The practice of critical thinking can be developed and refined during the college years but doesn't stop upon graduation. Critical thinking can serve us well in all endeavors and should be a lifelong pursuit.

In the 1990s the "Mozart effect"—an alleged increase in brain development in children when they listen to the music of Mozart—received wide coverage in the popular print and broadcast media. Since that time, the Mozart effect has taken on a life of its own. It's featured in publications offering parenting advice and educational goals, as well as music appreciation. Governors of several states started programs that give a Mozart CD to every newborn. Dozens of toys suddenly appeared proclaiming themselves "educational" because they played snippets of Mozart's "Rondo Alla Turca" rather than "Mary Had a Little Lamb." The Mozart effect has also been used to sell music lessons and music products. Moreover, claims have expanded: Classical music can not only increase a child's intelligence but also aid an adult's healing process. What caused this Mozart love fest?

The Mozart effect is an example of how science and the media can mix in our world. First, a scientific paper is published in a prestigious journal that reports a new and potentially important finding. The scientific study receives attention from the media, as it should. But next comes the oversimplification of the science. Sometimes reporters innocently misstate facts because of lack of scientific understanding. Other times, businesses may intentionally exaggerate a study's findings to promote their products and boost sales. Regardless of the cause, once these misstatements are embraced by the general public, what started as a trickle of misinformation can become a raging river of exaggeration that affects all in its flow—scientists and the general public alike.

In this case, Frances Rauscher and two colleagues (1993) from the Center for Neurobiology of Learning and Memory at the University of California–Irvine reported in *Nature* that listening to a composition of Mozart briefly increased scores among college students on a paper-folding task that measures spatial abilities. The increase in scores lasted only about 10 minutes. Nonspatial tasks measured on the same IQ test were unaffected by listening to the music. The boost in scores was widely reported, but the short-lived effect and narrow nature of the improvement received a lot less attention. The accuracy of the original findings was lost over the years as the Mozart effect morphed into the popular notion that "Mozart makes you smarter." This notion is, of course, a gross oversimplification. Does it really make sense to talk about being "smarter" if it only lasts 10 minutes?

Accuracy is needed in science *and* in the media. Too often, important research is trivialized and misrepresented in the popular media. The case of the Mozart effect can teach us several lessons. First, we should be careful not to abandon common sense when we read health-related news. If a claim seems a bit extreme or too good to be true, then this ought to be a warning flag that the news might be incomplete or distorted. Second, we should allow the data to speak for themselves. When findings are controversial, explore reputable websites for summaries, read the original report and the opinions of experts, and reach your own conclusions. Apply those critical thinking skills!

Consider critical thinking as a process that stresses an attitude of suspended judgment, incorporates logical inquiry and problem solving, and leads to an evaluative decision or action. In today's information age, critical thinking is more important than ever before. In addition to being an essential part of our intellectual health, critical thinking allows us to filter and analyze the maze of facts, claims, and hoaxes that surround health and medical issues. Critical thinking is what we must rely on if we are to successfully separate science from marketing and find solutions to complex questions.

### ✓ NEED TO KNOW

Health literacy is the knowledge and skills that enable us to successfully access, analyze, and interpret relevant information, to answer personal health questions, to provide guidance in dealing with a health condition, and to change a health behavior. Key aspects of health literacy include self-directed learning, effective communication, and critical thinking. These characteristics require related skills that must be developed. Health literacy also assumes a mindfulness and inquisitiveness that motivates continual learning.

## ➤ Concept of Risk

To fully appreciate the impact of our behaviors on our health, it's essential to understand what a health risk is and how to interpret it. Simply stated, a **health risk** or **risk factor** is the probability that an adverse event (an outcome) will occur if one engages in a certain behavior (exposure). For example, those who do not buckle up when riding in a car are at greater risk for a serious injury should an accident occur

A **health risk** or **risk factor** is any factor that increases susceptibility or has a strong association with the occurrence, onset, or progression of a disease or injury.

than those who do buckle up. The negative behavior (exposure) is not using a seat belt, and serious injury is the likely outcome if an accident occurs. The risk factors (behaviors and other factors) that are associated with specific diseases or injuries are established primarily by epidemiological studies.

**Epidemiology** is the study of the causes, distribution, and control of diseases in populations. Many medical findings reported in the popular media are based on epidemiological studies in which large numbers of people (hundreds or thousands) have been evaluated repeatedly over many years or decades. The goal of these studies is to investigate the links (associations) between the characteristics (including health behaviors) of the participants and the occurrence of specific outcomes across time (e.g., onset of diseases or death). Epidemiological studies help scientists sort through many, many factors and eventually identify those that are most highly related to a given disease.

Statistical correlations in population studies are based on observational data. That is, changes over time are observed and measured but no experimental treatment or intervention is being tested. As such, epidemiological findings by themselves cannot prove cause and effect. Just because variable A is highly related to variable B does not prove that A causes B. Does smoking cause cirrhosis of the liver? Probably not. Excessive consumption of alcohol is the likely cause. Yet, since heavy drinkers tend to be heavy smokers, the statistical association is there. More often than not, evidence from experimental research, such as controlled laboratory studies or clinical trials, is used in conjunction with epidemiological findings to support or refute potential causal relationships.

## RISK PERCEPTION

David Ropeik, a recognized expert and commentator on the subject of risk, has shown that risk perception is not a straightforward, logical process based on the best science. How we decide what to be afraid of and to what degree to be afraid is heavily influenced by psychological factors. Here are three examples of how we decide what's safe and what's risky:

1. People tend to be less afraid of risks that are natural than those that are human-made. There is greater fear of radiation from cell

---

**Epidemiology** is the scientific discipline studying the occurrence, distribution, control, and prevention of disease, infection, injury, and other health-related events in a defined human population. It includes the study of factors affecting the progress of an illness and, in the case of many chronic diseases, their natural history.

phones or power lines than from the sun, which presents a much greater risk.

2. People are less afraid of a risk they choose to take than one imposed on them. Smokers are less fearful of smoking than they are of asbestos or other indoor air pollutants in the workplace, over which they may have little control.

3. Most of us are less afraid of a risk that comes from people or organizations that we trust and more afraid if the risk comes from a source that we don't trust. We are more likely to accept the risk assessment of a drug's safety from a trusted physician than from the pharmaceutical company that makes it.

In his book *How Risky Is It, Really?* (2010) Ropeik provides evidence-based information to help put the risks in life in perspective. Researchers have found that Americans tend to over-estimate small risks and underestimate large risks, regardless of age, race, or socioeconomic status. When you are making decisions about health risks, be aware that perceptions can be shaped by emotions and feelings. Consider taking a step back and relying on careful objective analysis when a major health risk must be evaluated.

## RELATIVE RISK

Health risks are generally discussed in the language of medical statistics. **Relative risk** is a common way to quantify and report a health risk. Although statistics can be complex, relative risk is a straightforward concept and one we should know as medical consumers. Relative risk is the "times-greater chance" a person has of acquiring a specific negative health effect (e.g., a disease) based on the extent to which a certain variable (e.g., a characteristic or behavior) is present. Relative risk is the ratio of the rate of disease among those exposed to a variable compared to those not exposed or having limited exposure.

Article 1.3

To illustrate, the American Cancer Society reports that the annual death rate from lung cancer among people who smoke is approximately 50 deaths per 100,000 people per year while the death rate of people who don't smoke is only 2.5 deaths per 100,000 people per year. In this case, the relative risk—the ratio of the lung cancer death rates of those exposed (smokers) to those not exposed (nonsmokers)—is 20 (50 divided by 2.5). Put another way, relative risk is the ratio of

**Relative risk** is a measure of comparative risk of a health-related event such as disease or death between two groups. It is the chance that a person receiving an exposure will develop a condition compared to the chance that a nonexposed person will develop the same condition.

Smokers have both a greater relative risk and absolute risk of developing certain cancers than nonsmokers.

two absolute risks: The numerator is the absolute risk among those with the risk factor (50 deaths from lung cancer per 100,000 smokers), and the denominator is the absolute risk among those without the risk factor (2.5 deaths from lung cancer per 100,000 nonsmokers). A relative risk of 20 means that those who smoke have a 20-times-greater chance of dying from lung cancer than those who don't smoke. (Relative risk for smoking versus not smoking and death from lung cancer varies between 10 and 20 depending primarily upon the amount of smoking.)

Often a relative risk is reported by itself. A relative risk of 10 to 20 (as with smoking) is extremely high. Most relative risks are in the range of 1.5 to 3.0. Let's assume the absolute risk for developing a disease is 4 in 100 among people who exercise regularly, and the risk is increased 50 percent in those who do not exercise. The 50 percent relates to the absolute risk number, 4, so the increase in the risk is 50 percent of 4, or 2. Consequently, nonexercisers' absolute risk of developing the disease is 6 out of 100, and the relative risk is 1.5 for the nonexercisers compared to the exercisers (6 divided by 4). On the one hand, a 50 percent increase sounds alarming, but on the other, because the absolute risk is small, a 50 percent increase is not that significant overall—the risk only increased from 4 out of 100 to 6 out of 100. Consequently, when possible, find out both relative and absolute risks, and do your own calculation to determine the overall risk.

We believe that "knowing the numbers" is important. The trend in public health, however, is to not report any numbers when communicating risk, but simply to rate the risk of a behavior as low, moderate, or high. This may be fine for some risks but not for others. You must be the judge. When in doubt, continue to ask or research your questions until you completely understand the risks associated with a specific behavior, intervention, or treatment. From the examples presented, the value of using the concepts of absolute and relative risk should be evident. Interpreting results from epidemiological and clinical studies and applying them to individual situations will enable you to make more informed decisions.

✓ **NEED TO KNOW**

Health risk is the concept that relates specific health-compromising factors (exposures) to increased likelihood of developing diseases or higher death rates (outcomes). Conversely, from a proactive viewpoint, adopting health-enhancing or health-protective behaviors can reduce the probability of unwanted outcomes. Epidemiologists study the disease process in populations and quantify health risk in terms of absolute risk and relative risk.

## ➤ Advances in Public Health

The health concerns and health care services available when Lizzie Brown, the centenarian mentioned at the beginning of the chapter, was born in 1892 are vastly different from those that exist for a baby born today. A century ago, America was in the midst of the Industrial Revolution. Large numbers of people were migrating to the cities for jobs in factories. City housing was crowded, dirty, unheated, and unventilated. Clean water and proper sanitation (waste disposal) were limited, and food supplies were unreliable and often contaminated. These conditions allowed **infectious diseases** such as influenza, pneumonia, and tuberculosis to thrive.

Death rates fluctuated widely from year to year depending on disease (epidemics), severe weather (snowstorms, floods, hurricanes), and the harvest (varying from poor to bountiful). Infant mortality was high. In

An **infectious disease** is a medical condition typically resulting from a disease-causing organism—usually a bacterium, virus, or parasitic worm—known as a pathogen. Most infectious diseases are short-term or highly treatable illnesses, such as the common cold and strep throat. Other infectious diseases such as AIDS are long-term diseases for which no medical cure has yet been developed.

some cities, up to 30 percent of babies did not live to their first birthday. Many women died during childbirth. In short, life was hard. Under these conditions, it's understandable that good health would be thought of as being simply one step beyond the necessities for survival—that is, having adequate food and shelter and not being ill. The life expectancy for an American born in 1900 was less than 50. A century later, life expectancy was over 75.

## ADVANCES OVER THE PAST CENTURY

Several major public health advances contributed to the 50 percent increase in life expectancy over the past 100 years. Leading the way was the provision of clean water, improved sanitation (the building of sewer systems), and the development of vaccines and antibiotics—collectively these markedly improved the control of most infectious diseases. Other

President Franklin Delano Roosevelt contracted polio as an adult and was paralyzed from the waist down for the rest of his life. Polio epidemics are now practically unheard of in the developed world thanks to the discovery of vaccines.

notable public health achievements were safer and healthier foods, greater access to health care, and technologic improvements in health care. For example, since 1900, infant mortality has decreased 90 percent and maternal mortality has decreased 99 percent. Substantial reductions in disability (morbidity) and death (mortality) have also resulted from improvements in workplace safety (e.g., regulations in mining, manufacturing, and construction) and motor vehicle safety (e.g., better-engineered vehicles and highways and seat belt use). Most of these public health advances have been translated into public policy, such as school immunization policies and seat belt laws. Americans today can hardly imagine the difficulties their ancestors faced only four or five generations ago.

As infectious diseases were controlled with public health advances, the leading causes of death and disability in America shifted. In 1900 the three leading causes of death were pneumonia, tuberculosis, and diarrheal diseases. Today the three leading causes of death are not infectious diseases but chronic diseases—heart disease, cancer, and stroke. **Chronic diseases** are medical conditions that are prolonged, do not resolve spontaneously, and are rarely cured completely. And, just as with infectious diseases, chronic diseases impose huge human and economic costs.

As we once faced the scourge of infectious diseases, we now face a different challenge to our health, one that won't be solved solely by breakthroughs in medical technology or new drugs. Over the years, we've learned that the rise of chronic diseases, particularly over the second half of the 20th century, was due primarily to our lifestyle habits. Hence, chronic diseases are often referred to as "lifestyle diseases." As seen in Table 1.1, the first four causes of death, and six of the top 10, are chronic diseases attributed largely to daily habits associated with eating, physical activity, and tobacco use. National estimates indicate that about 50 percent of disease and premature deaths (i.e., death before age 65) are due to unhealthy lifestyles. Heart disease, cancer, stroke, and diabetes will be discussed in Part 3. As Pogo proclaimed in the 1970s, "We have met the enemy and he is us." (Walt Kelly's *Pogo*, a classic comic strip that ran from 1948 to 1975, provided social satire and laughs for both kids and adults.)

When considering lifestyle diseases, another approach is to consider deaths by actual causes as opposed to medical conditions. In Figure 1.4,

A **chronic disease** is a medical condition that is permanent, leaves a residual disability, is caused by a nonreversible pathological condition, and requires special training of the patient for rehabilitation or is expected to require a long period of supervision or care. Coronary heart disease and cancer are two common examples.

**TABLE 1.1    LEADING CAUSES OF DEATH**

| CAUSE | NUMBER OF DEATHS |
|---|---|
| Heart disease | 616,067 |
| Cancer | 562,875 |
| Stroke | 135,952 |
| Chronic lower respiratory disease | 127,924 |
| Unintentional injuries | 123,706 |
| Alzheimer's disease | 74,632 |
| Diabetes | 71,382 |
| Influenza and pneumonia | 52,717 |
| Kidney disease | 46,448 |
| Septicemia | 34,828 |

Source: CDC/NCHS. Health, United States, 2010.

tobacco use is shown to be the number one cause of mortality, responsible for an estimated 435,000 deaths per year. These tobacco-attributed deaths cut across several chronic diseases, including 90 percent of deaths from lung cancer and chronic lower respiratory disease

**FIGURE 1.4    ACTUAL CAUSES OF DEATH**

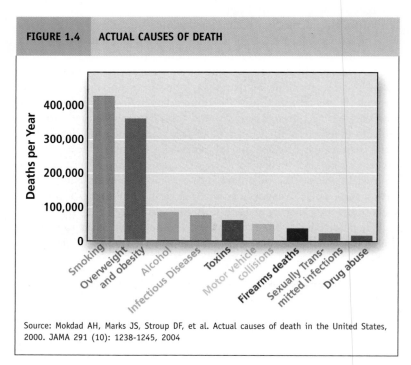

Source: Mokdad AH, Marks JS, Stroup DF, et al. Actual causes of death in the United States, 2000. JAMA 291 (10): 1238-1245, 2004

(chronic bronchitis and emphysema) and lower percentages of deaths from heart disease, stroke, and other cancers. Deaths due to poor diet and physical inactivity (400,000) combined with alcohol abuse (85,000) account for another 485,000 annual deaths. Findings from a major study confirm these preventable causes of death (Danaei, et al., 2009). Clearly, our habits regarding eating, exercise, and use of tobacco and alcohol have a major impact on individual health as well as population health.

Because most of you are young adults, let's consider the leading causes of death for your age groups. For the age group 15–24 (Figure 1.5), the leading cause of death is unintentional injury with the majority being motor vehicle accidents. The second and third leading causes of death are homicide and suicide. For the 25–44 age group (Figure 1.6), accidental death remains number one. However, cancer and heart disease are the second and third leading causes of deaths. These statistics highlight the importance of using seat belts, being alert to thoughts of suicide, screening for cancer (particularly melanoma) and heart disease, and behaving responsibly regarding alcohol, drugs, and firearms. In addition to personally minimizing these risks, consider the positive influence you might have with your peers. A few words of concern and caution from a friend can make a difference, a big difference.

While leading causes of deaths are important to discuss, it's equally important to step back and acknowledge that risky behaviors more often lead to serious injury than to death. The incidence of permanent

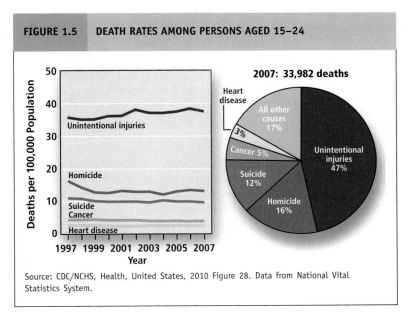

**FIGURE 1.5     DEATH RATES AMONG PERSONS AGED 15–24**

2007: 33,982 deaths

Source: CDC/NCHS, Health, United States, 2010 Figure 28. Data from National Vital Statistics System.

**FIGURE 1.6     DEATH RATES AMONG PERSONS AGED 25–44**

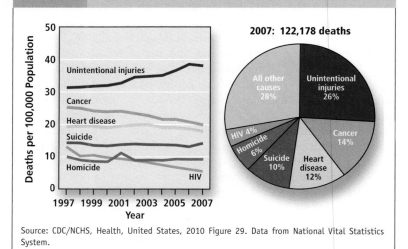

Source: CDC/NCHS, Health, United States, 2010 Figure 29. Data from National Vital Statistics System.

injuries resulting from accidents such as car crashes is often overlooked. The ratio of fatal to nonfatal but significant injuries is about 1 to 4. We all know of someone who survived a terrible accident yet sustained a life-changing injury such as brain damage or paralysis. The risk of death among young adults in America is low; the risk of disability somewhat higher. Both are tragic at a young age—especially when preventable. Most serious accidents are linked to alcohol and drug abuse. Simply taking the time to consider the possible dire consequences goes a long way in preventing dangerous situations. As my grandmother used to say, "Have fun but be careful!"

## HEALTHY PEOPLE 2020

Every ten years, the U.S. Department of Health and Human Services releases new national goals and objectives for health promotion and disease prevention. The most recent version, *Healthy People 2020* (www.healthypeople.gov), was released in December 2010. This comprehensive document is based on updated scientific and medical evidence as well as feedback from a wide range of government agencies, dozens of organizations, and the public. *Healthy People 2020* identifies the most significant preventable threats to public health and sets specific goals to reduce those risks. For example, health experts point out that the chronic diseases of heart disease, cancer, and diabetes are responsible for 7 of every 10 deaths among Americans each year and account for 75 percent of the nation's health spending. Since many of the risk factors that contribute to the development of these diseases are preventable, a major challenge is to help people take specific preventive actions to better reach their full potential for health.

The overarching goals of *Healthy People 2020* are:

1. Attain high-quality, longer lives free of preventable disease and premature death.
2. Achieve health equity, eliminate disparities, and improve the health of all groups.
3. Create social and physical environments that promote good health for all.
4. Promote quality of life, healthy development, and healthy behaviors across life stages.

The second goal is in response to known inequities due to race/ethnicity, socioeconomic status, gender, age, disability status, sexual orientation, and geographic location. The third and fourth goals are new and reflect a broader, more collaborative approach to improving the nation's health.

To progress toward these goals, the national plan uses an ecological approach focusing on both individual-level and population-level factors that influence health. This approach recognizes that health and health behaviors are determined by influences at multiple levels, including personal (biological and psychological), organizational/institutional, environmental (social and physical), and policy levels. In the past, individual-level health approaches were the mainstay. With *Healthy People 2020* though, an emphasis is placed on making our social and physical environments healthier. In Table 1.2, determinants of health are categorized and specific examples are provided for each category.

It's the interplay effect among factors such as those listed in Table 1.2 that determine individual and population health. Interventions that involve multiple determinants are most likely to be effective. The lesson here is that our health is influenced by a combination of factors beyond the boundaries of standard health care and public health. For example, harmful aspects of social and physical environments negatively impact us individually and collectively. Over the next decade, public health experts believe that establishing effective partnerships among different sectors of a community (e.g., education, housing, transportation, agriculture, business) will be instrumental to improving population health.

The 12 leading health indicators and 42 topic areas for *Healthy People 2020* are presented in Table 1.3. The leading health indicators represent the nation's most pressing public health issues. They are intended to help Americans—health professionals *and* consumers—understand

**TABLE 1.2    DETERMINANTS OF HEALTH: TYPES AND EXAMPLES**

**INDIVIDUAL BEHAVIORS**

- Diet
- Physical activity
- Alcohol, tobacco, and other drug use
- Hand washing

**BIOLOGY AND GENETICS**

- Age and gender
- Family history of heart disease
- Inherited conditions (e.g., hemophilia, cystic fibrosis)
- BRCA1 or BRCA2 mutation (higher risk for breast/ovarian cancer)

**HEALTH SERVICES**

- Lack of availability
- High cost
- Lack of insurance coverage
- Limited language access

**PHYSICAL ENVIRONMENT DETERMINANTS**

- Natural environment such as green space, weather, climate
- Worksites, schools, and recreational settings
- Housing, homes, and neighborhoods
- Exposure to toxic substances and other physical hazards

**SOCIAL ENVIRONMENT DETERMINANTS**

- Availability of quality schools
- Exposure to crime and violence
- Social support and social interactions
- Social norms and attitudes including discrimination

**POLICYMAKING**

- Food labeling laws
- Smoking bans in public places
- Gun control laws
- Auto safety standards (e.g., seat belts and air bags)

Source: *Healthy People 2020* (**www.healthypeople.gov**).

which areas we need to focus on the most to improve our health and the health of our families and communities. The 42 topic areas provide a comprehensive framework for goal setting across the spectrum of public health issues. Be sure to notice the 13 new topic areas—for example, genomics, global health, preparedness, and sleep health. Also, the health communication area has been expanded and now includes an emphasis on information technology to improve population health

| TABLE 1.3 | *HEALTHY PEOPLE 2020:* HEALTH INDICATORS AND TOPIC AREAS |
|---|---|

**LEADING HEALTH INDICATORS**

1. Healthy behaviors
2. Tobacco use
3. Substance abuse
4. Responsible sexual behavior
5. Mental health
6. Chronic disease
7. Injury and violence
8. Environmental determinants
9. Social determinants
10. Maternal and infant health
11. Access to care
12. Quality of care

**TOPIC AREAS (LISTED ALPHABETICALLY)**

1. Access to health services
2. Adolescent health*
3. Arthritis, osteoporosis, chronic back conditions
4. Blood disorders and blood safety*
5. Cancer
6. Chronic kidney disease
7. Dementias including Alzheimer's disease*
8. Diabetes
9. Disability and health
10. Early and middle childhood*
11. Educational and community-based programs
12. Environmental health
13. Family planning
14. Food safety
15. Genomics*
16. Global health*
17. Health communication and health information technology
18. Health care–associated infections*
19. Health-related quality of life*
20. Hearing and related disorders
21. Heart disease and stroke
22. HIV
23. Immunization and infectious diseases
24. Injury and violence prevention
25. Lesbian, gay, bisexual, and transgender health*
26. Maternal, infant, and child health
27. Medical product safety
28. Mental health and disorders
29. Nutrition and weight status
30. Occupational safety and health
31. Older adults*
32. Oral health
33. Physical activity
34. Preparedness*
35. Public health infrastructure
36. Respiratory diseases
37. Sexually transmitted diseases
38. Sleep health*
39. Social determinants of health*
40. Substance abuse
41. Tobacco use
42. Vision

*indicates new topic area in *Healthy People 2020*

Sources: Institute of Medicine (**www.iom.edu**) and *Healthy People 2020* (**www.healthypeople.gov**).

outcomes and health care quality. As society and the world changes, so too do our public health needs. Both the priority health indicators and wide-ranging topic areas underscore our role in making healthy choices—for ourselves and those close to us—about doctors, health insurance, health information, and a healthy lifestyle.

In *iHealth* you will find chapters, chapter sections, or selected articles on all 12 of the leading health indicators. As *iHealth* is purposely concise, all indicators do not have their own chapter. Rather, discussions on selected indicators—including injury and violence, environmental determinants, social determinants, and maternal and infant health—are featured in articles and intertwined as appropriate within related chapters.

The public health goal reflected by indicator 7 (and topic 24) is to reduce injuries, disabilities, and deaths due to injuries and violence. Most people sustain a significant injury at some time during their lives. Some mistakenly believe that injuries happen by chance and are the result of unpreventable accidents. Upon reflection, though, most of us know that is not the case. Most injuries are predictable and preventable. As noted previously, the leading cause of death among young adults is injury. Most injuries—unintentional and intentional—are associated with motor vehicle crashes, firearms, poisoning, falls, fires, and drowning, and the vast majority of these occur under the influence of alcohol or drugs.

Violence is also sometimes a factor in injuries. Date rape, spousal abuse, gang violence, and the mass murders at Virginia Tech in 2007 are all examples, from the more common to the rare. We all agree that such grievous incidents are unacceptable. Yet, what can we do? As you study the chapters on drugs, sexuality, stress, mental disorders, and personal health care, thoughtfully weigh the injury and violence issues and consider preventive actions you can take.

For public health indicators 8 and 9 (and topics 12 and 39), the goal is to promote well-being for all through healthy physical and social environments. The quality of the physical environment in which we live is a crucial factor. Examples include preventing or managing exposure to hazardous agents (biological, chemical, physical) in the air, water, soil, and food. Concerns about our physical environment also relate to our broader social environment and a range of diverse issues—from carpooling to city planning to the homeless. Our social and physical environments overlap and interact in many areas such as housing, land use, transportation, industry, agriculture, and safety. How can we give higher priority to protecting our living spaces and providing social networks and services that support healthy living?

Global environmental health issues also need to be faced. For instance, the effects of pathogens (disease-causing microbes) on food supplies and health are an increasing concern as world markets and international travel continue to expand. Then there are the calamities of natural disasters and the ever-present threat of bioterrorism. Less sensational but perhaps even more serious is the impact of

Article
1.4

overpopulation on health. Can we avert planetary overload and environmental degradation by controlling population growth and managing environmental resources? On all of these global issues, is multinational cooperation possible? Although it may be difficult to think of ourselves as members of a world community, it's becoming more of a reality every day and warrants our attention and action. Consider how our environment—both social and physical aspects—influences individual, community, and population health as you read the chapters on diet, stress, mental health, cancers, infections, and health care.

## PROSPECTS FOR THE 21ST CENTURY

Descriptions of today's achievements in science, technology, and medicine read like the science fiction of your grandparents' generation. What medical advances are on the horizon over the next decade? And, importantly, what are the implications for such progress? Selected health trends associated with key scientific concepts provide examples of what the future holds:

- Based on human genome research, the ability to screen for genetically based diseases and to tailor interventions will be greatly expanded. Issues associated with genetic counseling, patient privacy, and insurability will continue to be debated.
- Major advances will continue to be made in noninvasive medical imaging designed to screen for and diagnose cancers, heart disease, and neurological disorders such as depression and Alzheimer's disease. Sophisticated scanners will be faster, more accurate, and less burdensome on patients.
- The concept of racial blending will begin to replace the traditional racial-categories paradigm. Reducing health disparities among groups will no longer be based on race per se, but rather on economic, educational, and cultural factors.
- A grand melding of molecular biology, genetic engineering, and nanotechnology will strengthen the drug discovery and delivery process. Pharmacological research will develop drugs to treat every major disease.
- Advances in biomedical engineering will yield a new generation of tissue and organ replacements and improve the transplantation process. Growing and harvesting tissues in the laboratory will become a reality.

The examples listed above give a sense of the wondrous medical advances that are being made. Yet, such scientific and technological developments must be seriously considered and debated in light of ethical, social, and economic implications and the development of public policy.

Our health will continue to be influenced by a wide array of scientific advances, public health goals, changing societal expectations, and new and revised governmental policies. Yet, at the level of the individual and the family, it's ironic that the greatest potential benefit for the future health of Americans is not biomedical research. Rather, as prominent scientific and medical experts increasingly agree, the greatest promise for improved health lies with preventive medicine and a focus on understanding health as a consequence of human behavior.

Article 1.5

### ✓ NEED TO KNOW

Over the past century, tremendous gains have been made in the average lifespan and quality of life for Americans due largely to major advances in public health, drug discovery, and medical technology. Today the major causes of death are chronic diseases, not infectious diseases. Chronic diseases—such as heart disease, cancer, and diabetes (type 2)— are strongly tied to how we choose to live, to our daily habits. The nation's high-priority health issues are summarized in *Healthy People 2020*. They remind us that environmental factors (social and physical) also influence our health.

## ➤ Understanding Health Behaviors

Personal health texts focus primarily on knowledge and secondarily on contextual factors that influence our views and behaviors. However, a reminder is apropos—*knowledge by itself does not ensure positive decision making*. If it did, we would not see doctors and nurses who smoke or nutritionists who are overweight. Attitudes, beliefs, and values as well as knowledge underlie our decisions about health. This combination of influences makes it unlikely that a single factor is the basis of any given health decision. How can knowledge be separated from attitudes? Or attitudes from values? Decision making is clearly dependent on multiple factors.

The presentation of content is never done in a vacuum. Attitudes, beliefs, and values are shaped by our environment. The influence of family, friends, school, workplace, the media, and societal customs is substantial. Both formal and informal learning occur within these social and societal contexts. No individual makes decisions that are truly independent of all other persons and the society in which we live. The process by which we learn a new behavior or modify a current one is multifaceted. An appreciation of this is a prerequisite to understanding behavior.

Many of us have good intentions about changing an unhealthy habit (e.g., quitting smoking) or adopting a healthier behavior (e.g., eating more fruits and vegetables). The challenge is *how* to do it. As pointed out, our behaviors are complex, and from personal experience we know habits are not changed easily. So if we wish to change a behavior, we need a well-grounded plan. But before we can make a plan, we must first have a basic understanding of how people change.

To better understand health habits and behavior change, psychologists have developed **health behavior theories.** Briefly reviewing a few selected theories can be instructive because each theory takes a different approach to analyzing and explaining changes in health behaviors. Seeing the components of a behavior and the logic that connects them provide insights to our own behaviors. Three of the most practical theories are social cognitive theory, the health belief model, and the stages of change model. A brief overview of each theory is presented; more complete explanations are available in the online booklet *Theory at a Glance* (see Website Resources at the end of this chapter). These behavior-change theories will be referred to periodically throughout *iHealth* to illustrate their usefulness in formulating plans for translating good intentions into action.

## SOCIAL COGNITIVE THEORY

Albert Bandura's social cognitive theory is based on the principle that behavior is dynamic, depending on individual and environmental factors, all of which influence one another simultaneously. As illustrated in Figure 1.7, there is an ongoing interaction among a person's characteristics (biological, psychological, experiential), the environment within which the behavior is performed (social influences, physical environment, societal norms), and the specific behavior's characteristics.

A change in one component of the model will affect the others. To see how this works, let's use exercise as a behavior we wish to increase (target behavior). A personal characteristic such as confidence in being able to exercise for 30 minutes on a treadmill (an example of self-efficacy) will influence whether the person does, in fact, perform that behavior. Characteristics of the environment include available facilities (e.g., fitness center or exercise equipment) and associated factors such as affordability, convenience, and safety. The environment also includes

A **health behavior theory** is a conceptual framework of key factors or variables hypothesized to influence health behavior. An established theory is logical, supported by evidence, and underpins behavior change plans and strategies.

FIGURE 1.7    SOCIAL COGNITIVE THEORY

Source: Based on the work of Albert Bandura.

the social environment (e.g., the degree to which family and friends encourage and support the person's new exercise routine). Finally, the positive and negative characteristics of the behavior itself must be considered (e.g., whether the exercise was invigorating, challenging, and completed with a sense of accomplishment or exhausting, boring, and frustrating).

Social cognitive theory holds that the interactions among the individual, the environment, and the specific behavior are subtle and complex, but it provides a framework for understanding them. This ecological approach attempts to encompass all possible determinants of health behavior for individuals in their everyday lives. A key point is that success in changing a health behavior is just not a matter of self-determination. In addition to intention and commitment, an awareness of other potential intervening factors is necessary. The ecological framework for understanding population health (inclusion of environmental determinants, both social and physical) adopted by *Healthy People 2020* can be seen as an expansion of social cognitive theory.

## HEALTH BELIEF MODEL

Irwin Rosenstock's health belief model, one of the first theories of health behavior, was developed in the 1950s to explain why so few people participated in a national chest X-ray screening program for tuberculosis. The hypothesis was that many people hold mistaken beliefs about a disease or the screening process and that this keeps them from taking advantage of beneficial screening. In recent years, the health belief model has been used to improve participation in mammogram screening and to prevent the spread of sexually transmitted infections (STIs) and HIV.

The premise of the health belief model is that health-seeking behavior is influenced by a person's perception of a threat posed by a health problem and the value associated with actions aimed at reducing that threat. This involves a sequence from perception to assessment to action (or inaction). As seen in Figure 1.8, a person first forms a belief about the seriousness of and susceptibility to a medical condition. How dangerous is it? Will I get it? Cues to action (e.g., media campaigns, advice from others, illness of family member, doctor's explanation) can influence the person's perceived threat. A host of factors—both individual (e.g., age, gender, personality, personal experience) and socioeconomic (e.g., peer pressure, ethnicity, education, income)—play a role in both the perception of risk and the person's cost/benefit analysis (barriers to action versus benefits of action).

The model predicts that individuals will take action (e.g., screening, treatment) if: (1) they perceive themselves to be susceptible and that the condition will have serious consequences (high perceived threat), and (2) they believe a successful course of action to reduce susceptibility or minimize consequences is available and the benefits of taking action outweigh the barriers (positive cost/benefit analysis). The final step to take action is then dependent on the person's confidence to follow through (self-efficacy). The health belief model has been applied to sex education programs that aim to prevent STIs and HIV by increasing condom use, as well as in secondary prevention efforts to aid early detection of STIs or HIV. This model provides a framework

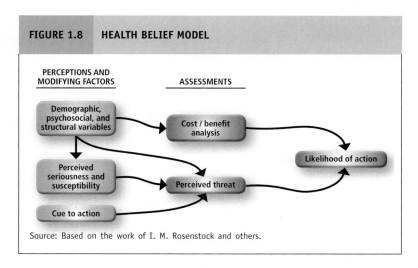

FIGURE 1.8    HEALTH BELIEF MODEL

PERCEPTIONS AND MODIFYING FACTORS

ASSESSMENTS

Demographic, psychosocial, and structural variables

Cost / benefit analysis

Perceived seriousness and susceptibility

Perceived threat

Likelihood of action

Cue to action

Source: Based on the work of I. M. Rosenstock and others.

for individuals, health care workers, and educators to use in understanding and intervening in the spread of these conditions.

## STAGES OF CHANGE MODEL

James Prochaska and Carlo DiClemente's stages of change model—technically known as the transtheoretical model—is often integrated with other theories (hence *trans-* or "across"). The central premise is that behavior change is a process, not an event and that individuals have varying levels of motivation or readiness to change. For most health behaviors, there appear to be five stages of change: (1) precontemplation—not thinking about change, (2) contemplation—thinking about change, (3) preparation—making small changes toward the desired behavior, (4) action—actually engaging in the desired behavior, and (5) maintenance—sustaining the new behavior over a prolonged period (Figure 1.9). The model predicts that individuals progress through these stages, but it also recognizes that setbacks occur. People can and do relapse to previous stages. This is accepted as a normal part of the change process.

The stages of change model was initially developed as a framework to understand smoking cessation programs. Over the years, the model has been adapted and used with a number of other health behaviors including eating and physical activity. The conceptual appeal of the stages of change model is that specific behavior-change strategies can be matched to specific stages. The type of information, counseling,

**FIGURE 1.9     STAGES OF CHANGE MODEL**

Source: Based on the work of J. O. Prochaska and C. C. DiClemente.

incentives, or reinforcement can be tailored to an individual's level of readiness or motivation (stage of change). Time frames may be associated with specific stages; for example, the "action stage" typically refers to the first six months of change, and the "maintenance stage" refers to continuing the behavior beyond six months. After several years, the target behavior becomes an established habit and part of one's lifestyle.

Across many different behavior-change theories, four factors appear to be necessary for successful change to occur: a *knowledge* or awareness of the benefit of the change, the *motivation* to take action, the *opportunity* in terms of resources and time, and the necessary *behavioral skills*. Your personal health course and *iHealth* are oriented toward increasing knowledge and assisting you in developing the requisite skill set (planning, organizational, and behavior-specific skills) to modify or adopt a target behavior. Increased motivation may be a byproduct of the class experience as well. When thinking about changing a health behavior, use the behavior-change models and keep the four common factors in mind: *knowledge, motivation, opportunity,* and *skills*.

## NEED TO KNOW

Behavior change is a complex process and often difficult to sustain. Developing healthy behaviors sometimes means competing against ingrained social and environmental practices. Information by itself is typically not enough. The benefits of behavior change must be compelling and outweigh the barriers. Three widely used health behavior models are social cognitive theory, the health belief model, and the stages of change model. Across models, four factors appear to be necessary for successful behavior change: knowledge, motivation, opportunity, and skills. Use conceptual frameworks and these four factors to guide you in making healthful lifestyle changes.

Website Resources

## connect Resources

 **ARTICLES**

1.1 "Aging Well: Toward a Way of Life for All People." *Preventing Chronic Disease* (CDC). This essay argues that creating a framework for dealing with aging issues will assist policymakers in meeting the needs of our growing older population.

1.2 "No Truth to the Fountain of Youth." *Scientific American*. While no anti-aging product has been proven to be a true cure, some products have been proven dangerous.

1.3 "Simple Tools for Understanding Risks: From Innumeracy to Insight." *British Medical Journal*. A psychologist and a medical professor discuss common pitfalls in medical decision making related to not understanding statistics.

1.4 "Global Warming: No Big Deal?" *The Atlantic*. How personal risk perception colors a person's worldview on broad issues such as global warming.

1.5 "Getting Serious about the Prevention of Chronic Diseases." *Preventing Chronic Disease*. Two public health experts talk about key strategies to include in the health reform movement.

 **SELF-ASSESSMENT**

1.1 Consider the Six Dimensions of Health

## Website Resources

Adbusters **http://adbusters.org**
Ad Council **www.adcouncil.org**
Centers for Disease Control and Prevention (CDC)
 **www.cdc.gov**
FamilyDoctor.org **www.familydoctor.org**
Health Communication, Health Literacy, and e-Health
 **www.health.gov/communication**
Health on the Net Foundation **www.hon.ch**
Healthfinder.gov **www.healthfinder.gov**
*Healthy People 2020* **www.healthypeople.gov**
*Issues in Science and Technology* **www.issues.org**
MayoClinic **www.mayoclinic.com**
MedlinePlus **http://medlineplus.gov**
Office of Minority Health (U.S. Department of Health and
 Human Services) **www.omhrc.gov**

Resources for Health Consumers (Medical Library Association)
**www.mlanet.org/resources/consumr_index.html**
*Theory at a Glance* (National Cancer Institute, NIH)
**www.cancer.gov/cancertopics/cancerlibrary/theory.pdf**
U.S. Census Bureau **www.census.gov**
WebMD **www.webmd.com**

## Knowing the Language

chronic disease, 25
epidemiology, 20
health, 3
health behavior theory, 35
health literacy, 11

health risk or risk factor, 19
infectious disease, 23
quality of life, 4
relative risk, 21

## Understanding the Content

1. Contrast the treatment model and the optimal health model.
2. What is meant by *health literacy*? What are the underlying factors that contribute to a person's health literacy?
3. What is epidemiology? Contrast the terms *absolute risk* and *relative risk*. As a young adult, what are your greatest risks for injury/illness and death?
4. Contrast the terms *infectious disease* and *chronic disease*. What is meant by the term *lifestyle disease*? What are the leading *actual* causes of disease in the United States?
5. Describe two behavior-change theories and how they could be used to help a person improve a health behavior.

## Exploring Ideas

1. Why should health be thought of as having different dimensions? How can this be helpful in improving our health or achieving personal goals?
2. To what degree do you have control over your current quality of life? Is it determined by your conscious decision making or by factors beyond your control?
3. How should one go about gathering information on a health topic? Select a health question, investigate it, and report on the process and your findings.

American Academy of Pediatrics, Committee on Public Education. Children, adolescents, and television. *Pediatrics* 107: 423–426, 2001.

American Cancer Society. Cancer Facts & Figures 2010. **www.cancer.org**

American College Health Association. ACHA–National College Health Assessment (NCHA) Data: Fall 2010. **www.acha-ncha.org/pubs_rpts.html**

*Atlanta Journal Constitution.* Lizzie Brown, 111, calm, kind, centenarian. Obituary section, January 6, 2003.

Bandura A. *Self-efficacy: The Exercise of Control.* New York: W. H. Freeman, 1997.

Centers for Disease Control and Prevention (CDC). *Health, United States, 2010.* **www.cdc.gov/nchs/hus.htm**

Corbett S. The long road from Sudan to America. *New York Times,* April 1, 2001.

Danaei G, Ding EL, Mozaffariah D, et al. The preventable causes of death in the United States: Comparative risk assessment of dietary, lifestyle, and metabolic risk factors. *PLOS Medicine* 6 (4): 2009.

Glanz K, Rimer BK, Viswanath K. *Health Behavior and Health Education: Theory, Research, and Practice* (4th ed.). San Francisco: Jossey-Bass, 2008.

Institute of Medicine (IOM). *Health Literacy: A Prescription to End Confusion.* Washington, DC: National Academies Press, 2004.

IOM. *Leading Health Indicators for Healthy People 2020.* Washington, DC: National Academies Press, 2011.

McMichael AJ. *Planetary Overload: Global Environmental Change and the Health of the Human Species.* New York: Cambridge University Press, 1993.

Medical Library Association. "Top Ten" Most Useful Consumer Health Websites. **www.mlanet.org/resources/userguide.html#5**

*Morbidity & Mortality Weekly Report (MMWR).* Ten great public health achievements—United States, 1900–1999. *MMWR* 48 (12): 241–243, 1999.

*MMWR.* Achievements in public health, 1900–1999: Healthier mothers and babies. *MMWR* 48 (38): 849–858, 1999.

Mokdad AH, Marks JS, Stroup DF, et al. Actual causes of death in the United States, 2000. *JAMA* 291 (10): 1238–1245, 2004.

National Institutes of Health (NIH). Understanding risk: *What do those headlines really mean?* July 2003. **www.nia.nih.gov/HealthInformation/Publications/risk.htm**

Prochaska JO, DiClemente CC. Stages and processes of self-change of smoking: Toward an integrated model of change. *Journal of Consulting and Clinical Psychology* 51: 390–395, 1983.

Prochaska JO, DiClemente CC, Norcross JC. In search of how people change: Applications to addictive behaviors. *American Psychologist* 47 (9): 1102–1114, 1992.

Rauscher FH, Shaw GL, Ky KN. Music and spatial task performance. *Nature* 365: 611, 1993.

Ropeik D. *How Risky Is It, Really? Why Our Fears Don't Always Match the Facts.* New York: McGraw-Hill, 2010.

Rosenstock IM, Strecher VJ, Becker MH. Social learning theory and the health belief model. *Health Education Quarterly* 15 (2): 175–183, 1988.

Schwartz B. *The Paradox of Choice: Why More Is Less.* New York: HarperCollins, 2004.

U.S. Census Bureau. **www.census.gov**

World Health Organization (WHO). Definition of health. **www.who.int/suggestions/faq/en/index.html**

It's difficult to think
anything but pleasant
thoughts while eating
a homegrown tomato.

— LEWIS GRIZZARD

# Chapter 2

## CHOOSE A HEALTHY DIET

In Chapter 2 we discuss food, a subject near and dear to all.
We present the basic vocabulary of nutrition and current recommendations for a healthy diet, and we discuss steps and strategies to improve our eating habits. We give special attention to the topic of weight control because it is of particular interest and relevance. Our aim is to separate the science from the advertising and show you how to navigate the gray areas.

A CENTURY AGO, the majority of Americans still lived on farms and raised their own food. Nearly every family had a vegetable garden and kept chickens for eggs. Working the garden and canning (and later freezing) the "produce" (vegetables and fruits) was standard practice. It was essential to stock the pantry to provide for food throughout the winter and into the spring. Many homesteads had a milk cow. Some also raised hogs or cattle for meat. Sausage and hams or beef cuts were bartered with neighbors in exchange for other goods. Grains were taken to a central stone mill to be ground into flour. The food supply was direct and simple; food was minimally processed. Agribusiness and the food industry were in their infancy.

Life was physically demanding, whether working on the farm or in a mill, mine, or factory. And the way people ate reflected the physical demands of how they lived. Breakfast, a hearty hot meal, included meat and eggs, not cereal out of a box. Dinner—the midday meal—was the largest meal of the day, with meats, vegetables, and bread or biscuits that were made from scratch every day. Lunch was a meal that evolved in the cities. The evening meal, known as supper, was a lighter meal, often simply leftovers from dinner.

Unlike today, an ample food supply was not a given. There were good years and lean years, depending on the weather, crop infestations, natural disasters, and human and animal epidemics. A plentiful harvest was celebrated, and hard times were endured. Think of the changes that your great-grandparents lived through and how those changes affected their eating patterns. Examples include transitioning from rural to city life, the development of refrigeration and modern appliances, new job opportunities not dependent on manual labor, and the ever-expanding grocery store.

Over the past century, dramatic changes have occurred in nearly every aspect of American life, including how and what we eat. Thanks to the scientific research of the past 30 to 40 years, we have an excellent understanding of the connections between nutrition and health. Without question, food resources and nutrition knowledge are far more extensive today than when your grandparents were your age. By considering the historical perspective, you can better appreciate the current food environment and understand the origins of the diet-related health challenges we now face. Your generation can share in the bounty of food choices available today but also must face pressing contemporary issues such as obesity, eating disorders, and dietary supplements. Keep this in mind as you study this chapter and learn to eat healthier.

## ➤ Nutrition Basics

Nutrition is the science of food and how the body uses it in health and disease. A nutrient is simply a substance found in food that is used by the body to support normal growth, maintenance, and repair. The six nutrient classes are carbohydrates, fats, protein, vitamins, minerals, and water. Nutrients can be broadly categorized based on the quantity that should be consumed. The **macronutrients**—carbohydrates, fats, protein, and water—are the main constituents of our food and form the bulk of what we eat every day. In contrast, the **micronutrients**—vitamins and minerals—are needed only in small quantities, and many are not required daily. Micronutrients occur naturally in many of our unprocessed foods such as fruits, vegetables, and whole grains. Nutrients are also categorized based on whether they are energy sources. Carbohydrates, fats, and protein are the energy nutrients. Vitamins, minerals, and water do not yield energy, but their presence in the body is necessary to aid in the proper use of the energy nutrients. Consequently, vitamins, minerals, and water are known as regulatory nutrients.

From a biological perspective, good nutrition is about providing both the right blend of nutrients and adequate fuel (energy) for the body's many needs. Balancing energy intake with energy expenditure is fundamental to maintaining a healthy weight. Weight control is a hotly debated and controversial topic that we address later in this chapter. In terms of basic nutrition, energy density and recommended energy intake by macronutrient are summarized in Table 2.1. At 9 Cal (Calories or kilocalories) per gram, fats have more than twice the energy (per weight) of carbohydrates and protein, which yield 4 Cal per gram. As we discuss carbohydrates, fats, and protein in turn, refer back to Table 2.1 to see what the recommended relative contributions should be.

For the sake of clarity, a comment about energy units is warranted. The common energy unit in the United States is the **Calorie (Cal),** or **kilocalorie (kcal).** (For the curious, the rest of the world uses the kilojoule, abbreviated kj.) Technically, 1 Cal, or kcal, is the amount of heat needed to raise 1 kg of water 1° Celsius. Yes, a Calorie (with a capital "C") is the same as a kilocalorie. Both terms are widely used: Food labels typically report Calories, while energy expenditure is often expressed in kilocalories. For example, a 12-oz. can of Coca-Cola contains 140 Cal, which is equivalent to the 140 kcal expended in walking 1.5 mi. To remove any confusion, our convention in *iHealth* is to use only Calories (Cal) when reporting energy intake or expenditure values. Last, a point on documentation in this chapter: Unless specifically

**Macronutrients** are the nutrients required in the greatest amounts, namely carbohydrates, fats, protein, and water. **Micronutrients** are nutrients that are required only in small amounts, the vitamins and minerals.

**Calorie (Cal),** or alternately the **kilocalorie (kcal),** is the standard unit of energy used in the United States to define and describe human energy intake and energy expenditure.

**TABLE 2.1** **RECOMMENDED ENERGY INTAKE BY MACRONUTRIENT**

| | | PERCENTAGE OF TOTAL DAILY CALORIES | |
| | | TARGET* | RANGE |
|---|---|---|---|
| **Carbohydrates** | 4 Cal/gram | 55% | 45–65% |
| | Emphasize complex carbohydrates | | |
| | Minimize sugars | [≤25%] | |
| **Fats** | 9 Cal/gram | 30% | 20–35% |
| | Emphasize unsaturated fats | | |
| | Minimize saturated fats | [≤10%] | |
| **Protein** | 4 Cal/gram | 15% | 10–35% |
| | | 100% | |

*Although percentages can vary within the given ranges, it is useful to have specific percentages to use as guidelines.

Source: Based on the *Dietary Guidelines* and the *Dietary Reference Intakes*.

cited otherwise, all recommendations that contain specific nutritional values or dietary intakes are based on two federal documents, either *Dietary Guidelines for Americans* (2010) or *Dietary Reference Intakes* (2006), both of which are available online.

## CARBOHYDRATES AND FIBER

The main function of **carbohydrates** is to provide energy. They are your body's main energy source, the primary fuel for your cells. Each gram of carbohydrate yields approximately 4 Cal, the same as a gram of protein. Carbohydrates should compose the largest percentage of daily caloric intake, at about 55 percent (within a range of 45–65 percent). Carbohydrates include both starches and sugars. Starches, or complex carbohydrates, are found in bread, rice, pasta, cereals, and vegetables. Sugars, or simple carbohydrates, are found in fruits, milk, and many processed foods and drinks that have added sugar, such as candy, pastries, desserts, and soft drinks.

In addition to supplying energy, complex carbohydrates and sugars from fruits and milk supply fiber, vitamins, minerals, and water. Consequently, they should be emphasized over sugars from candy, other sweets, and soft drinks. In addition, your body absorbs complex carbohydrates

**Carbohydrates** are organic compounds (i.e., they contain carbon, oxygen, hydrogen) divided into two types—simple and complex; they are generally known as sugars and starches.

more slowly than it absorbs sugars, providing more energy for a longer period. Remember that snacks and desserts with added sugar—such as candies, cakes, cookies, doughnuts, fruit drinks, and ice cream—provide many calories but offer negligible amounts of other nutrients. That is why typical junk foods are often referred to as having "empty calories," or as having low nutrient density. In the United States, soft drinks are the top source of added sugars.

Fiber—also referred to as roughage—is the indigestible part of plant-based foods. Nutritionists divide fiber into two types: soluble and insoluble. Soluble fiber may improve your cholesterol and blood sugar (glucose) levels. It's found in oats, dried beans, and some fruits. Insoluble fiber adds bulk to your stool and helps prevent constipation. It also reduces your risk of colorectal cancer. It's found mainly in vegetables, whole grains, and wheat bran. The average American consumes only 10 to 15 g (grams) of total fiber per day. Federal guidelines recommend 25 g per day for women and 38 g per day for men.

Self
Assessment
2.1

What's the best way to increase fiber? Eat a variety of whole grains, vegetables, legumes (peas, beans, lentils), and fruits. When buying bread, look for the word *whole* next to the name of the grain in the list of ingredients (e.g., whole wheat). Select bread with at least 3 g of fiber per slice and cereals with 3 g or more of fiber per serving. Try whole-wheat pasta—it typically has three times the amount of fiber as regular pasta.

To help encourage Americans to eat a variety of fruits and vegetables every day, the Centers for Disease Control and Prevention (CDC) and the Produce for Better Health Foundation administer an online public health initiative (**www.fruitsandveggiesmatter.gov).** This web page calculates how many fruits and vegetables you need and provides tips for adding more servings into your daily routine. As a general guide, most Americans should have five or more servings of fruits and vegetables every day.

## FATS AND CHOLESTEROL

**Fats,** or lipids, in the diet serve several purposes. They are the most concentrated energy source, yielding about 9 Cal per gram, more than twice that of carbohydrate or protein. Fats should constitute about 30 percent or less of total calories consumed each day (range: 20–35 percent). Fats satisfy hunger because of their slow absorption rate from the

**Fats,** or lipids, are organic compounds that provide the most concentrated source of calories in a diet. Saturated fats are found primarily in animal products, and unsaturated fats come from plants.

digestive system. Fats also play a role in many other functions, such as the maintenance and function of cell membranes and the absorption of the four fat-soluble vitamins (A, D, E, and K).

It is extremely important to understand the different kinds of dietary fats. Saturated fats are generally from animal sources such as meat, poultry, eggs, and dairy products (butter, cream, whole milk, cheese). Yet palm and coconut oils, which come from plants, are also saturated fats. Saturated fats are solid at room temperature. Diets high in saturated fats elevate blood cholesterol levels and risk of cardiovascular disease. *Trans* fats, which are vegetable oils chemically converted to a solid form, also raise blood cholesterol and should be minimized (refer to "Breaking It Down" for the full story). No more than 10 percent of total calories should come from saturated fats and *trans* fats.

Remember though, all fats do not get the thumbs down. Unsaturated fats are actually good for us. These fats are mainly plant-based and are liquid at room temperature. Polyunsaturated fats like corn, safflower, and sunflower oils are healthy choices. And monounsaturated fats like olive, peanut, and canola oils are even better, being the most healthful of the unsaturated fats. Also, substantial evidence indicates that omega-3 fatty acids—found in certain types of fish, such as salmon—bestow a variety of benefits, particularly to the maintenance of cardiovascular health.

Self Assessment 2.2

Cholesterol is a fatlike substance found throughout cells of the body. It is an essential substance that the body can obtain through diet or by production in the liver. Dietary intake should be less than 300 mg per day. All animal fats contain cholesterol, whereas fats from plant sources do not. Concentrated sources include eggs yolks (about 200 mg per yolk) and meats (60–100 mg per 3-oz. serving). Limit cholesterol; however, don't overemphasize its importance. Focus on reducing animal fats, and in turn, you will also be minimizing dietary cholesterol. Remember that the primary dietary determinant of high blood cholesterol has been shown to be saturated fats and *trans* fats, not cholesterol.

## PROTEIN

**Protein,** which is contained in every cell in your body, is necessary for tissue growth and maintenance. Protein is found in foods from animal and plant sources. Each gram of protein yields about 4 Cal, the same as

---

**Proteins** are complex organic compounds made up of amino acids that perform a wide variety of functions that include serving as structural components, enzymes, and signaling molecules.

The unusual story of *trans* fats deserves mention in any discussion of dietary fats. *Trans* fats are produced when unsaturated oils are partially hydrogenated (through the addition of hydrogen), a process that converts vegetable oils to more solid forms. This conversion increases shelf life and flavor stability. In 1911 Procter & Gamble introduced Crisco, a product of hydrogenation. It was the first solidified shortening product made entirely of vegetable oil. Crisco provided an economical alternative to lard (animal fat) and butter. In the 1940s stick margarines were introduced, followed by tub margarines and vegetable oil spreads in the 1960s. With a growing awareness of the health risks of saturated fats, the scientific community promoted the use of margarine—an unsaturated fat—as the healthy alternative to butter. The resulting increase in the use of *trans* fats occurred not only in our kitchens but also in restaurants and the fast-food and baking industries as hydrogenated vegetable oils replaced lard.

At that time, there was no way to know that the process of hydrogenation chemically altered vegetable oil in a detrimental way. Yet, by the 1990s, substantial evidence had come to light showing that *trans* fats are actually as harmful (or even more harmful) in increasing blood cholesterol levels as the saturated fats they were meant to replace. In recent years, the challenge has been to update the American consumer. In 2003, after further study and careful review, the Food and Drug Administration (FDA) mandated that by 2006 all food labels must report the amount of *trans* fats as well as saturated and unsaturated fats. Many food companies have already reduced or eliminated *trans* fats in their products. The bottom line: Check the food labels and eat as few *trans* fats as possible.

So we have come full circle. Vegetable shortening and margarine (*trans* fats from hydrogenation) were initially hailed as a healthy, practical option to lard and butter and widely accepted by the public. In the ensuing years, the effects of eating the new *trans* fats were studied, and they were found to be as dangerous as or worse than animal-based fats. What's the lesson? Creating new food products can have both upsides and downsides, and sometimes only time will reveal them.

carbohydrate. However, its role as an energy source is secondary to that of carbohydrate and fat. Poultry, seafood, meat, dairy products, legumes (beans, peas, peanuts, soy products), nuts, and seeds are the richest sources of proteins. About 15 percent of total daily calories should come from protein (range, 10–35 percent). There is some evidence that a higher protein intake (20–35 percent of total calories) may be beneficial for certain individuals. As more studies are published regarding this issue, dietary advice will evolve.

The basic components of proteins are amino acids. Of the 22 amino acids used in the body, only 9 are necessary in the diet and thus are known as the essential amino acids. The body has the ability to manufacture the remaining 13. Animal protein is complete, containing all 9 essential amino acids in sufficient amounts. In contrast, plant proteins are incomplete, lacking one or more of the essential amino acids. However, different plant foods can be eaten together to supply a complete protein, such as beans with rice or peanut butter on whole-grain bread. These complementary plant–protein relationships are especially important to vegetarians.

The amount of protein your body needs depends primarily on your body size. Recommended protein intake is 0.8 g per kg of body weight per day. For example, if you weigh 154 lb. (70 kg), then you should be consuming 56 g of protein per day. Most Americans typically consume far more protein than they need. What happens to those excess calories? If your body does not need the protein, it converts and stores those extra calories as fat. A final tip: Remember to choose your sources of proteins wisely. Many of the high-protein animal-based foods are also high in saturated fat and cholesterol. Emphasize meats that are lean, skinless, and nonfried, and consider obtaining some of your protein from plant sources.

## VITAMINS AND MINERALS

**Vitamins** (organic compounds) and **minerals** (chemical elements) are only found in small quantities in our food, yet these micronutrients have multiple and diverse roles in regulating and maintaining our bodies' functions. Many play special roles in the prevention and treatment of common chronic diseases. Federal standards for good nutrition (known as Dietary Reference Intakes) are available for 13 vitamins and 15 minerals and are organized by age, gender, and special conditions such as pregnancy. A link to these detailed tables is provided under Website Resources at the end of the chapter. Although a complete review of the micronutrients is beyond the scope of *iHealth,* we

**Vitamins** are a class of diverse organic substances that occur in many foods in small amounts and are necessary in trace amounts for the normal metabolic functioning of the body. **Minerals** are a group of inorganic elements that are essential to a variety of physiological processes and are obtained through the foods and beverages we consume.

Berries are examples of antioxidant-rich foods.

provide a brief overview to set the stage for further self-directed study.

Vitamins are either fat-soluble or water-soluble. The fat-soluble vitamins—A, D, E, and K—are necessary for the function or structural integrity of specific body tissues and membranes and are retained in the body. Most water-soluble vitamins are catalysts or coenzymes in metabolic processes and energy transfer and are excreted fairly rapidly. It is important to highlight the potential benefits of vitamins A, E, and C as antioxidants; antioxidants counter the harmful oxidative effects of free radicals and in so doing may protect body cells from damage. (For basic information on vitamins, including primary functions and food sources, see **http://kidshealth.org/teen/ misc/vitamin_chart.html;** for comprehensive descriptions, see the web page of the Micronutrient Information Center at the Linus Pauling Institute: **http://lpi.oregonstate.edu/infocenter/vitamins.html**.)

Calcium, iron, sodium, and potassium are four minerals familiar to many of us because they are linked to medical conditions. Low iron intake can lead to anemia (iron-deficiency anemia) in young women, and low calcium is related to osteoporosis. Conversely, high intakes of some minerals can be problematic. Excess iron intake (iron overload) in men increases risk for heart disease and cancer, and high sodium intake is related to hypertension. Temporary deficiencies may lead to acute conditions. For example, the nausea and weakness associated with heat illness is due in part to loss of potassium and sodium in sweat, as these minerals regulate water balance and nerve function. Accordingly, these minerals are put in sports drinks to aid recovery. As with vitamins, several minerals including selenium and manganese have been identified as antioxidants. (For basic information on minerals, see **http://kidshealth. org/teen/misc/mineral_chart.html,** and for comprehensive descriptions, go to **http://lpi.oregonstate.edu/infocenter/minerals.html**.)

## WATER

Water is the most essential nutrient. For many Americans though, water could just as well be called the forgotten nutrient as sweetened beverages dominate everyday fluid consumption patterns. People can ingest too few (or none) of the other nutrients for days or weeks before problems arise—not so with water. Insufficient water intake can result in symptoms ranging from lethargy to disorientation to death, depending on the degree of dehydration. Loss of water occurs primarily through urination, perspiration, and respiration (water vapor in the air we breathe out).

Women who appear to be adequately hydrated consume an average of about 90 oz. (2.7 liters [L])—from all beverages and foods—each day, while men average about 125 oz. (3.7 L) daily. About 80 percent of people's total water intake comes from drinking water and beverages—including caffeinated drinks—and the other 20 percent comes from food. Based on these estimates, women should be drinking about nine 8 oz. glasses of water and beverages per day (72 oz.), and men about 12–13 glasses (100 oz.). Due attention should be given to *what* we are drinking, however. The Beverage Guidance Panel reports that about 50 percent of Americans' excess calories come from sweetened (nondiet) beverages (Popkin et al., 2006). The panel recommends that water be the drink of choice and consumption of sweetened beverages be reduced.

Individual water needs may vary widely with body size, environmental conditions, and exercise patterns. Since the body's main method of cooling is by evaporation of perspiration, living in a hot climate or engaging in heavy physical activity can increase the body's water requirement substantially. Individuals can easily lose 1–3 percent of their body weight after several hours of exertion in the heat. Under these conditions, thirst alone may not be a good indicator of dehydration. Other measures for monitoring hydration are recommended: for example, checking body weight on a daily basis to ensure (water) weight is regained by drinking plenty of fluids in the hours following prolonged heat exposure or exercise. For more information, see "Dietary water and sodium requirements for active adults" (Kenney, 2004).

Article 2.1

---

✓ **NEED TO KNOW**

Nutrition is about understanding what types and how much food a person needs. To appreciate and apply nutrition principles, we must know that nutrients are composed of macronutrients (carbohydrates, fats, protein, water) and micronutrients (vitamins, minerals), and we must learn the basics about each type of nutrient. This fundamental knowledge serves as the foundation for making wise decisions about what we eat.

> Recommendations for Healthy Eating

The American public is under siege from an information blitz about nutrition and food. And much of the news is bleak. Obesity has become a major public health problem. As a society we eat too much and exercise too little. Many of the foods we eat are high in saturated fat, low in fiber, and stripped of naturally occurring vitamins and minerals. We live in a fast-paced, affluent society where convenience rules. Established restaurants regularly revamp menus, and new restaurants launch every day. Supermarkets are open round-the-clock. New food products are released on a regular basis. Today's large supermarkets carry over 200 fruits and vegetables in their fresh produce sections and stock over 20,000 items on their shelves. In our food and nutrition landscape, the choices are plentiful, affordable, and ever changing.

The challenge is to make smart choices and establish healthful habits. Doing so requires sorting the marketing from the science, but it can be difficult because the two are blended together. Should we be surprised that the average consumer is confused about nutrition issues? Yet, since the connection between what we eat and how we feel and function is indisputable, it's clearly worth the effort to be informed and to stay informed.

As part of public health policy, the federal government disseminates science-based dietary guidelines to aid the American consumer. Let's apply the basic nutrition terms and concepts reviewed in the previous section to the current guidelines. And let's look below the surface. The dietary guidelines deserve more than a superficial glance. These are not simply a list of "rules" to eat by. As self-directed learners, our aim is to develop a working knowledge of the recommendations—not only the *what* but also the *why* and the *how*.

Primarily through the U.S. Department of Agriculture (USDA), the government has provided nutrition information and advice to Americans for over a century. In 1994 the USDA bolstered its role in this regard by creating the Center for Nutrition Policy and Promotion. The formal establishment of the center came at a time when the American public was becoming increasingly aware of the importance of diet yet was receiving conflicting nutrition messages. Thus, a major role of the center is to serve as a trusted source to assure the public that nutrition information disseminated by the USDA is based on sound research and analysis. At its website—**www.cnpp.usda.gov/**—links are provided to the most recent *Dietary Guidelines for Americans* and the consumer-oriented ChooseMyPlate food guidance system. Become familiar with both.

The *Dietary Guidelines for Americans* are the cornerstone of federal nutrition policy and nutrition education activities. They are jointly issued by the U.S. Department of Health and Human Services (HHS) and the USDA. They were first released in 1980 and are updated every five years. The following questions and answers provide an overview of the *Dietary Guidelines* and insight on how they were developed. Key recommendations are then highlighted.

### What Are the Dietary Guidelines?

The *Dietary Guidelines* are based on what experts have determined to be the best scientific knowledge about diet, physical activity, and other issues related to what we should eat and how much physical activity we need. The *Dietary Guidelines* are designed to help Americans choose diets that meet nutrient requirements, promote health, support active lives, and reduce risks of chronic disease.

### Why Are the Dietary Guidelines *Important?*

The *Dietary Guidelines* allow government agencies to speak with one voice when presenting advice about proper dietary habits for healthy Americans. All federal dietary guidance for the public must be consistent with the *Dietary Guidelines*. They also influence the direction of government nutrition programs, including research, labeling, and promotion.

### How Are the Dietary Guidelines *Developed?*

The *Dietary Guidelines* are prepared in a three-stage process. In the first, an independent advisory committee of eminent scientists compile a report based on the best available evidence. In the second, government scientists and officials review the advisory committee's report and, based on the report and agency and public comments, develop the *Dietary Guidelines*. In the third stage, health communication specialists translate the *Dietary Guidelines* into meaningful messages for the public and educators. The latest consumer guide is ChooseMyPlate, which is presented in the next section.

### What Are the Key Recommendations of the 2010 Dietary Guidelines?

The *Dietary Guidelines* encompass two overarching concepts:

- *Maintain calorie balance over time to achieve and sustain a healthy weight.* People who are successful at achieving and maintaining a healthy weight do so through continued attention to consuming only enough energy from foods and beverages to meet their needs and by being physically active. To prevent obesity and

## Health & the Media The Milk Mustache Ad Campaign

Launched in 1996, the national "Got milk?" campaign, portraying celebrities wearing milk mustaches, has been one of the most enjoyed and recognized of any food product ad campaign. The print ads have featured dozens of celebrities over the years, each with a catchy story line linking his or her persona with the health benefits of drinking milk. Hugh Jackman, Spike Lee, Sheryl Crow, Jackie Chan, and Kermit the Frog are a few of the notables who have posed with a contented look, sporting the "milk mustache." This one features country pop singer-songwriter Taylor Swift. This ad campaign, which blends celebrity, creativity, and flair, has become a part of American pop culture. Funded by America's milk processors and dairy farmers, the milk mustache ads continue today. Who has been the latest athlete or entertainer urging us to drink our milk?

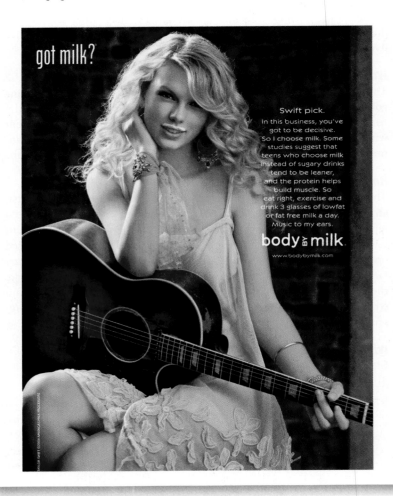

improve their health, many Americans must decrease the energy they consume and increase the calories they expend through physical activity.

- ***Focus on consuming nutrient-dense foods and beverages.*** A healthy eating pattern limits intake of sodium, solid fats, added sugars, and refined grains and emphasizes nutrient-dense foods and beverages—vegetables, fruits, whole grains, fat-free or low-fat milk and milk products, seafood, lean meats and poultry, eggs, beans and peas, and nuts and seeds.

Based on these two broad concepts, the *Dietary Guidelines* make key recommendations to the public in three main areas: balancing calories, foods to reduce, and foods to increase. The main recommendations for each area are listed below.

### *Balancing calories to manage weight:*

- Prevent and/or reduce overweight through improved eating and activity behaviors.
- Control energy intake to manage body weight (for those who are overweight, this means consuming fewer calories).
- Increase physical activity and reduce time spent in sedentary behaviors (i.e., sitting).
- Maintain appropriate calorie balance during each stage of life—childhood, adolescence, adulthood, pregnancy and breastfeeding, and older age.

### *Foods and food components to reduce:*

- Reduce daily sodium intake to less than 2,300 mg (about 1 tsp of salt) and, among African Americans, further reduce to 1,500 mg.
- Consume less than 10 percent of calories from saturated fats and less than 300 mg per day of cholesterol, and keep consumption of *trans* fats as low as possible.
- Reduce the intake of calories from solid fats and added sugars.
- Limit the consumption of foods that contain refined grains.
- If alcohol is consumed, it should be consumed in moderation—up to one drink per day for women and two drinks per day for men.

Regarding the recommendation to reduce sodium, the lower intake (1,500 mg per day) also applies to those with hypertension, diabetes, or chronic kidney disease and to everyone over the age of 50. As a result, the 1,500 mg recommendation should be followed by about half of the U.S. population, including children, and the majority of adults.

The recommendation on alcohol deserves further comment as excessive drinking on college campuses is a reality. A key is to resist peer pressure to overindulge. Also, remember that alcohol should not be consumed by some individuals, including those who cannot restrict their alcohol intake, women who are pregnant or lactating, children and adolescents, and individuals taking medications that interact with alcohol. And, of course, drinking and driving can be lethal. Bottom line—if you choose to drink, do so sensibly.

### Foods and nutrients to increase:

- Increase servings and variety of fruits and vegetables, especially beans, peas, and dark-green, red, and orange vegetables.
- Consume at least half of all grains as whole grains; replace refined grains with whole grains.
- Increase intake of fat-free or low-fat milk and milk products, such as milk, yogurt, cheese, or fortified soy beverages.
- Choose a variety of protein foods, which include seafood, lean meat and poultry, eggs, beans and peas, soy products, and unsalted nuts and seeds.
- Use vegetable oils (polyunsaturated and monounsaturated fats) to replace solid fats (saturated and *trans*).

For the complete list of recommendations, see Website Resources at the end of the chapter. These recommendations are also available in interactive and visual versions via the online ChooseMyPlate, which is discussed in the next section.

## USDA CHOOSEMYPLATE

Due to the enormous variability in both food preferences and food choices, learning to eat healthier—let alone maintaining the good habits we already have—can be quite a challenge. In June 2011, the USDA unveiled a new approach—ChooseMyPlate.gov—designed to make it easier for people to make better food choices. A plate-shaped image (Figure 2.1) replaces the long-used food pyramid. Lauded by nutrition experts as a solid step forward, the MyPlate icon is simple and intuitive. The five groups of fruits, vegetables, grains, protein foods, and dairy are represented using a familiar mealtime visual—a place setting.

The MyPlate website (**www.choosemyplate.gov**) features selected messages to help us focus on key eating behaviors that align with the key recommendations of the 2010 *Dietary Guidelines*.

- Enjoy your food, but eat less.
- Avoid oversized portions.
- Make half your plate fruits and vegetables.
- Switch to fat-free or low-fat (1%) milk.
- Make at least half your grains whole grains.
- Compare sodium in foods like soup, bread, and frozen meals—and choose foods with lower numbers.
- Drink water instead of sugary drinks.

**FIGURE 2.1    USDA MYPLATE ICON**

Source: U.S. Department of Agriculture.

The website features practical information on all five food groups with corresponding galleries of food images that depict serving sizes. Another handy resource is the *Ten Tips Nutrition Education Series* that provides easy-to-follow tips on a variety of topics—from "Build a Healthy Meal" to "Kid-Friendly Veggies and Fruits"—in a high-quality, printable format (1-page pdfs). These are excellent for posting in the kitchen or sharing with others. MyPlate also provides useful interactive tools, including the three highlighted below: *Food Tracker, Daily Food Plan,* and *MyFoodapedia.*

*Food Tracker* is a dietary assessment tool. After entering at least one day's worth of all food and beverage consumed, you will receive a report that includes total calories consumed and an analysis of macro- and micronutrients. A quality rating based on the types and amount of food you ate as compared to those recommended by the *Dietary Guidelines* is also generated. To get a representative picture of eating habits, input at least three days (two weekdays and one weekend day). As with any computerized analysis, the output is only as good as the input! Become familiar with the *Food Tracker* features, keep detailed written records of everything you eat and drink, and enter your information carefully. This will take time, but getting an accurate report is worth the effort. Try it and see how you score. A history function allows you to track progress over time, up to one year: **www.mypyramidtracker.gov.**

Some of you may want a food plan to get you started on the path to healthier eating. To meet this need, try the *Daily Food Plan*. This interactive tool personalizes a plan based on your age, gender, and physical activity level. After entering this information, a food plan is generated at the appropriate calorie level. The plan will specify daily amounts from each food group and a limit for discretionary calories (fats, added sugars, alcohol). Use the plan to set short-term goals and to compare with current eating patterns. To generate a customized plan, go to **www.choosemyplate.gov/myplate/index.aspx.**

Article
2.2

The *MyFoodapedia* interactive tool taps into a huge database and provides quick access to basic facts on nearly every food. Input the food (e.g., pizza) and it will query you for more information as necessary (e.g., type, condiments, portion size). Results will include the caloric content of the food and its contributions to the food groups. You can easily compare two foods as well: **www.myfoodapedia.gov.**

In closing this section, we should point out that the recommendations reviewed here are for the general adult population. Be aware that the *Dietary Guidelines* and MyPlate also contain recommendations for specific groups such as infants and young children, women who are pregnant and breastfeeding, and older adults. Since the majority of college students are young women, information on maternal and infant nutrition may be of special interest to many of you. A comment on breastfeeding is warranted, as few young people would have reason to know of its importance. *Healthy People 2020*, the Centers for Disease Control and Prevention, and the American Academy of Pediatricians all advocate the value of breastfeeding for its multiple health benefits to both the baby (e.g., protects from infections, reduces risk of sudden infant death syndrome, less likely to develop asthma or become obese) and the mother (e.g., decreased risk of breast and ovarian cancers and type 2 diabetes). Three out of four mothers start out breastfeeding (75%), but by six months the rate drops to under 50 percent. Programs and resources are in place to increase these rates. Mother's milk is a perfect nutrition, so encourage breastfeeding.

## ALTERNATIVE APPROACHES

Prior to the 2011 launch of the MyPlate icon, the standard USDA symbol used to teach healthy eating was a food pyramid. Nearly all of you learned your food groups (in primary and secondary school) using

**FIGURE 2.2** **HEALTHY EATING PYRAMID**
For more information go to www.thenutritionsource.org.

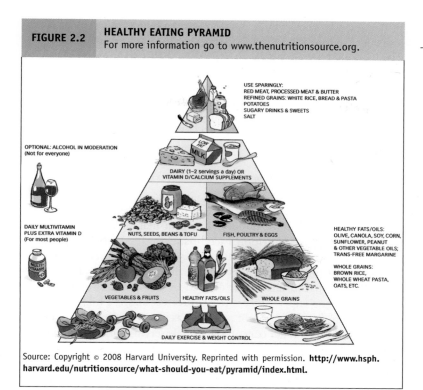

USE SPARINGLY:
RED MEAT, PROCESSED MEAT & BUTTER
REFINED GRAINS: WHITE RICE, BREAD & PASTA
POTATOES
SUGARY DRINKS & SWEETS
SALT

OPTIONAL: ALCOHOL IN MODERATION
(Not for everyone)

DAIRY (1–2 servings a day) OR
VITAMIN D/CALCIUM SUPPLEMENTS

DAILY MULTIVITAMIN
PLUS EXTRA VITAMIN D
(For most people)

NUTS, SEEDS, BEANS & TOFU      FISH, POULTRY & EGGS

HEALTHY FATS/OILS:
OLIVE, CANOLA, SOY, CORN,
SUNFLOWER, PEANUT
& OTHER VEGETABLE OILS;
TRANS-FREE MARGARINE

WHOLE GRAINS:
BROWN RICE,
WHOLE WHEAT PASTA,
OATS, ETC.

VEGETABLES & FRUITS      HEALTHY FATS/OILS      WHOLE GRAINS

DAILY EXERCISE & WEIGHT CONTROL

Source: Copyright © 2008 Harvard University. Reprinted with permission. **http://www.hsph. harvard.edu/nutritionsource/what-should-you-eat/pyramid/index.html.**

the food pyramid. A highly regarded alternative to the traditional USDA pyramid is the Healthy Eating Pyramid developed by Harvard's Department of Nutrition. Some nutrition experts and consumer advocates believe the Healthy Eating Pyramid better reflects the latest science (e.g., a plant-based diet is healthiest) and is free from corporate influence. Building on a foundation of regular exercise and weight control, the Healthy Eating Pyramid emphasizes eating more foods from the bottom part of the pyramid (vegetables, fruits, whole grains) and less from the top (red meat, refined grains, sugary drinks, salt) (Figure 2.2). It's a simple, general guide to how you should eat.

The Healthy Eating Pyramid is a variation of the traditional Mediterranean diet, identified by scientists decades ago as a model for eating patterns to promote lifelong good health. The Mediterranean diet is based on fresh fruits and vegetables, olive oil, whole grains, and fish, with little red meat and animal products. Features of the Mediterranean diet include reliance on locally grown and harvested food, minimal use of modern processed foods, and the enjoyment of good food with others.

Article
2.3

A vegetarian diet, which is followed by growing numbers of Americans, is a step beyond the Mediterranean diet. It's estimated that over 7 million people follow a vegetarian-based diet with another 23 million on a vegetarian-inclined diet. Most eat a vegetarian diet to improve overall health, and over half cite concerns about the environment and animal welfare as reasons for their choice. Both the American Dietetic Association and ChooseMyPlate.gov endorse the healthfulness of vegetarian diets and provide tips on developing nutritionally balanced plans. If you're interested in a vegetarian diet, see Website Resources for more information.

## FOOD LABELS

Reading food labels is an important step in making sound nutritional choices. By law the "Nutrition Facts" panel on food labels is standardized to give consumers easy access to key information. A sample food label is shown in Figure 2.3. A few of the key facts should be highlighted. Note that "a serving" is defined by the manufacturer—usually by size (e.g., one cup) or pieces (e.g., three cookies). While some manufacturers use the definition of a serving as given by the *Dietary Guidelines,* many do not. What constitutes a single serving can vary, sometimes widely, from one product line to another. Consider how many servings are in the food package, then ask yourself, "How many servings am I consuming?" Is it half a serving, one serving, or more? Note that serving size is always listed first, followed by the calories. In the calorie line (point 2), the fat percentage of the product can be calculated by simply dividing the calories from fat by the total calories. In this macaroni and cheese product, 44 percent (110/250) of the calories are from fat!

Grams for each of the energy nutrients are reported next, with additional information on the types of fat and carbohydrate. Under "Total Fat," a breakdown is given for saturated fat and *trans* fat. Under "Total Carbohydrate," a breakdown is given for dietary fiber and sugars. Saturated fat, *trans* fat, cholesterol, and sodium are nutrients that Americans generally need to limit, whereas dietary fiber, vitamins A and C, calcium, and iron are nutrients that most of us should aim to increase. With practice, using information from the "Nutrition Facts" label along with the list of ingredients will allow you to quickly determine the nutritional characteristics of the food. How healthy would you rate this macaroni and cheese product (Figure 2.3)?

In Figure 2.4, nutrition labels from two brand-name packages of one-serving chicken-pasta-broccoli frozen entrees are presented. Although both are essentially the same size (total weight: 10.5 vs. 9.5 oz.), the meal on the left has 41 percent more calories than the meal on the right (380 vs. 270 Cal). The difference in total energy is due almost

**FIGURE 2.3    UNDERSTANDING A FOOD LABEL**

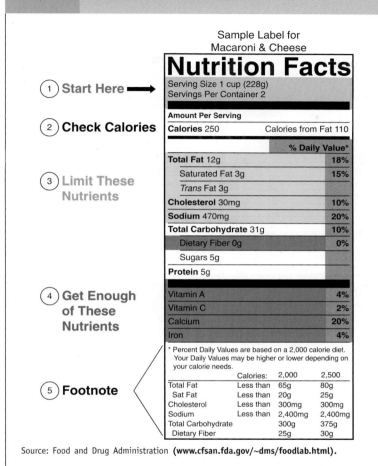

Sample Label for
Macaroni & Cheese

# Nutrition Facts

Serving Size 1 cup (228g)
Servings Per Container 2

**Amount Per Serving**

**Calories** 250          Calories from Fat 110

|  | % Daily Value* |
|---|---|
| **Total Fat** 12g | **18%** |
| Saturated Fat 3g | **15%** |
| *Trans* Fat 3g | |
| **Cholesterol** 30mg | **10%** |
| **Sodium** 470mg | **20%** |
| **Total Carbohydrate** 31g | **10%** |
| Dietary Fiber 0g | **0%** |
| Sugars 5g | |
| **Protein** 5g | |

| | |
|---|---|
| Vitamin A | 4% |
| Vitamin C | 2% |
| Calcium | 20% |
| Iron | 4% |

* Percent Daily Values are based on a 2,000 calorie diet.
Your Daily Values may be higher or lower depending on
your calorie needs.

| | Calories: | 2,000 | 2,500 |
|---|---|---|---|
| Total Fat | Less than | 65g | 80g |
| Sat Fat | Less than | 20g | 25g |
| Cholesterol | Less than | 300mg | 300mg |
| Sodium | Less than | 2,400mg | 2,400mg |
| Total Carbohydrate | | 300g | 375g |
| Dietary Fiber | | 25g | 30g |

(1) **Start Here** ➡

(2) **Check Calories**

(3) **Limit These Nutrients**

(4) **Get Enough of These Nutrients**

(5) **Footnote**

Source: Food and Drug Administration **(www.cfsan.fda.gov/~dms/foodlab.html).**

entirely to higher fat intake: 15 versus 6 g, more than twice as much. The saturated fat comparison is 6 g versus only 1.5 g—four times as much. Finally, the meal on the left has significantly more sodium, less fiber, and more sugar than the one on the right. It's easy to make the healthy choice between these two meals, especially since the costs are similar and the low-fat, low-calorie entree tastes just as good. In recent years, food scientists have developed many flavorful low-fat food products. Be ready to be surprised.

Use food labels to apply your nutrition knowledge and make informed choices. Review and compare the nutrition facts, critically analyze, and make your own judgments. For additional information

**FIGURE 2.4    COMPARISON OF TWO FROZEN ENTREES***

**Nutrition Facts**
Serving Size 1 package (10.5 oz)
Servings per Container about 1

**Amount per Serving**

**Calories** 380    Calories from Fat 140

| | % Daily Value* |
|---|---|
| **Total Fat** 15g | 23% |
| Saturated Fat 6g | 30% |
| **Cholesterol** 40mg | 13% |
| **Sodium** 1090mg | 45% |
| **Total Carbohydrate** 37g | 12% |
| Dietary Fiber 3g | 12% |
| Sugars 8g | |
| **Protein** 25g | |

*Percent Daily Values are based on a 2,000 calorie diet. Your daily values may be higher or lower depending on your calorie needs.

**Nutrition Facts**
Serving Size 1 package (9.5 oz)
Servings per Container about 1

**Amount per Serving**

**Calories** 270    Calories from Fat 50

| | % Daily Value* |
|---|---|
| **Total Fat** 6g | 9% |
| Saturated Fat 1.5g | 8% |
| **Cholesterol** 60mg | 20% |
| **Sodium** 550mg | 23% |
| **Total Carbohydrate** 34g | 11% |
| Dietary Fiber 5g | 20% |
| Sugars 6g | |
| **Protein** 19g | |

*Percent Daily Values are based on a 2,000 calorie diet. Your daily values may be higher or lower depending on your calorie needs.

*Stouffer's Chicken Fettuccine versus Lean Cuisine Bow Tie Pasta & Chicken.

Source: **www.foodfacts.com.**

on the nutrition facts panel as well as links to related nutrition labeling issues, go to the Food and Drug Administration (FDA) website: Food Labeling and Nutrition **www.cfsan.fda.gov/label.html.**

## FOOD SAFETY

"I was sick as a dog last night." This phrase conjures up images of a dog vomiting, its entire body convulsing with the effort—generally the result of a dietary indiscretion (eating garbage or worse). Or the saying might prompt a personal memory of a long, sleepless night in the bathroom combating nausea and dealing with gastrointestinal distress while hunched over the toilet. Thankfully, for most of us, these "bad food" experiences—although often intense, with symptoms of nausea, stomach cramps, diarrhea, vomiting, and fever—are generally short-lived.

But the fact remains that we are more likely to experience foodborne illness than nearly any other health risk. About one in four, or roughly 75 million Americans, suffers a bout of food poisoning every year. The consequence for the vast majority of those afflicted is a day or two of distress. However, foodborne illness also kills about 5,000 Americans a year. With prevention in mind, let's consider the primary risk factors and identify those people who are most vulnerable.

**Foodborne illness** or disease—routinely called "food poisoning"—is caused by consuming contaminated foods or beverages. Many different disease-causing microbes (pathogens) can contaminate foods as can poisonous chemicals. Most foodborne diseases are infections, caused by a variety of bacteria, viruses, and parasites. For example, *Salmonella* in chicken and eggs and *E. coli* (strain 0157:H7) in ground meat are bacterial pathogens that periodically receive media attention when identified as the "bugs" (microbes) responsible for outbreaks of foodborne illness. In nearly all cases, infections were preventable and resulted from inattention to safe food-handling practices. Unintended poisonings caused by harmful toxins or chemicals—accidentally eating poisonous mushrooms, for example—are less common.

Because it is the immune system that protects the body against pathogens, the most severe effects of foodborne diseases occur in the very young, the very old, or anyone with a compromised immune system. In newborns and infants, the immune system is not fully developed. Similarly, pregnant women and their fetuses are at higher risk. In the elderly the immune system is less robust due to age. And literally millions of others are immunocompromised because they are undergoing chemotherapy, taking steroidal or antimicrobial medication, or have an immune deficiency disease (whether genetically based or acquired, such as AIDS). Foodborne diseases in these vulnerable groups can cause serious complications and even death.

Although dozens of different "bugs" or pathogens are responsible for foodborne illnesses, several characteristics are common. They are carried by food that isn't handled carefully, washed adequately, cooked thoroughly, or stored properly. This simple knowledge and the associated food safety practices go a long way in reducing exposure. In addition, Americans now eat away from home between 30 and 50 percent of the time. This requires additional vigilance and precautions as you make choices about where and what you eat. For example, be observant and select carefully at salad bars, buffets, and those prolonged group picnics or summer reunions.

Restaurants are inspected routinely (or should be) by local health departments to make sure they are clean, have adequate kitchen facilities, and follow established food safety practices. Look at the score from the most recent inspection report (usually posted), and use that score to help guide your choice in where you eat. Some restaurants have specifically trained their staff in principles of food safety. Simple observation of the kitchen staff and servers in their handling of the

---

**Foodborne illness,** or "food poisoning," is an acute gastrointestinal disorder caused by the consumption of food contaminated with harmful microorganisms and, less often, toxic chemicals; it is marked by nausea, vomiting, and diarrhea.

food and cleaning of tables can reveal whether hygienic practices are being followed.

Whether the "food handler" is the cook at a restaurant or you at home, a few simple precautions can greatly reduce the risk of microbial foodborne diseases. Key recommendations regarding food safety from the *Dietary Guidelines* include

- *Clean hands, food contact surfaces, and fruits and vegetables.* Wash your hands with soap and water before and after preparing food. Don't be a source of foodborne illness yourself.
- *Separate raw, cooked, and ready-to-eat foods while shopping, preparing, or storing foods.* Avoid cross-contaminating by washing hands, utensils, and cutting boards after they have been in contact with raw meat or poultry and before they touch another food.
- *Cook foods to a safe temperature to kill microorganisms.* For example, cook ground beef to an internal temperature of 160° Fahrenheit. Eggs should be cooked until the yolk is firm.
- *Chill (refrigerate) perishable food promptly and defrost foods properly.* Bacteria can grow quickly at room temperature, so refrigerate leftovers within 4 hours.
- *Avoid raw (unpasteurized) milk or any products made from unpasteurized milk, raw or partially cooked eggs, raw or undercooked meat and poultry, unpasteurized juices, and raw sprouts.*

A comprehensive explanation of foodborne illness and food safety for the consumer is provided by the nonprofit Partnership for Food Safety Education: **www.fightbac.org.**

Lastly, remember to watch over the most vulnerable (e.g., infants and young children, residents in nursing homes or chronic care facilities, cancer patients) as they must depend on others to ensure that their food is wholesome and safe. In short, for most Americans the overall risk of food poisoning is high—about one out of four per year—but the consequences are relatively low—acute gastrointestinal distress for 6–48 hours—except for those in vulnerable groups. Yet even the healthiest among us should be smart about prevention. No one wants to be sick as a dog, not even for one night.

## DIETARY SUPPLEMENTS

As the name indicates, **dietary supplements** are intended to augment the diet. Most contain vitamins, minerals, or plant-based substances

> **Dietary supplements** are food products, added to the total diet, that contain vitamins, minerals, herbs, botanicals, amino acids, metabolites, constituents, extracts, or combinations of these ingredients.

(botanicals). Dietary supplements are intended to be taken as a pill, capsule, or liquid. The topic of dietary supplements is one of the most controversial and at times contentious in all of nutrition—an inevitable result when private enterprise, science, quackery, public health, politics, and the mass media get tangled together. From blatantly fraudulent to alluringly sophisticated, advertisements for dietary supplements are ubiquitous—on the Internet, on television, on the radio, and in magazines and newspapers.

The market for dietary supplements is huge: Annual U.S. sales now exceed $23 billion. Over half of all American adults use supplements, with the most common being the standard multivitamin/mineral supplement followed by calcium products, vitamin C, vitamin E, botanicals, and sports nutrition supplements. Yet, literally hundreds of different dietary supplements are promoted and sold. Claims for supplements are across-the-board—from treating the entire spectrum of medical conditions (from acne to cancer) to improving performance (sexual, sports, cognitive), to combating general malaise (low energy, poor appetite, insomnia). And the list goes on. Dietary supplements are available at grocery stores, pharmacies, and health food stores; they are also easily purchased over the phone or on the Internet.

Contrary to what the general populace believes, the federal government does not evaluate supplements before they are marketed. In 1994 the dietary supplement industry successfully lobbied Congress to pass legislation favorable to their products—the Dietary Supplement Health and Education Act. The definition of dietary supplement was broadened to include a wide array of products: vitamins, minerals, herbs, botanicals, amino acids, and other constituents and extracts of animal and plant origin. Based on this legislation—which is the law of the land—*there is no requirement for premarket review of dietary supplements* by the FDA.

The FDA must prove a supplement is unsafe *before* it can restrict consumer use. This can be a long uphill battle, as was shown in the case of ephedra, a supplement promoted for weight loss and improved athletic performance. After years of investigation, the FDA found that ephedra use was responsible for five deaths and similar numbers of heart attacks, strokes, and seizures. Clearly, ephedra posed an unreasonable risk. The FDA subsequently banned the sale of all ephedra supplements in 2004. Nutraceutical Corporation, one of the largest U.S. supplement companies, went to court, and a judge struck down the FDA ban in 2005. The next step was the U.S. Court of Appeals, which in 2006 ruled in favor of FDA and upheld the ban. The U.S. ban on the sale of dietary supplements that contain ephedra continues today. More recently, the FDA has taken steps to keep consumers safe from fraudulent, dangerous products with undeclared or mislabeled ingredients marketed as dietary supplements for weight loss, sexual enhancement, and bodybuilding.

These examples demonstrate that federal oversight of dietary supplements is limited. Action will be taken only in the most serious cases when a supplement has been shown to be unsafe or dangerous. Questions of effectiveness or truth in advertising are not routinely evaluated. Supplement manufacturers are not supposed to make unsubstantiated health claims, but often do with a caveat in small print. In stark contrast to the limited regulation of dietary supplements, the FDA has stringent approval guidelines for the development of new prescription drugs. For the pharmaceutical industry to get a new drug to market, the drug must be shown to be safe and effective *prior* to its release.

In summary, dietary supplements encompass hundreds of products. Some may be beneficial, many are not. For example, evidence supports the use of standard multivitamin/minerals and selected vitamins and minerals for some individuals, particularly those not eating a well-balanced diet or with known deficiencies. In general though, it's "buyer beware," since supplements with proven benefits make up only a small fraction of the entire dietary supplement market. Examine all advertising with skepticism. (See the section on complementary and alternative medicine [CAM] in Chapter 12.) Before buying any dietary supplement, do your research. The Office of Dietary Supplements within the National Institutes of Health provides an excellent consumer website: **http://dietary-supplements.info.nih.gov/Health_ Information/Health_Information.aspx**

✔ **NEED TO KNOW**

ChooseMyPlate is a web-based, consumer-friendly version of the *Dietary Guidelines*. Recommendations in MyPlate are communicated through practical messages and tools designed to educate and motivate Americans to improve their eating habits and overall health. Alternative approaches such as the Healthy Eating Pyramid are also available. An understanding of the related topics of food labels, food safety, and dietary supplements is also necessary to be a savvy consumer in today's food wonderland.

## ➤ Weight Control

News stories on obesity appear almost daily. The Centers for Disease Control and Prevention (CDC) report that obesity rates doubled among American adults between 1980 and 2010. The World Health Organization (WHO) documents similar trends in Canada, Britain, Australia, and other Westernized countries around the world. Based on recent health statistics, obesity is related to over 100,000 deaths per year in the United States alone.

How have we arrived at this current crisis with America's ballooning body weight? In large part, it can be understood as an unintended consequence of major technological advances over the past 50 years. Our 21st-century lifestyles require only minimal levels of physical activity, and our food choices are more plentiful and convenient than ever before. Sedentary living, combined with drive-through fast food and huge portions, has become the norm.

Given these conditions, it's not surprising that most Americans struggle with their weight. Moreover, the idealized body image advertisers promote to girls and women is to be thin while the message targeted at boys and men is to be muscular. Cumulatively, these conflicting factors negatively impact many people. At the one end of the weight continuum are those who are obese, and at the other end are those with eating disorders who are at risk of malnutrition and extreme thinness. Although much less prevalent than obesity, people with eating disorders, including anorexia and bulimia, have been increasing in numbers for several decades. Females in particular have fallen prey to societal pressures that equate thinness with beauty, success, and self-control.

The key to understanding weight control is the fundamental principle of energy balance—energy intake versus energy expenditure. The basic science and practical aspects of energy balance will serve as the link between our discussion of nutrition in the first part of this chapter and the material to be presented on physical activity in the next chapter.

In the following section, the primary focus is on understanding healthy weight. We start with the questions, What is it, and how is it measured? We will look at selected medical and scientific issues and key resources on obesity and eating disorders and then discuss energy balance. Learning about weight control can help you with your own weight management program and provide insights on weight-related health issues. The best approach to reducing prejudice and dispelling myths about those who are obese or have an eating disorder is to become informed.

## WHAT IS A HEALTHY WEIGHT?

A *healthy weight* simply refers to a body weight at which you feel good and physically function at a high level of well-being. Similar terms such as *optimal weight, ideal weight,* and *desirable weight* are also often used, but generally with reference to athletes where the focus is on the best body weight for competing in a particular sport. A healthy weight varies widely from one person to the next based on age and gender as well as body size, shape, and composition. We will limit our discussion of healthy weight to physically mature individuals from young adults to those in middle age.

As with most mammals, the male of the species *Homo sapiens* is on average significantly taller, heavier, and leaner than the female. Yet it's important to remember that large variability for height, weight, and leanness exists within each gender as well. Beyond the influence of gender, the basic body shape of a person (stockiness, tallness, roundness) is greatly influenced by heredity. These body characteristics can be assessed by measuring limb and torso dimensions and skinfolds. Individuals with extreme body shapes may be well suited to excel in specific sports—such as horse racing, gymnastics, basketball, football—but may not fare well in a world designed for average-sized people.

Although measurements of body size and shape can be used as indicators of a healthy weight, the aspect of physique that is most highly related to healthy weight is leanness or, more technically, body composition. The term *body composition* is used to describe the relative amounts of fat weight (adipose tissue) and lean weight (predominantly muscle and bone) and is reported as percent body fat (fat weight/body weight). A more popular approach to estimate healthy weight is to simply use height and weight and calculate body mass index.

### Body Mass Index (BMI)

**Body mass index,** or **BMI** is a ratio of body weight to height (kg/m$^2$). Instead of converting units and computing BMI, use Table 2.2 to determine your BMI. Find your height (in inches) in the left column and scan across to your weight, then follow the column up to find your BMI. Interpolate as necessary. For example if you are 65" (5'5") tall and weigh 144 lb., your BMI is 24. A BMI between 18.5 and 25 is considered healthy.

Many epidemiologic studies and systematic reviews have found that an increase in BMI is associated with an increase in risk of death. The mortality curve, described by a J-shaped curve (Figure 2.5), represents a continuum where the death rate begins to increase at a BMI of 25. This rise is similar for men and women and across racial groups. For a BMI above 25, the chances of dying early increase, mainly due to heart disease and cancer. For a BMI above 30, the chances increase even more steeply.

Based on this type of evidence, overweight is operationally defined as a BMI of 25 to 29.9, and obesity as 30 or higher. These are the federal standards used in surveillance studies that report on the prevalence of

---

**Body mass index,** or **BMI,** is a ratio of weight to height (kg/m$^2$) that is widely used as a measure of healthy weight (18.5–25), overweight (25–29.9), obesity (30 and above), and underweight (less than 18.5).

# TABLE 2.2    BODY MASS INDEX (BMI) CHART

| | NORMAL | | | | | | OVERWEIGHT | | | | | OBESE | | | | | | | | | |
|---|---|---|---|---|---|---|---|---|---|---|---|---|---|---|---|---|---|---|---|---|---|
| BMI | 19 | 20 | 21 | 22 | 23 | 24 | 25 | 26 | 27 | 28 | 29 | 30 | 31 | 32 | 33 | 34 | 35 | 37 | 39 | 41 | 43 |
| **Height (inches)** | | | | | | | | | | | Body Weight (pounds) | | | | | | | | | | |
| 58 | 91 | 96 | 100 | 105 | 110 | 115 | 119 | 124 | 129 | 134 | 138 | 143 | 148 | 153 | 158 | 162 | 167 | 177 | 186 | 196 | 205 |
| 59 | 94 | 99 | 104 | 109 | 114 | 119 | 124 | 128 | 133 | 138 | 143 | 148 | 153 | 158 | 163 | 168 | 173 | 183 | 193 | 203 | 212 |
| 60 | 97 | 102 | 107 | 112 | 118 | 123 | 128 | 133 | 138 | 143 | 148 | 153 | 158 | 163 | 168 | 174 | 179 | 189 | 199 | 209 | 220 |
| 61 | 100 | 106 | 111 | 116 | 122 | 127 | 132 | 137 | 143 | 148 | 153 | 158 | 164 | 169 | 174 | 180 | 185 | 195 | 206 | 217 | 227 |
| 62 | 104 | 109 | 115 | 120 | 126 | 131 | 136 | 142 | 147 | 153 | 158 | 164 | 169 | 175 | 180 | 186 | 191 | 202 | 213 | 224 | 235 |
| 63 | 107 | 113 | 118 | 124 | 130 | 135 | 141 | 146 | 152 | 158 | 163 | 169 | 175 | 180 | 186 | 191 | 197 | 208 | 220 | 231 | 242 |
| 64 | 110 | 116 | 122 | 128 | 134 | 140 | 145 | 151 | 157 | 163 | 169 | 174 | 180 | 186 | 192 | 197 | 204 | 215 | 227 | 238 | 250 |
| 65 | 114 | 120 | 126 | 132 | 138 | 144 | 150 | 156 | 162 | 168 | 174 | 180 | 186 | 192 | 198 | 204 | 210 | 222 | 234 | 246 | 258 |
| 66 | 118 | 124 | 130 | 136 | 142 | 148 | 155 | 161 | 167 | 173 | 179 | 186 | 192 | 198 | 204 | 210 | 216 | 229 | 241 | 253 | 266 |
| 67 | 121 | 127 | 134 | 140 | 146 | 153 | 159 | 166 | 172 | 178 | 185 | 191 | 198 | 204 | 211 | 217 | 223 | 236 | 249 | 261 | 274 |
| 68 | 125 | 131 | 138 | 144 | 151 | 158 | 164 | 171 | 177 | 184 | 190 | 197 | 203 | 210 | 216 | 223 | 230 | 243 | 256 | 269 | 282 |
| 69 | 128 | 135 | 142 | 149 | 155 | 162 | 169 | 176 | 182 | 189 | 196 | 203 | 209 | 216 | 223 | 230 | 236 | 250 | 263 | 277 | 291 |
| 70 | 132 | 139 | 146 | 153 | 160 | 167 | 174 | 181 | 188 | 195 | 202 | 209 | 216 | 222 | 229 | 236 | 243 | 257 | 271 | 285 | 299 |
| 71 | 136 | 143 | 150 | 157 | 165 | 172 | 179 | 186 | 193 | 200 | 208 | 215 | 222 | 229 | 236 | 243 | 250 | 265 | 279 | 293 | 308 |
| 72 | 140 | 147 | 154 | 162 | 169 | 177 | 184 | 191 | 199 | 206 | 213 | 221 | 228 | 235 | 242 | 250 | 258 | 272 | 287 | 302 | 316 |
| 73 | 144 | 151 | 159 | 166 | 174 | 182 | 189 | 197 | 204 | 212 | 219 | 227 | 235 | 242 | 250 | 257 | 265 | 280 | 295 | 310 | 325 |
| 74 | 148 | 155 | 163 | 171 | 179 | 186 | 194 | 202 | 210 | 218 | 225 | 233 | 241 | 249 | 256 | 264 | 272 | 287 | 303 | 319 | 334 |
| 75 | 152 | 160 | 168 | 176 | 184 | 192 | 200 | 208 | 216 | 224 | 232 | 240 | 248 | 256 | 264 | 272 | 279 | 295 | 311 | 327 | 343 |
| 76 | 156 | 164 | 172 | 180 | 189 | 197 | 205 | 213 | 221 | 230 | 238 | 246 | 254 | 263 | 271 | 279 | 287 | 304 | 320 | 336 | 353 |

Weight Control

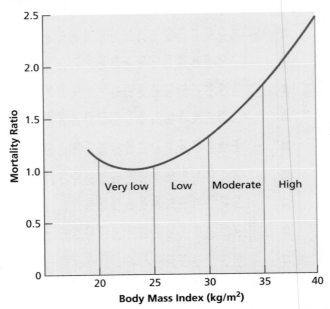

**FIGURE 2.5     RELATIVE RISK AND BODY MASS INDEX (BMI)**

Source: G. A. Bray, *Contemporary Diagnosis and Management of Obesity and the Metabolic Syndrome*, 3rd ed., Handbooks in Health Care, 2003, Fig. 6-3, p. 151. © 1997 George A. Bray. By permission of the author.

overweight and obesity among Americans. The BMI standards are the same for men and women. (The slight rise in death rate for underweight is associated with smoking and preexisting conditions.)

An optional additional measurement—waist circumference—is recommended for individuals in the overweight and obese categories (BMI ≥ 25) to further assess disease risk. Risk is lower for women with a waist size less than 35 in. and for men with a waist size less than 40 in. For a given BMI above 25, the lower the waist circumference, the better.

### Body Composition (percent fat)

As mentioned earlier, the preferred approach to estimating healthy weight is based on the concept of **body composition** in which the body is viewed

**Body composition** is the partitioning of body weight into fat (adipose tissue) and lean (primarily muscle and bone) components. Body composition is typically expressed as percent body fat (fat weight/body weight) and used to recommend a healthy weight range.

as consisting of different tissue components. The most common body composition model is a simple two-component one where the body is divided into fat weight (adipose tissue) and lean body weight (the remaining weight, primarily muscle and bone). The body composition approach is widely used in clinical and sports/fitness settings.

In individuals of normal weight, the majority of body fat is stored immediately beneath the skin—in the subcutaneous fat layer—with the remainder distributed in smaller quantities throughout other tissues and organs. Among obese individuals, large amounts of the excessive body fat can be found within nearly all tissues of the body. Conversely, having too little fat can also lead to an unhealthy state, because fat is an essential component of many tissues (e.g., cell membranes, nervous system). It's estimated that the amount of fat essential for normal physiological function (the lower limit) is equal to about 4 percent of body weight. In women, another 7 to 9 percent of body weight is gender-specific fat (located in breasts and hips) and is necessary to maintain reproductive function, pregnancy, and lactation. In addition to the essential fat (and gender-specific fat in women), another 8 to 10 percent of body weight as fat is considered to be within an acceptable range and normal for body functions such as insulation, protection, and energy storage.

Table 2.3 presents a set of body fat guidelines for adults. These body composition values reflect a general consensus from many studies, although there are in fact no universally accepted norms. Note the different standards for men and women due to differences in gender-specific fat. A healthy body composition for young adult women may range from 12 to 30 percent fat and for young adult men from 4 to 22 percent fat, with the majority of people in these larger ranges falling within the "moderate" subranges. After the age of 30, the norms can be adjusted upward at one percentage point per decade. For example, a 42-year-old man with a body composition of 24 percent would be at the upper end of the moderate range.

The challenge of using the body composition approach is that the measurement of percent fat is not straightforward like BMI where only height and weight are needed. Body composition measurements are

**TABLE 2.3    BODY COMPOSITION: % FAT GUIDELINES***

|  | TOO LEAN | LEAN | MODERATE | OVERFAT |
|---|---|---|---|---|
| Men | <4 | 4–12 | 13–22 | >22 |
| Women | <12 | 12–20 | 21–30 | >30 |

*Varies by age and goals.

categorized as either field-based or lab-based. Common field methods include skinfolds, circumferences, and bioelectric impedance. Field methods provide general estimates of percent fat (error ranges of ± 3–4 percentage points). Results from field methods should be used only as rough approximations. Laboratory measurements such as hydrostatic (or underwater) weighing or dual-energy X-ray absorptiometry (DXA) provide more accurate and reliable values. Although the DXA scan is used mainly for measuring bone mineral density (a measurement of skeletal health) to screen for osteoporosis (low bone density or brittle bones), it is increasingly being used to assess body composition.

Hydrostatic weighing involves submersion in water to determine relative body fatness. In contrast, DXA is an easier procedure for the subject, who merely lies supine on a scanning platform. DXA provides not only a percent fat value but also measures total bone mass. This added information about body composition is valuable as changes in eating and exercise patterns can selectively bring about changes in body fat, muscle mass, and bone mass. DXA scans will increasingly become available to the general public for body composition assessment.

### Body Fat Distribution

For people with excessive levels of body fat, the pattern of body fat distribution is another factor to be considered in determining the degree of risk—high or very high—for obesity-related cardiovascular and metabolic diseases. Researchers have shown that upper body fat (abdominal fat) may be more dangerous for long-term health than lower body fat (hips, buttocks). For example, two men—Mr. A and Mr. P—may have the same high BMI of 35 (e.g., 70", 243 lb.). This puts them well into the obese category. However, since Mr. A has more of an apple shape (upper body fat), he is at a higher health risk compared to Mr. P, who has more of a pear physique (lower body fat). This is the basis for the recommendation to measure waist circumference if one's BMI is in the overweight or obese categories. Although the apple shape is more common in men and the pear shape in women, both forms of body fat distribution occur within each gender.

### Limitations and Interpretation

BMI is calculated using only height and weight. Partly for this reason, it's widely used in public health and is the basis for the U.S. population statistics on the incidence and prevalence of overweight and obesity. As with most simple measures, there are limitations. What are the primary limitations in using BMI?

Since BMI is not a direct measure of body shape (e.g., stockiness vs. roundness) or body composition (leanness vs. overfatness), misclassification can result. Muscle and bone are more dense than fat, so an athlete or muscular person may have a high BMI but not be overfat. Yet, since few adults add muscle and bone after their early 20s, nearly all weight gained from young adulthood on is adipose tissue. Not surprisingly, weight gain during adulthood is an important predictor of many medical conditions.

To illustrate the use and interpretation of BMI and percent fat, let's consider three 30-year-old men—a professional football player, an Amish farmer, and a computer programmer—who have identical heights and weights (72", 221 lb.). The resulting BMI is 30, which is just into the obese category, a category associated with increased risk for multiple chronic diseases. Waist circumferences are 34, 37, and 41 in., respectively. And body composition assessments are 14, 20, and 28 percent fat. It's easy to visualize these three physiques.

Although categorized as obese based solely on their BMI, the football player and Amish farmer are not truly at an increased disease risk as indicated by their normal waist circumferences and percent fat values. They are exceptions. The football player is a muscular, highly trained professional athlete, while the farmer also has a relatively large lean weight and is physically conditioned from the routine manual chores he performs in working a farm. Yet most Americans with a BMI of 30 are much more like the computer programmer, who leads a sedentary lifestyle, spending most waking hours sitting. His large waist circumference and high percent fat confirm that he is overfat.

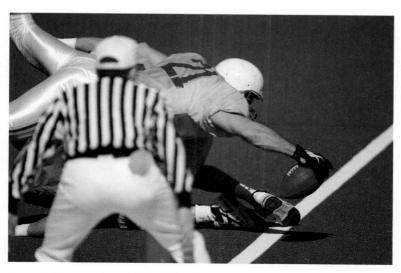

Some athletes may have higher BMIs due to more muscle mass than average, rather than from excess fat.

Knowing what each man's weight was at age 20 would provide added insight into interpreting or rating their current weights. However, be assured that as BMI rises to 30 and beyond, it's less and less likely that a person is simply a healthy exception with a large muscle mass, a normal waist circumference, and a healthy percent body fat. Are you at a healthy weight? Use the BMI approach as a first screening. If your BMI is higher than desired, check your waist circumference and perhaps also obtain a body composition assessment. And, remember that both BMI and body composition values are presented as recommended *ranges* for a reason. There is no evidence that a BMI of 21 is healthier than 23 or that a body composition of 20 percent fat for a young adult woman is healthier than 22 percent. Any fine-tuning of body weight within recommended ranges depends on individual preferences and circumstances.

## THE OBESITY EPIDEMIC

A recent national poll revealed that 30 percent of overweight people think their weight is fine, 70 percent of obese people feel they are merely overweight, and 39 percent of morbidly obese people think they are overweight but not obese. *Obesity* is a loaded word with many negative connotations. Being referred to as obese or fat is offensive to many people who simply think of themselves as big or large. Judgmental and prejudicial views of the obese by normal-weight individuals are not uncommon. Unless you have firsthand experience coping with excess weight, it's difficult to be sensitive to this issue. In *iHealth,* the term *obesity* is used only in the scientific or medical sense. We encourage you to be tactful when discussing obesity and to dispel unfounded characterizations of those who are obese, while at the same time recognizing the serious health consequences of obesity.

**Obesity** is the consequence of chronic energy imbalance in which the body stores excess energy in the form of adipose tissue. When a person consistently eats more calories than he or she expends, body fat storage will increase. Genetics also plays a role in the likelihood of developing obesity. Children of obese parents have a greater chance of becoming obese themselves than do children of parents who are not obese. Recent evidence also shows the influence (both negative and positive) of shared attitudes about body weight and size among family and friends. As illustrated in Figure 2.6, a person's potential for obesity is associated with high energy intake, low energy expenditure, genetic predisposition, and

**Obesity** is the storage of excessive amounts of fat that increases a person's risk for multiple chronic diseases. The accepted definition for obesity is a body mass index (BMI) of 30 or greater.

**FIGURE 2.6    KEY FACTORS CONTRIBUTING TO OBESITY**

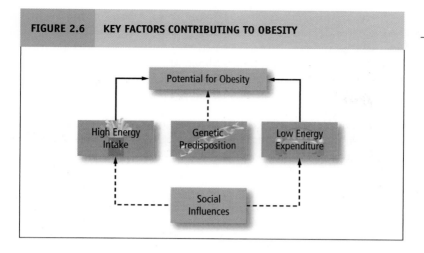

social factors that influence eating and activity patterns. Remember, though, regulation of body weight is predominantly determined by our eating and physical activity patterns. The underlying principle of energy balance is discussed more fully in a later section. A key point is that few of us are truly destined to be obese because it's written in our genes.

Public health officials view obesity as an extremely serious epidemic: The most recent data indicate that 34 percent of American adults meet the criteria for obesity (BMI $\geq$ 30). Perhaps even more serious is the fact that 17 percent of children and adolescents are obese. This percentage has increased twofold over the last 20 years. If the exponential rise in obesity continues, 99 percent of all American adults will be obese by the year 2053! While this statement seems preposterous to consider and the probability that such a rate will ever occur is (hopefully) unlikely, it highlights the phenomenal increase in the number of overweight Americans over the last three decades. This poses a grave health challenge to our society.

Obesity and overweight contribute to the development of many medical conditions and diseases. People who are obese have an increased rate of high blood pressure, lipid abnormalities, and diabetes—all factors that increase risk for cardiovascular disease and stroke. People with obesity are at increased risk for cancers, including colon cancer, breast cancer, gall bladder cancer, and uterine cancer. Obesity is associated with arthritis and mobility problems as well as sleep disturbances and breathing problems. Obesity is also linked to problems with childbearing, premature birth, learning disabilities, and other adverse outcomes for infants. Nationwide, obesity accounts for poorer health-related quality of life and higher health care costs than either smoking or problem drinking (Strum, 2002).

If we continue down the same path as we've been on for the past two to three decades, researchers believe that the generation in school now will be the first in American history to have a shorter life than its parents. Despite the bleak outlook, the tide can turn. Scientists know that obesity can be prevented with a two-pronged approach: (1) the right combination of individual lifestyle behaviors—namely, healthful eating and regular physical activity—*and* (2) supportive public policies that are accepted by American society. Let's do our part to embrace and promote both aspects for ourselves, our families, and our communities.

## EATING DISORDERS

With all the attention on the obesity epidemic, we must not overlook the serious health issues that occur at the other end of the body weight continuum. Extreme dieting to reach a body weight lower and leaner than needed for good health is implicitly promoted by the fashion industry and some sports groups. The National Eating Disorders Association reports that the average female model is 5'11" and weighs only 117 lb., which is thinner than 98 percent of American women. Is this idealized female image related to why 80 percent of American women are discontented with how they look? Some individuals—particularly teenage girls and young women—get caught up in the desire to meet unrealistic cultural expectations to be thin or succumb to pressures from family, coaches, or peers.

**Eating disorders** are one of the key health issues facing young women. More than 90 percent of those with eating disorders are female, and the number of Americans affected by these illnesses has doubled over the past three decades and continues to rise in the United States and worldwide. Eating disorders are a major concern among female athletes, particularly among elite athletes in appearance sports (e.g., gymnastics, diving, figure skating), endurance sports (e.g., distance running, triathlon), and weight-classification sports (e.g., judo). Eating disorders involve serious disturbances in eating behavior, such as extreme reduction of food intake or severe overeating, as well as feelings of distress or excessive concern about body image. More than likely, you have known someone who struggled with an eating disorder. Eating disorders occur across all socioeconomic, ethnic, and cultural groups. Heredity may play a part in why certain people develop eating disorders, but these disorders afflict many people who have no family history.

**Eating disorders** include a spectrum of clinical disorders involving disturbed eating patterns, with the two main types being anorexia nervosa and bulimia nervosa. These disorders are most common in adolescent girls and young women.

The exact causes of eating disorders are not clearly understood. However, their characteristics are well known. Eating disorders are complex psychological conditions that may begin with preoccupations about food and weight. But they are often about much more and serve as a way to focus control in one's life. People with eating disorders tend to be perfectionists who suffer from low self-esteem and are extremely critical of themselves and their bodies. They usually "feel fat" and see themselves as overweight, sometimes even despite life-threatening semi-starvation. An intense fear of gaining weight and of being fat may become all-consuming. In early stages of these disorders, patients often deny that they have a problem. Eating disorders often coexist with other psychological disorders like depression, anxiety, obsessive-compulsive disorder, and alcohol and drug abuse.

The two main types of eating disorders are anorexia nervosa and bulimia nervosa, commonly referred to as anorexia and bulimia. Anorexia is a dangerous condition in which people can literally starve themselves to death. Anorexia afflicts approximately 1 out of every 100 to 200 girls and young women. Patients with anorexia are usually extremely thin (BMI ≤ 18.5). They don't maintain a normal weight because they refuse to eat, often exercise obsessively, and sometimes force themselves to vomit or use laxatives to lose weight. Severe physical symptoms accompany starvation.

Although less life-threatening, bulimia is more widespread than anorexia, affecting about 1 out of every 30 to 100 girls and young women. Individuals suffering from bulimia follow a routine of secretive, uncontrolled binge eating—ingesting an abnormally large amount of food within a set period of time—followed by behaviors such as vomiting, using a laxative, or fasting to rid the body of food consumed. Individuals with bulimia can be slightly underweight, normal weight, or overweight. Because people with bulimia binge and purge in secret and are not excessively thin or heavy, they can hide the disorder for years. Multiple medical complications develop with repeated and chronic purging behaviors. The bulimia disorder may be constant or occasional, with periods of remission alternating with recurrences of binge eating. Bulimia can and often does occur independently of anorexia.

Eating disorders are not due to a personal failure in one's will or behavior. Rather, they are real psychological illnesses in which maladaptive patterns of eating take on a life of their own. The good news is that anorexia and bulimia are treatable conditions. Treatment teams generally consist of a psychiatrist or psychologist; a physician, who provides general medical care; and a nutritionist. As with most disorders, the earlier the condition is diagnosed, the more likely that treatment will be completely successful. If you know of someone who may have an eating disorder, persuade her or him to get counseling. Few who suffer with

**FIGURE 2.7    CONCEPT OF ENERGY BALANCE**

eating disorders seek professional help on their own, especially in the early stages. And remember that eating disorders can occur in boys and men (although less commonly) as well as girls and women. For more information on the mental health aspects of eating disorders, see Chapter 7 and refer to the websites of the National Eating Disorders Association (**www .nationaleatingdisorders.org**) and the American Psychiatric Association (**www.healthyminds.org/Main-Topic/Eating-Disorders.aspx**).

## ENERGY BALANCE

Calories do count. Despite compelling marketing to the contrary, the first law of thermodynamics cannot be broken. Energy is neither created nor destroyed; it only changes forms. Conservation of energy is a law of physics because it always works. As depicted in Figure 2.7, maintaining body weight is fundamentally a balance between energy consumed in the food we eat and energy expended throughout the day based on our body size and level of physical activity. If we eat fewer calories than we expend—known as negative energy balance—then the scale tips and we lose weight. If our energy consumption is consistently higher than our energy expenditure—positive energy balance—then the scale tips the other way and we gain weight. The goal, of course, is to strike a balance so weight is maintained. **Energy balance** is the essential principle of weight regulation, period.

This is not to say that innate biological variability in energy metabolism (efficiency of deriving energy from food and using it to fuel body processes and activities) does not exist from person to person. Individual differences are present in how we derive and use energy.

**Energy balance** is the relationship between energy input (caloric intake) and energy output (caloric expenditure). If input and output are matched, then a balance occurs and body weight is maintained.

But in the vast majority of cases, such differences amount to only negligible or very small differences in a person's overall energy balance. Occasionally, medical disorders have been shown to cause obesity; however, these cases are the exception, not the rule.

The principle of energy balance is easy to comprehend but difficult to implement because contemporary lifestyle encourages consumption of energy and discourages expenditure of energy. Think of the fast-food menus with portions referred to not just as large but as

Larger-than-needed meals are popular at restaurants, but they add to the problem of energy imbalance and weight gain.

giant, huge, and enormous or those omnipresent restaurants with the all-you-can-eat buffets. And consider the increase in time spent sitting (at work, at home, and in the car) and the decline in pedestrian-friendly suburbs and cities. (Did you walk or bicycle to school or to the store from your home?) Consequently, to achieve and maintain a healthy weight, we must be vigilant and determined. If we choose to remain intellectually and physically passive, the odds are against us; the calories will add up and pounds will be put on.

On the energy intake side of the equation, vigilance requires a familiarity with the caloric content of the foods and beverages that we consume. (Energy expenditure will be discussed in the following chapter on physical activity.) Knowing, for instance, that a medium piece of fruit (banana, apple, orange) is 50–100 Cal, a small soft drink (12-oz. can) 140 Cal, a small order of French fries about 250 Cal, and a standard fast-food burger (e.g., Big Mac, Whopper) 500–700 Cal is important to understanding the "energy currency" of foods and beverages. If the average American woman needs only 2,000 Cal per day to maintain her weight, then one "value-pack" meal (drink, burger, fries) will provide half the energy she needs for the day! Moreover, how often do we opt to get the larger size of this or that because it's only another dime or quarter? Or how many soft drinks or snacks do we consume throughout the day?

If a person consumes only 100 Cal more than needed every day for a year, this will amount to 36,500 surplus Cal that will be stored as body fat (adipose tissue). Since 1 lb. of body fat is equal to about 3,500 Cal, this small imbalance—only 100 Cal per day—will result in a 10-lb. gain! A slight but steady positive energy balance—less than the energy in a single soft drink, candy bar, or pack of snack crackers each day—can result in a significant weight gain in only a few months. And, conversely, cutting back by the same amount can result in a significant weight (fat) loss.

A more gradual increase in body weight of merely 1–2 lb. a year over many years is even easier to comprehend (an excess 10–20 Cal per day). This seemingly trivial energy imbalance results in the slow weight gain that the majority of Americans experience. This process known as creeping obesity is subtle. Several years pass and "suddenly" people notice that they are 5–10 lb. heavier. Continue the process for two to three decades, and the extra poundage becomes substantial.

This is why it's important to periodically consider everything you eat on a typical day and to assess how many calories are contained in those foods and beverages. Refer back and review the individual energy intake results you generated using the *Food Tracker* analysis tool. Interpret the results and plan accordingly. Make it a habit to read food labels. Knowledge of energy intake is a key to being nutrition savvy and achieving energy balance.

Understand, respect, and follow the principle of energy balance, and you will be able to reach and/or maintain a healthy body weight. Due to individual differences in physiology and eating behaviors, doing so will be more difficult for some and easier for others. Regardless though, basic knowledge, vigilance, and action are the keys to achieving a healthy weight.

✔ **NEED TO KNOW**

Maintaining a healthy weight in today's society is a challenge. Body mass index (BMI), simply a ratio of weight to height (kg/m$^2$), is a widely used method to define healthy weight. Body composition (% fat) is a more meaningful measurement for evaluating body weight but requires special equipment and expertise. The detrimental health consequences and lower quality of life due to obesity are underestimated by the American public. Although much less prevalent than obesity, eating disorders are also a significant health concern, particularly for teenage girls and young women. Energy balance is a concept fundamental to achieving a healthy weight and to treating weight-related problems.

## ➤ Translating Knowledge into Action

Article
2.4

If it were easy to eat well, we all would be doing it. For most of us, the next step is to translate our newfound nutrition knowledge into positive actions—to improve the everyday choices we make about food. This is no small challenge as we live in a society that gobbles up diet books in the search for the "one true diet" that produces results, whether it is losing body fat, gaining muscle, or removing supposed toxins. Of course, no one true diet exists. This is wishful thinking. At this point, we need to accept the fact that "dieting" is not an effective long-term solution. The dieting approach—"let's try the new X-week diet by celebrity Z"—promotes a temporary mind-set, which is counter to making lasting changes in lifestyle (developing healthier habits). Moreover, most special diets are restrictive, *not* without risk, and seldom successful (not to mention monotonous and illogical—the rice diet, the grapefruit diet, the detox diets).

We must remember that eating is one of our most basic human behaviors. As we eat multiple times every day, it should come as no surprise that we have developed eating habits that are resistant to change. Awareness and the desire to improve are important for change but often not sufficient. As discussed in Chapter 1, if we wish to change a behavior, the likelihood of success is much better if first we take the time to develop a sound plan.

As you map out a plan, consider these behavior-change strategies from the Mayo Clinic for achieving and maintaining a healthy weight. And be aware that these strategies are useful for those who are normal weight or underweight as well as those who aim to shed a few pounds.

1. **Make a commitment.** Be specific about what you are *willing* to do.
2. **Draw on support from others.** Rely on spouse, family, friends, professionals.
3. **Set a realistic goal.** Use the energy balance principle, monitor, be patient.
4. **Learn to enjoy healthier foods.** Explore healthy foods and dishes.
5. **Get active, stay active.** Engage in regular physical activity—more on this in Chapter 3.

The combination of these strategies will assist you in establishing a healthier lifestyle—moving you further along that positive health continuum.

For those who have struggled with their weight over many years, a general perception exists that almost no one succeeds in long-term maintenance of weight loss. However, this is not true. The National Weight Control Registry (**www.nwcr.ws**) estimates that 20 percent or more of overweight and obese people have been able to achieve lasting success. Established in 1994, the National Weight Control Registry enrolls and tracks individuals who have been successful not only in losing weight but also in keeping it off. In this program, long-term maintenance is defined as intentionally losing at least 10 percent of body weight and keeping it off for at least one year. Based on over 5,000 people in the

Exercise is important, but any physical activity, such as walking stairs rather than taking the elevator, helps maintain a healthy weight.

registry, three key characteristics are evident. Successful weight maintainers eat a low-fat diet (especially low in saturated fats and *trans* fats), engage in high levels of regular physical activity (about an hour per day), and monitor their food and weight. These findings are real-world evidence that support the *Dietary Guidelines*. If you are overweight or obese, incorporate these practices in your program.

Once you develop a personalized plan, use the following four questions as a final checklist to ensure that your plan meets the essential criteria for healthy eating and weight management. Again, these criteria apply equally to those who are normal weight or underweight as well as those who plan to lose excess weight.

1. **Is it based on wholesome, everyday foods?**
2. **Is it nutritionally balanced?**
3. **Is the energy content appropriate?**
4. **Does it include regular exercise?**

Affirmative answers to these questions dovetail nicely with recommendations of the *Dietary Guidelines*. Remember that good results depend on a good plan.

In this chapter we reviewed basic nutrition information and dietary guidelines and provided tools and strategies for choosing a healthy diet. In the final analysis, eating good food is one of the real pleasures in life. And remember that enjoying good food and healthy eating are fully compatible, so nourish your body with only the best. *Bon appétit.*

## ✓ NEED TO KNOW

Nutrition is about understanding what types and how much food a person needs and reconciling that with his or her eating habits. Even though our eating habits are ingrained, we can make changes. Using the ChooseMyPlate tools and the *Dietary Guidelines*, apply proven behavioral strategies to customize a plan that meets *your* needs and circumstances. No one size fits all. Give this plan due attention and integrate healthy eating into your lifestyle.

## connect Resources

 **ARTICLES**

2.1 "You Are Also What You Drink." *New York Times*. Jane Brody highlights beverage recommendations and shares some surprising findings about what we drink.

2.2 "How I Learned to Love Breakfast (Or at Least What to Eat for It)." *New York Magazine*. A piece that looks into the science behind the idea that breakfast is the most important meal of the day.

2.3 Ancel Keys, Acclaimed Researcher and Promoter of *Mediterranean Diet*. *iHealth* author Phil Sparling profiles the life of a remarkable scientist.

2.4 "Six Rules for Eating Wisely." *Time*. Michael Pollan translates the complex guidelines of healthy nutrition into easy-to-remember rules of thumb.

 **SELF-ASSESSMENTS**

2.1 Fruit, Vegetable, and Fiber Screener
2.2 Fat Intake Screener

## Website Resources

### GENERAL

American Dietetics Association **www.eatright.org**
Center for Science in the Public Interest
   **www.cspinet.org**
International Food Information Council Foundation
   **www.ific.org**
Nutrition for Everyone, CDC **www.cdc.gov/nutrition/everyone**
Rudd Center, Yale University **www.yaleruddcenter.org**

### HEALTHY EATING

*Dietary Guidelines for Americans* **www.health.gov/dietaryguidelines**
Dietary Reference Intakes **http://fnic.nal.usda.gov/interactiveDRI/**
Healthy Eating Pyramid **www.hsph.harvard.edu/nutritionsource**
Mediterranean Diet **www.oldwayspt.org/mediterraneandiet**
USDA ChooseMyPlate **www.choosemyplate.gov**
Vegetarian Diet **www.oldwayspt.org/vegetarian-diet-pyramid**

## FOOD LABELS

Nutrition Facts Label, FDA
**www.cfsan.fda.gov/~dms/foodlab.html**

## FOOD SAFETY

Federal Food Safety Gateway **www.foodsafety.gov**
Partnership for Food Safety Education **www.fightbac.org**

## DIETARY SUPPLEMENTS

Dietary Supplements, FDA
**www.cfsan.fda.gov/~dms/supplmnt.html**
Drugs, Supplements, and Herbal Information, Medline Plus
**www.nlm.nih.gov/medlineplus/druginformation.html**
Herbs at a Glance, NCCAM
**http://nccam.nih.gov/health/herbsataglance.htm**
Office of Dietary Supplements, NIH
**http://dietary-supplements.info.nih.gov**

## HEALTHY WEIGHT

Healthy Weight, CDC **www.cdc.gov/healthyweight**
National Weight Control Registry **www.nwcr.ws**
Weight Management Research to Practice Series, CDC
**www.cdc.gov/nutrition/professionals/researchtopractice**

## EATING DISORDERS

American Psychiatric Association
**www.healthyminds.org/main-topic/eating-disorders.aspx**
National Eating Disorders Association
**www.nationaleatingdisorders.org**

## Knowing the Language

## Understanding the Content

1. What are the six types of nutrients and their roles in the human diet?
2. What is the ChooseMyPlate guide, and how can it be used to tailor your diet?
3. What are three basic rules of food handling that minimize risk of illness?
4. What is body mass index, and how is it used to define overweight and obesity?
5. What is energy intake, and how would you measure it?

## Exploring Ideas

1. Why has the prevalence of overweight Americans increased so much over the past two decades?
2. How has the food industry changed its products to provide healthier options to the consumer? Identify three specific examples.
3. Why are so many Americans addicted to trying fad diets? Discuss the possible societal, social, psychological, and behavioral influences.
4. Why are dietary supplements so widely used by Americans? Discuss the pros and cons of dietary supplements.

## Selected References

American Dietetic Association. Position statement on weight management. *Journal of the American Dietetic Association* 109 (2): 330–346, 2009.

Bailey RL, Gahche JJ, Lentino CV, et al. Dietary supplement use in the United States, 2003–2006. *Journal of Nutrition* 141 (2): 261–266, 2011.

Berrington de Gonzalez A, Hartge P, Cerhan JR, et al. Body mass index and mortality among 1.46 million white adults. *New England Journal of Medicine* 363: 2211–2219, 2010.

Bray GA. *Contemporary Diagnosis and Management of Obesity and the Metabolic Syndrome* (3rd ed.). Newtown, PA: Handbooks in Health Care, 2003.

Centers for Disease Control and Prevention (CDC). Overweight and Obesity. **www.cdc.gov/nccdphp/dnpa/obesity**

Donnelly JE, Blair SN, Jakicic JM, et al. Appropriate physical activity intervention strategies for weight loss and prevention of weight regain for adults: American College of Sports Medicine position stand. *Medicine and Science in Sports and Exercise* 41 (2): 459–471, 2009.

FDA. Consumer Updates: Dietary Supplements. **www.fda.gov/ForConsumers/ConsumerUpdates/ucm153239.htm**

FDA. How to Understand and Use the Nutrition Facts Label. **www.cfsan.fda.gov/~dms/foodlab.html**

Finucane MM, Stevens GA, Cowan MJ, et al. National, regional, and global trends in body-mass index since 1980: Systematic analysis of health examination surveys and epidemiological studies with 960 country-years and 9.1 million participants. *Lancet* 377 (9765): 557–567, 2011.

Gidding SS, Lichtenstein AH, Faith MS, et al. Implementing American Heart Association pediatric and adult nutrition guidelines. *Circulation* 119: 1161–1175, 2009. **http://circ.ahajournals.org/cgi/content/full/119/8/1161**

Harmon K. How obesity spreads in social networks. *Scientific American,* May 2011. **www.scientificamerican.com/article.cfm?id=social-spread-obesity**

Harris Interactive Poll. Overweight? Obese? Or Normal Weight? Americans Have Hard Time Gauging Their Weight. September 2, 2010.

Heymsfield SB, Lohman TG, Wang Z, Going SB (eds.). *Human Body Composition* (2nd ed.). Champaign, IL: Human Kinetics, 2005.

Hill JO, Peters JC, Wyatt HR. Using the energy gap to address obesity: A commentary. *Journal of the American Dietetic Association* 109 (11): 1848–1853, 2009.

Katzen M, Willett WC. *Eat, Drink, and Weigh Less.* New York: Hyperion, 2006.

Kenney WL. Dietary water and sodium requirements for active adults. *Sports Science Exchange* 92, 2004. **www.gssiweb.com/Article_Detail.aspx?articleID=667**

Kumanyika SK, Obarzanek E, Stettler N, et al. Population-based prevention of obesity: A scientific statement from the American Heart Association. *Circulation* 118: 428–464, 2008. **http://circ.ahajournals.org/cgi/content/full/118/4/428**

Kushi LH, Byers T, Doyle C, et al. American Cancer Society guidelines on nutrition and physical activity for cancer prevention: Reducing the risk of cancer with healthy food choices and physical activity. *CA: Cancer Journal for Clinicians* 56: 254–281, 2006. **http://caonline.amcancersoc.org/cgi/content/full/56/5/254**

Lichtenstein AH, Appel LJ, Brands M, et al. Diet and lifestyle recommendations revision 2006: A scientific statement from the

American Heart Association Nutrition Committee. *Circulation* 114: 82–96, 2006.
http://circ.ahajournals.org/cgi/content/full/114/1/82

Mayo Clinic. Weight Loss: 6 Strategies for Success.
www.mayoclinic.com/health/weight-loss/HQ01625

National Eating Disorders Association. Information and Resources.
www.nationaleatingdisorders.org/information-resources

National Heart, Lung, and Blood Institute. Practical Guide: Identification, Evaluation, and Treatment of Overweight and Obesity in Adults, 2000. www.nhlbi.nih.gov/guidelines/obesity/practgde.htm

Nestle M. *What to Eat.* New York: Farrar, Straus and Giroux, 2006.

Olshansky SJ, Passaro DJ, Hershow RC, et al. A potential decline in life expectancy in the United States in the 21st century. *New England Journal of Medicine* 352 (11): 1138–1145, 2005.

Pollan M. *In Defense of Food: An Eater's Manifesto.* New York: Penguin, 2008.

Popkin BM, Armstrong LE, Bray GM, et al. A new proposed guidance system for beverage consumption in the United States. *American Journal of Clinical Nutrition* 83: 529–542, 2006.

Sparling PB. Obesity on campus. *Preventing Chronic Disease,* July 2007. www.cdc.gov/pcd/issues/2007/jul/06_0142.htm

Sturm R. The effects of obesity, smoking, and drinking on medical problems and costs. *Health Affairs* 21 (2): 245–253, 2002.

U.S. Department of Agriculture, Center for Nutrition Policy and Promotion. MyPyramid, 2005.

U.S. Department of Health and Human Services. *Dietary Guidelines for Americans* (6th ed.). Washington, DC: U.S. Government Printing Office, 2010.

Vegetarianism in America. *Vegetarian Times,* 2008.

Willet WC, Skerrett PJ. *Eat, Drink, and Be Healthy* (updated ed.). New York: Free Press, 2005.

World Health Organization (WHO). Obesity.
www.who.int/topics/obesity

# Chapter 3

## DEVELOP A FITNESS PROGRAM

The main topics in this chapter are health-related physical fitness, responses and adaptations to exercise, and exercise guidelines including national physical activity recommendations to improve health and prevent disease. Strategies are provided to assist you in developing an individualized plan that is enjoyable and sustainable.

THE HUMAN SPECIES was designed for movement. Until the mid-19th century, humans lived as gatherers, toolmakers, hunters, farmers, and artisans. For 99 percent of human history, physical tasks and manual labor were as much a part of daily life as eating and sleeping. Walking great distances, lifting and carrying loads, working with tools—muscular efforts of all types—were simply part of the everyday world. Our species not only survived but also flourished for several thousand generations prior to the advent of the automobile, television, and the Internet. Then abruptly—within only a few generations—the physical activity demands of work and domestic chores decreased so dramatically as to be nearly nonexistent in present-day urbanized societies. Most of our waking hours are spent sitting.

Without question, the nearly universal adoption of labor-saving technology has brought marvelous advances to nearly all facets of human living. Yet, it's increasingly evident that many of the chronic diseases we face today are associated with the resulting sedentary lifestyle. Physical *inactivity* is a risk factor for heart disease, diabetes, osteoporosis, and colorectal cancer, to name a few. These "diseases of inactivity" begin as early as the second and third decades of life. Moreover, the roots of obesity are at least as much in physical inactivity as in overeating.

From an evolutionary viewpoint, Dr. Thomas Rowland makes the case that habitual physical activity has a biological basis with a central neural control (not unlike hunger). In young children (and the young of most mammals), movement, which is central to growth and development, is often playful and spontaneous. The joy of movement in children is undeniable. Although the nature of this enjoyment—such as the discovery and mastery aspects—changes from childhood to adulthood, the enjoyment itself need not stop. If this natural drive for physical activity is severely limited, normal physiological function may be disturbed. In modern America, the design of our living spaces restricts physical activity, and most of our leisure pursuits are in fact sedentary. Do our physical environments and social norms subdue our innate biological drive to be physically active?

Article
3.1

To be clear, this is not a plea to return to the physical toil that our ancestors endured. Rather, it's a frank reminder that the pendulum has swung too far to the other side. Our bodies were designed and wired for movement, yet we live in an environment where physical activity is no longer needed and in many ways actually discouraged (e.g., fewer sidewalks, more drive-throughs).

Based on extensive evidence, public health researchers have identified physical activity as one of the key health behaviors that must be promoted. This is no small challenge. Across the country, rates of participation in fitness and exercise activities decline steadily during the teenage and young adult years—throughout high school, throughout college, and then even more steeply in the years immediately following college.

This widespread decline in physical activity is understandable. In the college setting, considerable time is spent in sedentary behavior (sitting in classes, studying, computer/Internet use). And, in nearly all cases, you are being educated for sedentary occupations. Sedentary patterns are being reinforced and are likely to persist through adult life unless *you* decide otherwise. On the positive side, colleges provide multiple exercise and fitness resources (i.e., extensive facilities, intramurals, sports clubs, credit and noncredit classes) and often a pedestrian- and bicycle-friendly campus. Most students have flexible schedules, making it easier to accommodate fitness and sports activities compared to what lies ahead with full-time jobs following graduation.

If our overall health and functioning are to be optimized, we need to be physically active on a regular basis. Nearly all colleges provide a wide range of exercise and fitness opportunities just waiting to be explored. It's important to note that in addition to the enjoyment and challenge of regular physical activity, exercise can relieve stress, alleviate anxiety and depression, and boost higher-level thinking. These are valuable benefits indeed, especially for college students. The key to reaping the benefits lies with your decision to take a proactive approach.

# ➤ Physical Activity, Exercise, and Physical Fitness

The terms *exercise* and *physical fitness* are probably spoken in every home in America. Although these and related terms actually have very specific meanings, the way in which they are used in everyday conversations varies widely among individuals and across groups. Let's eliminate any possible confusion by setting operational definitions for a few key terms at the onset.

## PHYSICAL ACTIVITY AND EXERCISE

We'll begin by defining two core terms: *physical activity* and *exercise.* These have similar but distinct meanings. Then we'll define *intensity* because it is a common descriptor used to characterize physical activity or exercise.

### Physical Activity

**Physical activity** is bodily movement produced by muscle contraction that increases energy expenditure above a resting level. Simply put, *physical activity* refers to moving around using our own muscle power. Physical

**Physical activity** is muscular movement of the body that results in significant energy expenditure above the resting metabolism.

activity includes all movement whether it is getting out of bed in the morning, getting dressed, preparing a meal, or walking to class. In recent years it has been shown that consistently incorporating physical activity into one's lifestyle (e.g., increasing incidental walking, commuting by foot or bike) can yield significant health benefits, particularly for those who have been sedentary. This active lifestyle approach may be more viable and appealing for many Americans who are not interested in playing sports or working out in a gym.

### Exercise

**Exercise** is a subcategory or type of physical activity. Exercise is physical activity that is planned and structured with the primary purpose of improving or maintaining one or more aspects of our physical capacity, commonly known as physical fitness (which will be defined in the next section). Thus, *exercise* refers to virtually all physical training and sports activities. Sports camps, physical education classes, and basic training in the military are all examples of exercise. Exercising regularly—whether it's training on a sports team or working out at the fitness center—improves health as well as physical capacity and performance.

### Intensity

**Intensity** is arguably the most important characteristic of physical activity or exercise, yet the concept remains fuzzy to many. *Intensity* refers to the physiological or perceptual effort given during a physical activity. Intensity is assessed with objective measurements (e.g., heart rate, energy expenditure) or subjective ratings (e.g., light, moderate, vigorous, all-out). Although intensity may be measured differently from setting to setting (e.g., health club, sports center, medical clinic), heart rate and perceived exertion are two widely used methods for gauging intensity. Both are reviewed in the section "Recommendations for Healthy Adults."

## PHYSICAL FITNESS

**Physical fitness** is a multifaceted concept whose definition has evolved over the past several decades. A generally accepted and enduring definition of physical fitness is "the ability to carry out daily tasks with

---

**Exercise** is structured physical activity that focuses on improving or maintaining physical capacity.

**Intensity** is the effort associated with physical activity and is typically measured using heart rate or subjective ratings.

**Physical fitness** is a developed physical capacity that enables people to perform routine physical tasks with vigor, participate in a variety of physical activities, and reduce their risk for multiple, inactivity-related chronic diseases.

vigor and alertness, without undue fatigue, and with ample energy to enjoy leisure time pursuits and meet unforeseen emergencies" (Clarke, 1971; U.S. Department of Health and Human Services, 2008). A succinct definition from the *Surgeon General's Report on Physical Activity and Health* is "a set of attributes that people have or achieve that relates to the ability to perform physical activity" (U.S. Department of Health and Human Services, 1996). In considering these definitions, three aspects of physical fitness should be noted. First, improved fitness implies an enhanced capacity to perform physical tasks of daily living as well as work-related and leisure-time physical activities. Second, as fitness improves so does physiological well-being, providing protection against numerous inactivity-related diseases. And, third, physical fitness is typically divided into two types or categories—health-related fitness and skill-related fitness—and each type has several components.

### Health-related Physical Fitness

Health-related physical fitness includes three fundamental components—cardiorespiratory or aerobic fitness, musculoskeletal or muscular fitness, and body composition (Table 3.1). The second, musculoskeletal fitness, is in turn composed of three subcomponents—strength, muscular endurance, and flexibility. These terms will be defined and discussed in detail in subsequent sections. For most of you, cardiorespiratory fitness, musculoskeletal fitness, and body composition are familiar concepts because they have long been included in school health and physical education classes.

The physical activity or exercise we engage in to develop health-related physical fitness protects against major threats to our health. Cardiorespiratory fitness lowers risk of dying prematurely, especially from heart disease and stroke. Musculoskeletal fitness increases bone density, muscle mass, and joint health and thereby lowers the risk of osteoporosis, low back pain, and degenerative joint conditions. Maintenance of a healthy weight (body composition) through physical activity and good nutrition protects against obesity, diabetes, and related

---

| TABLE 3.1 | PHYSICAL FITNESS: HEALTH-RELATED COMPONENTS |
|---|---|

Cardiorespiratory (or aerobic) fitness
Musculoskeletal (or muscular) fitness
    Muscular strength
    Muscular endurance
    Flexibility
Body composition

diseases including heart disease, arthritis, and some cancers. How many
of these diseases have you witnessed among family members and friends?
As we experience these events firsthand, the connection between physical
activity and health becomes more real and less abstract.

Body composition, which partitions body weight into lean tissue
(muscle and bone) and fat tissue, prescribes a healthy weight from
one's level of relative body fatness (% body fat). This health-related
fitness component is plainly dependent on *both* eating patterns and
physical activity, much more so than either cardiorespiratory or musculoskeletal fitness. As body composition answers to two masters, it is
sometimes discussed under the heading of diet and nutrition and
sometimes under exercise and physical fitness. Everyone must eat, but
physical activity is largely optional. For that reason, we provide our
main discussion of body composition and the importance of healthy
weight in Chapter 2; see the section on weight control to refresh your
understanding of this health-related fitness component.

When considering the health-related fitness components, it's natural
to think about the high end of sports performance. For elite endurance
athletes (e.g., Olympic marathoners or Tour de France cyclists) and
strength athletes (e.g., world-ranked Olympic weight lifters or power
lifters), the focus is necessarily narrow and specialized—to be faster or
stronger and have the best performance. The sole aim of the champion
endurance or strength athlete is to train relentlessly to improve performance in a single fitness component; any balance with other fitness components is only an afterthought. Such is the nature of national and
international sports competition.

Most elite athletes compete at the highest level for only a few years.
Upon retiring from competition, they dramatically reduce training
levels and (hopefully) transition toward general health and fitness
goals. For most of us, training and competing in sports and physically
challenging activities are enjoyable leisure-time pastimes, not our liveli-
hood or full-time pursuit. Thus, we are free to take a balanced approach
to our fitness programs. Regardless of our athletic abilities or sports interests, each of us can develop an exercise program that includes the three
components of health-related fitness—cardiorespiratory fitness, musculoskeletal fitness, and body composition—in a measured and meaningful way.

### Skill-related Physical Fitness

The second type of fitness is skill-related physical fitness. While there
are many skill-related components of physical fitness, the best known
are agility, speed, coordination, and balance. Skill-related components
are associated primarily with sport and motor skill performance and
only secondarily with improved health. (This view may be changing

Skill-related components of fitness, such as speed and agility, are mostly associated with sport performance rather than health.

because clinicians are increasingly citing the importance of balance to health; loss of balance is the major cause of falls for elderly people.) Among young adults, a finely tuned or specialized physical skill can translate into success in a variety of individual and team sports, from golf and tennis to baseball and basketball.

As many of us know from personal experience, components from both skill-related and health-related fitness intertwine in many sports. Soccer players must develop high levels of cardiorespiratory fitness in combination with soccer-specific skills, and gymnasts require high levels of musculoskeletal fitness to execute their skillful performances. Consider your favorite sports for other examples. As recreational athletes, many of us share a common goal—to develop the right combination of fitness components, both health-related and skill-related, to improve performance in our preferred sport(s).

> ## NEED TO KNOW

*Physical activity* refers to movement due to muscle contraction, which results in an increase in energy expenditure. Exercise is one type of physical activity; it involves planned, structured activity with a focus on physical fitness. *Physical fitness* is a multidimensional concept that relates to a person's ability to perform physical activity. Physical fitness includes both health-related and skill-related components. To counter the development of chronic diseases and to enhance overall quality of life, our personal fitness programs should emphasize the health-related components: cardiorespiratory fitness, musculoskeletal fitness, and body composition.

## ➤ How the Body Responds to Exercise

In miraculous fashion, the human body transforms the food we eat into our cells and tissues—blood, bone, muscle—and also uses food as fuel to supply the body's many energy needs. To understand how exercise can improve health and fitness, it's necessary to review the basic concept of energy metabolism, or how energy is produced for different types of physical activity.

## ENERGY PRODUCTION FOR MUSCLE CONTRACTION

Energy for physical activity is produced in the muscle cells through a complex series of reactions that converts chemical energy into mechanical energy, resulting in muscle contraction. The most immediate source of energy comes from the high-energy chemical bonds of adenosine triphosphate (ATP). However, ATP—the energy currency of cells—is stored in the muscle in very small amounts and can supply energy for only a few seconds. Only momentary movements such as picking up the phone or turning your head can be accomplished using stored ATP.

As movement is continued, ATP must be replenished from available macronutrients—primarily carbohydrate (glycogen) and fat. This is when the real work of energy production for muscular activity begins. Energy can be generated to replenish ATP via anaerobic or aerobic pathways. **Anaerobic metabolism** is the production of energy without oxygen present. This pathway of energy production is also relatively short-lived. It can provide a very high-energy output but only for about 30 seconds. Anaerobic metabolism is the predominant pathway for short-term, high-intensity activities such as weight lifting and sprinting. Lactic acid is a byproduct (see the "Breaking It Down" discussion on lactic acid).

Energy production in the presence of oxygen is called **aerobic metabolism.** This pathway can provide moderate energy output for many hours. Prolonged activities such as distance running, cycling, swimming, and other endurance sports rely on aerobic metabolism for continued energy production. Aerobic metabolism is dependent on the cardiorespiratory system to transport oxygen from the air we breathe to the working muscles, where energy for muscle contraction is released during the oxidation of carbohydrates and fats. Carbon dioxide is a byproduct. The oxygen transport and uptake processes are complex yet efficient.

Only a few types of exercise are purely anaerobic or aerobic. For example, performance in short-duration events such as a bench press, high jump, or 40-yard sprint is essentially completely dependent on the anaerobic pathway. In contrast, performance in events lasting several

---

**Anaerobic** (which means "without oxygen") **metabolism** refers to biochemical pathways that do not require oxygen to produce energy for muscle contraction.

**Aerobic** (which means "with oxygen") **metabolism** pertains to biochemical pathways that use oxygen to produce energy for muscle contraction.

Among athletes and coaches, it is widely accepted that the buildup of lactic acid in the muscles leads to detrimental effects such as muscle pain, fatigue, and soreness. But scientists have been suspicious of the lactic acid–soreness connection for many years and finally have shown with certainty that it just isn't so. In fact, we now know that a number of the performance limitations and side effects ascribed to lactic acid are simply not true. Let's take a quick look at how the lactic acid story arose.

In the early 1900s, prominent British researchers W. M. Fletcher and F. G. Hopkins found that isolated muscle fibers (from a frog) accumulated large amounts of lactic acid as they fatigued (when stimulated electrically). Following exercise, as the lactic acid dissipated, the muscle fibers recovered and were soon ready to contract again. This finding supported the hypothesis that a buildup of lactic acid causes muscle acidosis, which diminishes force production and in turn leads to fatigue. Good scientists always consider the most obvious or simplest explanation first. And that is what happened in this case. Follow-up studies appeared to support the hypothesis, so this research was readily published and widely disseminated over the next half century.

With better techniques and high-tech tools, our understanding of exercise physiology and energy production has advanced enormously, particularly since the 1970s. George Brooks, a professor at the University of California, Berkeley, led the way in furthering our understanding about lactic acid. For example, his findings show that the body can efficiently use lactic acid as a source of fuel on par with carbohydrates stored in muscle (glycogen) and sugar in blood (glucose). In fact, it appears that lactic acid plays a role in linking the two metabolic cycles—the oxygen-based aerobic pathway and the oxygen-free anaerobic pathway—previously thought to be distinct.

So what is the bottom line on lactic acid? First, lactic acid can serve as an important fuel when athletes work out and compete; lactic acid has an important role in physiological adaptations due to training. Second, although lactic acid may be responsible for some of the discomfort of intense exercise, its role in muscle fatigue remains unclear. The evidence is mixed; some shows lactic acid may prevent fatigue, and some indicates just the opposite. Third, lactic acid does not cause muscle soreness; there is simply no evidence or plausible mechanism. The likely explanation—with substantial evidence to support it—is that the muscle soreness we experience a few days following exercise is due to cellular-level disruption to muscle fibers and surrounding tissue.

Interestingly, these scientific revelations about lactic acid have had little impact on how coaches train athletes. Through trial and error, coaches know what works, and to a large degree, this coaching knowledge is independent of understanding the details of human physiology. Since these new scientific insights don't directly affect the actual training of athletes, the misconceptions persist. As with many aspects of human physiology and performance, the conventional wisdom is often a simplified version of early research and once established in popular thinking becomes difficult to revise or update. Now you know the real story about lactic acid, so spread the word and illuminate your friends. Let's set the record straight about lactic acid—it is more than just a byproduct of intense exercise.

hours such as running a marathon (26.2 miles) or cycling 50 miles is almost totally dependent on the aerobic pathway, which in turn reflects the capacity of the cardiorespiratory system to transport oxygen to the active muscles. For competitions that are intermediate in duration, such as events lasting 1–10 minutes, both aerobic and anaerobic pathways contribute proportionately, with the relative significance of each depending on the duration of the effort. Table 3.2 presents the relative contributions of energy from aerobic and anaerobic pathways to perform events of different durations.

Many physical activities and sports are "stop and go," or intermittent in nature. Tennis is a good example. For these activities, both aerobic and anaerobic systems are called on to varying degrees throughout the

**TABLE 3.2**  CONTRIBUTIONS OF AEROBIC AND ANAEROBIC METABOLISM TO ENERGY OUTPUT DURING MAXIMAL EXERCISE OF DIFFERENT DURATIONS

| DURATION | % ANAEROBIC | % AEROBIC |
|----------|-------------|-----------|
| 10 seconds | 95 | 5 |
| 30 seconds | 85 | 15 |
| 1 minute | 70 | 30 |
| 2 minutes | 50 | 50 |
| 4 minutes | 40 | 60 |
| 8 minutes | 30 | 70 |
| 12 minutes | 15 | 85 |
| 30 minutes | 5 | 95 |

Source: Adapted from Astrand PO, Rodahl K. *Textbook of Work Physiology*. New York: McGraw-Hill, 1977.

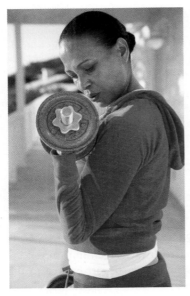

Weight lifting relies primarily on the anaerobic pathway.

game. Other factors being similar, the more continuous the activity, the greater the dependence on aerobic metabolism and thus the cardiovascular system. For instance, soccer and basketball, although not pure aerobic activities, are relatively more aerobic than baseball or volleyball.

## CARDIORESPIRATORY FUNCTION AND OXYGEN UPTAKE

*Cardiorespiratory function* refers to the integration of the heart, lungs, and blood vessels to transport oxygen in the blood to muscles and other tissues and to remove carbon dioxide, a byproduct of oxidation. Oxygen delivery to the working muscles is paramount to sustain physical activities.

To understand the circulation of blood through the body, remember that arteries are vessels carrying blood away from the heart, and veins are vessels carrying blood to the heart (refer to Figure 3.1). As blood circulates through the lungs, hemoglobin in the red blood cells binds oxygen. This freshly oxygenated blood (red) returns to the heart via the pulmonary veins, flows through the left side of the heart, and is then pumped through the aorta, the main artery from the heart, to the major parts of the body (systemic circulation).

Arteries distribute the oxygen-rich blood to the working muscles, where oxygen is removed (or taken up, thus the term *oxygen uptake*) and used for aerobic metabolism. Carbon dioxide is produced, and the veins return the oxygen-poor, carbon dioxide–rich blood (blue) back to the heart and then to the lungs, where carbon dioxide is released in exhaled air and exchanged for oxygen. And the cycle repeats with hemoglobin binding oxygen.

The heart is a special type of muscle (cardiac muscle), and like skeletal muscle, it must have an adequate oxygen supply to continue its work. Delivering oxygen and nutrients to the heart muscle is the role of the coronary arteries, which branch off the aorta back onto the heart's surface. If these vessels become narrowed with fatty deposits (atherosclerosis), blood flow can become restricted. This can lead to chest pain and heart attack.

## FIGURE 3.1    FLOW OF BLOOD THROUGH THE CIRCULATORY SYSTEM

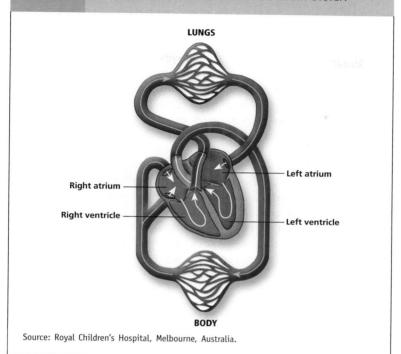

Source: Royal Children's Hospital, Melbourne, Australia.

Each beat of the heart can be felt as a pulse wherever an artery is close to the surface of the body, such as at the wrist or neck. Heart rate is expressed as beats per minute. The amount of blood ejected with each contraction (beat) of the heart is known as the stroke volume and is measured in milliliters per beat measured. The product of heart rate and stroke volume is cardiac output, which is the rate of blood flow in liters per minute. Cardiac output is directly proportional to oxygen transport: the greater the rate at which blood is being circulated, the greater the delivery of oxygen to the working muscles.

For most physical activities, the body responds in specific, predictable ways. As exercise begins—for example, going from sitting at your desk to walking across campus—the leg muscles need additional oxygen, so heart rate and stroke volume ramp up to deliver more blood. The elevation in heart rate is directly proportional to the demand for oxygen. Perhaps you are late for a class, so you walk quickly or jog. Again, your heart rate will increase proportionately as your exercise intensity increases. This is why heart rate is a widely used measure of exercise intensity.

Whether training or competing, if the exercise is demanding and prolonged, heart rate will continue to increase until the person's **aerobic capacity,** or maximal oxygen uptake, is reached. For example, this is the case for runners, cyclists, and triathletes during the final stages of their races. Aerobic capacity refers to one's maximal ability to produce energy aerobically during exhaustive exercise. It can be measured in the lab via a graded exercise test on a treadmill or a stationary bike (cycle ergometer), or it can be estimated from a field test such as a 2-mile run. Aerobic capacity is the single best measure of cardiorespiratory fitness and is the main determinant of endurance performance. This concept plays a central role in individualizing exercise programs and will be discussed in more detail later in this chapter.

For exercise that is focused on musculoskeletal fitness, such as weight training or calisthenics, the demand on the cardiorespiratory system is much less pronounced. As mentioned earlier, the physiological demands of different types of exercise vary widely. At one end of the continuum is cross-country skiing—a total-body form of exercise that requires the simultaneous use of the large muscles in the legs, trunk, and arms to sustain the high-energy output necessary to move one's body weight over a long distance. This type of exercise is clearly aerobic.

At the other end of the continuum is a one-arm bicep curl in which a relatively small muscle is producing force over a distance of only a few feet per repetition. The energy demand on the single muscle can be very high, but it is localized. Multiple repetitions take less than a minute. Relative to the energy required to move the entire body, the energy demand to move a dumbbell a short distance is small and short-lived. Consequently, muscular fitness training relies primarily on the anaerobic pathway. The contribution and interaction of aerobic and anaerobic systems vary depending on the duration, continuousness, and type of exercise.

## ADAPTATIONS TO PHYSICAL TRAINING

The physiological and performance changes that occur with regular training are collectively termed the **training effect.** A primary adaptation to aerobic exercise is improved oxygen delivery to the muscles. At the level of the lungs, training enhances the exchange of oxygen and carbon

---

**Aerobic capacity,** or maximal oxygen uptake, is the highest amount of oxygen the body can consume during exhaustive exercise. It is considered the single best measure of cardiorespiratory fitness.

The **training effect** is the physiological changes (adaptations) and improved fitness resulting from regular physical training.

dioxide at higher rates. Concurrently, as the heart strengthens, it can eject more blood with each beat. This increase in stroke volume results in the decrease in resting heart rate commonly observed after a few weeks of training. These cumulative pulmonary and cardiovascular changes account for the improved delivery of oxygen to the muscles.

Another fundamental adaptation that improves oxygen uptake and thus energy production takes place within the muscle cells themselves. Most of the cellular changes occur in the cell structure known as the mitochondrion, which is the actual site of aerobic metabolism—the conversion of food to usable energy in the presence of oxygen. Training causes the mitochondria to increase in size and number. The aerobic enzymes, catalysts in the aerobic pathway of energy production, also increase in quantity. Moreover, endurance is further improved by the enhanced ability of the muscles to use fats as fuel, sparing muscle carbohydrate stores (glycogen).

Resistance or weight training to improve musculoskeletal fitness can bring about significant increases in muscle size (hypertrophy), strength, muscular endurance, and flexibility. Improvements in muscle tone and force production are induced in several ways. A program of resistance training coupled with flexibility exercises improves blood flow to and neural control of muscle fibers, allowing for more efficient energy production, fiber recruitment, and muscle recovery. Over the same period, concentrations of anaerobic and/or aerobic enzymes are increased in the muscle cells, depending on the energy pathways being challenged. In addition, resistance/flexibility training maintains healthy joints and connective tissues such as tendons, ligaments, and cartilage, and it is protective against musculoskeletal injury.

A balanced exercise program develops or maintains both cardiorespiratory and musculoskeletal fitness. Such a program improves performance whether in specific fitness tests, sports competitions, or challenging physical tasks in daily life. A balanced exercise program also yields direct health benefits modulated through the body's multiple biological systems. Primary health benefits include

- Improved metabolism (namely, normalized blood lipids and glucose) and lower risk for heart disease and diabetes
- Improved body composition and weight control and lower risk for obesity
- Maintenance of healthy bones, muscles, and joints and lower risk for osteoporosis, joint diseases, and low back pain
- Improved psychological health and reduced risk for anxiety and depression

A dose-response relationship is evident for both cardiorespiratory and musculoskeletal exercise. That is, the more you exercise, the greater the improvements in health and fitness. If a pill could bring about this impressive combination of benefits, it would be hailed as a wonder drug. Moreover, regular physical activity has few unwanted side effects, and costs are easily minimized. As top researcher Steven N. Blair succinctly affirms, exercise will make you feel better, function better, look better, and live longer. A final point to remember about the training effect: Improved fitness and associated health benefits are reversible and diminish with inactivity. We can't store up fitness. The key is to establish exercise as a habit.

✓ **NEED TO KNOW**

Energy for most physical activity is provided via aerobic metabolism, which is dependent on the cardiorespiratory system to transport oxygen to the working muscles. Aerobic capacity (maximal oxygen uptake) is the single best measure of cardiorespiratory fitness. The *training effect* refers to both the physiological adaptations and performance improvements that occur as a consequence of regular training. A balanced physical activity program to promote health and fitness includes both cardiorespiratory and musculoskeletal training.

## ➤ Recommendations for Healthy Adults

The physical activity recommendations presented in this section focus on the amounts and type of exercise known to improve health. These recommendations are based on the *Physical Activity Guidelines for Americans, 2008* and position statements from leading scientific and public health organizations including the American College of Sports Medicine, the American Heart Association, and the Centers for Disease Control and Prevention.

For those who lead a sedentary lifestyle, these guidelines provide a reasonable goal. For those who are fit and engage in more advanced training programs, these guidelines serve as a benchmark to check the balance of the exercise program. You can glean tips to adjust your current program and insights on how to assist a friend in starting or maintaining a program.

First, we'll review the basic principles of exercise training as a prelude to presenting the physical activity recommendations for cardiorespiratory fitness followed by those for musculoskeletal fitness. Then we'll present the physical activity continuum to illustrate where the recommendations fall within the broad spectrum of physical activity levels.

Exercise training is based on four principles: overload, reversibility, specificity, and individual differences. Consider each principle when planning an exercise program.

### Principle of Overload

To improve a physiological system, it must be exposed to a stimulus greater than it is normally accustomed to—such as a faster pace or a heavier weight. This is the fundamental principle upon which all exercise training is based. Repeated exposure over time to progressively greater amounts of exercise results in responsive changes by the lungs, heart, muscle, and connective tissue—structural and functional adaptations from the molecular to the system level. These adaptations include enhanced capacity and efficiency in cardiorespiratory and/or musculoskeletal function. This translates into improved fitness.

### Principle of Reversibility

This principle is simply the converse of the principle of overload. When one stops exercising and the training overload is removed, the previously developed physiological systems will over time return to pre-training levels. To maintain fitness, one must continue to exercise. Fitness cannot be stored.

### Principle of Specificity

Many training effects are specific to the type of exercise, the particular muscles involved, and the intensity. For example, if the goal is to run a 5-kilometer (5K) race at a 7-minute-per-mile pace, then the principle of specificity suggests that the person should focus on *running* and include training sessions *at the goal pace*. If all training is done at an 8- to 9-minute-per-mile pace, it will be difficult to shift gears on race day, because the body has not been exposed to the specific demands of running at the faster pace. Moreover, swimming and cycling, although excellent aerobic exercise, will do little to improve running performance because the muscles are used in different ways for each activity. Training specificity is critical for reaching performance goals.

### Principle of Individual Differences

There is tremendous variability from one person to the next in both natural fitness level and in the rate of improvement that occurs with exercise training. Due to different genetic endowments, each of us begins at a different point on the fitness continuum. This is no different from variability among individuals in height or hair color. What is not as apparent though is the variability among individuals' responses to a similar training program. A standard exercise dose may be just right for many people but too hard for others and not enough for some.

For best results, customize your exercise program as you learn how your body responds. The exercise recommendations that follow should be used as a *guide*. The fine-tuning is left up to each of us individually.

## CARDIORESPIRATORY FITNESS

**Cardiorespiratory fitness,** also known as aerobic fitness or cardiorespiratory endurance, is the ability of the respiratory and circulatory systems to supply oxygen to the working muscles during sustained physical activity. For most people, being fit or in shape means having good cardiorespiratory fitness. Due to the potent beneficial effect that cardiorespiratory fitness has on lowering chronic disease risk, particularly heart disease, many scientists believe this fitness component is the most important.

### The FITT Acronym

Four factors constitute an exercise plan: frequency, intensity, time (duration), and type. Conveniently, the first letters of these four factors form the acronym FITT, which is an easy way to remember them. Recommendations for cardiorespiratory fitness follow.

### Frequency: How Often?

The recommended exercise frequency is at least three and up to seven days per week. One should consider frequency relative to both intensity and duration. For example, those who enjoy vigorous exercise should consider training every other day, while those who prefer moderate intensity activity could probably exercise most days of the week (e.g., hard running three to four days per week vs. brisk walking five to six days per week).

### Intensity: How Hard Do I Have to Push Myself?

Exercise intensity should be within 50–85 percent of aerobic capacity, with **moderate intensity** defined as 50–59 percent and **vigorous intensity** as 60–85 percent. For most young adults, a moderate-intensity activity is similar to brisk walking (about 4 miles per hour), and a vigorous-intensity activity is like jogging/running. (A lower threshold of 40 percent

**Cardiorespiratory fitness** is a health-related component of physical fitness that relates to the ability of the circulatory and respiratory systems to supply oxygen to the working muscles during sustained physical activity.

**Moderate-intensity physical activity** is brisk walking or similar activities that require 50–59 percent of one's aerobic capacity (equivalent to 50–59 percent of one's heart rate training range using the heart rate reserve method).

**Vigorous-intensity physical activity** is running and similar sweat-producing activities that require 60–85 percent of one's aerobic capacity (equivalent to 60–85 percent of one's heart rate training range using the heart rate reserve method).

of aerobic capacity may be appropriate for older, chronically sedentary people.)

**Heart Rate (HR) as a Measure of Intensity.** Since oxygen uptake and heart rate are highly correlated, heart rate can be used to gauge intensity. There are several approaches to using heart rate to calculate training zones (ranges). Although it is common to take a straight percentage of a person's estimated maximal heart rate, we prefer the heart rate reserve method because it takes into account resting heart rate and is directly proportional to increases in oxygen uptake (energy expenditure). The heart rate reserve is simply the difference between the resting heart rate ($HR_{rest}$) and the maximal heart rate ($HR_{max}$). Maximal heart rate is estimated by subtracting age from 220. To calculate the training heart rate range, determine the lower and upper limits as follows:

$$HR \text{ at } 50\% \text{ intensity} = [(HR_{max} = HR_{rest}) \times 0.50] + HR_{rest}$$
$$HR \text{ at } 85\% \text{ intensity} = [(HR_{max} = HR_{rest}) \times 0.85] + HR_{rest}$$

For example, using these equations, the heart rate training range (from 50–85 percent intensity) for a 20-year-old with a resting heart rate of 70 would be 135–181 beats per minute. As this is a large range, the next step would be to decide whether to train in the moderate or vigorous part of the range. The training heart rate zone for different ages is plotted in Figure 3.2.

| FIGURE 3.2 | TRAINING HEART RATE ZONE BY AGE, USING THE HEART RATE RESERVE METHOD |

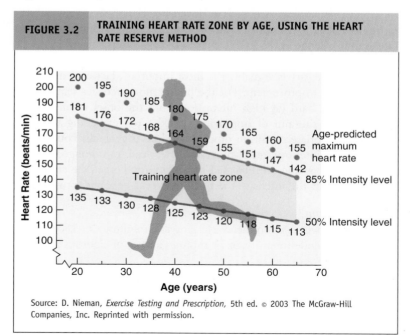

Source: D. Nieman, *Exercise Testing and Prescription,* 5th ed. © 2003 The McGraw-Hill Companies, Inc. Reprinted with permission.

**How to Measure Heart Rate.** Measuring heart rate is easy to learn. Take your pulse on the inside of the wrist (at the radial artery) by placing the tips of your first two fingers about an inch below the base of the thumb. When you feel the pulse, count the beats for 10 seconds and then multiply the 10-second count by six to determine your heart rate in beats per minute. To measure your resting heart rate, check your pulse after sitting quietly for at least 10 minutes or upon waking in the morning. To estimate your exercise heart rate, count your pulse immediately after exercise. Take time to practice so you can reliably measure the higher heart rates. An option is to use a heart rate monitor that displays heart rate continuously. Heart rate monitors that consist of a chest strap (transmitter) and watch (receiver) are reliable, durable, and relatively inexpensive.

**Perceived Exertion as a Measure of Intensity.** Another approach for monitoring intensity is to use the **rating of perceived exertion (RPE)** scale developed by Professor Gunnar Borg. This scale links a person's subjective rating of physical exertion to a number between 6 and 20 using verbal descriptors (Table 3.3). For example, if the exercise effort feels "very light," the rating would be a 9; "somewhat hard" would be a 13; and "extremely hard" a 19. The RPE scale correlates well with heart rate and is commonly used during exercise testing and in exercise classes. The scale is useful in teaching people how *hard* or *easy* to work to achieve an appropriate exercise intensity. For most young adults, ratings from 12 to 14 correspond to about 50–60 percent of the heart rate training range (HR reserve method), and ratings from 15 to 18 correspond to 60–85 percent.

Exercise intensity is arguably the most important factor in determining the rate of improvement. For the highly motivated, it's tempting to work out very hard (at high intensities) from the onset of an exercise program with the aim of improving quickly. Yet, exercising too hard without appropriate transition time to build up is generally counterproductive. High-intensity starter programs often lead to prolonged fatigue, extreme soreness, and an increased risk of injury. Forget the crash programs and limit the intensity the first few weeks of a new program.

### Time: How Long?

Consensus guidelines recommend engaging in a minimum of 150 minutes a week of moderate-intensity, or 75 minutes a week of vigorous-intensity

**Rating of perceived exertion (RPE)** is a subjective measure of the strenuousness of a physical activity, based on one's overall perception of effort; it is widely used as a measure of exercise intensity. The RPE scale ranges from 6 to 20 with accompanying verbal descriptors (e.g., light, hard).

**TABLE 3.3    RATING OF PERCEIVED EXERTION: BORG RPE SCALE®**

| | |
|---|---|
| 6 | No exertion at all |
| 7 | Extremely light |
| 8 | |
| 9 | Very light |
| 10 | |
| 11 | Light |
| 12 | |
| 13 | Somewhat hard |
| 14 | |
| 15 | Hard (heavy) |
| 16 | |
| 17 | Very hard |
| 18 | |
| 19 | Extremely hard |
| 20 | Maximal exertion |

Source: © Gunnar Borg, 1970, 1985, 1994, 1998. Reprinted with permission of Gunnar Borg.

# Instructions to the Borg RPE Scale®

While exercising, we want you to use this scale to rate your perception of exertion. How heavy and strenuous does the exercise feel to you, combining all sensations and feelings of physical stress, effort, and fatigue? Do not concern yourself with any one factor, such as leg pain or shortness of breath, but try to focus on the total feeling of exertion.

6 "No exertion at all," means you don't feel any exertion whatsoever— no muscle fatigue, no breathlessness or difficulty breathing.

9 "Very light" exertion, such as taking a short walk at your own pace.

13 "Somewhat hard" work, but it still feels OK to continue.

15 "Hard" and tiring, but continuing isn't terribly difficult.

17 "Very hard" means very strenuous work. You can still go on, but you really have to push yourself and you are very tired.

19 "Extremely hard" is for most people the strongest exertion they have ever experienced.

Try to appraise your feeling of exertion as honestly as possible, without thinking about what the actual physical load is. Try not to underestimate and not to overestimate your exertion. It's your own feeling of effort and exertion that is important, not how it compares with other people's. Look at the scale and the expressions and then give a number.

Source: © Gunnar Borg, 1985, 1994, 1998, 2006. Reprinted with permission of Gunnar Borg.

aerobic activity, or an equivalent combination. Intensity and duration generally balance each other—the higher the intensity, the shorter the duration, and vice versa. For moderate-intensity aerobic activities like brisk walking, the guideline is at least 30 minutes per day, five days per week. Durations as short as 10 minutes can be accumulated throughout the day. Because of the dose-response relationship between physical activity and health, more is better: 45–60 minutes per day is preferable, and 60–90 minutes may be necessary for weight control (refer to Chapter 2).

### Type: Which Activities?

The type or mode of activity should stress the cardiorespiratory, or aerobic, system. Such activities use major muscle groups, are rhythmic, and can be done continuously. The most common aerobic activities are walking, running, cycling, and swimming, but many other activities meet the criteria as well. Most important though is to select an activity that you like. If the activity is not fun or enjoyable, it's unlikely that you will continue. A word of caution for beginning exercisers or older people: avoid high-impact activities like running and aerobic dance as initial choices because of their higher injury rates.

## MUSCULOSKELETAL FITNESS

**Musculoskeletal fitness,** or muscular fitness, is composed of three intertwined elements: muscular strength, muscular endurance, and flexibility. **Muscular strength** is a muscle or muscle group's maximal capacity to exert force against an external resistance—that is, the most weight you can lift one time (e.g., one-repetition maximum, 1RM), such as with the arm curl for the biceps muscle or the leg extension for the quadriceps. **Muscular endurance** is slightly different. It refers to the muscle's ability to sustain a submaximal force or to persist at some relative level—for example, the number of repetitions you can complete at a resistance equal to 50 percent of 1RM. **Flexibility** is the functional

---

**Musculoskeletal fitness,** a health-related component of physical fitness, refers to the combination of muscular strength, muscular endurance, and flexibility.

**Muscular strength** is the maximal force that a muscle (or muscle group) can exert against a resistance.

**Muscular endurance** is the ability of a muscle (or muscle group) to apply a submaximal force repeatedly or to sustain a muscular contraction over an extended period.

**Flexibility** is the range of motion available in a joint (or group of joints).

range of motion in a joint or group of joints. Flexibility varies from joint to joint and depends on the muscles, tendons, and ligaments at the involved joint(s).

Musculoskeletal fitness is demonstrated in nearly all sports. To varying degrees during a competition, muscles are called on to exert peak force, resist fatigue, and perform well through multiple ranges of motion. Musculoskeletal fitness is certainly related to our health status, too. It enables us to perform demanding physical tasks—both routine and unplanned—that arise in everyday situations as well as helping to combat osteoporosis, low back pain, joint disease, loss of mobility, and frailty.

To develop musculoskeletal fitness, we must engage in some form of **resistance training.** Although it is better known as strength training or weight training, *resistance training* is the preferred term for several reasons. First, strength *and* muscular endurance are usually developed in combination. Second, "resistance" can be applied to the muscles using iron weights (dumbbells, barbells, weight stacks), but it can also be accomplished using muscle- and movement-specific equipment with pneumatic, hydraulic, and computer-controlled resistance, as well as simply body weight (e.g., calisthenics—sit-ups, push-ups, pull-ups). Resistance training coupled with appropriate attention to flexibility exercises is the basis for improving musculoskeletal fitness.

Compared to the hundreds of scientific studies on cardiorespiratory fitness, far fewer have been conducted to determine what constitutes a sufficient (health-promoting) exercise dose for developing strength and muscular endurance. Yet, enough solid research is available to provide guidance with confidence. An adequate evidence base for recommending flexibility exercises is another matter though. Although stretching exercises have proven effectiveness in regaining range of motion during rehabilitation from musculoskeletal injury or surgery, there is little quality research on the health benefits of flexibility for people with no physical limitations. Among the many official statements on physical activity recommendations from scientific organizations, only the American College of Sports Medicine provides commentary and suggestions on flexibility. Although of less overall importance than either aerobic or resistance training, flexibility training is certainly important as a complementary component and should be included as part of a balanced program of physical activity.

---

**Resistance training,** commonly known as weight training or strength training, is exercise that develops strength and muscular endurance using free weights, machine weights, body weight (calisthenics), or some combination.

Using the FITT acronym's categories, we present recommendations for achieving a healthy level of musculoskeletal fitness.

## Frequency: How Often?

The recommended training frequency for resistance training is two or more nonconsecutive days per week. Training three days per week will result in greater benefits. The standard practice is to allow two days of rest between resistance training sessions to give muscles time to recover and adapt (e.g., work out on Monday and Wednesday).

## Intensity: How Hard Do I Have to Work?

Intensity is a function of the resistance (e.g., amount of weight lifted). The recommendation is to complete at least one set of 8–12 repetitions of 8 to 10 exercises that condition the major muscle groups. Through trial and error, you will learn to select the proper resistance for each exercise—that is, a weight that results in substantial muscle fatigue during the final 1–2 repetitions of the set. The RPE scale can also be used to gauge intensity. In Table 3.4, we provide a sample program of 10 exercises.

## Time: How Long?

As a practical matter, the time or duration is the length of the entire workout session. This includes the actual time exercising (e.g., lifting weights) and the recovery time between exercises, which should be kept to 1–2 minutes. A duration of 20–30 minutes is a reasonable estimate for the total time needed to complete one set of 8 to10 exercises.

| TABLE 3.4 | STANDARD RESISTANCE EXERCISES AND ASSOCIATED MUSCLE GROUPS |
|---|---|
| **EXERCISE*** | **MUSCLE GROUP** |
| 1. Bench press | Chest (pectoralis, triceps) |
| 2. Leg press | Legs, buttocks (quadriceps, gluteals) |
| 3. Shoulder press | Shoulders (deltoids, triceps) |
| 4. Leg extension | Front of thigh (quadriceps) |
| 5. Pull down | Back (latissimus dorsi) |
| 6. Leg curl | Back of thigh (hamstrings) |
| 7. Triceps extension | Back of arm (triceps) |
| 8. Heel raise | Calves (gastrocnemius) |
| 9. Arm curl | Front of arm (biceps) |
| 10. Curl-ups | Abdomen (abdominals) |

*These or very similar exercises can be done with free weights or on exercise machines. Also, note that all the major muscle groups can be developed with calisthenics (e.g., push-ups, pull-ups, bar-dips, curl-ups, heel raises, bench stepping with added weight).

## Type: Which Activities?

In contrast to training for cardiorespiratory fitness, the options for improving or maintaining muscular fitness are more limited. Such training must involve resistance exercise whether it is traditional weight training, calisthenics, or newer variations of resistance-based exercise. Regardless of the type of equipment or specific program, the overall goal is the same: to condition all the major muscles, not just a couple specific muscles. Website Resources at the end of the chapter provide detailed information on resistance exercises and programs for different levels (novice, intermediate, advanced).

To maintain range of motion with the involved joints, flexibility exercises should be included as part of a musculoskeletal training program. Although flexibility training per se is not included in the physical activity position statements of all organizations, it is an accepted component for individual exercise plans. Stretching should focus on muscle/tendons groups at major joints (e.g., ankle, knee, hips, back, neck, shoulder, elbow, wrist). Stretches should be slow and steady (static), maintained at a position of mild discomfort for about 30 seconds, and repeated two or three times. Refer to the Website Resources at the end of the chapter for descriptions and illustrations of flexibility exercises.

Article 3.2

## PHYSICAL ACTIVITY CONTINUUM

It's easy to categorize everyone into two groups: exercisers and nonexercisers. Yet, this oversimplification neglects a fundamental fact: Physical activity levels vary tremendously across a broad continuum, from no physical activity beyond the routine activities of daily living to enormous amounts of training required for high-level sports competition. In Figure 3.3, the physical activity (PA) continuum is depicted as three overlapping spheres representing low, moderate, and high activity. Within each sphere, multiple levels exist. During various periods in our lives, we shift among levels within a sphere and from one sphere to another.

Many college students may find themselves in the low-activity sphere in which the sedentary lifestyle rules. They engage in few if any physical activities other than those required to get through the day. These students are plainly falling short of achieving recommended levels of physical activity. Some may be taking incremental steps toward incorporating more activity into daily routines (e.g., walking across campus instead of taking the bus), which moves them closer to the next sphere in the continuum.

Those who are achieving recommended levels of physical activity for both cardiorespiratory and muscular fitness are in the middle sphere of the continuum. The recommendations allow wide latitude

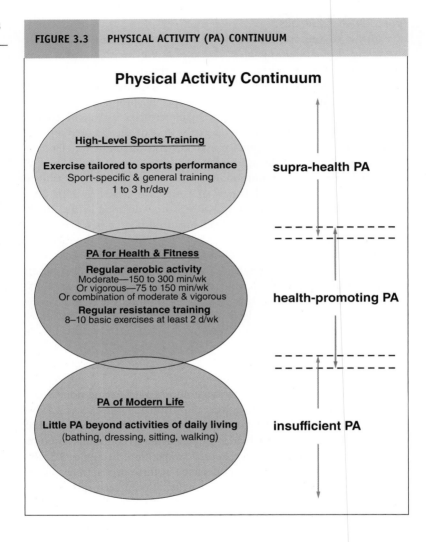

FIGURE 3.3    PHYSICAL ACTIVITY (PA) CONTINUUM

**Physical Activity Continuum**

**High-Level Sports Training**

**Exercise tailored to sports performance**
Sport-specific & general training
1 to 3 hr/day

**supra-health PA**

**PA for Health & Fitness**

**Regular aerobic activity**
Moderate—150 to 300 min/wk
Or vigorous—75 to 150 min/wk
Or combination of moderate & vigorous
**Regular resistance training**
8–10 basic exercises at least 2 d/wk

**health-promoting PA**

**PA of Modern Life**

**Little PA beyond activities of daily living**
(bathing, dressing, sitting, walking)

**insufficient PA**

in developing programs to meet individual needs and preferences. For example, some people prefer vigorous aerobic exercise, while others find moderate-intensity physical activity more to their liking. Similar options exist for meeting recommendations for muscular fitness. Lifting weights and stretching at a fitness center is a popular choice, but others may prefer a home-based program of calisthenics and flexibility exercises. This sphere is expansive and includes those who are expending 800–1,000 Cal per week (e.g., briskly walking 2 miles per session five days per week) up through those who may be expending twice that amount through a variety of daily activities (e.g., a combination of running, swimming, basketball, and soccer). Approaches are variable: Some may choose lifestyle physical activity such as accumulating multiple 10-minute walks throughout the day, while others opt for structured hour-long exercise classes. Within this middle sphere, regardless of the approach, the greater the total physical activity, the greater will be the health benefits.

The top sphere of the continuum is the realm of high-level exercise and sports training. Many of you have been in this sphere, perhaps as an age group or high school athlete. And some of you are in this sphere now, enjoying the challenge of advanced training on a sports team or for personal fitness. Competing at a high level requires a commitment to training, often several hours a day most days of the week. The goals at this level are focused on performance, not on health. Health benefits derived from training at this level are small compared to health gains achieved from training in the middle sphere. Yet, remember that successful training at this level depends on a solid fitness base and robust health developed in the middle sphere.

Throughout this section, physical activity recommendations have been presented as ranges for frequency, intensity, time, and type of activity. The public health standard—equivalent to 30 minutes of brisk walking at least five days per week—imparts significant health benefits, particularly for those who have been sedentary. If the entire population could achieve this activity threshold, it would significantly improve the nation's health. However, this level of physical activity is the minimal, *not* the optimal—it's the lowest level within the middle sphere. Let's be clear on this point. In general, greater amounts of physical activity result in greater health benefits. People who can maintain an exercise program that is of longer duration and/or more vigorous and encompasses cardiorespiratory and musculoskeletal components (a high level within the middle sphere) will derive greater health benefits as well as improve fitness.

✓ **NEED TO KNOW**

The physical activity "dose" needed to impart significant health benefits is known. Exercise is prescribed in terms of frequency, intensity, time, and type (FITT) for both aerobic and musculoskeletal conditioning. The basic training principles of overload (and reversibility), specificity, and individual differences can guide you in applying the various exercise recommendations. The physical activity (PA) continuum has three spheres: physical activity of modern life (insufficient PA), physical activity for health and fitness (health-promoting PA), and training for high-level performance (supra-health PA).

Developing a fitness program involves linking the recommendations to individual goals—such as to increase stamina, gain strength, improve muscle tone, lose body fat, add muscle mass, control weight, relieve stress, or improve sports performance. What are your goals? Since many exercise goals are related to losing body fat or gaining muscle mass, we'll review the energy expenditure side of the energy balance equation in this section.

From time to time, each of us are drawn to try a new sport or special event but may be wary of the physical demands—perhaps a local 10K road race or a vacation trip centered on downhill skiing, ocean kayaking, mountain biking, or scuba diving. Use this as a goal and devise a fitness plan to prepare accordingly. The more fit you are, the more enjoyable the experience will be, and the more you will be able to do. List your main short-term goals and a few long-term goals too. In the latter part of this section, key practical points are shared to help you develop an exercise program that works.

### ENERGY BALANCE: ENERGY EXPENDITURE

One of the primary reasons people exercise is for weight control—that is, to help keep a balance between energy intake and energy expenditure. In Chapter 2, the *energy intake* or food consumption side of the energy balance equation was discussed. Now let's take a closer look at the *energy expenditure* side. Understanding how physical activity contributes to energy expenditure is critical to preventing unwanted weight gain and to successful long-term weight management.

#### Estimating Daily Energy Expenditure

Three factors determine a person's daily energy expenditure: (1) resting metabolic rate, (2) the thermic effect of food, and (3) the amount of physical activity. Resting (or basal) metabolic rate is a function of body size and accounts for the majority of one's daily energy expenditure (about 60–75 percent). Plainly, the larger your mass (the more you weigh), the more energy you need to keep all physiological functions operating at the resting level (e.g., sleeping or sitting quietly).

The *thermic effect of food* refers to the energy associated with digestion. This is that slight but noticeable warm-up many people can feel one or two hours after a large meal. This energy expenditure component is relatively small (5–10 percent) and generally included as part of the resting metabolic rate.

The third factor is the amount of physical activity. This is the only factor that we control. Physical activity is highly variable among people and within an individual. It may account for as little as 25 percent of daily energy expenditure in sedentary folks whose only physical activity is that required by daily living—such as dressing, bathing, and necessary walking. Or physical activity can account for as much as 40 percent or more among highly active people who get an hour or more of exercise every day.

Daily energy expenditures for a moderately active 121-lb. woman and a moderately active 154-lb. man would be about 2,000 and 2,500 Cal, respectively. Your energy expenditure will vary accordingly based on your weight and activity level (see the assessment in Connect Resources at the end of the chapter).

### Additional Caloric Expenditure Through Physical Activity

Average calories burned for different types of moderate and vigorous physical activities are shown in Table 3.5. Note that the energy expended during resistance training is quite a bit lower than what is expended for aerobic activities. This should be clear from the earlier discussion on energy pathways and the different energy demands of aerobic training versus resistance training.

A second point to highlight is the trade-off between intensity and duration among aerobic activities. If your primary aim is to expend calories, you have a choice between exercising at a higher intensity for a shorter period of time or longer at a lower intensity. The total energy required to move a mass—in this case, a person's body weight—over a given distance is not substantially affected by the speed at which it occurs. The energy expended by running 2 miles in 15 minutes (about 200 Cal) is only about 10 percent more than is expended by walking the same distance in 30 minutes (about 180 Cal). For a beginning exerciser or a high-BMI person though, the preferable option is to extend duration and go at a moderate pace.

When considering healthful levels of physical activity, the recommended target range for energy expenditure is 150–400 Cal per day. This is above the minimal energy expenditure from activities of daily living. The lower end of the range represents a minimal caloric threshold of about 1,000 Cal per week, which equates to the public health physical activity recommendation of 30 minutes of brisk walking five days per week. Based on the positive dose-response relationship between physical activity and health, gradually moving toward the 300–400 Cal per day level is encouraged. Intentional energy expenditure at 2,000 Cal per week and higher (60–90 minutes per day) has been shown to be successful for both initial weight loss and weight maintenance.

Self Assessment 3.1

## DEVELOPING AN EXERCISE PLAN

It's time to translate the cardiorespiratory and musculoskeletal guidelines into a specific exercise prescription based on your goals. Alternatively, if

| TABLE 3.5 | ENERGY EXPENDITURE FOR INTERMITTENT AND CONTINUOUS ACTIVITIES |
|---|---|

| INTERMITTENT ACTIVITIES | CAL EXPENDED IN 30 MINUTES |
|---|---|
| Resistance training—light | 100 |
| Volleyball | 100 |
| Golf—walking | 150 |
| Resistance training—vigorous | 150 |
| Aerobic dance | 215 |
| Basketball | 220 |

| CONTINUOUS ACTIVITIES | CAL EXPENDED IN 30 MINUTES |
|---|---|
| Walking at 4 miles/hour | 200 |
| Bicycling | 245 |
| Swimming | 255 |
| Stair climbing | 300 |
| Jogging at 6 miles/hour | 310 |
| Running at 8 miles/hour | 440 |

**These are estimates of total energy expended in 30 minutes for a 154-lb. person.** Those who weigh more will expend more, and those who weigh less will expend less. These values are approximations that allow for relative comparison among different activities. Actual calories expended can vary depending on the intensity and continuousness of the activity.

Source: Compendium of physical activities. **https://sites.google.com/site/compendiumofphysicalactivities/**

you are already a regular exerciser, take the time to assess your program in light of the current recommendations. To help with the translation process, consider the following points.

### Physical Activity or Exercise?

Most people in their 20s still have moderate to high functional capacities simply due to their youth. Relying solely on moderate-intensity physical activity, such as brisk walking, may not be sufficiently challenging unless you have been very sedentary—in that case, moderate-intensity activity *is* the appropriate choice. The majority of college students report that they *prefer* exercise that is more vigorous whether it's recreational sports, basic fitness training, or a combination.

Since nearly all college students have good-to-excellent sports and exercise facilities available on campus, it's truly a once-in-a-lifetime opportunity to explore different types of classes. The variety of college physical education and campus recreation classes taught by high-caliber instructors is impressive. High school offerings pale in comparison, and your choices following college will be more restricted due to fewer choices, higher cost, and less accessibility and time. Develop an exercise program based on activities and sports you enjoy, and, at least once a year, take the plunge and try a new exercise/activity class for a semester.

## Initial Screening and Risks of Exercise

For nearly all apparently healthy young adults, it is safe to begin or intensify an exercise program. In fact, some experts contend that you put yourself *at greater risk for medical problems if you remain physically inactive.* However, as a precaution to identify individuals who may need medical clearance, you should take the seven-question Physical Activity Readiness Questionnaire (PAR-Q). This form is available online **(www.csep.ca/CMFiles/publications/parq/par-q.pdf).**

Every year a few sudden deaths occur among high school and college athletes during training or competition. There is always immediate speculation as to the cause of death because the official explanation is typically not known for several weeks pending medical tests. At that point, the official cause of death receives only back-page coverage. Nearly all confirmed causes of sudden deaths in young athletes are attributable to inherited cardiac abnormalities, heat stress, drug or supplement use, or a combination of these factors.

A sensible program of exercise is very safe, especially for young people. The greatest exercise risk for college students is simply overdoing it—too much, too fast. As shown in Figure 3.4, low-to-moderate levels of training impart many benefits with minimal risks. In contrast, as training levels increase beyond those recommended for health and

**FIGURE 3.4** **RELATIONSHIP OF BENEFITS AND RISKS TO INCREASING LEVELS OF PHYSICAL ACTIVITY**

fitness, the benefits diminish while the risks increase. This rise in risk is most notably due to overtraining—exercising too hard, too long, and/or too often. This results in a cumulative overload that exceeds the body's capacity to adapt. Overtraining commonly results in musculoskeletal injuries or respiratory infections (e.g., common cold, flu). These "breakdowns" are highly treatable with rest, medical management, and common sense.

### Initial Fitness Level

One's initial fitness level is the foundation upon which the exercise prescription (frequency, intensity, time, type) is built. If you don't already know your fitness level, consider using standard fitness tests to see where you stand; for example, time yourself in a 1-mile walk or a 2-mile run to assess cardiorespiratory fitness and use push-up, sit-up, and trunk-flexion tests to assess muscular fitness. A variety of fitness tests with instructions and scoring are available online (**www.topendsports. com/testing/tests**). How you rate against normative scores may be of interest. The true value of assessment though is in using the results as a baseline for tailoring your exercise plan. Be honest in your self-appraisal and carefully set the initial training level to your current condition. One of the main reasons the exercise recommendations are presented as ranges is to accommodate the wide variability of initial fitness levels.

Equally important is how to gauge the rate of progression for increasing the exercise overload. Rate of progression is dependent on the principle of individual differences in which you learn your dose-response curve through trial and error. Envision an exercise program as having three stages: an initial conditioning stage, which lasts a few weeks; an improvement stage, which can be highly variable in length; and a maintenance stage, which goes on indefinitely. A systematic increase in overload is applied during the second stage. Small, steady increments in the exercise dose (5–15 percent) every week or two is a reasonable rate of progression. Ramping up too quickly is often counterproductive.

### Anatomy of the Exercise Session

The format for an exercise session or workout is a warm-up period, the main conditioning phase that involves aerobic and/or resistance training, and a cool-down period. In Figure 3.5, this format is illustrated for a 30-minute aerobic workout in which heart rate is plotted against time. Warm-up facilitates the transition from rest to exercise, and cool-down allows gradual recovery and transition back to the resting level.

When feasible, aerobic training and resistance training should be performed on alternate days, although both activities can be combined into the same workout. If combined, the training you wish to

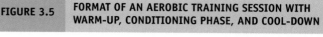

**FIGURE 3.5** | **FORMAT OF AN AEROBIC TRAINING SESSION WITH WARM-UP, CONDITIONING PHASE, AND COOL-DOWN**

Note: 200 is the estimated maximal heart rate for a 20-year-old.

*HRR = Heart Rate Reserve.

emphasize (aerobic or resistance) should be done first. Stretching is typically done during the cool-down, as stretching is more effective when the muscles are warm. However, flexibility exercises are also often included as part of a warm-up and are sometimes done at a separate time altogether.

Aerobic, resistance, and flexibility training are the components of a complete fitness program. There is wide latitude in how you choose to mix or blend these activities. For example, participation in sports such as basketball, soccer, and tennis can be a core element of your fitness program or simply be included for competitive and social pleasures. Yet, regardless of the specific sport or fitness activity, it's wise to follow the exercise session format and include a warm-up and a cool-down.

## CONSUMER ISSUES

Many consumer issues can arise when developing an exercise program or moving from one setting to another (e.g., new school, new job, new living arrangement). Three common topics of interest are fitness centers, personal trainers, and home exercise equipment.

### Fitness Centers

Most colleges have very good sports facilities for their students. Having a state-of-the-art fitness center is increasingly viewed as not just important but necessary. A modern, well-equipped facility also provides an edge with student recruitment. These fitness centers are usually well staffed, open long hours, and conveniently located. There is often no monthly fee as they are supported from mandatory student fees paid with tuition.

You may also want to investigate what's available at a community health/fitness club as an alternative to using a campus facility. Fitness programs can be categorized as for-profit health clubs (e.g., 24 Hour Fitness, Gold's Gym, LA Fitness), not-for-profit centers (e.g., YMCAs, YWCAs, Jewish Community Centers), and hospital-affiliated fitness centers. Fitness/health clubs vary widely in their size and equipment, breadth and quality of programs and services, and costs. Make sure you carefully consider your options before joining one. To help in making a wise decision, use guidelines available from trusted sources such as the American College of Sports Medicine and *Consumer Reports.*

### Personal Trainers/Expert Instructors

Campus fitness centers usually offer a number of classes and individualized training sessions at reasonable rates by well-qualified instructors and personal trainers. Depending on your particular exercise plan, it may be smart (and fun) to use these services. For example, if you are ready to start a resistance-training program, consider getting a personal trainer to work with you for the first few sessions so that you become familiar with the proper technique and use of the resistance-training equipment. Exercise equipment—both resistance and aerobic—can vary widely from one center to another.

Article
3.3

A personal trainer provides expert instruction, immediate feedback, and motivation. This individualized coaching can be most helpful, particularly for novices but also for those who have been away from exercise for an extended period or who simply want reassurance and guidance in getting started.

Before hiring a personal trainer, be sure to first check the trainer's qualifications and experience—having a good body is *not* enough! For example, does the trainer have a college degree in the fitness field (e.g., exercise science, kinesiology, physical education) or certification by a nationally recognized organization such as the American College of Sports Medicine or the National Strength and Conditioning Association?

### Home Exercise Equipment

For most college students, home exercise equipment is not a pressing consumer issue. Yet, for those considering such a purchase, begin by asking these key questions:

- Will the equipment help me reach my goals?
- Will I really use the equipment regularly?

- Is the equipment well made?
- Do I have room for the equipment?
- Can I afford a quality piece of equipment?

Remember that health-related fitness can be developed without any special equipment. Moreover, high-quality equipment for cardiorespiratory training (e.g., treadmills, stationary bicycles, elliptical trainers) or resistance training is expensive. Refer to *Consumer Reports* and Website Resources at the end of the chapter for reviews of exercise equipment, and take your time in making a decision to buy.

## ✓ NEED TO KNOW

Developing an individualized exercise plan involves tailoring the physical activity recommendations to meet your goals, with due consideration of initial fitness level, rate of progression, and available campus resources (i.e., facilities, programs, personal trainers). Selected websites listed at the end of the chapter provide additional guidance, expertise, and detail on specific types of exercise training.

## ➤ Establishing the Exercise Habit

Article
3.4

Motivated to lose weight and get in shape, a friend joined a health club several months ago. I asked him how it was going and he said, "Paid my $250 bucks but haven't lost a pound. Guess you actually have to go and work out!" His comeback quip was a humorous way to describe an unsuccessful effort to begin an exercise program. And he is not alone. During the last two decades, the year-by-year growth in the number of health clubs mirrored the increase in obesity in the United States with a near perfect correlation (>0.9). Although the growth in health clubs is obviously not causing America's obesity epidemic, it is intriguing that the increase in fitness facilities appears to have no impact on helping Americans reach or maintain a healthy weight. This ironic finding shows that for many, many people facilities alone are not sufficient to make the transition from couch potato to regular exerciser.

When it comes to changing a health behavior, we often have good intentions but poor results. This is especially true regarding exercise because it's voluntary, time-consuming, and requires effort. Let's examine some of the factors that influence change in physical activity and consider strategies that may enable you to successfully implement and maintain your exercise program.

## Health & the Media A Sport for Every Body

Can you identify these sports legends nattily attired in white tuxedos? This photo by portrait photographer Annie Leibovitz is from a 1987 American Express print ad. Basketball star Wilt Chamberlain towers above champion jockey Willie Shoemaker. Chamberlain—who once scored 100 points in a game—was 7'1" and weighed over 300 lb., while Shoemaker—winner of over 9,000 races—was 4'11" and weighed less than 100 lb. The contrast in body size and dimensions is striking and wondrous. This image should remind us that there is no single ideal form when it comes to sport. Every person can find a sport that matches his or her physique. Clearly, body size does not have to interfere with the innate enjoyment of exercise and one's quest to become physically fit.

© Annie Liebowitz/Contact Press Images.

The large majority of college students report that they enjoy exercise and sports activities, and over 80 percent indicate that they know how to set up a fitness program (Sparling, 2002). Yet, according to the Centers for Disease Control and Prevention, only about one in three engage in recommended levels of exercise. Why does this large gap exist?

An assessment of self-motivation can be useful in determining likelihood of exercise adherence. Take the assessment in Connect Resources and calculate your "dropout" score. Do the results agree with your past exercise experiences?

Also, note that a BMI of 30 or higher is associated with discontinuing exercise. If your self-motivation score or your BMI indicates that you are likely to drop out, view this as a challenge to remain active. Remember these are simple predictors about groups of people and not necessarily true for every individual within a group. Consider your results in light of insights about modifying your approach to improve consistency with your exercise routine from this point forward.

Self
Assessment
3.2

Readiness to change as described in the stages of change model (see Chapter 1) provides another baseline measure that is useful in putting an exercise plan into action. Most students find themselves in one of the three middle stages—contemplation, preparation, or action. Ten to 15 percent are already in maintenance, and a smaller percentage are in pre-contemplation.

To determine your current stage, select the statement in the following list that best reflects your recent physical activity pattern. Note that *exercise* refers to jogging or similar vigorous activities lasting at least 20 minutes at a time, and *walk* refers to brisk walking or similar moderate activities lasting at least 30 minutes at a time.

1. I don't exercise or walk regularly and don't intend to start.
2. I don't exercise or walk regularly, but I have been thinking of starting.
3. I'm trying to begin exercising or walking.
4. I exercise or walk but not on a regular basis (vigorous less than three days per week or moderate exercise less than five days per week).
5. I have been exercising or walking regularly for the last few months (vigorous three or more days per week or moderate exercise five or more days per week).
6. I have been exercising or walking regularly for more than six months.

If you chose 1, you're in the pre-contemplation stage; 2 is contemplation; 3 is preparation; 4 is action; 5 is maintenance; and 6 is when exercise has become an established behavior. For example, perhaps you are stuck in the preparation stage; you play soccer or run a couple times per week but can't seem to get beyond that. Identifying your current stage can help you see what you need to do to reach the next stage—in this case, to add the third session per week.

There are many barriers to adopting or maintaining an exercise program. Americans often report lack of time and limited access to facilities and equipment. Yet, for most college students these are not significant barriers. In fact, just the opposite—a flexible schedule, fewer family responsibilities, and an accessible campus fitness center provide an opportunity. So let's focus on other variables that are more likely to influence exercise adherence. Each can be viewed as a negative or a positive. Consider the following list in relation to your current or planned exercise routine:

- Boring versus enjoyable
- Disapproval versus encouragement by close friends, family
- Injuries, physical limitations versus injury free, no limitations
- Haphazard schedule versus regular routine
- Inadequate instruction versus expert instruction
- Previous experience versus complete novice

The combination of negative factors often outweighs that of positive factors. Consequently, it's important to take stock of key variables and work at turning each negative into a positive whenever possible. Also, despite a sound plan and your best efforts, know that interruptions can occur at all stages. If you have to discontinue exercise for a short time, don't let that stop you from starting again. Relapses are a natural part of the long-term process of establishing a new behavior.

## STRATEGIES FOR INCREASING EXERCISE ADHERENCE

The aim is to leverage every feasible strategy to establish exercise as a permanent habit. If we don't, then exercise will frequently lose out to the many other interests that compete for our time. Consider the following practical strategies to tip the scale—the balance between the pros and cons—in the right direction.

- Make exercise fun.
- Schedule your exercise.
- Set specific long-term and short-term goals.
- Keep a log and include periodic testing to monitor your progress.
- Reward yourself for consistency and milestones.
- Minimize injuries by starting out with a moderate program.
- Try something new from time to time.
- Be patient but consistent—remember, the tortoise beat the hare.
- Exercise to feel better.

Apply as many of these suggestions as possible, especially if you are in the contemplation, preparation, or action stage. Another useful strategy is to exercise with a friend. Although some people prefer to exercise by themselves as a time break away from everything and everybody, most of us enjoy the camaraderie of exercising with others. Why should all social time with family and friends revolve around eating and other sedentary activities? Physical activity—whether simply a long walk or sports and fitness activities—provides an excellent opportunity to share time together.

The aim of applying behavioral strategies to our physical activity behavior is to make it difficult to *not* exercise. A sensible, individualized program of exercise can directly improve quality of life. Only by engaging in a long-term exercise routine can we experience this health enhancement. The natural consequence is that the value of exercise is elevated, and the behavior becomes more ingrained. Eventually, a behavior repeated over months and years becomes a lifelong habit. Follow your individualized plan, apply the most helpful strategies, and with time and commitment you will establish the exercise habit.

## THE NATIONAL PHYSICAL ACTIVITY PLAN

Establishing the exercise habit is not just an individual goal, it's a societal goal. The vision of the National Physical Activity Plan—a large-scale, private–public collaboration—is that one day, all Americans will be physically active and will live, work, and play in environments that facilitate regular physical activity.

Launched in 2010, the National Physical Activity Plan provides a comprehensive set of initiatives and policies to increase physical activity across America, from the large cities to the small towns. Recommendations are organized by key sectors including education, business, health care, recreation/sports, transportation/land use, and public health. For example, city planners are encouraged to prioritize and integrate infrastructure (sidewalks, bikeways) and green space for active commuting within larger transportation projects.

Look for and support the National Physical Activity Plan initiatives and programs in your communities. The ultimate aim is to create a national culture that supports physically active lifestyles, and in turn improve health, prevent disease, and enhance quality of life.

### ✓ NEED TO KNOW

Integrating a fitness program into your lifestyle is not just a matter of choice. Becoming a regular exerciser requires a plan and perseverance. By identifying barriers and incentives and applying strategies that fit your situation, you stack the odds in your favor. Exercise empowers living. And it's a metaphor for life. You get out of it what you put into it. Enjoy the good feelings and positive health that come with fitness.

**connect** Resources

 **ARTICLES**

3.1 "The Play of the Year." *Sports Illustrated*. The benefits from engaging in sports aren't just in the records set. This story captures a special moment that reflects the goodness in people and transcends a single event in a single game.

3.2 "Should Athletes Stretch Before Exercise?" Gatorade Sports Science Institute. Surprisingly little scientific evidence supports the idea that stretching before exercise prevents injuries and improves performance. The article reviews the science and summarizes unanswered questions.

3.3 "Body Image: Are You Imagining the Wrong Image?" *ACSM's Health and Fitness Journal*. An article written for personal trainers and group exercise leaders that examines how to help a client improve his or her body image.

3.4 *The Courage to Start: A Guide to Running for Your Life*. Fireside Press. The author shares how he went from an out-of-shape klutz to a marathon runner—albeit a slow one. He shows us that the fun of running is not limited to the swift.

 **SELF-ASSESSMENTS**

3.1 Assessment of Daily Energy Expenditure
3.2 Self-Motivation Assessment for Exercise

## Website Resources

### PHYSICAL ACTIVITY RECOMMENDATIONS

National Physical Activity Plan **www.physicalactivityplan.org**
Physical Activity Guidelines for Americans
   **www.health.gov/paguidelines**
Progression Models in Resistance Training (ACSM) **www.ms-se.com/ pt/pt-core/template-journal/msse/media/0309progression.pdf**

### EXAMPLES OF EXERCISE RESOURCES

Fitness Facilities and Equipment (ACSM brochures)
   **www.acsm.org/AM/Template.cfm?Section=Brochures2**
Fitness Tests from Topend Sports **www.topendsports.com/testing/tests**
Resistance Exercises from Exercise Prescription on the Net
   **www.exrx.net/Lists/Directory.html**

Stretching Exercises from the Mayo Clinic
**www.mayoclinic.com/health/stretching/SM00043&slide=1**

## STRATEGIES TO INCREASE PHYSICAL ACTIVITY AMONG THE SEDENTARY

America on the Move **www.americaonthemove.org**
Be Active Your Way (U.S. Department of Health and Human Services)
**www.health.gov/paguidelines/adultguide/default.aspx**
President's Challenge **www.presidentschallenge.org**
Smallstep (U.S. Department of Health and Human Services)
**www.smallstep.gov**

## GENERAL

American College of Sports Medicine (ACSM) **www.acsm.org**
Centers for Disease Control and Prevention (CDC): Physical Activity
**www.cdc.gov/physicalactivity**
Gatorade Sports Science Institute **www.gssiweb.com**
National Strength and Conditioning Association **www.nsca-lift.org**

## Knowing the Language

aerobic capacity, 106
aerobic metabolism, 101
anaerobic metabolism, 101
cardiorespiratory fitness, 110
exercise, 97
flexibility, 114
intensity, 97
moderate intensity, 110
muscular endurance, 114

muscular strength, 114
musculoskeletal fitness, 114
physical activity, 96
physical fitness, 97
rating of perceived
    exertion (RPE), 112
resistance training, 115
training effect, 106
vigorous intensity, 110

## Understanding the Content

1. Contrast and define the following terms: *physical activity, exercise,* and *physical fitness.*
2. What are the three primary components of health-related physical fitness? How are they related to our health?
3. What are the minimum levels of aerobic activity and resistance training recommended to improve and maintain health for adults?
4. An exercise session has three phases. Name and describe them and illustrate with an example.

## Exploring Ideas

1. Physical activity and health have a dose-response relationship. Explain this concept and comment on the advantages and limitations of prescribing exercise as a medicine.

2. Approximately how many calories should one burn in intentional physical activity (per day or week) to improve and maintain health? Where does this level of energy expenditure fall within the physical activity continuum? Explain.

3. How do the basic principles of exercise training—overload, specificity, and individual differences—relate to tailoring an individual exercise plan? Explain with examples.

4. Most of us enjoy exercise and know it's beneficial. Yet, only a small percentage of Americans exercise regularly. Explain this quandary and suggest strategies to enable folks to become more active.

## Selected References

ACSM. *ACSM's Guidelines for Exercise Testing and Prescription* (8th ed.). Baltimore: Lippincott Williams & Wilkins, 2009.

ACSM. Position stand: Progression models in resistance training for healthy adults. *Medicine and Science in Sports and Exercise* 41: 687–708, 2009.

ACSM. Position stand: Quantity and quality of exercise for developing and maintaining cardiorespiratory musculoskeletal, and neuromotor fitness in apparently healthy adults. *Medicine and Science in Sports and Exercise* 43: 1334–1359, 2011.

ACSM/ADA. Joint position statement: Nutrition and athletic performance. *Medicine and Science in Sports and Exercise* 41: 709–731, 2009.

ACSM/AHA. Joint position statement: Exercise and acute cardiovascular events: Placing the risks into perspective. *Medicine and Science in Sports and Exercise* 39: 886–897, 2007.

ACSM/AHA. Physical activity and public health: Updated recommendation for adults from the American College of Sports Medicine and the American Heart Association. *Circulation* 116: 1081–1093, 2007.

Ainsworth BE, Haskell WL, Herrmann SD, et al. 2011. Compendium of Physical Activities: a second update of codes and MET values. *Medicine and Science in Sports and Exercise* 43: 1575–1581, 2011. **https://sites.google.com/site/ compendiumofphysicalactivities/**

AHA. Resistance exercise in individuals with and without cardiovascular disease, 2007 update: A scientific statement from the American Heart Association. *Circulation* 116: 572–584, 2007.

American Heart Association (AHA). Scientific statement: Interventions to promote physical activity and dietary lifestyle changes for cardiovascular risk factor reduction in adults. *Circulation* 122: 406–441, 2010.

Anderson B. *Stretching.* Bolinas, CA: Shelter Publications, 2010.

Borg G. *Borg's Perceived Exertion and Pain Scales.* Champaign, IL: Human Kinetics, 1998.

Bouchard C, Blair SN, Haskell WL. *Physical Activity and Health.* Champaign, IL: Human Kinetics, 2007.

Brooks GA, Fahey TD, Baldwin KM. *Exercise Physiology. Human Bioenergetics and Its Applications* (4th ed.). New York: McGraw-Hill, 2005.

Brown DW, Brown DR, Heath GW, et al. Associations between physical activity dose and health-related quality of life. *Medicine and Science in Sports and Exercise* 36: 890–896, 2004.

Centers for Disease Control and Prevention. Prevalence of self-reported physically active adults—United States, 2007. *Morbidity and Mortality Weekly Report* 57 (48): 1297–1300, 2008.

Clarke HH (ed.). Basic understanding of physical fitness. *Physical Fitness Research Digest.* Washington, DC: Presidents Council on Physical Fitness and Sport, July 1971.

Fields KB, Burnworth CM, Delaney M. Should athletes stretch before exercise? *Sport Science Exchange* #104, Gatorade Sports Science Institute, June 2007.

Gladden, LB. Personal communication with PB Sparling on the lactic acid–muscle performance relationship. May 2011.

Herbert RD, de Noronha M. Stretching to prevent or reduce muscle soreness after exercise. *Cochrane Database of Systematic Reviews* 4: 2007. **www.cochrane.org/reviews/en/ab004577.html**

Hertzog C, Kramer AF, Wilson RS, et al. Fit body, fit mind? Your workout makes you smarter. *Scientific American,* July 2009.

Kolata G. Lactic acid is not muscles' foe, it's fuel. *New York Times,* May 16, 2006.

Leslie E, Sparling PB, Owen N. University campus settings and the promotion of physical activity in young adults: Lessons from research in Australia and the USA. *Health Education* 101: 116–125, 2001.

Marcus BH, Forsyth L. *Motivating People to Be Physically Active,* 2nd ed. Champaign, IL: Human Kinetics, 2009.

McArdle WD, Katch FI, Katch VL. *Exercise Physiology: Energy, Nutrition, and Human Performance* (7th ed). Baltimore: Lippincott Williams & Wilkins, 2009.

Owen N, Sparling PB, Healy GN, et al. Sedentary behavior: Emerging evidence for a new health risk. *Mayo Clinic Proceedings* 85 (12): 1138–1141, 2010.

Powell KE, Paluch AE, Blair SN. Physical activity for health: What kind? How much? How intense? On top of what? *Annual Review of Public Health* 32: 349–365, 2011.

Powers SK, Howley ET. *Exercise Physiology: Theory and Application to Fitness and Performance* (7th ed.). New York: McGraw-Hill, 2009.

Ratey JJ, *Spark: The Revolutionary New Science of Exercise and the Brain.* New York: Little, Brown, 2008.

Rowland TW. The biological basis of physical activity. *Medicine and Science in Sports and Exercise* 30 (3): 392–399, 1998.

Shiroma EJ, Lee IM. Physical activity and cardiovascular health: Lessons learned from epidemiological studies across age, gender, and race/ethnicity. *Circulation* 122: 743–752, 2010.

Sparling PB. College physical education: An unrecognized agent of change in combating inactivity-related diseases. *Perspectives in Biology and Medicine* 46: 579–587, 2003.

Sparling PB, Snow TK. Physical activity patterns in recent college alumni. *Research Quarterly for Exercise and Sport* 73: 200–205, 2002.

U.S. Department of Health and Human Services. *Physical Activity and Health: A Report of the Surgeon General.* **www.cdc.gov/nccdphp/sgr/sgr.htm**

U.S. Department of Health and Human Services. *Physical Activity Guidelines for Americans, 2008.* **www.health.gov/paguidelines**

Voss MW, Nagamatsu LS, Liu-Ambrose T, et al. Exercise, brain, and cognition across the lifespan. *Journal of Applied Physiology* (e-pub ahead of print), April 2011.

There are people who strictly deprive themselves of each and every eatable, drinkable, and smokeable pleasure which has in any way acquired a shady reputation. They pay this price for health. And health is all they get for it.

— MARK TWAIN

# Chapter 4

## AVOID DRUG ABUSE

In Chapter 4 we provide a foundation for an understanding of the principles regarding drug use, misuse, and abuse. The chapter begins with an overview of the scope of drugs in society today and then explains key language and terminology. The chapter moves on to explain various categories of drugs and ends with a discussion of drug testing and drug abuse treatment options. The goal is to provide a grounding in the concepts integral to understanding the risks associated with drugs.

# Chapter 4 | AVOID DRUG ABUSE

DRUG USE, misuse, and abuse not only alter an individual's body chemistry and perception of reality, but drugs have widespread economic and social costs. Murder, child abuse, drowning, rape, assault, suicide, spousal abuse, and traffic fatalities all too often have improper use of controlled substances as a contributing factor. And substance abuse among young adults is especially common. According to the National Center on Addiction and Substance Abuse at Columbia University (CASA, 2007), college students have higher rates of drug dependence than the general public, with almost 23 percent of them classified as substance dependent. Alcohol abuse is especially common and costly in this age group, with about 30 percent of students meeting the criteria of alcohol abusers. About one in four college students also reports missing classes, falling behind in courses, or doing poorly on schoolwork due to their alcohol consumption. Additionally, each year in the United States among 18- to 24-year-old college students, there are the following alcohol-related incidents (Hingston et al., 2002):

- 1,400 deaths from accidents
- 500,000 injuries
- Over 600,000 physical assaults
- Over 100,000 occasions when students were unsure if they consented to sex
- Over 70,000 sexual assaults
- 400,000 instances of unprotected sex

Instances of drug misuse and abuse among other groups in the United States are also quite high. The United States consumes a whopping 60 percent of the world's supply of illicit drugs. Over 77,000 two- and four-year college students completed the Core Institute's Alcohol and Other Drug Survey in 2008. (The Core Institute manages the nation's largest database on college students' drinking and drug use.) Some of the key findings included:

- 84.3 percent consumed alcohol in the past year (86.9 percent at least once in their life)
- 71.7 percent consumed alcohol in the past 30 days (21.8 percent three times a week or more)
- 65.4 percent of those students under 21 consumed alcohol in the previous 30 days
- 46.1 percent reported binge drinking in the previous two weeks
- 31.1 percent used marijuana in the past year (45.1 percent at least once in their life)
- 17.3 percent used marijuana in the previous 30 days
- 11.9 percent used an illegal drug other than marijuana in the past year

- 5.6 percent used an illegal drug other than marijuana in the previous 30 days

To complicate matters 37.1 percent reported being involved in public misconduct at least once during the past year, 22.3 percent drove a car while under the influence, 28.1 percent missed a class, 62 percent had a hangover, 20.8 percent performed poorly on a test or important project, 36 percent did something they later regretted, 34.7 percent had a memory loss, and 9.5 percent had been taken advantage of sexually.

It is clear that drug use behavior does not begin in college. What the Core Institute data is to college students, the Monitoring the Future (MTF) survey is to high school students. MTF has been used annually since 1975. MTF results show that alcohol continues to be the drug of choice among high school students (41.2 percent of 12th-graders reporting using alcohol in the past 30 days). The most recent data released show that among high school students, alcohol use has decreased and marijuana and illicit drug use has increased.

## ➤ Drug Administration and Terminology

Drug administration and absorption are key issues that influence safety in drug doses. For any drug to have an effect, it must enter the blood, where it can potentially affect any cell in the body within minutes. There are five types of drug administration:

1. **Oral administration** is when the drug, normally in pill or liquid form, is swallowed and absorbed through the stomach and intestines. This is the most common way to administer drugs, but it is also the least efficient because of differences in rates of digestion between people.
2. **Parenteral administration** is the injection of a drug with a needle. Types of injection include intravenous (into the vein), intramuscular (into muscle), and subcutaneous (under the skin). The effects of parenteral administration are quick since the drug is absorbed into the bloodstream almost immediately.
3. **Inhalation administration** is when a drug is inhaled into the lungs as a gas or snorted into the nose as a powder. Again, there is an almost immediate effect, as blood vessels in the lungs and nose aid quick absorption.

**Oral administration** is the taking of a drug by mouth in pill or liquid form. **Parenteral administration** refers to injected drugs. **Inhalation administration** is breathing in a drug as a gas or vapor.

A nicotine patch, used to help smokers deal with cigarette withdrawal symptoms while quitting, is an example of a drug that uses transdermal administration.

4. **Rectal administration** is the insertion of suppositories into the rectum. As the suppository melts, the drug enters the many blood vessels that support the lower digestive system.
5. **Transdermal administration** takes place when a drug is contained in an adhesive patch that is affixed to the skin. The drug diffuses into the bloodstream via the skin.

## DRUG TERMINOLOGY

It is important to understand some basic drug terminology. **Drug use** refers to taking a drug for its intended purpose, such as swallowing an antihistamine capsule to treat symptoms of allergy. **Drug misuse** is the taking of a drug for a reason other than that for which it was intended—for example, taking an antihistamine to feel a "buzz." **Drug abuse** is the chronic, long-term, and consistent taking of a drug for a reason other than the intended use. If someone regularly takes antihistamines to achieve a high, that is considered abuse. These terms can also be applied to alcohol consumption: having a drink to relax is

**Rectal administration** is used for drugs in suppositories that are absorbed through rectal membranes. **Transdermal administration** refers to drugs given through adhesive patches put on the skin.

**Drug use** is using a drug for its intended purpose. **Drug misuse** is using a drug for a reason other than the intended use. **Drug abuse** is chronically using a drug for a reason other than the intended use.

considered drug use, drinking enough to get drunk is misuse, and getting drunk regularly, by definition, is considered abuse.

There are also factors beyond the frequency of use that can influence the effect of drugs. **Set** is a powerful variable that refers to a person's expectations regarding how a drug will be experienced. If people believe a drug has a certain effect before they take it—for example, that it causes hallucinations—then there is a good chance that they will experience what they expect while under the influence of the drug. The placebo effect is an example of a set variable. In this case, people take a placebo (sugar pill) rather than a real drug but still display the effect of the drug they thought they took.

The **setting,** or environment in which a drug is taken, also influences the effect. For example, alcohol is a depressant and should induce drowsiness when consumed. If someone drinks in a quiet environment, then the most likely result is sleepiness. But if the same amount of alcohol is consumed in an environment where there is a festive atmosphere and social interaction, chances are that the user will feel stimulated.

Dependence is another important concept related to drug use. **Physical dependence** is when the body learns to require a certain drug in order to function normally. When the drug is removed from the dependent person's body, he or she will have withdrawal symptoms, or physical reactions that can range from a headache to seizures, depending upon the type of drug and the extent of dependence. Withdrawal symptoms eventually subside over time if the drug remains out of the person's system, but they will also subside if the person immediately consumes more of the drug. To become physically dependent, a person usually needs to take a drug for a long period of time. However, drugs such as methamphetamines are capable of reinforcing a craving very quickly, so physical dependence on them can develop in a short period of time.

**Psychological dependence** is an emotional attachment to a drug that develops in the person taking it. If the user does not take the drug at regular intervals, then withdrawal symptoms such as anxiety or irritability result. In this case, the drug fulfills an underlying emotional need in the user. Many drugs result in both physical and psychological

Article
4.1

---

Set is the mental expectation regarding the effects of a drug. The **setting** is the environment in which a drug is consumed, which can influence its effect.

**Physical dependence** occurs when the body requires a drug, and withdrawal symptoms occur if the drug is not administered and absorbed. **Psychological dependence** is an emotional attachment to a drug.

dependency. For example, a person who usually smokes a cigarette after dinner each night may feel irritable and anxious if he or she is prevented from doing so, even when wearing a patch that prevents nicotine levels from dropping to the point where physical cravings are triggered. Drugs that cause both physical and psychological dependence tend to be the hardest for users to stop taking.

Last, there are a few concepts relating to the amount of drugs taken. An **effective dose** of a drug is the amount of the substance it takes to achieve the therapeutic or desired effect. A **lethal dose** is the amount of drug that will overwhelm the body's systems and result in death.

Normally, effective doses and lethal doses are expressed with respect to the percentage of people experiencing the effect at that dose. For example, if we say the effective dose for 50 percent of people (ED50) for a certain drug is 10 mg, that means that 50 percent of people will experience the desired therapeutic effect after taking 10 mg. But it also indicates that the other 50 percent of people will need more or less of the drug to achieve the intended effect. The same concept holds true for the lethal dose—the amount of a drug that may cause one person to die may even be an effective dose for another person.

The effect of different doses varies depending on body mass and underlying health, as well as tolerance. **Tolerance** is a condition that occurs when a drug is taken repeatedly over time, and the effects at the original dose diminish. To get the same original effect, the user must take increasingly larger doses. A person who has established a tolerance has probably taken the drug over an extended period of time, and the body has adapted to certain levels of the drug in the blood.

### NEED TO KNOW

Drugs can be administered orally, transdermally, rectally, and parenterally, as well as via inhalation. Taking a drug for its intended purpose is called *drug use*. *Drug misuse* is the taking of a drug for a reason other than the one for which it was intended, and *drug abuse* is the chronic, long-term, and consistent taking of a drug for a reason other than the intended use. Set and setting are perhaps as important in determining a drug's effect as the actual physical action of the drug itself because mental expectations and environment influence one's behavior.

**Effective dose** is the dose necessary to produce a desired effect. **Lethal dose** is the dose capable of causing the user's death. **Tolerance** is a condition in which a person needs an increased amount of a drug to achieve the desired effect.

# CLASSIFYING DRUGS

In the United States, the Drug Enforcement Administration (DEA) is in charge of regulation and classification of controlled substances. It "schedules" drugs according to five categories (I, II, III, IV, and V) that describe effects, legal availability, and potential for abuse (Figure 4.1). The drug schedule weighs the negative risks and effects of various drugs against their possible beneficial uses and then assigns penalties and use parameters accordingly. Drugs with the fewest accepted medical uses and the most negative or dangerous effects are often banned outright and carry the highest penalties for improper trafficking and distribution. Drugs that are dangerous under most circumstances but still have therapeutic medical uses are made available only under strict controls and with high penalties for misuse or improper possession. At the other end of the scheduling spectrum are drugs deemed as having little chance for misuse, abuse, and dependency. These drugs are more readily available, and the penalties for abuse tend to be lower.

According to the DEA, Schedule I drugs are the ones with the highest potential for abuse and dependency and are not currently acceptable for medical use. Examples of Schedule I drugs include heroin, marijuana, and LSD. Possessing or taking these drugs is banned outright in the United States. The government also considers Schedule II drugs highly addictive, but these drugs have widely accepted medical uses. Examples of Schedule II substances include morphine, cocaine, and methamphetamines.

Schedule III drugs have common uses in medical treatment, and they include anabolic steroids, most barbiturates, and the antinausea drug Marinol. Like Schedules I and II drugs, these drugs are addictive, and they may cause moderate physical or high psychological dependence.

Finally, Schedules IV and V drugs have medical uses but low potential for abuse and the risk of only limited physical or psychological dependence. The anti-anxiety drug Xanax and the sedative

## ✓ NEED TO KNOW

There are two types of drug dependence: physical and psychological. Effective and lethal doses of drugs can vary according to many factors, including body mass and tolerance. Tolerance of a drug can develop over time, requiring larger doses to achieve the desired effect. The government regulates the selling and taking of all drugs and classifies use and penalties under a system of "schedules." Penalties regarding unlawful use and trafficking of controlled substances are severe and aggressively prosecuted by state and federal governments.

**FIGURE 4.1    DRUG SCHEDULES AND LEGAL PENALTIES**

A new class of substances was created by the Anti-Drug Abuse Act of 1986. Controlled substance analogues are substances that are not controlled substances but may be found in the illicit traffic. They are structurally or pharmacologically similar to Schedule I or II controlled substances and have

### SCHEDULE I

- The drug or other substance has a high potential for abuse.
- The drug or other substance has no currently accepted medical use in treatment in the United States.
- There is a lack of accepted safety for use of the drug or other substance under medical supervision.
- Examples of Schedule I substances include heroin, lysergic acid diethylamide (LSD), marijuana, and methaqualone.

### SCHEDULE II

- The drug or other substance has a high potential for abuse.
- The drug or other substance has a currently accepted medical use in treatment in the United States or a currently accepted medical use with severe restrictions.
- Abuse of the drug or other substance may lead to severe psychological or physical dependence.
- Examples of Schedule II substances include morphine, phencyclidine (PCP), cocaine, methadone, and methamphetamine.

### SCHEDULE III

- The drug or other substance has less potential for abuse than the drugs or other substances in Schedules I and II.
- The drug or other substance has a currently accepted medical use in treatment in the United States.

Source: Drug Enforcement Administration, *Drugs of Abuse,* 2005 **(www.justice.gov/dea/pubs/abuse/1-csa.htm#Analogues).**

*(Continued)*

**FIGURE 4.1    DRUG SCHEDULES AND LEGAL PENALTIES (*continued*)**

no legitimate medical use. A substance that meets the definition of a controlled substance analogue and is intended for human consumption is treated under the Controlled Substances Act (CSA) as if it were a controlled substance in Schedule I. [21 U.S.C. 802(32), 21 U.S.C. 813]

◈ Abuse of the drug or other substance may lead to moderate or low physical dependence or high psychological dependence.

◈ Anabolic steroids, codeine and hydrocodone with aspirin or Tylenol®, and some barbiturates are examples of Schedule III substances.

## SCHEDULE IV

◈ The drug or other substance has a low potential for abuse relative to the drugs or other substances in Schedule III.

◈ The drug or other substance has a currently accepted medical use in treatment in the United States.

◈ Abuse of the drug or other substance may lead to limited physical dependence or psychological dependence relative to the drugs or other substances in Schedule III.

◈ Examples of drugs included in Schedule IV are Darvon®, Talwin®, Equanil®, Valium®, and Xanax®.

## SCHEDULE V

◈ The drug or other substance has a low potential for abuse relative to the drugs or other substances in Schedule IV.

◈ The drug or other substance has a currently accepted medical use in treatment in the United States.

◈ Abuse of the drug or other substances may lead to limited physical dependence or psychological dependence relative to the drugs or other substances in Schedule IV.

◈ Cough medicines with codeine are examples of Schedule V drugs.

barbital are examples of Schedule IV drugs. Mixtures having small amounts of codeine, such as a prescription cough syrup, are examples of Schedule V drugs.

Now we will turn to the second way drugs are classified—by their effect—and discuss some of the major types of drugs that medical professionals and regulators are concerned with today.

## ➤ Depressants

Depressants are drugs that decrease or slow down body processes. These drugs include opioids, sedative-hypnotics, and the number one drug of use, misuse, and abuse in the United States—alcohol.

### ALCOHOL

The major forms of alcoholic beverages are beer, wine, and distilled liquor. Generally beer has a 3–6 percent concentration of ethyl alcohol, wines have 10–14 percent, and distilled liquors such as whisky and bourbon have 35–40 percent. The term *proof* is used to designate the amount of alcohol in a beverage. One-half of the proof number equals the percentage of alcohol. For example, a 90-proof beverage contains 45 percent alcohol. In terms of standard serving sizes, a can or bottle of beer is usually 12 oz., a glass of wine is 4 oz., and a mixed drink contains one shot (1–1.5 oz., depending on the proof of the liquor). It is interesting to note that although the concentration of alcohol in each type of beverage is different, the standard size adjusts total volume so that in the end, one serving of beer, wine, or liquor each contains 0.5 oz. of ethyl alcohol. This guide can be a handy measure for monitoring your alcohol consumption. Just be aware that certain mixed drinks such as margaritas and Long Island iced teas contain more than one shot of alcohol, so they count as more than one serving.

Because alcohol is a liquid, it quickly absorbs into the bloodstream, where it moves on to affect the nervous, circulatory, endocrine, and digestive systems. The higher the dose, the greater the effect. In the central nervous system, alcohol's depressant effect is most noticeable in the cerebrum, cerebellum, and medulla areas of the brain. Alcohol affects memory, awareness, and reasoning—collectively, these are what we call *judgment*—and it diminishes balance and coordination. Heart rate and breathing are also slowed. With smaller doses of alcohol, such as 1–2 drinks in an hour, the main effect felt is relaxation—hence alcohol's reputation as the social lubricant. With high doses, such as 7–8 drinks in one hour, the user would have impaired judgment, movement, and balance, and decreased heart rate and breathing. With extremely high doses of alcohol, say 15–20 drinks in one hour, loss of consciousness and death can result because in addition to the continuing depression of the cerebrum and cerebellum, the medulla is being depressed to a point where it no longer instructs the heart to beat or the lungs to breathe (Figure 4.2).

Alcohol causes blood vessels to expand, so the drinker feels very warm and sweats. The more alcohol in the system, the longer the vessels will dilate, and the longer one will feel uncomfortably warm or hot. Alcohol also increases urination, so it is easy to become dehydrated while drinking too much alcohol.

The digestive system is affected in two ways. First, alcohol is a gastric irritant that causes food to move through the system quicker, so there is poor absorption of nutrients, and constipation, diarrhea, or both can result. People who have digestive problems such as ulcers or gastric reflux should abstain or significantly limit drinking and never drink on an empty stomach. Second, alcohol also affects the liver, which is chiefly responsible for breaking down alcohol in the body in a process called *oxidation,* in which alcohol, as it cycles through the liver, is eventually broken down into water and carbon dioxide. The liver oxidizes the amount of alcohol in a standard size drink (half an ounce) in about one hour. Oxidizing alcohol is hard on the liver, and prolonged excessive drinking will damage it. But most experts agree that 1–2 drinks per day won't cause a negative impact on the liver of an otherwise healthy person.

### Blood Alcohol Level

The effects of alcohol are directly related to the amount of alcohol in the blood, referred to as *blood alcohol level* (BAL) or *blood alcohol concentration* (BAC). Figure 4.2 shows the effects of alcohol at selected blood alcohol concentrations.

The higher the level of alcohol in the blood, the greater the effect: from relaxation (.01) to death (.40). Four variables influence blood alcohol concentration: (1) the amount of alcohol consumed in a given time period, (2) the weight of the drinker, (3) the gender of the drinker, and (4) the amount of food in the stomach. Figures 4.3 and 4.4 bring together the first three variables. Here we can see that blood alcohol levels are influenced by the amount consumed as well as the weight and gender of the drinker. When they consume the same number of drinks, a person who weighs less will have a higher BAL than a person who weighs more. In addition, if a man and a woman consume the same number of drinks and they also weigh the same, the woman will still have a higher blood alcohol level than the man. This is because women normally have less of a digestive enzyme called *gastric acetaldehyde,* and as a result they digest less alcohol than men. Another reason is that women have a lower percentage of body water

## FIGURE 4.2  BLOOD ALCOHOL CONCENTRATIONS AND BEHAVIORAL EFFECTS

### 0.01 – 0.03 BAC

- slight euphoria, loss of shyness
- depressant effects are not apparent
- mildly relaxed and maybe a little light-headed

### 0.04 – 0.06 BAC

- euphoria
- feeling of well-being, relaxation, lower inhibitions, sensation of warmth
- minor impairment of reasoning and memory
- lowering of caution
- exaggerated behavior
- intensified emotions

### 0.07 – 0.09 BAC

- 0.08 is legally impaired, and it is illegal to drive at this level
- slight impairment of balance, speech, vision, reaction time, and hearing
- euphoria
- reduced judgment and self-control
- impaired caution, reason, and memory
- belief that they are functioning better than they really are

### 0.10 – 0.125 BAC

- significant impairment of motor coordination
- loss of good judgment
- speech may be slurred
- impaired balance, vision, reaction time, and hearing
- euphoria

### 0.13 – 0.15 BAC

- gross motor impairment and lack of physical control
- blurred vision
- major loss of balance
- severely impaired judgment and perception

Source: Greater Dallas Council on Alcohol and Drug Abuse.

(Continued)

◆ reduced euphoria
◆ dysphoria (anxiety, restlessness) beginning to appear

### 0.16 – 0.19 BAC

◆ dysphoria predominant
◆ nausea may appear
◆ drinker has the appearance of "sloppy drunk"

### 0.20 BAC

◆ feeling dazed, confused, and otherwise disoriented
◆ may need help to stand or walk
◆ if injured, may not feel the pain
◆ nausea and vomiting
◆ impaired gag reflex—drinker can choke if they vomit
◆ blackouts—drinker may not remember what has happened

### 0.25 BAC

◆ severely impaired mental, physical, and sensory functions
◆ increased risk of asphyxiation from choking on vomit
◆ increased risk of serious injury by falls or other unintentional accidents

### 0.30 BAC

◆ stupor
◆ little comprehension of where they are
◆ may pass out suddenly and be difficult to awaken

### 0.35 BAC

◆ level of surgical anesthesia
◆ coma is possible

### 0.40+ BAC

◆ onset of coma
◆ possible death due to respiratory arrest

## FIGURE 4.3 BLOOD ALCOHOL CONCENTRATION ESTIMATE FOR MEN

| Drinks[a] | Body Weight in Pounds | | | | | | | | Influence[b] |
|---|---|---|---|---|---|---|---|---|---|
| | 100 | 120 | 140 | 160 | 180 | 200 | 220 | 240 | |
| 1 | .04 | .03 | .02 | .02 | .02 | .02 | .02 | .02 | Possibly Impaired |
| 2 | .08 | .06 | .05 | .05 | .04 | .04 | .03 | .03 | |
| 3 | .11 | .09 | .08 | .07 | .06 | .06 | .05 | .05 | Impaired |
| 4 | .15 | .12 | .11 | .09 | .08 | .08 | .07 | .06 | |
| 5 | .19 | .16 | .13 | .12 | .11 | .09 | .09 | .09 | DUI |
| 6 | .23 | .19 | .16 | .14 | .13 | .11 | .10 | .09 | |
| 7 | .26 | .22 | .19 | .16 | .15 | .13 | .12 | .11 | |
| 8 | .30 | .25 | .21 | .19 | .17 | .15 | .14 | .13 | |
| 9 | .34 | .28 | .24 | .21 | .19 | .17 | .15 | .14 | |
| 10 | .38 | .31 | .27 | .23 | .21 | .19 | .17 | .16 | |

[a]One drink is 1.25 oz. of 80-proof liquor, 12 oz. of beer, or 5 oz. of wine.
[b]Subtract .01 for each hour of drinking.

Source: Greater Dallas Council on Alcohol and Drug Abuse.

## FIGURE 4.4 BLOOD ALCOHOL CONCENTRATION ESTIMATE FOR WOMEN

| Drinks[a] | Body Weight in Pounds | | | | | | | | Influence[b] |
|---|---|---|---|---|---|---|---|---|---|
| | 90 | 100 | 120 | 140 | 160 | 180 | 200 | 220 | |
| 1 | .05 | .05 | .04 | .03 | .03 | .03 | .02 | .02 | Possibly Impaired |
| 2 | .10 | .09 | .08 | .07 | .06 | .05 | .05 | .04 | |
| 3 | .15 | .14 | .11 | .10 | .09 | .08 | .07 | .06 | Impaired |
| 4 | .20 | .18 | .15 | .13 | .11 | .10 | .09 | .08 | |
| 5 | .25 | .23 | .19 | .16 | .14 | .13 | .11 | .10 | DUI |
| 6 | .30 | .27 | .23 | .19 | .17 | .15 | .14 | .12 | |
| 7 | .35 | .27 | .23 | .19 | .17 | .15 | .14 | .12 | |
| 8 | .40 | .36 | .30 | .26 | .23 | .20 | .18 | .17 | |
| 9 | .45 | .41 | .34 | .29 | .26 | .23 | .20 | .19 | |
| 10 | .51 | .45 | .38 | .32 | .28 | .25 | .23 | .21 | |

[a]One drink is 1.25 oz. of 80-proof liquor, 12 oz. of beer, or 5 oz. of wine.
[b]Subtract .01 for each hour of drinking.

Source: Greater Dallas Council on Alcohol and Drug Abuse.

than men. Because of enzyme and body water differences, women absorb more alcohol than men.

As a general rule, an average-size man's BAL will rise approximately .025 per drink per hour. An average-size woman's BAL will rise approximately .030 per drink per hour. The liver oxidizes one drink each hour, so BAL will drop .025 per drink per hour for both genders. This is a general approximation of oxidation rates, including the fact

## Health & the Media *Alcohol Advertising and Behavior*

It has been reported that by age 18 the typical American youth has seen or heard over 100,000 alcohol advertisements on television, in print, and on the radio. Billions of dollars are spent each year on alcohol advertising. In a 2006 *Archives of Pediatrics and Adolescent Medicine* study, researchers reported that underage youth viewed, on average, 23 alcohol ads per month. The study also found that such advertising contributes to an increase in drinking among underage youth, and that for each additional dollar per capita spent on alcohol advertising in a local advertising market, young people drank 3 percent more. Does alcohol advertising work? The short answer is yes.

that women tend to process alcohol in their system more slowly than men. A more precise, individualized measure can be obtained with a breathalyzer, a machine that analyzes alcohol content when a person exhales into it. The concentration of alcohol in the breath is an excellent indication of the concentration of alcohol in the blood, and it is legally defensible, as in the case of a Driving Under the Influence (DUI) or Driving While Intoxicated (DWI) legal charge.

### Alcohol-related Problems

Alcohol is a caustic substance that over time can lead to debilitating conditions such as deterioration of the heart muscle and cirrhosis of the liver. But perhaps the most common alcohol-related problem is the headache, nausea, dehydration, and light-headedness collectively referred to as a *hangover.* A number of factors come into play with a hangover. The expansion of cerebral blood vessels can cause the headache. Furthermore, the first step in the liver's breaking down of alcohol produces a toxic chemical that, in abundance, can also cause nausea and headache. Finally, the dehydration that comes with excessive drinking can also cause symptoms such as headache, nausea, and light-headedness.

Hangovers are for the most part self-limiting—their symptoms pass after the body oxidizes the alcohol, and systems have cycled back to normal. There is no cure for a hangover except time. Hangover symptoms can be treated, but one must be careful, because certain common over-the-counter medications, such as acetaminophen (Tylenol) and ibuprofen (Advil), can interact with alcohol and damage the liver. People who take too much pain reliever medication after a hangover can experience profound liver problems, including liver failure.

Another alcohol-related problem is drinking and driving. Driving Under the Influence (**DUI**) or Driving While Intoxicated (**DWI**) are the most common legal terms describing one who is driving after having consumed alcohol. "Under the influence" and "while intoxicated" are defined as driving while having a .08 BAL or above. If you recall (see Figures 4.3 and 4.4), it doesn't take a huge amount of alcohol to reach a .08 level, and people with a high tolerance may not even appear to have been drinking but have a .08 BAL. Tolerance is individual and subjective, but the laws governing drinking are fairly universal and black and white. A .08 BAL can impair judgment and driving reflexes in most people, so it is now the main criteria for a DUI or DWI conviction in almost all states.

In most states conviction of a DUI or DWI is a Class I misdemeanor, which means that the person will have a criminal record forever. Conviction can also mean that the person will not be eligible for certain occupations, especially those that require a security clearance, since these organizations will not hire someone with a criminal record. Also, car insurance premiums can increase 200–400 percent (assuming that the driving record other than the DUI or DWI is good) for 2–3 years. Finally, legal representation, fines, and court costs can total thousands of dollars. Thomas von Hermet of the Thomas Jefferson Area (Virginia) Community Criminal Justice Board estimated that the financial costs of a DUI could be as high as $20,000. A DUI/DWI is a serious offense with lifelong implications.

Article 4.2

DUI stands for "driving under the influence." DWI stands for "driving while intoxicated."

Another alcohol-related problem is drinking while under the legal age of consumption, which is 21 years old in all 50 states. The fake ID is a popular way for underage people to misrepresent their age and be allowed to purchase alcohol and attend nightclubs or parties where alcohol is served. Possessing a fake ID is legally considered fraud, and depending on the context of use, it can result in a Class I misdemeanor conviction and criminal record for life. To compound matters, a fake ID Class I misdemeanor can be considered a "crime of moral turpitude," which means that the person convicted is a dishonest person who committed fraud. Many employers, organizations, and segments of the general population view this as a character flaw with far-reaching implications. So the legal and societal penalties related to fake ID convictions can be surprisingly harsh.

### High-risk Drinking

In recent years much attention has been directed at what is termed **binge drinking,** which is defined as four or more drinks for a female and five or more drinks for a male in one setting. There is no time limit inherent in binge drinking, although some researchers attach a two-hour period for consumption of these drinks. Binge drinking is a concern on college campuses, but what is of more concern is consumption of even higher amounts of alcohol in a short period of time, which is referred to as "high-risk drinking."

Much high-risk drinking is done in a game context, such as the "power hour"—21 shots in an hour during a 21st birthday celebration. As blood alcohol levels rise, judgment gets more impaired, personal safety can be compromised, and blood alcohol content can rise to lethal levels. High-risk drinking is certainly a problem; it can range being episodic (for festive events) to something done by an inexperienced underage drinker with limited access to alcohol.

Self
Assessment
4.1

Problem drinking, in a clinical context, usually refers to alcohol abuse and alcohol dependence. *Alcoholism,* although a commonly used term, is not typically used in clinical contexts. **Alcohol abuse** is defined as "continued drinking despite recurring social, interpersonal, and legal problems." **Alcohol dependence** is predicated on the presence or absence of tolerance and withdrawal symptoms. How would one know if he or she is a normal drinker or a problem drinker heading toward alcohol abuse, alcohol dependence, or both?

> **Binge drinking** is having four drinks in one occasion for a woman and five drinks for a man.
>
> **Alcohol abuse** is continued drinking despite recurring social, interpersonal, and legal problems. **Alcohol dependence** is predicated on the presence of withdrawal symptoms.

## Help for Problem Drinkers

A typical model for assisting a problem drinker involves three steps: detoxification, counseling, and support groups. Detoxification is a medically supervised effort that removes the alcohol from a person's system and helps reduce the related cravings. It is important that the detoxification be medically supervised because of potentially serious withdrawal symptoms, including tremors, rapid heart beat, confusion, nausea, anxiety, and convulsions. Medications can be used to help limit the severity of symptoms.

Once detoxification is over, people should undergo counseling to deal with the issues that drove them to use alcohol in the first place. Counseling can be individual, family, or group. The counseling effort also focuses on coping skills other than the use of alcohol. In addition, emotional support is also important to help people stay clean and sober. Without this, it is more likely that the user will relapse. Support groups are made up of people who are also trying to stay clean and sober. In every community there are numerous support groups that meet daily, and in these groups people hold one another accountable in the effort to stay clean and sober. Perhaps the best example of a support group is Alcoholics Anonymous (AA).

Article
4.3

> ✓ **NEED TO KNOW**
>
> The amount of alcohol in a standard-size drink is the same in a glass of wine, a shot of liquor, or a glass of beer. Nothing can be done to speed up the oxidation of alcohol by the liver. Women digest alcohol slower than men, so even if they weigh the same, women will have a higher blood alcohol level than men after the same number of drinks. It takes women longer than men to rid their body of alcohol due to differences in levels of certain digestive enzymes between men and women. Taking too many pain relievers (such as Tylenol or Advil) after drinking heavily can lead to liver damage. Excessive alcohol consumption is a high-risk behavior that can have disastrous consequences. DUI and fake ID convictions are economically costly and have lifelong implications in regard to security clearances for certain jobs. Finally, help for problem drinkers usually involves three steps: medically supervised detoxification, counseling, and support groups.

## OPIOIDS

Another class of depressant drugs is called *opioids*. This name refers to natural products of crude opium, semi-synthetic products containing some natural crude opium, and synthetic opiates, which react in the body in the same manner as opiates but are made without natural products.

Collectively, opioids are a very important class of drugs due to their effectiveness at treating pain. But they also have a high potential for dependence and abuse, and their use is highly regulated. The range of effects includes euphoria, including a dreamlike state of significant relaxation; drowsiness; respiratory depression; nausea; and constipation.

Crude opium is a product of a poppy that grows wild in Asia and other parts of the world. For centuries opium was used to treat pain, diarrhea, and coughs. It was also used recreationally to induce euphoria or a sense of well-being. In the early 1800s, morphine, the active ingredient in crude opium, was isolated, and later that century heroin, a semi-synthetic drug, was also created. Codeine, another active ingredient in crude opium, was isolated in the 1930s. All of these opiates were used medically for decades. There were originally no laws regarding their sale or use, and it was not until the Civil War, when thousands became morphine addicts after receiving drugs for treatment of war injuries, that the downsides to opiates became widely known in the United States. In the early 1900s the government passed the first legislation to control distribution and use of opium, morphine, heroin, and other drugs referred to as *narcotics*.

Heroin is a Schedule I narcotic, meaning it is illegal and considered to have no medical use. It continues to be widely abused, causing many personal and societal problems. Most heroin addicts do not live long because the habit is expensive, and they often have to turn to crime to pay for drugs. Further, heroin addicts often share needles and eventually expose themselves to bloodborne infections such as HIV and hepatitis.

Many other semisynthetic opioids have medical uses, so they are listed as Schedule II narcotics. These include Demerol, Dilaudid, and Darvon. In recent years two other opioids, methadone and Oxycontin, have received much publicity.

Methadone is primarily used in heroin rehabilitation. So-called methadone maintenance is designed to determine the stabilization dose of methadone necessary to eliminate the craving for heroin. Once that dosage is reached, the heroin addict can undergo both personal and vocational counseling in order to reintegrate back into society as a productive member. Methadone maintenance is controversial, mostly because one drug (methadone) is substituted for another (heroin). There is conflict between the view that drug addiction is a poor life choice (a "disorder of the will") and that it is a disease. However, the two views do intersect. At first, the person is making a choice to modify his or her mood (an act of the will), but after time, if tolerance, physical dependence, and psychological dependence are established, the user has little control, and stopping the drug will lead to withdrawal symptoms requiring medical intervention. There is no easy answer to this conflict, as both views of addiction have merit.

A more recent controversy involves the drug **Oxycontin,** a time-released opioid normally prescribed to people in significant pain, such as cancer patients. It is a powerful opioid, and like many powerful drugs, has become a popular illicit drug because of the euphoria it can produce. Patients taking Oxycontin must be monitored closely because of the potential problems of drug interactions, tolerance, and dependence and the possibility of dosages reaching a lethal level. Recreational abuse of Oxycontin has particularly been a problem in Appalachia (southwest Virginia and eastern Kentucky), where it is has been referred to as *hillbilly heroin.* Other opioids that are prescribed and popularly abused include Vicodin, Lortab, and Tussionex.

Vicodin and Lortab are prescription drugs used to treat pain and coughs. The generic name is hydrocodone, and it is an effective pain reliever. Because the drug produces a euphoric effect, it is an attractive recreational drug. Side effects of Vicodin and Lortab include upset stomach, nausea, and dizziness.

Dextromethorphan or DMX is an over-the-counter cough suppressant drug. DMX works on the cough center in the brain, and when the recommended dose is taken, it produces little or no euphoria. When taken in higher than recommended doses, a heightened euphoria results. Since it is readily available and a "cheap high," DMX is abused. Long-term effects of abuse are similar to most other depressants: sensory changes, agitation, paranoia, and in some cases hallucinations.

## SEDATIVE-HYPNOTICS

**Sedative-hypnotic** drugs are a category of depressants normally used to induce sedation and sleep (hypnotic). These drugs are medically prescribed and include barbiturates, which are classified as ultra-short, intermediate, and long-acting. Ultra-short barbiturates such as thiopental are used to induce anesthesia; intermediate ones such as Seconal are used to induce sleep; and long-acting ones such as butalbital and phenobarbital are used to treat headaches and prevent seizures, respectively. Of the three types of barbiturates, the intermediate drugs have been the most problematic, since at one point they were popularly used to treat insomnia. Seconal dependence can occur fairly rapidly, and Seconal combined with alcohol can be toxic and result in death. Further, withdrawal from barbiturates can cause serious problems and even be life-threatening.

**Oxycontin** is a time-released opioid similar to morphine and extremely potent.

**Sedative-hypnotic** drugs are capable of producing sedation and sleep.

Nonbarbiturate sedative hypnotics also exist. Meprobamate (Miltown) has the same effect as an intermediate barbiturate, but the risk of dependence is not as serious. With the introduction of minor tranquilizers in the 1960s, there has been less need for barbiturates and non-barbiturates as sedative-hypnotics.

## INHALANTS

Inhalants are solvents and solutions that are used in hair spray, gasoline, paint, glue, and other commonly used items. *Huffing* is the term used to describe use of inhalants. The effects from huffing include euphoria, light-headedness, and lack of coordination. The chemicals in the solvents can interfere with the amount of oxygen reaching the brain and other tissues, resulting in a condition called *hypoxia,* a dangerously low level of oxygen. Inhalant use can introduce toxic levels of the solvent into the system, and brain damage can result.

Nitrous oxide, or "laughing gas," is a popular inhalant. Nitrous oxide is used medically as an anesthetic. Inhaling nitrous oxide results in relaxation and a loosening of inhibitions often resulting in uncontrolled laughter. The amount of nitrous oxide administered for medical purposes must be closely monitored. Recreational users find items such as $CO_2$ cartridges containing nitrous oxide used in baking and inhale the nitrous oxide right from the cartridge. This is extremely dangerous because of the freezing temperature in the cartridge. Frostbite of the nose and lung damage from freezing can result.

---

✔ **NEED TO KNOW**

Other depressants include opioids, sedative-hypnotics, and inhalants. Drugs in the opioid category include morphine, codeine, Vicodin, and Oxycontin. These drugs are powerful and have a high potential for abuse. Sedative-hypnotics is a broad category of depressants with a wide variety of uses ranging from anesthesia to prevention of seizures. Inhalants also have medical uses, but like other depressants, they can be abused, especially by adolescents who have easy access to glue, household chemicals, and other common substances that when inhaled can deprive the brain of oxygen and induce a euphoric effect.

---

## ➤ Stimulants

Stimulants are a large category that includes powerful drugs such as cocaine, crack, and amphetamines and milder cerebral stimulants such as nicotine and caffeine. *Speed* is a term used to describe stimulants, particularly amphetamines. All stimulants have the capability to increase functional activity of the nervous system. This can have a significant effect on thought processes to the point where thinking becomes so scrambled that it is difficult for people to focus their thoughts. Sometimes this can serve as a catalyst for creativity, such as in stand-up comedy, but it can also lead to a split from reality involving the personality called a *psychosis*.

## COCAINE AND CRACK

Cocaine is a drug found in the leaves of the coca bush, which grows wild in parts of Bolivia, Colombia, and Peru. Ancient civilizations such as the Incas integrated cocaine into their culture through chewing coca leaves for the stimulant effect. Cocaine also has local anesthetic properties. What the common pick-me-ups caffeine and nicotine are to current society, cocaine was to the ancient Incas.

Cocaine has an interesting history that includes Sigmund Freud, who at first espoused the use of cocaine to treat morphine addiction, then renounced it as a scourge when he became addicted himself. The fictional detective Sherlock Holmes is known for his "7 percent solution," the special formula he used in preparing his cocaine. Inventor John Pemberton used cocaine in his original formula for Coca-Cola. In low doses cocaine can increase heart rate and blood pressure, decrease fatigue, and increase mental alertness and sociability. But in high doses it can cause dizziness, blurred vision, and tremors, as well as repress heart enzymes and cause convulsions and death. The cocaine experience is short-lived. After snorting it, users experience a euphoric high for 15–30 minutes. After that they "crash," becoming light-headed and nauseated. The only ways for users to resolve the experience are to wait out the crash or to snort more cocaine to alleviate it. Snorting more cocaine will reinforce the craving—this is why cocaine is considered so addictive.

Recreational use of cocaine ebbs and flows in popularity. When it was extremely popular to abuse in the 1980s, a new, purer form called *crack* was created. Crack is about 10 times more powerful than regular cocaine, in terms of both its euphoric high and the painful crash afterward. As such, it is even more addictive than cocaine.

Cocaine, a stimulant drug derived from the leaves of the coca plant, has been used by humans for at least a thousand years.

Interestingly, cocaine is not a Schedule I drug. The DEA placed it in Schedule II because it is a powerful local anesthetic used to numb the eyes or nasal passages for surgery.

## AMPHETAMINES

Amphetamines are powerful prescription stimulants used to treat narcolepsy, low blood pressure, and attention-deficit/hyperactivity disorder (ADHD). Amphetamines are similar to cocaine in experience, but their effect lasts much longer, up to 10 or more hours. The crash from amphetamine use is also more prolonged. Because amphetamines have such a long duration, they are popularly taken to help people stay awake for long periods of time. Some students use them to stay awake all night to cram for an exam, and some truck drivers use them to drive for longer periods of time. Unfortunately, the effects of the amphetamines can be scary and even life-threatening. Extreme restlessness, anxiety, confusion, paranoia, high blood pressure, convulsions, and cardiac arrest can result from excessive doses or extended use.

In a medically supervised context, amphetamines improve quality of life. Attention-deficit/hyperactivity disorder (ADHD) is a case in point. The stimulant Ritalin is prescribed for children, but adults who are diagnosed with ADHD can also be prescribed the drug. A person with ADHD has a short attention span, has difficulty concentrating, and is easily distracted. Learning is compromised. How Ritalin works is not entirely clear, and it does seem like a paradox that a hyperactive person would find relief from a prescription stimulant, but true ADHD patients receive tremendous benefit from Ritalin. They can take the drug without experiencing euphoria. People who take Ritalin who do not have ADHD will experience an amphetamine high, though. For that reason, Ritalin has become a drug of abuse in non-ADHD populations.

Article 4.4

In recent years a form of amphetamine called *methamphetamine* has become a serious problem, especially in communities where the rave culture is prominent. Methamphetamine use has increased in popularity. There was a 50 percent increase in emergency room visits between 1995 and 2002 due to methamphetamine-related emergencies. In its oral form, the drug is often called *speed* or *meth,* and in smokeable form, *ice* or *crystal.* Both forms are normally made in illegal laboratories from ingredients in common over-the-counter drug products such as appetite suppressants, decongestants, and allergy products. There were over 10,000 methamphetamine lab incidents in 2010. Methamphetamines generally have a much more intense effect on the nervous system than prescription amphetamines, and the addictive potential is more profound.

Methamphetamines are extremely dangerous, and increased use can result in delusions and hallucinations, as well as heart problems. Smoking methamphetamine allows the administration and absorption to be quicker than taking it in tablet form, and the effects are more intense because the drug is getting to the brain quicker. The long-term effects of methamphetamine use include aggressive and violent behavior, weight loss, and psychosis. In addition to these effects, people who smoke methamphetamines can develop "meth mouth" when the teeth become destroyed and look like they are rotting away.

## NICOTINE

Nicotine is another naturally occurring stimulant. Found in tobacco, nicotine is highly addictive. Once absorbed into the blood, it exerts a cerebral stimulant effect that is both pleasurable and short-lived. The smoker must inhale again and again to obtain more of the pleasurable feeling, and over time that produces cravings and addiction. Unfortunately, in addition to the nicotine, a smoker inhales tars and carbon monoxide, which starve tissue of oxygen. This is why smokers are at higher risk of both cancer and heart disease. The health hazards associated with any form of tobacco use are documented and well known. And for the approximately 29 percent of the population who smokes, tobacco use is an expensive habit. A pack-a-day cigarette habit will cost most smokers well over $1,000 each year.

In addition to the health hazards associated with smoking, those who are exposed to cigarette smoke are also at risk for health problems. Secondhand smoke (the smoke that people around a smoker inhale) contains carbon monoxide and carcinogens and can cause heart disease or even cancer in nonsmokers who spend large amounts of time in the company of smokers.

Getting dependent on nicotine is easy. Quitting tobacco use is hard. The withdrawal symptoms of nicotine include headache, nervousness, fatigue, poor concentration, and sleep disturbances. But users who have a desire to quit have numerous options. First, there is the classic "cold turkey" withdrawal, whereby the user quits tobacco, overcomes the withdrawal symptoms, and stays tobacco free. Second, there are gums that contain nicotine. They provide enough of the drug to reduce the craving for tobacco gradually. Third, there are nicotine patches, which release the drug into the blood at a steady rate through the skin and reduce the craving for nicotine. Finally, there are prescription medications, such as the antidepressant Zyban, which reduce the craving for nicotine and can be effective in helping people quit.

In the continuing effort to educate people of the health effects of cigarette smoking, the FDA sponsored the development of new cigarette warning labels that are very graphic and depict the health effects of smoking. Cigarette companies are required to place the labels on cigarette

## TABLE 4.1 OVER CAFFEINATED: EXAMINING CAFFEINE AND ITS AFFECTS

| | 8 OZ | 12 OZ CAN | PER/OZ |
|---|---|---|---|
| **Caffeine in Coke Products** | | | |
| Coke Classic | 23 mg | 34.5 mg | 2.875 mg |
| Coke Zero | 23 mg | 34.5 mg | 2.875 mg |
| Vanilla Coke | 23 mg | 34.5 mg | 2.875 mg |
| Diet Coke | 31 mg | 46.5 mg | 3.875 mg |
| Diet Vanilla Coke | 31 mg | 46.5 mg | 3.875 mg |
| Barq's Root Beer | 15 mg | 22.5 mg | 1.875 mg |
| Tab | 31 mg | 46.5 mg | 3.875 mg |
| Pibb Xtra | 27 mg | 40.5 mg | 3.375 mg |
| **Caffeine in Pepsi Products** | | | |
| Pepsi | 25 mg | 37.5 mg | 3.125 mg |
| Diet Pepsi | 24 mg | 36 mg | 3 mg |
| Pepsi One | 36 mg | 54 mg | 4.5 mg |
| **Caffeine in Mountain Dew** | | | |
| Mountain Dew | 36 mg | 54 mg | 4.5 mg |
| Diet Mountain Dew | 36 mg | 54 mg | 4.5 mg |
| Code Red | 36 mg | 54 mg | 4.5 mg |
| **Misc. Sodas** | | | |
| Surge | 53 mg | 70.5 mg | 6.625 mg |
| Jolt | 47 mg | 70.5 mg | 5.875 mg |
| Mello Yellow | 35 mg | 52.5 mg | 4.375 mg |
| Sunkist | 27 mg | 40.5 mg | 3.375 mg |
| Dr. Pepper | 27 mg | 40.5 mg | 3.375 mg |

| | CAFFEINE IN ENERGY DRINKS | | |
|---|---|---|---|
| | 8 OZ | 12 OZ CAN | PER/OZ |
| **Caffeine in Energy Drinks** | | | |
| MDX | 47 mg | 70.5 mg | 5.875 mg |
| Diet MDX | 50 mg | 75 mg | 6.25 mg |
| Amp Energy Drink | 71 mg | 106.5 mg | 8.875 mg |

packs, cartons, and advertisements. Only time will tell how effective this new approach will be in reducing cigarette smoking.

## CAFFEINE

Caffeine is the most common cerebral stimulant. It is found in coffee, chocolate, tea, soft drinks, and many over-the-counter drugs from analgesics to weight-loss products. The highest amounts of caffeine are found

| TABLE 4.1 | OVER CAFFEINATED: EXAMINING CAFFEINE AND ITS AFFECTS *(continued)* | | |

| | 8 OZ | 12 OZ CAN | PER/OZ |
| --- | --- | --- | --- |
| No Fear | 83 mg | 124.5 mg | 10.375 mg |
| SoBe Adrenaline Rush | 75 mg | 112.5 mg | 9.375 mg |
| Adrenaline Sport | 35 mg | 52.5 mg | 4.375 mg |
| Red Bull | 80 mg | — | 10 mg |
| Atomic Rush | 100 mg (7 oz) | — | 14.29 mg |
| Bawls Guarana | 67 mg (10 oz) | — | 6.7 mg |

| | CAFFEINE IN COFFEE AND OTHER HOT DRINKS | | |
| --- | --- | --- | --- |
| | 8 OZ | 12 OZ CAN | PER/OZ |
| **Coffee, Espresso, and Tea** | | | |
| Espresso | *2 oz | 100 mg | 50 mg |
| Coffee, Instant | 75 mg | 112.5 mg | 9.375 mg |
| Coffee, Decaffeinated | 3 mg | 4.5 mg | .375 mg |
| Coffee, Brewed | 135 mg | 202.5 mg | 16.876 mg |
| Tea, Green | 15 mg | 22.5 mg | 1.875 mg |
| Tea, Leaf or Bag | 50 mg | 75 mg | 6.25 mg |

| | CAFFEINE IN FOODS | | |
| --- | --- | --- | --- |
| | MG | SERVING SIZE | MG PER/OZ |
| **Chocolate** | | | |
| Hershey's Special Dark Chocolate | 31 mg | 1 bar (1.5 oz) | |
| Hershey's Milk Chocolate | 10 mg | 1 bar (1.5 oz) | |
| Chocolate Milk | 5 mg | 7.5 mg | .625 mg |

| | TABLET | | |
| --- | --- | --- | --- |
| | MG | SERVING SIZE | MG PER/OZ |
| **Tablets** | | | |
| Caffeine tablet (Vivarin) | 200 mg | 1 tablet | — |
| Caffeine tablet (NoDoz) | 200 mg | 1 tablet | — |
| Excedrin tablet | 65 mg | 1 tablet | — |

Source: Data from **OverCaffeinated.org.**

in coffee, where the dose can range from 75 mg per cup for instant coffee to 150 mg per cup for drip coffee. In soft drinks the caffeine can range from 37.5 mg in a 12-oz. can of Pepsi to 70 mg in extra-caffeinated drinks like Jolt Cola. Other energy drinks contain 120 mg or more. Table 4.1 shows the caffeine content in popular beverages.

Ingesting caffeine results in a higher level of alertness and mild euphoria. A dose of caffeine can exert this effect for about an hour and then it gradually wears off. People can become dependent on

Caffeine is a popular, legal stimulant most commonly found in coffee, sodas, and teas.

caffeine, and this can lead to a craving. The most common withdrawal effect is a headache.

Sometimes caffeine users over-caffeinate themselves and induce a state of **caffeinism.** The symptoms include tremors, restlessness, agitation, confusion, light-headedness, and anxiety. Abstaining from coffee for a few hours will cause the symptoms to subside. Although it is not pleasant, caffeinism is not generally harmful or dangerous. However, people should be aware that caffeine is rather caustic and can aggravate ulcers and acid reflux disease, so those who have digestive problems should not use it. Individuals with anxiety disorders and women who are pregnant should also avoid excessive caffeine in their diets.

✓ **NEED TO KNOW**

Stimulants make people feel energetic or euphoric, and they may have numbing or pain-relief qualities. Medical uses include anesthesia and treatment of ADHD (hyperactivity). Stimulants are widely abused and can induce dependence quickly, due to both the high and the unpleasant low that comes as the drug leaves the body. Whether it is caffeine, nicotine, cocaine, or amphetamines, all stimulants produce an up-and-down cycle, but their effects differ in degree and intensity.

## ➤ Hallucinogens

Hallucinogens are a category of drugs capable of inducing hallucinations, which is a perception of sights, sounds, physical senses (touch), or taste with no basis in reality. Similar to a hallucination is a delusion— a misinterpretation of something real. For example, a person who looks at a car and sees a dog instead of the vehicle is having a delusion, while a person seeing a car when nothing is there is having a hallucination.

**Caffeinism** is an outcome of an excessive dose of caffeine.

# LSD

LSD was accidentally discovered in the late 1930s when a Swiss chemist was working with ergot, a fungus that grows on rye, in an attempt to find a cure for migraine headaches. LSD proved not to have any headache-relief properties despite numerous experiments to find a medical use for the drug. In the 1960s LSD became popular as a part of the counterculture movement. It is a colorless, odorless, and tasteless drug. A small dose, called a *microdot,* can induce an 8- to 12-hour psychoactive experience that includes hallucinations. This experience can be framed by anxiety, and the beginning, several hours of hallucinations, can be followed by several hours of depression. Like any other drug, the intensity of these effects varies.

There has been no documentation of physiological damage among LSD users. However, some users have experienced a post-hallucinogenic sensory disorder and have hallucinations years after using LSD. Also, during the hallucinogenic phase of the LSD experience, safety can be compromised if the false perception involves a potentially dangerous situation. For example, a person could be unaware of his or her surroundings and walk in front of oncoming traffic or fall out a window. Like cocaine, LSD popularity ebbs and flows. Much of the current LSD use is tied to rave culture.

## PSILOCYBIN

Psilocybin is a hallucinogenic drug found in *teonanacatl,* a type of mushroom native to the United States and Mexico. The term *shrooms* is sometimes used for these psilocybin-containing mushrooms. Shrooms are usually eaten, and the effects can last from 3 to 8 hours. Small doses of psilocybin induce a tranquil euphoric state, and higher dosages can induce hallucinations. The shroom experience is similar to LSD, but normally not nearly as intense or potent.

## MESCALINE

Mescaline is a hallucinogenic drug found in peyote, a growth or "button" found on a small cactus that grows in Mexico and the southwestern United States. Mescaline produces a total psychoactive experience for about 10 hours, with hallucinations lasting about 2 hours. Although not a very powerful hallucinogen, mescaline can still pack a punch depending on the size and frequency of doses. Unlike many other hallucinogens, mescaline has medical uses; it is prescribed as a respiratory stimulant and as a treatment for heart problems.

## PCP AND KETAMINE

Phencyclidine (PCP) was originally developed as a dissociative anesthetic (one capable of keeping patients awake but pain free during surgery and other procedures). The early trials of PCP as an anesthetic found it to be effective, but the patients experienced mood swings, hallucinations, and displayed violent behavior, all symptoms that indicated a narrow margin of safety, so the FDA never approved PCP for human use. However, it was approved for use as a veterinary anesthetic and tranquilizer. Consequently, it was easy to divert to human populations.

The effects of PCP are very unpredictable, causing some experts to characterize PCP as the most dangerous illicit drug. It can induce profound mood swings, delusions, violent primal behavior, and hallucinations. This experience can last for hours, and users may endanger themselves and others while under the influence. To complicate matters, when users are hurt, they do not feel the pain because of PCP's anesthetic properties. So users can continue violent and destructive behavior for much longer than would be possible for anyone who is not under the influence of PCP.

Like PCP, ketamine is a dissociative anesthetic and is used in veterinary medicine. Not as powerful as PCP, ketamine is also used as an anesthetic for humans. It can induce a PCP-like experience, and when used illicitly, it is sometimes called Special K. Often ketamine is marketed as PCP.

## KHAT AND SALVIA

Khat is a naturally occurring stimulant that comes from a shrub common to Africa and the Middle East. Cathinone is the active ingredient in khat, and while khat is not scheduled by the DEA, cathinone is, and it is a Schedule I drug. Similar to amphetamines, khat can be effective in eliciting a euphoric effect and increased alertness for about 1–3 hours, after which the user experiences depression, anorexia, and difficulty in sleeping. Long-term use of khat can result in periodontal disease, gastrointestinal problems, and cardiovascular problems.

Salvia is an herb commonly found in Mexico and throughout Central and South America. Salvinorin A is the active ingredient in salvia. The salvia leaves are usually chewed, smoked, or consumed in liquid form. The effects of salvia begin within 1 minute after it enters the blood and last for about 30 minutes. Effects include hallucinations and mood swings. Since salvia is an herb, it is not scheduled by the DEA and is readily available in the United States. Of concern is that in the 2009 MTF, 5.7 percent of high school seniors reported using salvia the previous year, more than reported using Ecstasy.

Hallucinogens are powerful drugs with unpredictable effects. PCP and ketamine are particularly dangerous due to the unpredictable, sometimes violent behavior they can cause users to exhibit. Khat and salvia are two newly popular hallucinogens derived from plants and herbs. Khat produces similar effects to amphetamines, and salvia produces hallucinations and mood swings.

## ➤ Marijuana

*Marijuana* is the name for products from the cannabis plant that are dried and prepared for smoking. Cannabis has been referred to as a weed because it does grow wild in many areas of the world. A resin called tetrahydrocannabinol (THC) is the chief agent responsible for the physical and psychological effects associated with marijuana.

### FORMS AND EFFECTS OF MARIJUANA

How cannabis impacts someone relates to the concentration of THC in the final product. Ganja, the tops and leaves of the cannabis plant, generally contains 3–5 percent concentration THC. Sinsemilla, or "without seeds," refers to a form of marijuana with an 8–10 percent concentration of THC. Hashish is a more concentrated form that is usually smoked in small, square blocks and contains a 14–16 percent THC concentration. Finally, the most potent form is hash oil, which can contain up to 60 percent THC. Hash oil will induce an LSD-like experience. The other forms of marijuana are less potent and can induce significant sedation and possibly delusions but not hallucinations.

Because smoking is the chief method of administration, the effects are felt almost immediately. The psychological effects of THC include relaxation, relief from anxiety, euphoria, laughter, and if the concentration of THC is high enough, impaired judgment and short-term memory. Physical effects of marijuana include dry mouth, increased appetite, bloodshot eyes, coughing, and decreased muscle coordination. Often the effects of marijuana are compared to alcohol, particularly by those who want to see marijuana legalized. Long-term effects of marijuana use include the development of amotivational syndrome, impaired immunity, respiratory problems, and increased cancer risk.

Physical dependence and tolerance to marijuana have not been shown. Psychological dependence can be related to anything, so it is safe to say that users can become psychologically dependent on marijuana.

# MARIJUANA'S SAFETY AND THE QUESTION OF LEGALIZATION

Self
Assessment
4.2

Due to its common illicit use since the 1960s, some people feel that using marijuana in moderation is as safe as alcohol or cigarettes and ought to be legalized. Just how safe is marijuana use?

Although THC and alcohol may both be used for relaxation, alcohol is not smoked, so the method of administration is not comparable. Smoking marijuana puts one at risk of the same kinds of conditions that cigarette smokers are at risk for, including heart disease and cancer. **Cannabinoids** are tars in cannabis, many of which are cancer causing. Further, marijuana smoke, like cigarette smoke, contains high levels of carbon monoxide. Thus tissues become oxygen starved when marijuana is used. The dangers that may come with marijuana smoke have not been studied as closely as the dangers of cigarette smoke, so the long-term impact of marijuana use is not as well understood. See "Breaking It Down" for more information on the legalization controversy.

## Breaking It Down Should More Drugs Be Legalized?

The United States spends billions of dollars on drug regulations, prohibitions, and enforcement. High-profile people such as former Secretary of State George Shultz and the late Nobel laureate Milton Friedman have stated that making drugs illegal leads by default to the involvement of organized crime. If drugs were legal, the argument goes, the government could control sales and tax the products. This would generate large amounts of revenue now lost to the government because they cannot currently track illegal sales. Further, if drugs were legal, organized crime might be reduced because people seeking drugs could do so legally. Without the involvement of organized crime in drug trafficking, there might be fewer homicides and other types of violent crime surrounding drug use and sales. There would also be fewer incarcerations and possibly fewer health problems such as overdoses, because if the government enforced quality control of drugs, people would be able to ascertain the exact substance they had and know the safer dose levels. Finally, most of those who favor legalizing some or all drugs feel that drug use is a personal choice and should not be subject to government interference.

**Cannabinoids** are tars in cannabis and marijuana, some of which are carcinogenic.

In contrast, opponents of legalizing some or all drugs, such as Lee P. Brown, director and spokesperson of the Office of National Drug Control Policy and Drug Enforcement, argue that legalization of drugs is immoral. People who are against legalizing drugs also tend to believe that the stiff penalties for drug use deter many from trying drugs in the first place, and that saves lives. Opponents feel legalization would only increase social problems like addiction and the violent crimes that are committed by people under the influence.

Although the idea of legalizing heroin or cocaine is not widely accepted in the United States, a growing number of Americans seem to feel that the classification of marijuana as a Schedule I drug should be changed. They point out that Marinol, an antinausea drug used by cancer patients, is derived from marijuana, so the government's claim that marijuana is a Schedule I drug without any accepted medical uses is inconsistent and incorrect. Many states—including California, Alaska, Colorado, Hawaii, Maine, Montana, Nevada, New Mexico, Oregon, Rhone Island, Vermont, and Washington—have passed laws in the past decade that remove state-level penalties for possessing or growing marijuana if it is intended to be used as a treatment for depression, chronic pain from illnesses such as cancer, or for the treatment of glaucoma. Furthermore, another 10 states (plus the District of Columbia) have statutes that symbolically support the idea of medical marijuana use but do not specifically provide users protections under state laws.

Despite widespread public support for medical marijuana use, the Bush administration maintained a desire for federal prosecution of anyone possessing marijuana for any reason. Opponents of legalization claim that the pro-legalization camp is disingenuous about its motives and simply wants to relax the bans and make the recreational use of marijuana easier for everyone. Opponents point out that although the psychological effects of THC are similar to alcohol, the long-term effects of chronic use of marijuana are more similar to smoking cigarettes. Marijuana smoke has high levels of carbon monoxide and carcinogenic tars. Collectively these substances can starve the tissues of oxygen, leading to cardiovascular disease as well as cancer. So significant health risks are associated with marijuana. Further, marijuana dependence does occur in some people, and marijuana can impair driving performance.

There seems to be more controversy and less support for the total legalization of marijuana because opinions on its general safety vary, and there may be wisdom in restricting recreational use. But continuing the ban on medical use of marijuana is much more up in the air. The prosecution of medical marijuana cases, both at the federal and the state level, appears to be an issue in flux.

## SPICE AND K2

Spice and K2 are together a mixture of herbs with psychoactive properties that has been successfully marketed as an incense substitute for marijuana. Since it is an incense, it is commonly available through numerous outlets—health food stores, head shops, convenience stores, and the Internet. Spice and K2 is usually smoked but can be prepared in liquid form and consumed. In addition to the mostly marijuana-like effects, users can also experience rapid heart rate, vomiting, agitation, confusion, and hallucinations. Because of the immediate dangers associated with Spice and K2 use, the DEA was able to effect emergency scheduling, making Spice and K2 a Schedule I drug and essentially banning it.

> ✔ **NEED TO KNOW**
>
> Marijuana is a popular recreational drug. The concentration of THC in the marijuana induces the psychoactive effect. The higher the concentration of THC, the more intense the effect. Street-grade marijuana today is much more powerful than it was in the 1960s and 1970s. Use of marijuana carries health risks that are similar to the health risks associated with smoking. The common comparison to alcohol holds true only for THC ingested in some way other than smoking. Spice and K2 are herbs that have been promoted as substitutes for marijuana, and as a result the DEA has banned both.

## ➤ Psychotherapeutic Drugs

Psychotherapeutic drugs treat mental and emotional problems that range from anxiety to depression. For many, this category of drugs represents a medical miracle—these substances can enable users to continue with their life in a healthful way and be free from symptoms of mental illness. Further, the effectiveness of these drugs confirms the biological basis of anxiety and depression, which previously had been subject to debate. The most common psychotherapeutic drugs include antidepressants, minor tranquilizers, and major tranquilizers.

### ANTIDEPRESSANTS

Clinical depression has a biological basis. Abnormalities in the level of neurotransmitters, specifically serotonin, can result in depression. Antidepressants as a category of drugs have improved the lives of millions of people because they "adjust" the neurotransmitters to a point where depression is prevented. Common antidepressants today are selective serotonin reuptake inhibitors (**SSRIs**). These drugs allow serotonin to stay in the synapse longer and prevent depression. Examples of SSRIs include Prozac, Zoloft, and Paxil. Another category is the selective serotonin norepinephrine reuptake inhibitors (**SSNRIs**). These drugs allow both serotonin and norepinephrine to stay in the synapse longer to prevent depression. Examples of SSNRIs include Cymbalta and Effexor.

A person diagnosed with depression and who is prescribed an antidepressant should see some improvement within just a few weeks. The hopelessness and despair should be significantly lessened. This improvement should give the person a clearer perspective on life and life's events.

Not only are antidepressants popular in treating depression, but some such as Paxil are popular in treating generalized anxiety feelings, including fear, over-worry, over-concern, and panic. And since antidepressants influence neurotransmitters, they are often prescribed for conditions other than depression. Many people are able to prevent migraine headaches with antidepressants, and many others with chronic pain feel antidepressants decrease the intensity of pain they regularly experience.

Long-term use of antidepressants appears to be safe. On occasion a news article has focused on a bad side effect with Prozac or Zoloft, but upon further evaluation, there has not been enough evidence to pull the drug off the market. This doesn't mean that it won't eventually happen; it just means the problem that was observed could not be related to the use of antidepressants, or the effect happens in such a small number of users that closer patient monitoring is needed rather than pulling the drug from the market.

## MINOR TRANQUILIZERS

Minor tranquilizers have been referred to as "anti-anxiety drugs." **Benzodiazepines** are the most commonly prescribed minor tranquilizers and include such drugs as Valium, Xanax, and Tranxene. These drugs are designed for short-term medication of anxiety and insomnia. They should not be used long term. If long-term medication is needed for anxiety, most physicians will cycle the person through the SSRIs to determine which one works best.

Minor tranquilizers are generally taken in pill form. The effects last a short time, and tolerance to these drugs can build quickly. When taken in conjunction with alcohol, the effect can be toxic.

An **SSRI** is a selective serotonin reuptake inhibitor, which is used to treat depression. **SSNRI** is a selective serotonin and norepinephrine reuptake inhibitor also used to treat depression.

**Benzodiazepines** are minor tranquilizers and include drugs such as Xanax, Valium, and Tranxene.

## MAJOR TRANQUILIZERS

Major tranquilizers are termed *antipsychotic drugs* because they can be effective in medicating people with serious conditions such as schizophrenia. Drugs from a category of major tranquilizers called *phenothiazines,* such as Thorazine, have made a positive difference in the lives of millions. Before the introduction of phenothiazines, most people who suffered from schizophrenia had to be institutionalized.

Lithium is another major tranquilizer. It is used to treat serious bipolar disorder, which has also been called *manic depression.* The benefits of major tranquilizers far outweigh the side effects.

## DATE RAPE DRUGS

The common scenario for a date rape begins with a man dropping a drug into a woman's drink. About 20 minutes after consuming the drugged beverage, the woman feels light-headed and wants to go home. The man who put the drug in her drink assists her, but his motive is to rape her. Shortly after the onset of symptoms, she lapses into unconsciousness or dissociates herself from the environment, meaning that she is awake but not processing environmental stimuli. In this state, he rapes her, and later when she is conscious, she has no memory because the drug has induced amnesia.

A drug commonly used in date rapes is Rohypnol, a minor tranquilizer from the benzodiazepine group. Rohypnol is similar to Valium but 10 times more powerful. Rohypnol is illegal in the United States but is available in many other countries, so there are multiple sources for the drug.

Another date rape drug is gamma-hydroxybutyrate, or GHB. GHB was originally developed as a dissociative anesthetic, and like PCP, it was found to have negative side effects and so was never marketed. The precursor to GHB contains chemicals commonly used by bodybuilders, so smart chemists can purchase these chemicals at health food stores and cook up GHB. The effects of GHB include significant muscle relaxation, nausea, vomiting, and amnesia. A high dose can cause hallucinations, respiratory distress, seizures, and possible coma. When combined with alcohol, the effects are enhanced and potentially life-threatening.

✓ **NEED TO KNOW**

It is easy for a drug such as Rohypnol or GHB to be put into a drink. Always make sure that there is no possibility for someone to add something to a drink. Trust your instincts—if you feel unusually or excessively drowsy or light-headed after a drink, then be sure to have friends take you home.

# ➤ Designer and Club Drugs

Designer drugs and club drugs are not categories of drugs like stimulants. **Designer drugs** are those made a certain way, and **club drugs** are those used in nightclubs or raves. Designer drugs are chemical analogues—that is, drugs that are very similar chemically to another drug but not exactly the same.

For example, fentanyl is a pain reliever more powerful than morphine. In many cities, the heroin that is marketed is actually a designer drug derived from fentanyl that is processed to look like heroin. Just about any drug distributed in the illegal market could be a designer drug.

A more common designer drug is the amphetamine analogue called Ecstasy. Its effect is similar to an amphetamine in that it increases heart rate and respiration. Some users experience mild distortions of perception, interpreted as a tranquil effect, which often progresses to a feeling of trust in their social interactions. This has led to Ecstasy being referred to as the *love drug*.

There have been two waves of Ecstasy popularity—one in the mid-1980s and one currently. After the wave of use in the mid-1980s, the drug was discovered to destroy serotonergic neurons, those neurons that produce serotonin, and brain damage can result. For this reason, Ecstasy is considered a dangerous drug.

In addition to its negative effect on neurons, Ecstasy can throw off the body's thermostat, resulting in dehydration and, potentially, cardiac arrest. People do die from Ecstasy use because of this. Ecstasy users trying to game the system have been known to "front load" their water, or drink gallons of water before or immediately after consuming

## ✓ NEED TO KNOW

Ecstasy is an extremely powerful chemical. It destroys nerve cells and disrupts the body's thermostat, resulting in extreme dehydration. People under the influence of Ecstasy don't feel thirsty yet they need fluids. This loss of fluids can result in a heart attack. Some users recognize this and drink excessive amounts of water before experiencing the effects of Ecstasy. This also has some dangers because consuming excessive amounts of water can cause body tissues to swell, and if swelling occurs in the brain, brain damage or death can result.

**Designer drugs** are chemical analogues of other drugs. **Club drugs** are powerful drugs used in the nightclub scene or raves.

Ecstasy, so that they will not become dehydrated. This behavior can also be life-threatening because it can produce a condition called *hyponatremia,* in which too much water causes tissues to swell. In extreme cases death can result.

Ecstasy is also considered a club drug. Other club drugs include LSD, shrooms, and marijuana. These are drugs that have long-lasting effects, are used in club or rave settings, and are used to maximize the club or rave experience.

## ➤ Drug Testing and Drug Treatment

Drug testing is a common practice to determine if a person has used certain drugs. The most common drugs tested for are opiates, cocaine, amphetamines, marijuana, Ecstasy, and barbiturates. Traces of these substances remain in urine for varying times after use. The typical window of time for a person's urine sample to test positive after use of opiates, cocaine, amphetamines, Ecstasy, and barbiturates is 24–48 hours. Marijuana can be detected for one week up to two months, depending on frequency of use, because THC is stored in the fat and released slowly.

### DRUG TESTING PROTOCOLS AND PROCEDURES

There are three major drug testing protocols: random, for cause, and condition of employment. Random drug tests can be carried out at any time without a particular reason or suspicion. Most random drug screens are done in professions with a strong public-good emphasis where the employees should be drug-free, such as medicine, law enforcement, airlines, and the military. For-cause drug tests are given to employees because a problem or incident at work provokes suspicion of substance abuse. Drug testing as a condition of employment is done to screen out drug-using candidates before they are hired.

A urine test is the most common procedure in testing for drugs. It is simple and inexpensive. The urine sample is divided into two separate samples. The first one is subjected to an **immunoassay** test, where antibodies react to the drug being tested for. If the person tests positive, the second sample is subjected to a confirmation test, such as gas chromatography or mass spectrometry. This confirmation test is expensive, but it is precise in terms of confirming the immunoassay. There is also a possibility of a false positive, so the confirmation test is very important.

**Immunoassay** is the most basic drug test used as a part of the urine screen.

Another drug test uses hair samples. Not currently as popular as urine, the hair-sample test adds another dimension to testing because a drug is contained in the hair for a long time after ingestion, whereas urine tests only detect what has been in the system for a short period.

## FALSE POSITIVES AND FALSE NEGATIVES

Drug testing is usually very accurate. However, some substances can interfere with the tests and make the results inaccurate. When a person tests positive to a drug but has not used it, this is called a *false positive*. Benadryl, a common antihistamine, can cause a false positive for amphetamines. Ibuprofen, an over-the-counter analgesic, can cause a false positive for marijuana. Poppy seeds can cause a false positive for opiates. This is why the confirmation test is so important. A gas chromatography or mass spectrometry will be able to determine if the person used Benadryl or amphetamines.

When a person has used a drug and tests negative, this is called a *false negative*. Generally a false negative results when the urine has been adulterated with a chemical that can deceive the immunoassay. Many products are sold in counterculture magazines and on the Internet that claim a false negative will result if the product is ingested before a drug test. The most common way for a false negative to occur is if the urine is diluted to a point where the immunoassay cannot react to the drug.

## STANDARD DRUG TREATMENT MODEL

The standard treatment model for substance dependence is detoxification, counseling, and support groups. This model was discussed earlier in the chapter with respect to treatment for alcohol dependence. The components are similar no matter what drug dependence is being treated. What is important for treatment is a three-pronged approach: medical detoxification, psychological counseling, and support groups that give reinforcement for staying clean and sober. If all three elements are not in place, then a person will be at high risk for relapse.

Unfortunately, too few drug treatment programs are available in the United States. Many more

Certain foods, such as the poppy seeds on a roll or over-the-counter drugs such as Benadryl, can cause false-positive results in certain drug tests.

resources are allocated to law enforcement than to treatment. Beyond the physical and mental difficulties of breaking from addictive behaviors, the cost of treatment is also a major hurdle. People who want to become clean and sober but who don't have good health insurance can find treatment and recovery a difficult road to navigate.

**NEED TO KNOW**

Drugs can circulate through the body for long periods of time. Most drugs have about a 24- to 48-hour window of being detectable in the system. Marijuana (THC) is different—it is stored in the fat and slowly released into the blood. So THC can be detected for much longer periods of time—weeks or months depending on the extent of use. Drug testing will be a part of everyone's future—whether it be a condition of employment or health insurance.

## ARTICLES

4.1 "How We Get Addicted." *Time.* This article highlights current thinking on the nature of addiction, including biological and psychosocial factors.

4.2 "A Host of Trouble." *U.S. News & World Report.* When party hosts allow or excuse excessive drinking, they might be legally responsible for any problems that occur.

4.3 "Screening and Brief Intervention for Underage Drinkers." *Mayo Clinic Proceedings.* This piece gives contemporary information on alcohol-related screening, intervention, and referral for treatment for underage drinkers.

4.4 "American's Most Dangerous Drug." *Newsweek.* The addictive and destructive properties of methamphetamine make it America's most dangerous drug.

## SELF-ASSESSMENTS

4.1 Is Alcohol a Problem in Your Life?
4.2 How Much Do You Know about Marijuana?

## Website Resources

CASA—The National Center on Addiction and Substance Abuse at Centers for Disease Control and Prevention
   **www.cdc.gov**
Columbia University
   **www.casacolumbia.org**
DanceSafe—Promoting Health and Safety Within the Rave and Nightclub Community
   **www.dancesafe.org**
Drug Enforcement Administration
   **www.usdoj.gov/dea/index.htm**
Drug Policy Alliance
   **www.drugpolicy.org**
National Clearinghouse for Alcohol and Drug Information
   **http://ncadi.samhsa.gov/**
National Institute on Drug Abuse
   **www.nida.nih.gov**
National Organization for the Legalization of Marijuana
   **www.norml.org**

Office of National Drug Control Policy: Media Campaign
   **www.mediacampaign.org**
Substance Abuse and Mental Health Administration
   **www.samhsa.gov**

## Knowing the Language

alcohol abuse, 154
alcohol dependence, 154
benzodiazepines, 171
binge drinking, 154
caffeinism, 164
cannabinoids, 168
club drugs, 173
designer drugs, 173
drug abuse, 141
drug misuse, 141
drug use, 141
DUI, 153
DWI, 153
effective dose, 143
immunoassay, 174

inhalation administration, 140
lethal dose, 143
oral administration, 140
Oxycontin, 157
parenteral administration, 140
physical dependence, 142
psychological dependence, 142
rectal administration, 141
sedative-hypnotic, 157
set, 142
setting, 142
SSNRI, 171
SSRI, 171
transdermal administration, 141
tolerance, 143

## Understanding the Content

1. Distinguish between the different methods of drug administration and absorption.
2. Define the following terms: *drug use, drug misuse, drug abuse, set, setting, physical dependence, psychological dependence,* and *tolerance.*
3. Describe the effects of alcohol on the cerebrum, cerebellum, and medulla.
4. What are the differences between the different forms of marijuana?
5. What are the major dangers in designer and club drugs?
6. Describe the components of the standard drug treatment model.

## Exploring Ideas

1. Use of alcohol, including underage drinking, is considered a rite of passage in college. At age 18, one can legally vote and serve in the military. Should the drinking age be lowered to 18? Why or why not?

2. How does someone know he or she may have a drug problem? What kinds of signs and symptoms should the person look for?
3. Some professionals feel that the more punitive the measures, the more compliant people will be with the law. With that in mind, should college students be randomly drug tested to determine the extent of drug use in this population?

## Selected References

American Psychiatric Association. *Diagnostic and Statistical Manual of Mental Disorders* (4th ed.). Washington, DC: APA, 1994.

Centers for Disease Control and Prevention. Alcohol attributable deaths and years of potential life lost—United States, 2001. *Morbidity & Mortality Weekly Report* 53 (37): 866–870, September 24, 2004.

Drug Enforcement Administration (DEA). Drug Schedules. **www.usdoj.gov/dea/pubs/scheduling.html**

DEA. Federal Trafficking Penalties. **www.usdoj.gov/dea/agency/penalties.htm**

Haroz R, Greenberg MI. New drugs of abuse in North America. *Journal of Laboratory and Clinical Medicine* 26: 147–164, 2006.

Harrison PM, Allen JB. *Bureau of Justice Statistics: Prisoners in 2002.* Washington, DC: U.S. Dept. of Justice, July 2003, p. 10.

Johnston, LD, O'Malley, PM, Bachman, JG, & Schulenberg, JE (2010). Monitoring the future national survey results on drug use, 1975–2009. Volume I: Secondary school students (NIH Publication No. 10–7584). Bethesda, MD: National Institute on Drug Abuse, 734 pp.

Kinney J, Leaton G. *Loosening the Grip: A Handbook of Alcohol Information* (7th ed.). New York: McGraw-Hill, 2003.

Maxwell JC. *Patterns of Club Drug Use in the U.S., 2004.* Austin, TX: Center for Excellence in Drug Epidemiology, 2004.

National Center on Addiction and Substance Abuse at Columbia University (CASA). *Wasting the Best and Brightest.* New York: Columbia, March 15, 2007.

National Institute on Drug Abuse. *Community Drug Alert Bulletin (Club Drugs).* Bethesda, MD: National Institute on Drug Abuse, May 2004.

National Institute on Drug Abuse. *Methamphetamine Abuse and Addiction.* Research Report Series. Bethesda, MD: National Institute on Drug Abuse, September 2006.

Office of Applied Studies, Substance Abuse and Mental Health Services Administration (SAMHSA). *Prevalence of Substance Use Among Racial and Ethnic Subgroups in the U.S.,* 2005.

Office of Applied Studies, Substance Abuse and Mental Health Services Administration. Substance use among past year Ecstasy users. *The NSDUH Report,* April 29, 2005. **www.drugabusestatistics.samhsa.gov/NHSDA/Ethnic/ethn1006.htm**

Office of National Drug Control Policy. *Drug Data Summary.* Rockville, MD: Drug Policy Information Clearinghouse, March 2003.

Ruhm CJ. Alcohol policies and highway vehicle fatalities. *Journal of Health Economics* 15 (4): 435–454, 1996.

SIUC/Core Institute. Core Alcohol and Drug Survey, Long Form, Executive Summary. May 11, 2010.

Snyder LB, Milici FF, Slater M, Sun H, Strizhakova Y. Effects of alcohol advertising exposure on drinking among youth. *Archives of Pediatrics and Adolescent Medicine* 160: 18–24, 2006.

Substance Abuse and Mental Health Services Administration (SAMHSA). *Results from the 2001 National Household Survey on Drug Abuse.* Rockville, MD: SAMHSA, September 2002.

U.S. Department of Health and Human Services. *Alcohol Alert, Economic Perspectives in Alcoholism Research.* Rockville, MD: U.S. Department of Health and Human Services, 2001.

Familiarity breeds
contempt—and
children.

— MARK TWAIN

# Chapter 5

## RESPECT SEXUALITY

In Chapter 5, we cover a wide variety of topics related to both the physical and psychosocial aspects of human sexuality. Probably no other topic is as misunderstood as sexuality, from the details of reproductive anatomy to the range of behaviors. Most misunderstandings result from questionable sources of sexuality information. Friends, family, and media often communicate incomplete or incorrect information, and ignorance about the facts can lead to high-risk decisions. This chapter reviews the basics of sexual anatomy, reproduction, and contraception. It also discusses selected aspects of sexual dysfunction, sexual identity, sexual behavior, and relationships.

## Female and Male: Genetics and Hormones

**THE FEMALE REPRODUCTIVE SYSTEM**

**THE MALE REPRODUCTIVE SYSTEM**

**DISORDERS**

## Conception, Pregnancy, and Childbirth

**FIRST TRIMESTER**

**SECOND TRIMESTER**

**THIRD TRIMESTER**

**COMPLICATIONS OF PREGNANCY AND CHILDBIRTH**

## Contraception

**HORMONAL METHODS**

**BARRIER METHODS**

**SURGICAL METHODS**

**NATURAL METHODS**

**EMERGENCY CONTRACEPTION**

**TERMINATION OF PREGNANCY**

**THE ABORTION CONTROVERSY**

## Sexual Behavior

**THE HUMAN SEXUAL RESPONSE MODEL**

**SEXUAL DYSFUNCTION**

## Gender Identity and Sexual Orientation

## Healthy Relationships

**COMMITTED RELATIONSHIPS AND MARRIAGE**

**HEALTHY AND UNHEALTHY RELATIONSHIPS**

**COMMUNICATION AND CONFLICT RESOLUTION SKILLS**

CONCEPTION, PREGNANCY, AND CHILDBIRTH are integral forces in the world. Having some control over births is central to control of property, wealth, and lineage—in other words, power—for both individuals and societies. Before contraception existed, the only way to control births was to discourage certain segments of the population, such as the very young and the unmarried, from having sex. Abstinence was the only reliable birth control. Relatedly, the main activity of women was childrearing, and families tended to be large.

The rules by which society operated changed with the development of reliable contraception methods in the 20th century. Especially after the birth control pill became widely available in the 1970s, consequences for various behaviors became different. In turn, so did the behaviors of many Americans. People could engage in sexual activity without a baby being a near-automatic part of the relationship. Women could delay reproduction, have fewer children, or avoid motherhood altogether. This created opportunities for women to enter educational, professional, and social circles that had once been exclusive to men. This so-called sexual revolution in the late 20th century sometimes encouraged good outcomes, such as more equality among men and women, but it also contributed to new challenges, such as the rise of AIDS and other sexually transmitted infections (STIs).

Today sexuality is defined as much more than just fertility. It is something that begins before birth and continues throughout life, influencing and shaping relationships at every age. In addition to anatomy, physiology, sexual development, and reproduction, sexuality includes sexual orientation, gender identity, and people's values and beliefs regarding these issues. To make good decisions regarding health and relationships, adults must be educated in the full range of these issues.

## ➤ Female and Male: Genetics and Hormones

Healthy people are born with 46 chromosomes arranged in 23 pairs. It is the 23rd pair of chromosomes that determines sex—females have an XX pair, and males have an XY pair. Sexual development is genetically programmed to occur when children reach the age of 12 or 13, and signs of maturation begin well before that. During puberty, the reproductive system matures, secondary sex characteristics appear, and masculine and feminine body features become refined.

Chemical messengers called **hormones** bring about puberty and rule sexuality. The most important sexual hormones are estrogen, progesterone,

**Hormones** are chemical messengers.

## FIGURE 5.1    FEMALE REPRODUCTIVE SYSTEM

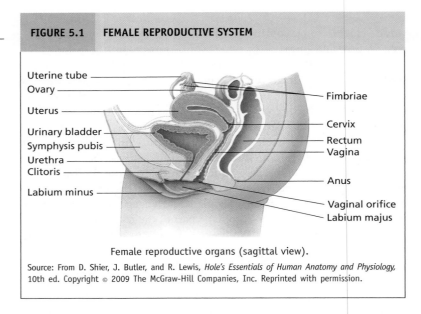

Uterine tube
Ovary
Uterus
Urinary bladder
Symphysis pubis
Urethra
Clitoris
Labium minus

Fimbriae
Cervix
Rectum
Vagina
Anus
Vaginal orifice
Labium majus

Female reproductive organs (sagittal view).

Source: From D. Shier, J. Butler, and R. Lewis, *Hole's Essentials of Human Anatomy and Physiology*, 10th ed. Copyright © 2009 The McGraw-Hill Companies, Inc. Reprinted with permission.

and testosterone. **Estrogen** controls female secondary sex characteristics such as breast development and also plays a part in menstruation and ovulation. **Progesterone** is responsible for building up the endometrial tissue lining a woman's uterus, a key step of the female fertility cycle. In males, **testosterone** is responsible for both primary and secondary sex characteristics, such as a deepening voice and sperm production. We tend to classify estrogen as female and testosterone as male, but women actually have small amounts of testosterone in their bodies, and men have small amounts of estrogen. In addition to being important for secondary sex characteristics, estrogen and testosterone are necessary for brain functions, including the sex drive.

## THE FEMALE REPRODUCTIVE SYSTEM

The female reproductive system includes both internal and external organs (Figure 5.1). The internal organs are the ovaries, fallopian or uterine tubes, uterus, cervix, and vagina. The **ovaries** are the female

**Estrogen** is a female hormone responsible for female secondary sex characteristics.

**Progesterone** is a female hormone responsible for the development of endometrial tissue.

**Testosterone** is a male hormone responsible for male secondary sex characteristics.

reproductive glands that produce ova (eggs), the female sex cells. They also produce estrogen and progesterone. When an ovary releases an egg, it is swept into the nearby **fallopian tube,** where fertilization can take place, if the egg meets up with a sperm cell.

Whether fertilized or not, an egg travels down the fallopian tube and ends up in the **uterus,** an elastic, muscular organ designed to stretch to accommodate a growing baby. At the bottom of the uterus is a round, thick muscle called the **cervix.** The cervix connects the uterus to the **vagina,** where sperm are deposited during intercourse. The vagina is also the route through which a woman's endometrial tissue sloughs off during menstruation, and it is the canal through which a baby enters the world during birth.

The external female genitalia, collectively referred to as the *vulva,* include the clitoris, labia majora, labia minora, and Bartholin's glands. The **clitoris** contains a dense nerve network that when stimulated results in an orgasm, the heightened pleasurable sensation that is the climax, or culmination, of sexual stimulation. The labia majora and labia minora are folds of tissues that cover the opening to the vagina. The Bartholin's glands, located inside the labia minora, secrete a lubricating substance during sexual arousal that results in less skin friction during intercourse.

The menstrual cycle (or fertility cycle) is typically about 28 days long (Figure 5.2). The first day of the menstrual cycle, or "period," is usually counted as day 1, with the menstrual period lasting about five days. After menstruation ends, the pituitary gland secretes follicle-stimulating hormone (FSH), which causes an ovum to ripen in an ovary. FSH also signals the ovary to secrete more progesterone, so the endometrial tissue in the uterus builds up in preparation for a potential pregnancy. The ovum reaches maturity around halfway through the cycle (approximately day 14), and at that point the pituitary gland secretes luteinizing hormone (LH), signaling the ovary to release the ripe egg into the fallopian tube. This is called **ovulation.**

**Ovaries** are glands that produce ova and the hormones estrogen and progesterone. **Fallopian tubes** are the structures into which a ripe ovum is released and where it is fertilized by a sperm.

The **uterus** is the organ in which a fertilized ovum implants and develops into a baby. The **cervix** is the neck of the uterus, opening into the vagina. The **vagina** is the passage between the cervix and the external sex organs and the female structure for sexual intercourse; it is also referred to as the *birth canal.*

The **clitoris** is composed of a dense nerve network and is important in female arousal and orgasm.

**Ovulation** is the release of a mature or ripe ovum.

**FIGURE 5.2**    **MENSTRUATION HORMONES**

Source: From D. Shier, J. Butler, and R. Lewis, *Hole's Essentials of Human Anatomy and Physiology*, 10th ed. Copyright © 2009 The McGraw-Hill Companies, Inc. Reprinted with permission.

An egg in a fallopian tube can survive 48–72 hours. If the ovum is not fertilized by a sperm during that time, it will break down and be reabsorbed into the body. At around day 28 of the cycle, a new period begins.

Some women experience physical and emotional discomfort before menses, referred to as premenstrual syndrome (PMS). Common PMS symptoms include acne, breast swelling and tenderness, bloating, headache, backache, tension, irritability, and anxiety or depression. If a woman is bothered by these symptoms, her physician may prescribe synthetic estrogen or progesterone to provide relief.

If fertilization occurs, cell division begins immediately. The fertilized egg leaves the fallopian tube and implants in the endometrial tissue in the uterus (Figure 5.3).

## FIGURE 5.3    FERTILIZATION

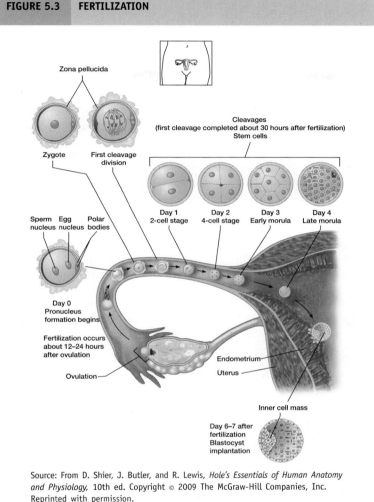

Source: From D. Shier, J. Butler, and R. Lewis, *Hole's Essentials of Human Anatomy and Physiology,* 10th ed. Copyright © 2009 The McGraw-Hill Companies, Inc. Reprinted with permission.

Females usually become fertile around age 13, when they get their first period. Women usually lose the ability to get pregnant in their late 40s or 50s. **Menopause** is the term for the process by which ovaries stop releasing eggs and monthly periods end. Menopause is a gradual process, but as the ovaries produce less and less progesterone and estrogen, many

**Menopause** is the cessation of the menstrual cycle.

**FIGURE 5.4    MALE REPRODUCTIVE SYSTEM**

Urinary bladder
Pubic bone
Vas deferens
Urethra
Corpus cavernosum
Corpus spongiosum
Penis
Glans penis
Prepuce

Large intestine
Ureter
Seminal vesicle
Ejaculatory duct
Prostate gland
Bulbourethral gland
Anus
Epididymis
Testis
Scrotum

Source: From D. Shier, J. Butler, and R. Lewis, *Hole's Essentials of Human Anatomy and Physiology*, 10th ed. Copyright © 2009 The McGraw-Hill Companies, Inc. Reprinted with permission.

physical and emotional symptoms can occur as the body adjusts to the changes. Common symptoms include hot flashes, irritability, loss of libido, depression, muscle aches, and sleep problems.

## THE MALE REPRODUCTIVE SYSTEM

Like the female system, the male reproductive system includes both internal and external organs (Figure 5.4). The internal organs are the testes, vas deferens, bulbourethral glands, prostate gland, urethra, and the glans penis. The external organs are the penis and the scrotum.

**Testes** are glands that produce sperm, the male sex cells, and the hormone testosterone. The epididymis is attached to the testes and is the place where sperm mature and are stored. Surrounding the testes is a sac of skin called the **scrotum.** The scrotum not only protects the testes but also maintains a lower-than-core-body temperature in the organs inside it, which is important for healthy sperm production.

After sperm are produced in the testes, they move to the **vas deferens,** where sperm are stored and provided with a route to the urethra, where

**Testes** are glands that produce sperm and the hormone testosterone. The **scrotum** is the sac of skin that protects the testes.

**Vas deferens** are structures that receive sperm from the testes and provide a route for the movement of sperm.

during orgasm they will be ejaculated. As sperm travel down the vas deferens, they collect fluids from three major glands: the **seminal vesicles,** the **bulbourethral glands,** and the **prostate gland.** The seminal vesicles secrete a nutritive substance so that sperm can thrive. The bulbourethral glands (also called *Cowper's glands*) secrete a lubricating substance that is believed to lubricate the urethra to facilitate the passage of sperm. The prostate gland secretes an alkaline substance that neutralizes the acidic environment in the vagina. Collectively, secretions from all these glands and the sperm are referred to as *semen.*

The urethra in males is located in the penis and transports both urine and semen, though not at the same time. (In females, the urethra is not part of the reproductive system; its sole purpose is to carry urine from the bladder.) The penis is the male external reproductive organ that contains the majority of the urethra. The head of the penis (or **glans penis**) has a dense nerve network that when stimulated can result in orgasm, inducing the involuntary ejaculation of semen.

During sexual activity, sperm move from the testes to the vas deferens and then pass through the seminal vesicles, bulbourethral glands, and prostate gland. The semen travels down the urethra, and if orgasm occurs, it is ejaculated. If ejaculation occurs during vaginal intercourse, sperm in the semen will attempt to move up through the cervix, uterus, and fallopian tubes. If the sperm comes into contact with a mature ovum in the fallopian tubes, then fertilization can occur.

## DISORDERS

A variety of common disorders can affect both the female and the male reproductive systems. Effects of these disorders can range from mild discomfort to infertility.

### *Female Disorders*
Several fairly common irregularities can affect female fertility. **Menorrhagia** is heavy menstrual bleeding, or an excess flow of endometrial tissue. It is often caused by hormonal imbalances and can be

---

Seminal vesicles secrete a nutritive substance so that sperm can survive. The **bulbourethral glands** secrete a lubricating substance to help sperm pass through the urethra. The **prostate gland** secretes an alkaline substance that neutralizes the acid medium normally present in the vagina.

The **glans penis** is the head of the penis and is a dense nerve network and the focal point for orgasm.

**Menorrhagia** is excessive menstruation.

treated with synthetic estrogen and/or progesterone (in the form of birth control pills). Less often it is caused by uterine fibroids, which are benign tumors of the uterus.

**Amenorrhea** is the absence of menstruation. If the woman is not pregnant or breastfeeding, amenorrhea is usually caused by stress, being extremely underweight, or having an extremely low percentage of body fat. Excessive exercise and participation in rigorous sports can lead to amenorrhea, as can eating disorders such as anorexia nervosa.

**Dysmenorrhea** is painful menstruation, characterized by severe cramping. It can be caused by high levels of body chemicals called *prostaglandins;* when this is the case, symptoms can often be relieved simply with ibuprofen. It can also have other causes, including *endometriosis,* a condition where endometrial tissue becomes implanted in the abdominal cavity outside the uterus; *ectopic pregnancy,* when a fertilized egg implants in the wrong location in the uterus or in the fallopian tube or ovary; and *pelvic inflammatory disease* (PID), a widespread infection of tissue in the pelvic area.

Menstrual problems require a physician's evaluation, and once the cause is identified, there are usually interventions available to treat the condition. Medical interventions can range from occasional use of pain relievers or taking birth control pills (which tend to make women's periods lighter) to, in severe cases, a surgery called *dilation and curettage* (D&C), which removes the endometrial tissue from the uterus.

### Male Disorders

Several disorders for males are also relatively common. A hernia is a protrusion of an organ through a structure that contains it. Hernias can result from too much pressure or straining when lifting heavy objects. An inguinal hernia occurs when a loop of intestine has broken through the abdominal wall located above the scrotum (called the *inguinal wall;* Figure 5.5).

Hernias can be serious because the intestinal loop can push its way into the scrotum, causing a bowel constriction or even sterility. Physicians conducting physical exams on male patients typically will place the index finger up under the pubic bone in the top part of the scrotum and ask the patient to cough. The coughing usually can exert enough pressure for the physician to feel if a hernia exists. Sometimes surgery is needed to pull the loop of intestine back to where it belongs and suture the damaged inguinal wall.

**Amenorrhea** is the absence of menstruation.

**Dysmenorrhea** is painful menstruation.

## FIGURE 5.5   HERNIA

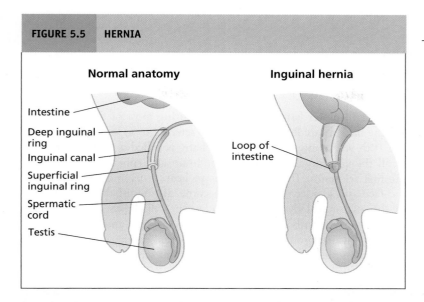

Normal anatomy

Intestine
Deep inguinal ring
Inguinal canal
Superficial inguinal ring
Spermatic cord
Testis

Inguinal hernia

Loop of intestine

Prostate problems are most common in older males, but infections such as STIs can cause prostate problems in younger men. If the prostate becomes infected, a man may have difficulty urinating or have a continual urge to urinate. The prostate is checked through a digital rectal exam whereby the physician inserts a finger into the rectum and feels the prostate for enlargement and for growths.

In addition to some prostate problems, STIs can also cause pelvic inflammatory disease (PID) or infertility. Many of these problems are discussed in Chapter 11.

### ✓ NEED TO KNOW

Hormones are chemical messengers that represent the most basic language of sexuality. The female hormones include estrogen and progesterone. Estrogen and progesterone are the major hormones produced by the ovaries and are responsible for secondary sex characteristics in females. Testosterone is the major hormone produced by the testes and is responsible for secondary sex characteristics in males. Secondary sex characteristics begin to develop during puberty. The female and male reproductive systems are different in structure but similar in function: production of hormones and of female ova or male sperm. Some common problems in the reproductive systems are menstrual problems such as dysmenorrhea, menorrhagia, and amenorrhea in females and hernia and prostate problems in males. Medical interventions are available to treat these problems.

# ➤ Conception, Pregnancy, and Childbirth

Pregnancies typically last about 40 weeks and are divided into three phases of about three months (13 weeks) each, referred to as **trimesters.**

### FIRST TRIMESTER

The first trimester lasts 12–13 weeks. During most of the first trimester, the ball of rapidly dividing cells is referred to as an **embryo.** From the 10th week onward, the unborn baby is called a **fetus.** Formation of all the vital organs, including the brain and spinal cord, occurs in the first trimester. The heart begins to beat, arms and legs grow, and the face and gender of the baby become distinguishable. In addition to the anatomical development, an organ called the *placenta* grows. Placentas allow unborn babies to obtain oxygen and nutrients and exchange waste products with their mother. At the end of the first trimester the baby is about 2–4 in. long and weighs 1–2 oz.

A 3-D ultrasound image of a male fetus aged 5 months.

**Trimesters** are the three phases of pregnancy, each about three months long.

An **embryo** is an unborn baby from conception through the eighth or ninth week of pregnancy.

A **fetus** is an unborn baby from about the 10th week of pregnancy to birth.

Weeks 14–26 are the second trimester of pregnancy. The organs that formed in the first trimester become more specialized and functional. The baby can swallow and digest, has waking and sleeping periods, and moves. Hair grows. At the end of the second trimester the baby is about 15 in. long and weighs 2–2½ lb.

## THIRD TRIMESTER

Weeks 27–40 are the final phase of pregnancy. During this period the fetus grows rapidly. Toward the end of the trimester the baby begins to change position in preparation for birth. Fetal lungs mature to the point that they will be ready to breathe air after birth, when the placenta stops providing oxygen. At birth an average baby weighs about 7–8 lb. and measures over 14 in. long. The third trimester culminates in labor and childbirth.

## COMPLICATIONS OF PREGNANCY AND CHILDBIRTH

Although most pregnancies culminate in the birth of a healthy baby, complications can sometimes occur. For instance, gestational diabetes is a form of diabetes that occurs only during pregnancy. The pregnancy affects the woman's pancreas, which produces insulin, so that levels of blood sugar become uncontrolled. (For more information on diabetes, see Chapter 10.) Urinary tract infections are also common during pregnancy, and if undiagnosed and untreated, they can cause premature labor.

When a fertilized egg implants in a location other than the uterus, such as in the fallopian tube or on the ovary itself, the result is an **ectopic pregnancy.** In some cases, the body rejects the embryo and the pregnancy ends naturally, but in other cases the embryo may rupture the fallopian tube, causing life-threatening problems, including massive hemorrhaging. The embryo and sometimes the fallopian tube need to be removed surgically to save the mother's life.

Normally placentas develop above the cervix inside the uterus, but occasionally a placenta will cover the cervix as it grows. This condition is called *placenta previa,* and it can cause severe bleeding beginning at the end of the second trimester. Treatment for placenta previa can range from bed rest during pregnancy to blood transfusions. Vaginal delivery is considered too dangerous due to risk of hemorrhaging. So, if the

**Ectopic pregnancy** occurs when a fertilized egg implants somewhere other than the uterus, usually in a fallopian tube.

mother has placenta previa at the end of pregnancy, the baby will be delivered via caesarian section (C section).

*Placental abruption* occurs when the placenta separates from the uterine wall before delivery, potentially depriving the baby of oxygen. Once the condition is diagnosed, depending on its severity, the treatment can include bed rest, hospitalization, or a caesarian section.

*Preeclampsia* is a condition characterized by high blood pressure, edema (the swelling of tissue from excess fluid), headaches, dizziness, vision problems, and stomach pain in the pregnant woman. It can also cause fetal distress and even fetal death. If not treated, preeclampsia can progress to *eclampsia,* which is characterized by seizures, coma, and sometimes death. If preeclampsia is severe enough, labor may be induced or an emergency C section may be performed to protect both mother and baby.

Premature labor is labor that occurs before 37 weeks of gestation. If premature labor cannot be stopped with bed rest and other means, medications may be prescribed to stop the contractions.

Postpartum depression is normally a mild depression that occurs three days to two weeks after delivery. Most times the depression ends naturally; however, there are some extreme cases where the depression requires counseling and medication.

Miscarriage is the expulsion of the embryo or fetus from the uterus before the middle of the second trimester. In most cases, a miscarriage is due to a problem with a lack of progesterone being produced during the first and second trimesters. During the first and second trimesters of pregnancy, significant amounts of progesterone are produced until the placenta matures. However, if the production of progesterone decreases before the placenta is mature, then a miscarriage can result.

## ➤ Contraception

Unless you are actively trying to have a baby or would not object to an unexpected pregnancy, it is very important to use contraception whenever you engage in sexual activity. Table 5.1 details each of the contraceptive methods by type, failure rates, risk, availability and convenience.

### HORMONAL METHODS

**Hormonal contraceptives** such as injections, implants, birth control pills, and the contraceptive patch or ring are made from estrogen and/

---

**Hormonal contraceptives** introduce progestin and/or estrogen into a woman's body in order to suppress ovulation.

| TYPE OF CONTRACEPTIVE | DESCRIPTION | FAILURE RATE (number of pregnancies expected per 100 women per year) | SOME RISKS | PROTECTION FROM SEXUALLY TRANSMITTED DISEASES (STIs) | AVAILABILITY |
|---|---|---|---|---|---|
| Male Condom Latex/Polyurethane | A sheath placed over the erect penis blocking the passage of sperm. | 11–16 | Irritation and allergic reactions (less likely with polyurethane) | Except for abstinence, latex condoms are the best protection against STIs, including gonorrhea and AIDS. | Nonprescription |
| Female Condom | A lubricated polyurethane sheath shaped similarly to the male condom. The closed end has a flexible ring that is inserted in the vagina. | 20 | Irritation and allergic reactions | May give some STI protection; not as effective as latex condom. | Nonprescription |
| Diaphragm with Spermicide | A dome-shaped rubber disk with a flexible rim that covers the cervix so that sperm cannot reach the uterus. A spermicide is applied to the diaphragm before insertion. | 15 | Irritation and allergic reactions, urinary tract infection. Risk of toxic shock syndrome, a rare but serious infection, when kept in place longer than recommended. | None | Prescription |
| Spermicide Alone | A foam, cream, jelly, film, suppository, or tablet that contains nonoxynol-9, a sperm-killing chemical. | 20–50 (studies have shown varying effectiveness rates) | Irritation and allergic reactions, urinary tract infections | None | Nonprescription |

*(Continued)*

**TABLE 5.1    CONTRACEPTIVE DEVICES AND APPROACHES BY TYPE, FAILURE RATE, RISKS, AND AVAILABILITY (continued)**

| TYPE OF CONTRACEPTIVE | DESCRIPTION | FAILURE RATE (number of pregnancies expected per 100 women per year) | SOME RISKS | PROTECTION FROM SEXUALLY TRANSMITTED DISEASES (STIs) | AVAILABILITY |
|---|---|---|---|---|---|
| Oral Contraceptives— -combined pill -Progestin-only minipill -91-day regimen (Seasonale) | A pill that suppresses ovulation by the combined actions of the hormones estrogen and progestin. A chewable form was approved in November 2003. | 5 | Dizziness; nausea; changes in menstruation, mood, and weight; rarely cardiovascular disease, including high blood pressure, blood clots, heart attack, and strokes | None | Prescription |
| Patch (Ortho Evra) | Skin patch worn on the lower abdomen, buttocks, or upper body that releases the hormones progestin and estrogen into the bloodstream. | 5 Appears to be less effective in women weighing more than 198 pounds. | Similar to oral contraceptives— combined pill | None | Prescription |
| Vaginal Contraceptive Ring (NuvaRing) | A flexible ring about 2 inches in diameter that is inserted into the vagina and releases the hormones progestin and estrogen. | 5 | Vaginal discharge, vaginitis, irritation. Similar to oral contraceptives—combined pill | None | Prescription |
| Postcoital Contraceptives (Preven and Plan B) | Pills containing either progestin alone or progestin plus estrogen | Almost 80 percent reduction in risk of pregnancy for a single act of unprotected sex | Nausea, vomiting, abdominal pain, fatigue, headache | None | Prescription |

| Method | How it works | Failure rate | Risks | STDs | How to obtain |
|---|---|---|---|---|---|
| Injection —Depo-Provera —Lunelle | An injectable progestin that inhibits ovulation, prevents sperm from reaching the egg, and prevents the fertilized egg from implanting in the uterus. | Less than 1 | Irregular bleeding, weight gain, breast tenderness, headaches | None | Prescription |
| IUD (Intrauterine Device) | A T-shaped device inserted into the uterus by a health professional. | Less than 1 | Cramps, bleeding, pelvic inflammatory disease, infertility, perforation of uterus | None | Prescription |
| Periodic Abstinence | To deliberately refrain from having sexual intercourse during times when pregnancy is more likely. | 20 | None | None | Instructions from health care provider |
| Transabdominal Surgical Sterilization—female —Falope Ring, —Hulka Clip, —Filshie Clip or —Essure System | The woman's fallopian tubes are blocked so the egg and sperm can't meet in the fallopian tube, preventing conception. | Less than 1 | Pain, bleeding, infection, other postsurgical complications, ectopic (tubal) pregnancy | None | Surgery |
| Surgical Sterilization—male | Sealing, tying, or cutting a man's vas deferens so that the sperm can't travel from the testicles to the penis. | Less than 1 | Pain, bleeding, infection, other postsurgical complications | None | Surgery |

Note: Failure rates are based on information from clinical trials submitted to the U.S. Food and Drug Administration (FDA) during product reviews. This number represents the percentage of women who become pregnant during the first year using a birth control method. For methods that the FDA does not review, such as periodic abstinence, numbers are estimated from published literature. For comparison, about 85 out of 100 sexually active women who wish to have a child and do not use contraception become pregnant within one year of first trying to conceive.

Source: Food and Drug Administration, April 2010.

or progesterone (sometimes called by its synthetic form, progestin). These contraceptives biologically simulate pregnancy in the woman's body, thus suppressing ovulation. In addition, some of the hormonal methods thicken cervical mucus, which impedes the movement of sperm. Hormonal methods of contraception are very effective, with a failure rate of only 1–5 percent depending on the type of hormonal method used. In the United States they are available only by prescription. Usually a physician conducts a comprehensive physical evaluation to ensure that the woman does not have risk factors that would rule out their use.

**Birth control pills** come in a variety of dosages and strengths and are taken either daily or for three weeks each month, depending on the type of pill. Side effects include high blood pressure, headaches, diabetes, elevated cholesterol levels, and blood clots.

**Contraceptive implants** are surgically placed under the skin of the upper arm. The implants contain progestin and can suppress ovulation for up to five years. Implanon, consisting of a single capsule and providing protection for three years, was approved by the FDA in 2006 and is now available.

Injectable contraceptives are administered via a shot in the arm or buttocks and provide protection for approximately 14 weeks. The best known injectable is **Depo-Provera,** but others are under development. Each injection is generally effective for three months.

The vaginal ring is a flexible plastic ring that contains low levels of hormones. It is inserted into the vagina and left in place around the cervix for approximately three weeks and then removed for one week for menstruation. A new ring is inserted every month.

The contraceptive patch contains hormones that slowly absorb into the body through the skin. The patch can be placed on the buttocks, upper arm, or upper torso and is changed once a week for three weeks and then not worn one week during menstruation.

Hormonal methods of contraception have the advantage of providing long-term, highly effective protection against pregnancy with little effort on the part of the woman. However, hormonal methods are not for all women because some of the side effects mentioned earlier can be significant and result in medical emergencies.

---

The **birth control pill,** commonly known as "the pill," is a hormonal method of contraception in pill form.

**Contraceptive implants,** such as Implanon, are surgically inserted under the skin and can provide hormonal contraception for up to five years.

**Depo-Provera** is a hormonal method of contraception delivered in an injection.

## BARRIER METHODS

Barrier methods of contraception include the intrauterine device (IUD), condom, sponge, diaphragm, and cervical cap. These methods work by blocking sperm from traveling through the cervix and into the uterus and fallopian tubes. Some of the barrier methods—such as the sponge, diaphragm, and cervical cap—also use a chemical that kills sperm (spermicide), making them even more effective.

Intrauterine devices (IUDs) must be placed in a woman's uterus by a trained medical professional. They can remain in place and provide highly reliable contraception for 1 to 10 years.

An **IUD** is a small, T-shaped, plastic or copper device that is inserted into the uterus by a physician. Depending upon the type, the IUD can be left in place for 1 to 10 years. There are two types of IUDs: copper (brand name ParaGard) and hormonal (brand name Mirena). In addition to being "T" shaped, they both release either a metal or a hormone, and the resulting action is a bit different. The copper released by ParaGard prevents sperm from reaching and fertilizing an egg. The progestin released from Mirena prevents the ovary from releasing an egg. ParaGard can stay in the uterus 5 to 10 years, and Mirena can stay in the uterus for up to 5 years. The effectiveness of the IUD as a contraceptive method is high, with a failure rate of only 1–2 percent. Some relatively rare side effects of IUDs include uterine perforations, cramping, and heavy bleeding.

A **diaphragm** is a thick, flexible concave rubber structure with a hard but flexible outer ring. It is inserted into the vagina and placed over the cervix, forming a barrier to sperm. A small amount of spermicide is placed in the diaphragm and around the rim to kill any sperm that penetrate the physical barrier. For maximum effectiveness, the diaphragm must be inserted before intercourse and be left in place for six hours

An **IUD** (intrauterine device) is a barrier method of contraception in which a small plastic or copper unit is placed in the uterus. It is thought to function by affecting the movement of sperm and/or egg or preventing fertilization.

A **diaphragm** is a concave latex "cup" that is inserted into the vagina and serves as barrier method of contraception.

afterwards. The failure rate for the diaphragm can be as high as 15 percent. If the diaphragm is left in place for an extended period of time, there is a small risk of toxic shock syndrome, a dangerous bacterial infection.

The **cervical cap** is a small, flexible cap that is inserted into the vagina and placed over the cervix to form a barrier to sperm. Like the diaphragm, it is used with spermicide. It can be left in place for longer— up to 48 hours. The failure rate can be as high as 22 percent. As with the diaphragm, there is a slight risk of toxic shock syndrome if the cervical cap is left in place too long.

**Sponges** are round soft foam devices that contain a spermicide. It is inserted into the vagina and covers the cervix. It can be worn up to 30 hours and can be inserted 24 hours before sex. Failure rates are between 16–32 percent.

**Condoms** are the most common and popular type of barrier contraception because they do not require a prescription, are available in many stores, and are fairly inexpensive and simple to use. Condoms are made and marketed for both males and females, but the more popular ones are male condoms.

The male condom is a tightly rolled latex sheath that is worn by unrolling it down over an erect penis. During intercourse, semen is ejaculated into the condom, thus preventing sperm from entering the vagina. The failure rate is approximately 15 percent. Male condoms not only help prevent pregnancy, but they also provide protection against sexually transmitted infections (STIs). They are available in a wide variety of brands, colors, and styles, with and without lubricants and spermicides. Condoms that contain the spermicide nonoxynol-9 (N-9) in some cases have been found to increase tissue irritation, which can increase the likelihood of STI transmission. (See this chapter's "Breaking It Down.")

The female condom is a polyurethane sheath with a flexible ring on each end. The ring on the closed end is inserted into the back of the vagina and the other ring remains outside the vagina. During intercourse, the sheath creates a barrier to sperm. The failure rate for female condoms is 20 percent, more than that for male condoms.

**Spermicides** are chemicals marketed in many forms: gels, foams, suppositories, and jellies. These chemicals are inserted into the vagina before intercourse. In theory, when sperm are ejaculated into the

**Cervical cap** is similar to the diaphragm but smaller.

**Sponges** are a soft foam-like barrier method of contraception.

**Condoms** are latex devices that either cover the penis (male condom) or line the vagina (female condom) and serve as a barrier to sperm.

**Spermicides** are chemicals that kill sperm.

vagina, the spermicide kills them. To be effective, the spermicide should be placed in the vagina one hour before intercourse, and if intercourse is repeated, more spermicide should be used. The failure rate is 20–30 percent.

Combining barrier methods can significantly decrease failure rate. For example, use of both spermicides and condoms can be 95 percent effective in preventing pregnancies.

## SURGICAL METHODS

Vasectomy for men and tubal ligation for women are the two most common surgical methods of contraception. Neither procedure should have an effect on sex drive.

The **vasectomy** is a simple surgical procedure in which the vas deferens in each testis is cut, and the exposed ends are sealed by cauterization (burning with special instruments). After cauterization the exposed end is folded back and tied. Sperm are still produced and released but are not able to progress past the cauterized, tied end of the vas deferens. The vasectomy takes about 20–30 minutes and can be done in a physician's office under local anesthesia.

**Tubal ligation** is usually done in a surgical facility under general anesthesia, but the principle is similar. An incision is made in the lower abdomen, and the fallopian tubes are cut, cauterized, and tied back. Mature ova are still produced, and menstruation still occurs, but the egg that is released into the fallopian tube will travel only as far as the cauterized, tied end of the fallopian tube. Sterilization implants (brand name Essure) and the procedure are relatively new and involve placing a thin tube into each fallopian tube. After about three months scar tissue forms in the fallopian tube, which prevents movement of both the egg and sperm, resulting in sterilization.

Vasectomy, tubal ligation, and sterilization implants should be considered permanent. Although the procedures can be reversed in some cases, there is no guarantee that reversal will be successful.

Self
Assessment
5.1

## NATURAL METHODS

Of course, the most natural method of birth control—complete abstinence from sexual intercourse—is also the most effective. But another

---

**Vasectomy** is a surgical method of contraception for men, where the vas deferens are cut, cauterized, and tied to block movement of sperm.

**Tubal ligation** is a surgical method of contraception for women, where the fallopian tubes are cut, cauterized, and tied to block movement of both sperm and ova.

Nonoxynol-9 (N-9) has been used as a spermicide since the early 1980s. Because N-9 had demonstrated an ability to kill HIV in a laboratory setting, condoms containing N-9 were recommended as one of the key public health interventions to prevent the spread of HIV/AIDS. For about 15 years most public health prevention messages emphasized use of condoms containing N-9. But now studies have found that N-9 is not only ineffective at stopping the spread of HIV, but it has actually increased risk of disease transmission. How could this have occurred?

The problem originated because officials and product manufacturers made a critical error: They assumed that if N-9 killed HIV in the laboratory, it automatically must be effective in real-world situations involving sex. Unfortunately, this proved untrue. The evidence against the effectiveness of N-9 was highlighted in a 2000 study of N-9 use among sex workers in South Africa and Thailand. A chief finding of this study was that the incidence of HIV was higher among women using N-9 than among those using a similar product without N-9. Even worse, some people who used N-9 frequently had problems with tissue damage. This led the Centers for Disease Control and Prevention and the World Health Organization to the following conclusions:

- N-9 is ineffective at killing the HIV virus and other STIs.
- When used vaginally multiple times a day, N-9 can cause genital lesions that may increase a woman's risk of acquiring HIV.
- Condoms lubricated with a small amount of N-9 are no more effective in preventing pregnancy than are lubricated condoms without N-9.

The case against N-9 was so strong that major condom manufacturers like Johnson & Johnson discontinued production of condoms containing N-9. The Planned Parenthood Federation of America also recommended that production of condoms containing N-9 be stopped.

N-9's plunge in popularity reflects an important principle in science and health. When new information from scientific studies discredits a "sound" prevention approach, then industry and society respond, and in this case they responded appropriately. It also shows how important it is for us to keep our health knowledge current. "Best practices" in all areas of health continue to evolve. What may have been the gold standard in treatment last decade could turn out to be less than optimal as scientific evidence builds up.

**natural method** of birth control that is used by some sexually active women is referred to as *fertility awareness* or *periodic abstinence*. This method requires a woman to accurately predict when she is ovulating on the basis of body temperature and other signs and determine "safe" versus "unsafe" days for intercourse. Accurately monitoring body temperature is key—body temperature drops slightly just before ovulation and rises slightly afterward. A woman using the fertility awareness method takes her temperature with a special thermometer (called a *basal body temperature thermometer*) every morning before she gets out of bed. When her temperature drops and then rises, she can assume that ovulation is taking place. She abstains from intercourse on the 10–12 days per month she is fertile (from about 7 days prior to ovulation to about 3 days after). Since so much effort is required and the margin for error is great, periodic abstinence has a failure rate of 14–47 percent.

Withdrawal is also considered a method of natural birth control. With this method, at the point of orgasm the penis is removed from the vagina so that ejaculation occurs outside the vagina. But withdrawal is very ineffective for two reasons: first, some sperm are in the pre-ejaculate fluid, and second, withdrawal requires a significant amount of self-discipline.

## EMERGENCY CONTRACEPTION

Emergency contraception can be used after unprotected sex or when contraception fails (such as a condom breaking). Emergency contraception usually consists of a "morning after" pill that contains enough hormones to cause a woman's period to come early. This "restarts" a woman's monthly fertility cycle, so that pregnancy does not occur.

Plan B One-Step is a widely available emergency contraception. The pill is taken no more than 72 hours after unprotected intercourse. It is available over the counter to women 18 years of age and older. Women under 18 need a prescription.

Ulipristal is another emergency contraceptive drug. It can be taken up to 5 days after sexual intercourse.

---

**Natural methods** of birth control are methods that are designed to reinforce abstaining from sexual intercourse. They include fertility awareness, or determining the days a women is most fertile (i.e., releasing an egg) and, if pregnancy is not desired, abstaining from intercourse on these days. Another method is withdrawal, or removing the penis from the vagina just before orgasm.

## TERMINATION OF PREGNANCY

In everyday language the term **abortion** usually refers to ending a pregnancy by choice. But medically speaking, the word *abortion* is more generic, describing both "natural" losses, when the body rejects a developing embryo or fetus, as well as surgical or medical procedures that interrupt pregnancy. *Miscarriage* is the common term for a **spontaneous abortion** that occurs in the first half of a pregnancy. Death of a fetus after week 20 in a pregnancy is often referred to as *stillbirth*. And medically speaking, ending a pregnancy by choice is usually referred to as **artificial abortion.**

Pregnancies end via spontaneous abortion about 20 percent of the time, usually within the first 90 days of pregnancy. Many of these pregnancy losses are due to genetic problems in the developing fetus or from problems in the uterine environment. Often, levels of progesterone, which must be high the first 90 days of pregnancy until a placenta develops fully, decline suddenly and significantly. When levels get too low, the pituitary gland secretes a chemical called oxytocin, which causes the uterus to contract and expel the embryo or fetus.

Methods for terminating a pregnancy by choice differ based largely on the stage of pregnancy during which they are performed. During the first trimester, a surgical procedure called dilation and curettage (D&C) may be used to remove the embryo from the uterus. The cervix is dilated, and a suction curette, a hollow tube, is inserted into the uterus; the contents of the uterus are then suctioned out. Another surgical procedure used during the first trimester is *manual vacuum aspiration*. This method is similar to suction curettage but can be performed earlier in pregnancy. Both procedures are performed under local anesthetic at a clinic or medical facility.

Drugs called *abortifacients* may also be used during the first trimester. They cause a change in the balance of hormones in the body and lead to uterine bleeding and expulsion of the embryo. RU-486, consisting of the two drugs mifepristone and misoprostol, is an example of an abortifacient.

The most common second trimester abortion method is *dilation and evacuation* (D&E), a procedure somewhat similar to a D&C. Other options include labor and hysterotomy. In labor induction abortions, which are performed rarely, saline solution and prostaglandins are injected into the uterus, killing the fetus and inducing labor. The fetus is delivered 2 to 4 days after the procedure. Hysterotomy is a

---

**Abortion** is the expulsion of an embryo or fetus from the uterus before it has fully developed. **Spontaneous abortion,** often called miscarriage, is the body's rejection of the embryo or fetus. **Artificial abortion** is a medical procedure that is used when a woman chooses to terminate her pregnancy.

surgical procedure in which incisions are made in the lower abdomen and uterus and the fetus is surgically removed.

According to the Guttmacher Institute (2008), a prominent non-profit organization that focuses on sexual health and public education, more than 1 million artificial abortions are performed in the United States each year. The typical profile of a woman who has an abortion is a never-married white woman, under 25 years of age. Further, 89 percent of abortions are done during the first trimester, and fewer than 1 percent are performed after the 20th week of pregnancy.

Although there can be physical complications with abortions, the risk is minimal, especially if done early in the pregnancy. Psychological and emotional consequences are difficult to measure because it is such a deeply personal issue and very much grounded in morality and religious beliefs. Long-term, scientifically sound studies, while difficult, should be conducted to determine psychological and emotional consequences of abortion.

## THE ABORTION CONTROVERSY

Abortion has become one of the most highly charged issues of modern times in American politics and society. Opponents of abortion, the so-called pro-life camp, base their opposition on the belief that human life begins at the moment of conception. According to this view, ending that life at any time, for any reason, is morally wrong and ought to be illegal. On the other side, the so-called pro-choice camp believes that women should have the right to choose the circumstances under which they have children. According to this view, the decision regarding

✓ **NEED TO KNOW**

Pregnancy can be prevented. Knowing the options regarding contraceptive methods and how those methods work is important in making the best individual choice. Abstinence is the only method of contraception that is 100 percent effective. Hormonal methods biologically simulate pregnancy through use of synthetic hormones, but they can have side effects. Barrier methods block movement of the sperm and prevent them from reaching the ovum. Surgical methods—vasectomy and tubal ligation—are invasive and should be considered permanent. The fertility awareness method requires careful body monitoring to determine the unsafe days for intercourse. When contraception fails, it is mostly due to human error. Choosing to terminate a pregnancy through abortion is a deeply personal and difficult decision. The invasiveness of the procedure depends on when in the pregnancy it is performed.

Contraception

## Health & the Media Pregnancy Prevention

Since 2000, the National Campaign to Prevent Teen Pregnancy has sponsored an annual contest with cash prizes for 13- to 21-year-olds to design a public service announcement (PSA). The assignment is to create a compelling magazine ad with a catchy slogan and image to spread the message of teen-pregnancy prevention. The top PSAs appear in magazines nationwide. This winning PSA reflects a realistic view of a teenager speaking to other teenagers. It suggests abstinence but also emphasizes contraception for those who have sex. The message clearly communicates responsibility without being preachy. The National Campaign is working to build a more coordinated and effective grassroots movement and to influence cultural values by teaming with the entertainment media and other influential sectors in society.

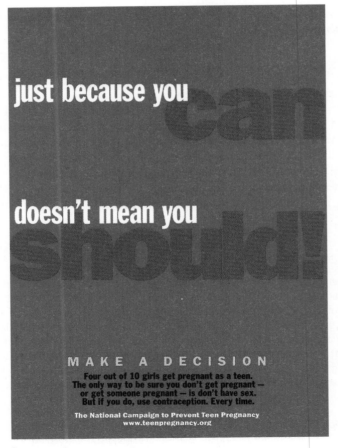

just because you can

doesn't mean you should!

MAKE A DECISION

Four out of 10 girls get pregnant as a teen.
The only way to be sure you don't get pregnant —
or get someone pregnant — is don't have sex.
But if you do, use contraception. Every time.

The National Campaign to Prevent Teen Pregnancy
www.teenpregnancy.org

Source: **www.teenpregnancy.org**

whether to continue a pregnancy or end it is a personal one that (within certain limits) should stay a private matter that is not interfered with by the government.

Fetal viability, or the age at which a fetus can survive outside the uterus, has become a key issue in the abortion debate. By 24 weeks gestation, there is a 40 percent chance for survival outside the uterus, whereas by week 28 in a pregnancy (near the beginning of the third trimester), the chance of survival is 90 percent.

## ➤ Sexual Behavior

Hormones influence not only reproductive processes but also how people experience and express their sexuality. Humans have a biological urge for sexual activity known as the *sex drive* (or libido), driven primarily by testosterone. The sex drive also has cognitive and emotional components. For example, a person can become sexually aroused just by thinking or fantasizing about sex and sexual images.

Article 5.1

The sex drive usually becomes intense in both boys and girls at puberty. The libido is highest for men in their late teens and early 20s and for women in their mid-20s into their 30s.

The Centers for Disease Control and Prevention (CDC) have surveyed sexual behavior among Americans and have reported the following findings for adults aged 25–44 (Chandra et al., 2011):

- 97 percent of men and 98 percent of women have had vaginal intercourse.
- 90 percent of men and 89 percent of women have had oral sex with an opposite-sex partner.
- 44 percent of men and 36 percent of women have had anal sex with an opposite-sex partner.
- 12 percent of women and 5.8 percent of men ages 25-44 reported any same-sex contact in their lifetime.

The survey also showed there is a high percentage of sexual activity in younger age groups. Roughly 40 percent of adolescents report having sex for the first time between ages 15 and 17. Seventy percent of 18- and 19-year-olds reported having sex with the opposite sex.

Sexual behaviors are influenced by a variety of factors, including individual biology and personality, personal values and beliefs, family and cultural influences, and the media. People often wonder if they are normal in terms of what is sexually arousing to them, how frequently they engage in sexual activity, how they express themselves sexually (e.g., through masturbation, intercourse, etc.), and so on. For better or worse, there is no real answer to the question, What is normal sexual behavior? Sex drive and sexual behavior are deeply personal matters, and although

Article 5.2

there are some universals, there is also tremendous variation. Further, sex drive varies significantly over the course of the lifespan. To try to establish norms and benchmarks is misleading and ultimately meaningless.

## THE HUMAN SEXUAL RESPONSE MODEL

Although scientists have long understood human reproduction, the physiology of the human sexual response was not well understood until the 1970s, when William Masters and Virginia Johnson conducted their groundbreaking clinical research on sexuality. Masters and Johnson studied the physiological changes that occur during sexual activity and identified four major stages in human sexual response: excitement, plateau, orgasm, and resolution. They also identified differences between the sexual response of men and women, adding to the body of knowledge about men's and women's sexual health.

According to the **human sexual response model** (Figure 5.6), the first phase is excitement, when both males and females become sexually aroused. Signs of arousal include erection of the penis in men and vaginal lubrication and swelling of the clitoris in women. Heart and breathing rates increase. As arousal intensifies, there is a transition to the plateau stage, a leveling off of sensation just before orgasm. Muscle tension increases, the penis increases in size, and the upper part of the vagina expands. The third phase is orgasm, a reflex involving a massive discharge of nerve impulses, causing muscle contractions in the genital area, sensations of intense pleasure, and, in men, the ejaculation of semen. The last phase is resolution, a return to a relaxed, pre-arousal state.

During the resolution phase, men experience a refractory period, during which blood vessels are constricted and the penis is flaccid so they are not able to experience another orgasm. The refractory period can last from minutes to hours. Women do not experience a refractory period.

As mentioned previously, women and men experience the sexual response differently. For example, the excitement and plateau phases tend to be longer for women than men—it generally takes women longer than men to become aroused. Another difference is that men experience one orgasm, and women can experience multiple orgasms. These are normal differences between the sexes that may or may not make any difference in a relationship.

When a sexual problem does occur in a relationship, it may take the form of a man experiencing excitement, plateau, and orgasm while the woman is still experiencing excitement. As a result he is sexually satisfied

---

The **human sexual response model** is a four-stage model of the physiology of sexual response; the four stages are excitement, plateau, orgasm, and resolution.

## FIGURE 5.6 HUMAN SEXUAL RESPONSE

Note: A, B, and C represent three different female sexual responses.
Source: From William H. Masters and Virginia E. Johnson, *Human Sexual Response,* Figures 1-1 & 1-2, p. 5. Copyright © 1966 by William H. Masters and Virginia E. Johnson. Boston: Little, Brown and Company.

while she is still only aroused. The solution generally recommended is that there be more foreplay to increase the woman's arousal level. It is more natural physiologically for men to extend the excitement and plateau phases than for women to try to shorten these phases. Issues involving the human sexual response are often issues affecting couples, and couples need to work together to deal with them. Good communication skills are essential to satisfying sexual relationships.

## SEXUAL DYSFUNCTION

At some point in their lives, most people experience sexual problems or dysfunctions. **Sexual dysfunctions** are usually categorized as disorders of desire or arousal, orgasm disorders, and pain disorders.

Sexual desire disorders, or lack of interest in sex, can affect both men and women, as can sexual arousal disorders. Both disorders can be related to hormone levels, the ability to relax, and to a certain extent, wellness— that is, how well a person is functioning physically, mentally, and socially. Low levels of testosterone in men and estrogen in women can reduce desire and arousal, as can high levels of stress, emotional problems, worries and anxiety, and problems in the relationship. Certain medical conditions can also affect arousal, such as back pain, heart problems, endocrine disorders, or an enlarged prostate. Interventions for sexual

**Sexual dysfunctions** are common sexual disorders including sexual desire disorders, sexual arousal disorders, orgasm disorders, and sexual pain disorders.

desire and sexual arousal disorders include medications, relaxation techniques, and, if appropriate, counseling and education.

Sexual arousal disorder in men can result in erectile dysfunction (ED), also known as *impotence*. ED is the inability to achieve and/or maintain an erection long enough to have intercourse. ED is both a symptom of a condition and a condition itself. The causes of ED can range from low testosterone levels to depression and anxiety or vascular disease, including coronary artery disease. Sometimes medications that are used to treat a variety of conditions—including high blood pressure, diabetes, and depression and anxiety—can also cause ED as a side effect. The anxiety associated with ED can be emotionally damaging and can exacerbate the condition.

There are interventions that treat the symptom of erectile dysfunction and allow a man to achieve and maintain an erection long enough for intercourse without treating the underlying problem. Medications like Viagra act directly on the blood vessels that carry blood to the penis. When these blood vessels relax and dilate, they allow the erectile tissue in the penis to become engorged, producing an erection. Viagra allows a man to have an erection even in the midst of anxiety.

In women, sexual arousal disorders can result in the inability to relax vaginal muscles long enough to allow intercourse, to produce enough vaginal lubrication, or to attain orgasm. Intercourse can then be painful or undesirable. Unlike ED, sexual arousal disorders in women are not easy to treat with a drug. However, the symptoms can be treated with a lubricant to make vaginal penetration by a penis less painful and with muscle relaxants or minor tranquilizers to induce relaxation of vaginal muscles and allow orgasm to occur.

Both women and men can experience orgasm disorders, although such problems are more common in women. The chief symptom is delayed or absent orgasm. In many cases, lack of orgasm is due to timing differences between men and women, as described earlier, and the issue is more likely one of couple communication. Other causes of orgasm disorder include psychological or emotional problems, lack of knowledge, problems in the relationship, and the use of drugs or medications.

Sexual pain, or pain during or after intercourse, known as *dyspareunia,* is an unusual disorder that can affect both men and women. In women, dyspareunia may be caused by vaginismus, involuntary contractions of the vagina that make penetration painful, or by lack of vaginal lubrication. Vaginismus can have physical causes (e.g., pelvic inflammatory disease), which should be treated by a physician, or psychological causes, which may call for relaxation techniques or counseling. Lack of vaginal lubrication can be addressed with longer foreplay or with commercial lubrication products. In men, dyspareunia is generally related to infections of the urethra or inflammation of the urethra or foreskin, in some cases caused by a sexually transmitted infection. Men experiencing pain during or after intercourse should see their physician.

## ✓ NEED TO KNOW

Human sexual response consists of excitement, plateau, orgasm, and resolution. This response is different for males and females. Males have shorter excitement and plateau phases, one orgasm, and resolution. Women experience longer excitement and plateau phases, can have multiple orgasms, and have a slower resolution. These natural biological differences can become problematic in a relationship, particularly for a woman, so good communication is needed to ensure mutual sexual satisfaction. Sexual dysfunctions can have physiological or psychological origins, and most are a combination of both. Sexual arousal disorders, erectile dysfunction, orgasm disorders, and sexual pain are examples of sexual dysfunctions that most often require medical intervention, which can range from medication to counseling or be a combination of the two. The dysfunctions are common and treatable.

## ➤ Gender Identity and Sexual Orientation

Up to this point this chapter has focused on the anatomy and physiology of human sexuality. The second half of the equation is how people express their sexuality. As noted at the beginning of the chapter, biological sex is determined at the chromosomal level and physically manifested in the appearance of the external genitals. Gender, on the other hand, is a concept defined more by a particular culture. Gender consists of the traits that a culture ascribes to males and females, contributing to what are considered "masculine" and "feminine" attributes and behaviors. **Gender identity** is the sense a person has that he or she is male or female.

Self Assessment 5.2

By 18–30 months of age, children have a clear sense of whether they are boys or girls. Between the ages of 5 and 7, children solidify their sense of gender identity and strive to be consistent with their identity by employing stereotypes as rules. Between the ages of 7 and 12, children achieve gender stability, which is the cognitive understanding that gender is permanent. Both gender identity and stability are normally well formed prior to puberty.

**Gender identity** is a person's sense of being male or female.

In rare instances and for mostly unknown reasons, some individuals experience a conflict between their biological sex and their gender identity. Boys or girls may feel they are "really" the opposite sex, rather than the gender that their body has. Individuals who experience this sense of gender dysphoria may be considered to have gender identity disorder and may be referred to as *cross-gender identified* or *transgendered*. Gender identity is not the same as sexual orientation. In other words, a transgendered person may either be homosexual or heterosexual.

**Sexual orientation** is commonly defined as an enduring emotional, romantic, and sexual attraction to members of one's own sex or of the opposite sex. It is generally recognized that sexual orientation exists along a continuum, with interest in romantic relationships exclusively with members of the same sex at one end of the continuum (homosexuality) and interest in romantic relationships exclusively with members of the opposite sex on the other end of the continuum (heterosexuality). Being attracted to and interested in members of both sexes falls in the middle of the continuum (bisexuality).

People can fall anywhere along this continuum, although social pressures encourage most people to identify themselves as heterosexual. The National Center for Health Statistics (2005) reported that among men aged 18–44, about 90 percent think of themselves as heterosexual, 2.3 percent say they are homosexual (gay), 1.8 percent report being bisexual, 3.9 percent "something else," and 1.8 percent did not answer the question. Among women in the same age group, about 90 percent say they are heterosexual, slightly over 1 percent identify as homosexual (lesbian), and almost 3 percent say they are bisexual.

It is not clear what causes a person's sexual orientation, but it is most likely an interaction of environment and individual biology, including genetics and hormonal factors. People do not choose their sexual orientation, although they can choose to express it or conceal it. Gay men and lesbians are often the targets of homophobia (fear of homosexuality) and may experience prejudice, discrimination, and even violence. Sometimes people experience so much conflict about their sexual orientation that they conceal it from themselves, which can lead to depression and other psychological problems.

Homosexuality is not a mental illness. Rather, it is a normal variation in one aspect of human experience. Abundant research indicates that gay men and lesbians are as mentally healthy as their heterosexual counterparts and equally competent at citizenship, parenting, and relationships.

**Sexual orientation** is emotional, romantic, and sexual attraction to people of the same or the opposite sex.

## ✓ NEED TO KNOW

Gender identity and sexual orientation are different. Gender identity is one's sense of being male or female. A person who experiences a conflict between his or her biological sex and gender identity may be said to have gender identity disorder. Sexual orientation is enduring emotional, romantic, and sexual attraction to members of one's own or the opposite sex. Sexual orientation exists along a continuum from exclusive hetero-sexuality through bisexuality to exclusive homosexuality. Sexual orientation is influenced by both biological (genetic, hormonal) factors and environmental (family, societal, cultural) factors. People do not choose their sexual orientation.

# ➤ Healthy Relationships

Sexuality is an integral part of adult intimate relationships, but it is just one facet of relationships. Healthy relationships meet many more human needs than the sexual one. In his hierarchy-of-needs model, Abraham Maslow identified love and belonging as basic human needs; these needs can be met only in relationships. Besides love and belonging, intimate relationships offer such comforts as emotional intimacy, affirmation and acceptance, companionship, connection to others, and security for the future. Healthy relationships are central to wellness.

Article
5.3

## COMMITTED RELATIONSHIPS AND MARRIAGE

Most Americans meet their emotional needs in committed partnerships, whether marriage or cohabiting relationship. As a highly sanctioned social institution, marriage offers a great number of benefits, including economic benefits. Approximately 74 percent of Americans marry at least once in their life, reflecting the importance placed on marriage by the majority of the population. Research studies indicate that marriage is also good for your health—married people live longer than unmarried people, score higher on assessments of mental health, have lower rates of certain illnesses, and report being happier. Strong and supportive relationships of all kinds can offer some of the same benefits.

It has been reported that about half of all couples marrying today in the United States will eventually divorce. This statistic can be misleading, however; a more realistic percentage may be 40 percent. According to a U.S. Census Bureau report, marriages "are most susceptible to divorce in the early years of marriage. After 5 years approximately ten percent of marriages are expected to end in divorce, and another ten percent divorce by the tenth anniversary" (Kreider & Fields, 1996). The remaining 20 percent of all divorces happen between the 11- and 50-year mark.

This shows that after a couple's 10th anniversary, the likelihood of divorce greatly decreases.

## HEALTHY AND UNHEALTHY RELATIONSHIPS

The most important elements of a healthy relationship are respect, trust, support, honesty, accountability, and shared responsibility. Respect is expressed by not constantly negatively criticizing or judging your partner's beliefs and actions and by performing helping behaviors that make his or her life easier. Trust, honesty, and support involve sharing open communication, willingness to admit mistakes, and the ability to take responsibility for your behavior. Shared responsibility means that work in the relationship, both emotional work and physical work, is shared equally.

In an unhealthy relationship, on the other hand, power is often unequal, and one partner tries to dominate or control the other. The Iowa Coalition Against Violence developed criteria to assess relationships. The following seven points summarize this criteria. In a healthy relationship, most answers will be yes.

Article
5.4

1. I can explain what I like and admire about my partner.
2. My partner is glad I have other friends, and has other friends himself/herself.
3. My partner is happy about my interests, accomplishments, and ambitions.

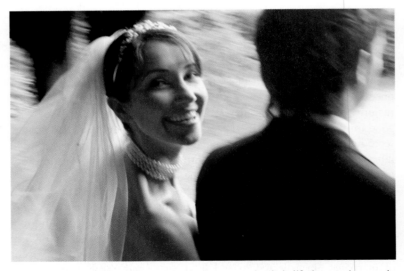

About 74 percent of Americans marry at least once in their lifetime, and research indicates people in committed relationships enjoy improved overall health compared to those who are not in committed relationships.

4. My partner has interests, accomplishments, and ambitions outside of me.
5. My partner has a good relationship with his/her family.
6. My partner takes responsibility for his/her actions and doesn't blame others for failures.
7. My partner talks about feelings, listens to me, and respects my opinions.

## COMMUNICATION AND CONFLICT RESOLUTION SKILLS

One way to improve relationships is by developing better communication and conflict resolution skills. Communication is key in both avoiding and resolving conflict. Conflict is simply disagreement between two people. Clear, open, and honest communication between people can cut down on conflict in relationships. Although some conflict is inevitable because people think and feel differently about things, it is very important not to allow conflict to become a contest where one must win at all costs. Differences in opinions are not contests. There is not a winner and a loser.

All the approaches to resolving conflict are intended to have a win-win outcome. In resolving conflict, it is important to (1) make sure communication is not hostile; (2) try to keep your emotions in check so that they don't get in the way of hearing what the other person is saying; (3) accept differences in opinions and feelings; (4) learn that it is OK to disagree; (5) listen to what is being said—don't be too quick to defend yourself; and (6) communicate in such a way that both of you feel that you have resolved the disagreement—even if you are not necessarily in agreement.

# connect Resources

## ARTICLES

5.1 "Hooking Up and Hanging Out: Casual Sexual Behavior Among Adolescents," University of Florida, IFAS Extension. This article examines current trends in adolescent and young adult sexual behavior.

5.2 "I Got Your Back: Friends' Understandings Regarding College Student Spring Break Behavior." *Journal of Youth Adolescence.* This piece examines the understanding of peers regarding high-risk sexual behaviors during spring break.

5.3 "Speed Dating." *Current Directions in Psychological Science.* Speed dating as a type of romantic attraction is trendy and might just lead to meaningful relationships.

5.4 "A Longitudinal Perspective on Dating Violence Among Adolescent and College Age Women." *American Journal of Public Health.* An analysis of physical assault in dating relationships and its co-occurrence with sexual assault from high school through college.

## SELF-ASSESSMENTS

5.1 Sexual Health Assessment
5.2 Sexually Transmitted Infections Assessment

## Website Resources

Alan Guttmacher Institute **www.guttmacher.org**
American Society for Reproductive Medicine **www.asrm.org**
Centers for Disease Control and Prevention (CDC) **www.cdc.gov**
CrisisPregnancy.com **www.crisispregnancy.com**
MSN Health Center **http://health.msn.com**
National Men's Health Network **www.menshealthnetwork.org**
National Women's Health Network **www.womenshealthnetwork.org**
Planned Parenthood **www.plannedparenthood.org**
Sexuality Information and Education Council of the United States
    **www.siecus.org**
WebMD (Pregnancy) **www.webmd.com/baby/**

## Understanding the Content

1. Identify and briefly describe the structures in the male and female reproductive systems that have similar functions.
2. Discuss how each of the following methods of contraception work: hormonal, barrier, vasectomy and tubal ligation, and fertility awareness/periodic abstinence.
3. What is the difference between spontaneous abortion and artificial abortion? What are the major issues inherent in artificial abortion?
4. What are the implications of the phases of human sexual response for men and women?
5. Identify and briefly describe the major types of sexual dysfunction in both men and women.

## Exploring Ideas

1. What is the relationship between physiology and sexuality? How can acknowledgment of this relationship help in making low-risk choices with respect to sexual issues?
2. What major issues should be considered in contraception?
3. Is it better to treat the symptoms of sexual dysfunction or to try to treat the causes of sexual dysfunction?

## Selected References

Basson R. Are our definitions of women's desire, arousal and sexual pain disorders too broad and our definition of orgasmic disorder too narrow? *Journal of Sex and Marital Therapy* 28 (4): 289–300, 2002.

Blum D. *Sex on the Brain: The Biological Differences Between Men and Women.* New York: Viking Press, 1998.

Chandra A, Mosher WD, Copen C, Sionean C. *Sexual Behavior, Sexual Attraction, and Sexual Identity in the United States: Data from the 2006–2008 National Survey of Family Growth.* Bethesda, MD: National Center for Health Statistics, 2011.

Guttmacher Institute. Facts on Induced Abortions in the United States, 2008. **www.guttmacher.org/pubs/fb_induced_abortions.html**

Kinsey A, Pomeroy W, Martin C. *Sexual Behavior in the Human Female.* Bloomington: Indiana University Press, 1948.

Kinsey A, Pomeroy W, Martin C. *Sexual Behavior in the Human Male.* Bloomington: Indiana University Press, 1948.

Kreider RM, Fields JM. Number, timing, and duration of marriages and divorces: 1996. *U.S. Census Bureau Current Population Reports,* February 2002.

Masters W, Johnson V. *Human Sexual Response.* Boston: Little, Brown, 1966.

Masters W, Johnson V. *On Sex and Human Loving,* Vol. 1. Boston: Little, Brown, 1988.

National Center for Health Statistics. *Sexual Behavior and Selected Health Measures: Men and Women 15–44 Years of Age, United States, 2002.* Bethesda, MD: National Center for Health Statistics, 2002.

Nelson A, Hatcher R, Zieman M, Watt A, Darney P, Creinin M. *A Pocket Guide to Managing Contraception.* Dawsonville, GA: Bridging the Gap Foundation, 2005.

Oriel J. Sexual pleasure as a human right: Harmful or helpful to women in the context of HIV/AIDS. *Women's Studies International Forum* 5 (28): 392–404, 2005.

Potts A, Gaven N, Grace V, Vares T. The downside of Viagra: Women's experiences and perspectives. *Sociology of Health and Illness* 25 (7): 697–719, 2003.

Savin-Williams RC. Who's gay? Does it matter? *Current Directions in Psychological Science* (15): 1, 40–44.

Wincze J, Carey M. *Sexual Dysfunction* (2nd ed.). New York: Guilford, 2001.

Wolf N. *Promiscuities: A Secret History of Female Desire.* London: Chatto and Windus, 1997.

In the middle
of difficulty lies
opportunity.

— ALBERT EINSTEIN

# Chapter 6

## MANAGE STRESS

Stress is part of life. Too much can be harmful, yet too little stress is unhealthy. In this chapter, we focus on understanding the concept of stress and how to recognize and deal with excessive stress. We describe a variety of proven stress management techniques and suggest new ways to think about stress.

# Chapter 6 | MANAGE STRESS

"THERE IS NEVER ENOUGH TIME, unless you're serving it," quipped Malcolm Forbes, the flamboyant business-magazine publisher. This quotation captures the modern view of stress in several ways. It reflects the sentiment that life is hectic, and people continually rush about trying to do everything that needs to be done. It is also a joking reference to life behind bars, which in reality would be fraught with difficulties. Forbes's tongue-in-cheek comment shows how easily stress can be found in all aspects of life. For some people, common incidents like waiting in line or being stuck in traffic can be stressful. Yet, in the larger picture these are just minor inconveniences that pale in comparison with truly grave or consequential situations, such as those involving unrelenting pain, mental anguish, or debilitating illness.

Stress is certainly part of our common conversational language. This is particularly true in recent years due to the Great Recession; many Americans have faced bleak economic times and uncertainty about the future. Hardly a day goes by when we don't hear someone say, "I'm under a lot of stress" or "I'm really stressed out." As college students, you can easily list your top stresses. They often arise from the challenge of balancing coursework and financial pressures with social life and family relationships. Many students have jobs too, which adds another significant factor to the equation. Successfully coordinating all these activities requires self-management skills. As we found with eating and exercise, a proven approach for improving a desired lifestyle behavior is to learn the basic concepts, chart a plan, and then develop the necessary skills and take action. In this case, the aim is to improve your ability to manage stress in a positive way.

Plainly, stress is part of living but highly variable. Much of the time we can control and manage the many demands and pressures in our lives. But it can be difficult. College students rank "dealing with stress" as a top concern. In this chapter, we examine the concept of stress through a broad, objective lens. You will find that stress can be a positive influence in your life, a force to be understood and reframed to your benefit, not simply something to be dreaded or avoided. We also review how to recognize excessive stress, and we present effective coping strategies.

## ➤ The Nature of Stress

The origin of the word *stress* can be traced to its use in physics, where it refers to the amount of force, pressure, or strain (load) put on an object to bend or break it. For example, when building a bridge or an airplane, engineers need to know the level of stress that component materials (woods, metals, plastics) can withstand before they break or fail. Decades ago, researchers in biology and medicine borrowed the term and applied it to the tensions and pressures that living organisms experience.

## DEFINING AND DESCRIBING STRESS

At the onset, let's define a few basic terms, because *stress* and related words have multiple meanings even across the biological and social sciences. **Stress** refers to the collective psychobiological responses that occur when a person's natural balance is disrupted. Throughout the animal kingdom, organisms inherently strive to maintain physiological balance, or homeostasis. Any factor or force that disrupts homeostasis is technically known as a stressor.

A **stressor** can be physical or psychological, and both types are wide-ranging. Imagine that you decide to go for a run on a cold day and inadvertently trip over a curb and land squarely on your knee. (It's easy to imagine the pain and see the bloody gash!) In this scenario, several physical stressors can be identified: the exertion of exercise, exposure to a low temperature, and the tissue damage from the impact of the fall. There is also the momentary psychological stressor of the fall itself when you know you can't catch yourself and you're going down.

Let's extend the story. Later that day you complete a difficult math assignment, participate in a group meeting that turns argumentative, and finally return to your dorm room for a quiet break—only to discover that your roommate has invited a few friends over. The psychological stressors include the mental challenge of the math assignment and the emotional frustrations that can arise when working or living with others. And, as in these examples, stressors are often multiple and overlapping, not just occasional, isolated events.

Stressors that deplete energy and cause a decline in performance or function lead to **distress,** or a negative stress condition. The word *stress* is typically used in this negative context, but technically, the correct term is *distress.* Conversely, stressors can also be positive. Stressors that motivate and result in improved performance or function lead to **eustress,** or a positive stress condition. Examples of eustress are a nice bonus for completing a specific project or the potential of exploring a new relationship with a person you find attractive. Knowing that stressors can lead to either distress or eustress, you can more easily see that stressors are not

---

**Stress** refers to a person's collective psychobiological responses to challenging situations, such as those which are tiring, threatening, exciting, or new. The situation, event, or factors that cause the stress response are known as **stressors.** Stressors disrupt a person's natural state of balance (homeostasis) and can be positive as well as negative.

**Distress,** or negative stress, is created by stressors that deplete energy and result in impaired performance.

**Eustress,** or positive stress, is created by stressors that motivate and result in improved performance.

limited to threatening or unpleasant situations but also include those that are exciting or simply new.

Stress also can be categorized by its duration; we describe stress as acute, episodic, or chronic. Acute stress is brief but intense. Examples include being called on unexpectedly in class by a professor or losing control of your car and narrowly avoiding an accident. Episodic stress is regular or predictable but intermittent. Final exams and class projects at the end of every semester or a difficult family situation that you have to deal with during visits home are examples of episodic stress. Last, chronic stress is prolonged and continuous. New military recruits experience this during boot camp, where they are challenged physically and mentally with no letup over several months of basic training. Another example is a job that is unpleasant or unfulfilling but necessary to make a living. A high-stress job is often one in which you have responsibility for outcomes but little or no control over them. Arguably the most difficult chronic stress situations are those in which people must deal with constant discomfort or pain due to a health condition. The degree of distress is magnified if no viable options are available.

Before we review techniques for balancing and managing the stressors in our lives, let's briefly consider the concept of stress from two viewpoints—one biological, the other psychological. This background material will allow us to better understand the basis and rationale for different stress management techniques.

## THE BIOLOGY OF STRESS: PHYSIOLOGICAL RESPONSES

The biological perspective is based on the principle that our responses to stress are regulated by the brain, which controls all body functions. The urge to act when threatened is rooted in our neurological and endocrine systems, whose coordinated stress responses provide the extra strength and energy needed to cope. These collective physiological responses—including an increase in heart rate and breathing, a tensing of muscles, and a focusing of attention—are known as the *fight-or-flight response*. The fight-or-flight response evolved as a survival mechanism in the early development of our species. Let's take a closer look.

Hans Selye, M.D. (1907–1982), known as the father of stress research, developed a model called the **general adaptation syndrome** to describe how animals, including humans, respond to stress. He defined a stressor as anything that disrupts homeostasis (physiological balance). In turn, he described the stress response as the body's adaptations designed to reestablish homeostasis.

> The **general adaptation syndrome** is a model that describes the body's physiological responses to stressors in three stages: alarm, resistance, and exhaustion.

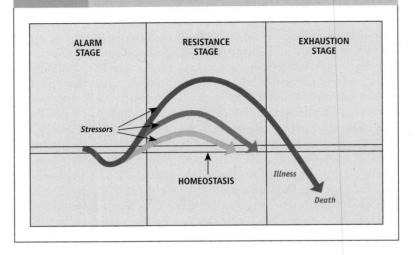

**FIGURE 6.1    GENERAL ADAPTATION SYNDROME**

In Figure 6.1, the general adaptation syndrome is shown as the time course of the body's resistance to a stressor (adaptive capacity). The baseline is the person's stable level of physiological balance (homeostasis). The three predictable stages are *alarm* (resistance is briefly lowered), *resistance* (the body mobilizes resources to increase resistance), and *exhaustion* (extreme or prolonged stress overrides the body's ability to adapt, leading to illness and sometimes death). This classic three-phase response to overwhelming stressors is represented by the red line. In general, though, our bodies readily adapt to stressors and return to homeostasis during the resistance stage (illustrated with dark orange and light orange lines). The specific time course of the stress response depends on the magnitude of the stressor and the individual's ability to adapt.

Let's take a closer look. In the alarm stage, the brain's initial response to a stressor is to signal the **fight-or-flight response** throughout the systems of the body. This is achieved via the autonomic (involuntary) nervous system, the neuroendocrine system, and the voluntary nervous system. These complex systems can be thought of as a communication network that coordinates multiple physiological processes, some of which are activated while others are inhibited. For example, nutrients

The **fight-or-flight response** is the acute stress response in which the autonomic nervous system triggers a set of physiological changes that ready the body for action. The fight-or-flight response corresponds to the alarm stage of the general adaptation syndrome.

are released from energy stores to provide fuel for action, while blood vessels to the skin and digestive tract constrict to allow more blood to go to the muscles. Many of these changes are mediated through the release of chemical messengers (neurotransmitters) such as epinephrine (adrenaline) and cortisol. These chemical messengers are commonly referred to as *stress hormones*. All physiological changes heighten awareness and ready the body for action—fight or flight. Routine sensations and feelings such as hunger, comfort, joy, and sorrow are simply overridden. The effect is rapid and intense.

If the stressor continues, the body goes into the resistance stage and will continue to mobilize energy and biochemical resources (chemical messengers) as needed to withstand the threat. During this stage, the body's physiological processes are aimed at both adapting to the stressor and regaining homeostasis. If additional stressors occur during this phase, the body will likely not be able to meet the challenge because all resources are already being allocated to withstand the initial stressor. The cumulative stressors would overcome the body's capacity to adapt. In this sense, the body is particularly vulnerable during the resistance stage. If the body can successfully adapt to the stressor, there is a return to homeostasis. If, however, the stressor is too great or persists too long, the body moves into the exhaustion stage. In this stage, the stressor overcomes the body's capacity to adapt, with subsequent exhaustion, illness, and eventually death.

Visualize a lion stalking a gazelle and consider the biological alarm and cascade of effects that occur within the gazelle as it senses the presence of the lion (alarm stage). Due to a quick response and great speed, the gazelle may elude the lion. Alternatively, after a brief encounter, the gazelle may escape with wounds that will heal (resistance stage), or despite its best efforts to escape, the gazelle may in the end become exhausted and fall prey to the lion (exhaustion stage).

The fight-or-flight response (alarm stage of the general adaptation syndrome) is logical and purposeful as a means for dealing with short-term physical stress. Our ancestors regularly confronted wild animals. Just as with the gazelle, their ability to activate an innate emergency system was a key survival mechanism. Although this system has equipped humans for dealing with short-term physical stress, how well does it equip us for the stressors of modern life? How does it help us accommodate the mental or emotional stressors that are chronic or uniquely human?

## THE PSYCHOLOGY OF STRESS: MENTAL AND EMOTIONAL RESPONSES

Psychologists point out that although a biological perspective of stress is critical to our understanding, it alone does not present the complete picture. A limitation of the biological model is that it does not explain the individual variability that we see in responses to stress. Research has shown that individuals do in fact respond differently to the same stressor because of differences in how they *perceive* and *interpret* the stressor.

Richard Lazarus, Ph.D. (1922–2002), a leading researcher on cognition and emotion, was among the first to propose that the interpretation of stressful events is more important than the events themselves. The ability of people to think about and assess future events—both the potential harms and challenges—makes them vulnerable in ways that other animals are not. Dr. Lazarus's research was primarily with humans, whereas Dr. Selye's work focused on laboratory animals. Research has confirmed that humans, due to their higher-level cognitive abilities, experience a wider range of mental and psychosocial stresses than do other animals.

Dr. Lazarus and his colleague Susan Folkman, Ph.D., defined stress as a particular relationship between the person and the environment that is appraised by the person as taxing or exceeding his or her resources and endangering his or her well-being. This definition is the basis of their **transactional model of stress and coping,** in which stressful experiences are seen as person–environment interactions (transactions). Two fundamental transactions are a person's judgment about the significance of the stressor and the person's self-appraisal of his or her ability to successfully cope with the stressor. This psychological perspective on stress allows opportunities for management at several points: during the initial appraisal of the stressor, during self-assessment of one's ability to control or cope, and during implementation of coping behaviors. We will discuss specific stress management approaches in the last section of this chapter.

These psychological concepts of stress were dramatically brought to life during the classic Stanford Prison Study, conducted by Stanford University researcher and social psychologist Philip Zimbardo and his colleagues in 1971. The intent of this experiment was to study the psychology of imprisonment by randomly assigning college men to roles as either prisoners or guards and then observing their interactions and behaviors for two weeks in a simulated prison environment. The unexpected occurred, conditions got out of control, and the study had to be shut down after only six days. Even though the college

---

The **transactional model of stress and coping** views stress as a transactional (person–environment) phenomenon dependent on the meaning of the stressor to the perceiver. The impact of the external stressor is first mediated by the person's appraisal of the stressor and then by the social and cultural resources at his or her disposal.

students knew they were subjects in a study, the "prisoners" soon lost the ability to cope, with some showing signs of depression and extreme stress. Some "guards" became ruthless in their positions of authority. These surprising and controversial findings highlighted the importance of perception, control, and coping and demonstrated that the interactions between the person and the environment are malleable and dynamic. (For complete documentation on this classic study, go to **www.prisonexp.org.**)

✓ **NEED TO KNOW**

The nature of stress is highly variable. Stressors can be physical or psychological, and they can occur acutely, episodically, or chronically. Dr. Hans Selye, a pioneer in stress research, used animal studies to develop the general adaptation syndrome, a model depicting the biological effects of stress. His basic concepts are still used today to understand the broad array of stress-related disorders. Dr. Richard Lazarus, a leading psychologist of the 20th century, conducted complementary research with humans, examining the role of cognition and emotion on the experience of stress. He and other psychologists have shown that individual responses to stressful events not only are highly variable but also depend on one's perceptions both of the stressors and of one's ability to cope. Integrating biological and psychological perspectives provides a holistic view of the complex relationships among stress, behavior, and health.

## ➤ Stress and Illness

The role of stress, particularly chronic stress, in causing or contributing to illness and disease is one of the most studied topics in medical science. Although parts of the puzzle remain unsolved, fundamental knowledge about the sources of stress and resulting signs and symptoms of excessive stress are well established. An update on type A behavior as a risk factor for heart disease, the potential link of stress to obesity, and recent insights on the connection between socioeconomic level and well-being are highlighted to show the varied pathways in which stress may influence our health.

### SOURCES OF STRESS

The main sources of stress in America today are associated with changes in personal relationships and occupation. (Of course, as a student your "job" is to make progress in school and eventually earn your degree.)

Article
6.1

## TABLE 6.1    EXAMPLES OF STRESSFUL EVENTS

| LIFE EVENT | POINT VALUE |
| --- | --- |
| Death of a spouse | 119 |
| Divorce | 96 |
| Fired from work | 79 |
| Major injury or illness | 74 |
| Pregnancy | 67 |
| Birth of a child | 66 |
| Parents' divorce | 59 |
| Marriage | 50 |
| Change residence to different city or state | 47 |
| Breakup of close personal relationship | 47 |
| Beginning or ending college | 38 |
| Making a major purchase | 37 |
| General work troubles | 28 |
| Change in personal habits | 26 |
| Vacation | 24 |

Source: From Mark A. Miller and Richard H. Rahe, "Life changes scaling for the 1990s," *Journal of Psychosomatic Research* 43 (3): 279–292. Copyright © 1997, Elsevier. Reprinted with permission.

Self Assessment 6.1

Some changes in life are traumatic, such as failing in school, enduring the breakup of a close personal relationship, experiencing a major injury or illness, losing a job, or experiencing the death of a family member. As we now know, positive changes can also be stress-filled, such as graduating, getting married, having a child, or getting a job promotion.

In an effort to quantify the amount of stress a person is experiencing and the corresponding increased risk for stress-related illness, psychologists Thomas Holmes and R. H. Rahe developed their now-well-known Social Readjustment Rating Scale. Using a statistical analysis of responses from a large, diverse group of adults, they were able to assign values to a variety of events based on their perceived stressfulness. The resulting values indicate the relative impact of stressful events on health and give a sense of the wide range of stressors in our lives. In Table 6.1, a few different events are listed to illustrate their findings. The events listed are representative. You could add items, many of them likely to carry high values.

Our environment also encompasses multiple sources of stress, many of which are seemingly omnipresent. Most Americans are city dwellers and encounter crowding, pollution, and noise in their daily lives. Separately, and even more so in combination, these stressors have been shown to harm health, particularly mental health. Collectively referred to as *urban press,* such negative environmental stressors are often beyond personal control. Conversely, positive environmental stressors can be found in the community via the arts, sports, museums, and parks. These can be sought out for excitement and enjoyment by individuals and groups.

## SIGNS AND SYMPTOMS OF EXCESSIVE STRESS

Recognizing major life-changing events, such as those at the top of the stress scales, is not a problem. However, recognizing our *responses* to these events is not always so straightforward. Identifying the more subtle combination or accumulation of less dramatic daily or episodic stressors and our responses to them requires a higher level of awareness and analysis. We should be alert to clues. The following 10 questions capture common signs and symptoms of excessive stress.

- Have you become anxious and easily depressed?
- Have you become indecisive and generally apathetic?
- Have you become irritable and easily angered?
- Have your memory and concentration deteriorated?
- Have you experienced an increase in headaches or digestive problems?
- Has your blood pressure become elevated?
- Has your sleep pattern changed (insomnia/excessive sleep)?
- Have your eating habits changed (appetite loss/binge eating)?
- Have you increased your use of alcohol or drugs?
- Have you developed any nervous habits or phobias?

If you answered yes to one or more of these questions, reassess the stressors in your life. First, can you identify them? Is it likely that they are causing the signs and symptoms? And if so, are you taking the time to address both the stressors and your responses to them? (See "Breaking It Down" on sleep as a primal need.) A discussion of stress management, including practical strategies and techniques, is provided later in this chapter.

If you currently face demanding or distressing situations that tax your ability to make it through the day, or if you show signs of stress that are not subsiding, see a counselor or health specialist at your counseling center or student health center. These professionals are there to assist you, so don't hesitate to make an appointment and meet with them.

## CHRONIC STRESS AND HEALTH

As we now know, the body's response to stress can be both helpful and harmful. From an evolutionary perspective, it equips us for survival—to face emergencies with speed and strength. But in the 21st century,

The need for sleep is as fundamental to life as the need for food and water. We literally cannot live without sleep. In fact, forced sleep deprivation is used as a means to break down prisoners during interrogation. Despite extensive research, scientists have yet to understand why sleep is so vital—this essential question remains a mystery. However, they do know a great deal about the characteristics of sleep—for example, the types (shallow vs. deep sleep) and structure (sequence, organization) of sleep and how these aspects change from infancy to old age. Of particular interest is how normal sleep patterns are affected by sleep disturbances such as insomnia, sleep apnea (breathing interruptions during sleep), and narcolepsy (daytime "sleep attacks"). Sleep-related problems affect about one out of five Americans of all ages, races, and socioeconomic classes. More and more physicians are being trained in sleep medicine, a specialization offered through the American Boards of Internal Medicine, Pediatrics, Otolaryngology (ear, nose, throat), and Psychiatry and Neurology. Patients with sleep problems can see a specialist at over 1,000 accredited sleep centers spread throughout the United States.

Both science and personal experience tell us that the relationship between sleep and stress is reciprocal. Stressors can definitely disrupt sleep—we've all had nights when emotional turmoil or a major deadline has kept us up. And, conversely, not getting enough sleep is also a stressor, so the potential for a vicious cycle exists. For college students, the effects of inadequate sleep on learning are especially relevant. The evidence shows that sleep loss results in impairment in learning capacity—that is, in higher cognitive functions such as attention, memory, and problem solving. Studies in which sleep was actively restricted or optimized showed a corresponding worsening or improvement in learning and academic performance. Establishing a healthy sleep routine is often a matter of recognizing and then eliminating or minimizing sleep disrupters:

*Caffeine consumption*—avoid coffee, sodas, pills, and, yes, chocolate too within a few hours of bedtime.

*Exercise*—by all means engage in regular exercise, but complete your workout a few hours before bedtime.

*Indigestion*—avoid problem foods and have antacids on hand just in case.

*Reaction to medicines*—be aware of active ingredients that may interfere with sleep, and find substitutes.

Other sleep disrupters—such as pain, emotional upset, or illness—can be more difficult to deal with but are still generally manageable, and in most cases these are short-lived. If you have recurring or chronic sleep problems, see a health care professional at your student health or counseling center. Depending on your specific situation, you may be referred to a sleep medicine specialist for a complete sleep-disorder evaluation. Even though today's high-tech world seemingly runs 24/7, humans are still subject to the biological control of circadian (daily) rhythms that dictate our need for regular restful sleep. Sleep deprivation interferes with our ability to learn and function, and in that sense it becomes an added stressor that further hinders our ability to cope. The opposite is true as well: maintaining healthy sleep habits goes a long way in helping us deal with stressors that are beyond our control. For more information about the science and medicine of sleep and tips for getting restful sleep, go to

National Sleep Foundation
   **www.sleepfoundation.org**

American Academy of Sleep Medicine
   **www.sleepeducation.com**

the stressors we face are more often psychosocial than physical, and more typically chronic than acute. Long-term activation of the stress response resulting from the interplay between the nervous system and stress hormones can have detrimental effects on the body's major systems. When anxiety and worry about work and relationships don't let up, stress hormones continue to circulate throughout the body in high levels, never leaving the blood and tissues.

Simply put, persistent stress can damage the same physiological systems activated or affected by the stress response in the first place. At the head of the list are the nervous, endocrine, cardiorespiratory, metabolic, immune, and gastrointestinal systems. Over time, unrelenting stress and the accompanying biochemical turmoil translate into an increased risk for a vast array of disorders and diseases. Stress can both cause diseases and worsen existing ones. Heart disease, obesity, and depression are three of the most common stress-related conditions.

Stress can accelerate the aging process too. Think of our three most recent Presidents—Bill Clinton, George W. Bush, and Barack Obama—and how they aged during their terms. Aging expert Michael Roizen of the Cleveland Clinic believes the nonstop and often high-pressure demands of being president of the United States or a top CEO ages a person at about twice the normal rate. In Figure 6.2, the toll of the presidency is captured in the face of Barack Obama. Moreover, in 2004 former president Bill Clinton, at age 58, was diagnosed with heart disease (significant blockage of the coronary arteries) and subsequently underwent bypass surgery.

### Stressful Behavior: Type A Behavior and Hostility

Nearly 50 years ago, two cardiologists, Meyer Friedman and R. H. Rosenman, developed the concept of **type A behavior** and identified it as a psychological risk factor for heart disease. They found that people with classic type A personality continually put themselves in stressful situations, which over time resulted in far more heart attacks than happened to people who were not type A. Today we are all familiar with type A behavior and easily recognize it in others. Type A individuals are competitive, aggressive, and time-driven; they never seem to miss a step. In contrast, type B individuals are methodical, move at a slower pace, and are generally easygoing. In reality, most of us fall somewhere in between the classic type A (driving, impatient) and type B (unhurried, calm) dispositions.

Further research on type A behavior and heart disease has yielded additional important findings. It turns out that type A traits can be broken down into three components—excessive competitiveness, time-urgency, and **hostility**—and the hostility component is the primary

Self Assessment 6.2

Type A behavior is characterized by excessive competitiveness, time-urgency, and hostility. People with this profile tend to engage their stress response systems on a chronic basis. The **hostility** component has been identified as the primary trait that puts people at risk for the development of heart disease and other stress-related medical conditions.

culprit behind the continual activation of the stress pathways that lead to disease. Hostility—a combination of anger, aggression, and cynicism—may be a better predictor of heart disease than traditional risk factors like cigarette smoking, hypertension, and high cholesterol. See the 10-question hostility questionnaire in Connect Resources.

## Stress and Obesity

Connections between chronic stress and seemingly unrelated conditions continue to be uncovered. The role of chronic stress in the current obesity epidemic is one example. As researchers unravel how the body's stress response system is regulated, the details of the actions and interplay between the brain and multiple chemical messengers are becoming clearer. It is now known that caloric input, energy stores, and body weight are intertwined with the chronic stress response network.

The details of these interactions are exceedingly complex and require specialized training to fully understand. However, the essence is that problematic eating behaviors, including the overconsumption of so-called comfort foods (pleasing foods typically high in carbohydrates and fat), may be stimulated by elevated levels of stress hormones. At the metabolic level, these surplus calories tend to be stored in the abdominal area and over time result in abdominal obesity, which is strongly related to type 2 diabetes, heart disease, and stroke. In other words, stress can make us put on fat more easily, especially if we seek consolation in snack foods. This chronic stress–obesity connection offers another example of the dynamic interactions among physiological systems, emotions, and coping methods.

## Social Standing and Health Status

It's no surprise that the most disadvantaged in society face more stress-related illness due to the continual struggle for life's necessities (food, clothing, housing). Discrimination and limited access to health care compound the difficulty of their situation. Government and private-sector agencies work diligently to reduce these inequities.

Article
6.2

Recent research in public health has produced a related new finding with wide-reaching implications. It appears that certain psychosocial factors are at work not just among the poor but across the entire socioeconomic spectrum. Based on longitudinal analysis of demographic, psychological, and health variables in large population studies, a British research team led by Michael Marmot, M.D., professor of public health at University College, London, found that it's not socioeconomic level that determines health (quality of life, longevity) but the underlying and related factors of individual autonomy and social participation.

Dr. Marmot labels this the **status syndrome.** Higher status usually affords more opportunities for individual control and meaningful relationships. Lower status means that external forces are more likely to determine one's fate. In other words, a person's health appears to be tied to his or her place in the social gradient above and beyond income, level of education, health behaviors, and genetic predisposition. Evidence from psychosocial research also supports the central proposition that explains the status syndrome: individual control and opportunities for social engagement are critical for lessening the risk of stress-related disorders and maximizing well-being and longevity.

## STRESS—THE "BIG PICTURE"

This is an opportune time to step back and reconsider the "big picture" about stress and disease. As alluded to earlier, there are two complementary views on this issue. The first is the mainstream medical view rooted in biology: stress triggers specific physiological changes that make us more vulnerable to illness and disease via molecular, cellular, and genetic mechanisms. The second is anchored in a mind–body view, in which the excessive stress–poor health connection is due to psychosocial factors such as stress perception, coping abilities, individual autonomy, social support, and modern-day environmental stressors. Each view is incomplete without the other. A recent finding illustrates the convergence of the biological and psychological viewpoints.

In the year 2000, researchers reported that women appear to display an alternative stress response that they dubbed the **tend-and-befriend response.** It turns out that the classic fight-or-flight stress response was based largely on studies of male laboratory animals. When similar studies were conducted with female animals, their stress responses—which are in part mediated by sex-specific hormones—were, not surprisingly, somewhat different from the stress responses of males.

The **status syndrome,** a recent concept in public health, refers to the effect of social position on a person's quality of life and longevity beyond that accounted for by education and income; it appears that risk for stress-related health problems are mediated through the opportunity for, or lack of, individual autonomy and social participation.

The **tend-and-befriend response** is a behavior pattern of protecting and caring for offspring and seeking social support exhibited by humans (and some other animals) when under threat. This type of stress response appears to have both biological and psychological underpinnings.

Females demonstrated an added dimension of protecting offspring and seeking the companionship of others. When stressed, females—both lab animals and humans—exhibit nurturing-of-children behavior and seek social support, especially from other females. Indeed, clinical and social psychologists know that women are more likely than men to seek out and provide social support when facing difficult situations. Researchers are careful to note that the tend-and-befriend response is not a universal female phenomenon but rather is a general gender-related behavioral tendency. The tend-and-befriend finding is another step forward in understanding variability in how we

When stressed, women often display "tend-and-befriend" behavior as a way of coping.

respond to stressors. Moreover, it illustrates the power of understanding stress from a holistic perspective that unifies biological and psychosocial knowledge.

Finally, let's not forget the essential role of stress in living a full life. Because uncontrolled chronic stress is clearly linked to a variety of health problems, it's easy to forget that stress is primarily a positive force in our lives. Think of stress in the context of excitement, challenges, and new experiences. Stress is not just good or bad but an undulating blend of positive and negative stressors. This motley assortment of forces and events that we dub stress is not optional. Rather it's an unavoidable part of living and personal growth. In times of high stress, we often say we long for a stress-free life, when in fact we actually mean a life with a manageable level of stress. Certainly, after a prolonged period of hard work or difficulty, a few days of carefree living are welcomed and can be restful and restorative—but then it's back to a routine with roles, responsibilities, and expectations. In a matter of days or weeks, a truly stress-free life would become boring, as many people discover when they retire. As long as our lives focus on goals and challenges, a healthy level of stress will be part of the equation. The key is to recognize stress and manage it to our benefit when we can. In many situations, we can use stress to reach our goals, whether at school or work or with family or friends.

# ➤ Managing Stress

Many adults are quick to tell college students to enjoy themselves; they often add that their college years were the best times of their lives. Whether this is selective memory or wistful longing for a time with fewer responsibilities is open to speculation. What we do know is that for increasing numbers of students today, the college years are not carefree, joyful times but rather full of anxiety and stress.

Along with many positive societal changes in recent decades, there have been negative trends too. Mass media and particularly television continually bring news of violence, illness, death, wars, and natural disasters into our daily lives. At the same time, we have become more separated from families and neighbors who might be able to help if these events were to actually directly impact us. For many college students, family support systems are unstable (more parents are separated, divorced, and remarried), financial worries are commonplace (college costs and student loans are mounting, more students are working to help pay for school), and the employment situation after graduation is bleak for many majors. Add these to the traditional sources of student distress—homesickness, difficulty making friends, poor grades, broken romances, easy access to drugs and alcohol, and sleep deprivation—and you have a situation that can be challenging to even the most resilient students.

Despite these challenges, colleges are still filled with opportunities. With planning, exploration, and follow-through, you can find your place, succeed in college, and have fun along the way.

Now that you have some background on the biology and psychology of stress, as well as the signs and symptoms of chronic stress, let's consider how you can manage the stress in your life. There are three key aspects to successful stress management. The first relates to the importance of using time management to reach your goals and avoid unnecessary stress. The second focuses on understanding your own personality and temperament and how you perceive and respond to stress. And the third deals with identifying healthy coping strategies—including specific stress management techniques—that meet your needs.

## TIME MANAGEMENT

The transition from high school to college presents various challenges. For many students, the greatest challenge is learning to manage their time effectively. Going to college means greater personal independence and less parental oversight of day-to-day activities. With increased freedom comes more responsibility for routine tasks previously handled by parents, such as meal planning and cooking, keeping the home organized and clean, and scheduling appointments. When these new duties are suddenly added to a student's normal college activities—attending classes and labs, completing assignments, studying for tests, making new friends, and participating in extracurricular activities—it's easy to become overwhelmed. Commuting and part-time jobs are often part of the mix as well. Even for the best prepared, the transition to college life requires adjustment and flexibility. Given these factors, it should come as no surprise that poor time management is a root cause of many stressors college students face.

Article 6.3

**Time management** simply means the planned efficient use of one's time. It is the prioritization, scheduling, and execution of responsibilities to one's personal satisfaction. Everyone has the same amount of time in a day, so it's up to each of us to make the best use of it. We certainly don't want to squander time, the very currency of life. The good news is that time management does not have to be complicated. It can be boiled down to three steps: perform a time audit, prioritize activities, and develop an action plan.

### Perform a Time Audit

Analyze how you use your time. Write down all your activities on several representative days and make a chart showing the time allocation over the 24-hour periods. Next, categorize your activities into committed time (e.g., classes, work, family), maintenance time (e.g., personal hygiene, eating, exercising, necessary chores, sleeping), and discretionary time, which is free time to use as you wish. Identify

---

**Time management** is the prioritization, scheduling, and execution of responsibilities to one's personal satisfaction.

blocks of time that could be better used. For example, are small blocks of time being lost that could be rearranged to be used more efficiently?

### Prioritize Your Activities

First things first. Organize your activities by importance and urgency into four categories: (1) urgent and important, (2) not urgent but important, (3) urgent but not important, and (4) not urgent or important. For example, studying for an exam may be both urgent and important, whereas spending time with family and friends is not urgent but important. Attending a sale may be urgent but not important, while watching TV soap operas is not urgent and not important. Prioritizing is not always straightforward, but it is critical. It is time well spent. Not prioritizing leads to many stressful situations because the most important activities are not given the special consideration they deserve.

### Develop an Action Plan

Create a plan and execute. Based on your time audit and prioritization of activities, you can develop a schedule and to-do list. Many students use print versions of daily planners/organizers or handheld PDAs (personal digital assistants). Both are fine because they allow you to translate the first two steps into action by having a planned schedule and a timeline for tasks and projects. Execution is the final phase—the act of carrying out or completing the tasks you set out to accomplish. All the analysis and planning is for nil if you don't roll up your sleeves and actually do the work. A large part of time management is the drive to get tasks done and do them well. When you reach this point, your system for time management is in place. With time and practice, the steps will eventually become second nature.

Few of us learn time management as part of our formal education, yet it is fundamental to being productive and preventing negative stressors. Indeed, poor time management is recognized as a primary factor contributing to low graduation rates (only 5 in 10 college students graduate within six years). Colleges now recognize the importance of time management to student success and routinely cover this topic in first-year student seminars. Other noncredit, short courses are often offered periodically through Student Services. If you feel your time management skills need sharpening, investigate what's offered on campus and get a refresher course.

### KNOW THYSELF

How we view our level of personal control in the world can have a major bearing on our response to stress. To better understand this personal control–human behavior connection, clinical psychologist

Julian Rotter, Ph.D., developed the concept of **locus of control** and devised a scale to measure it. Locus of control is simply a set of beliefs about the relationship between behavior and subsequent outcomes. These beliefs are described in one of two ways—an **internal control orientation** or an **external control orientation.** For most people, one orientation dominates their view and approach to living. (Take the locus-of-control survey in Connect Resources to see how you rate.)

Those with an internal control orientation believe that outcomes of their actions depend on what they do. These "internalizers" presume that they chart their own course and control their destiny. They believe that they are autonomous and, as masters of their fates, also bear responsibility for what happens to them. In contrast, those with an external control orientation believe that outcomes are based on events outside their personal control and that they have little influence. That is, outcomes are determined by powerful others, by luck or fate, or are simply unpredictable. These "externalizers" believe they are subject to external forces, and their actions often show that they feel little or no responsibility for what happens to them.

Self Assessment 6.3

A major difference between these attribution styles is that people with an internal locus of personal control know how to act to get their desired outcomes, whereas people with an external locus of personal control seem not to have this knowledge. Rather, externalizers tend to wait passively for whatever comes their way. Yet, we should be mindful that various factors may shape our sense of autonomy—it's not simply a matter of choice. For example, those who face discrimination—because of poverty, lack of education, race, religion, gender, age, or other factors—may have learned from experience that what they do doesn't have much effect.

Locus of personal control plays a major role in our motivation, expectations, self-esteem, and risk-taking behavior, and in so doing can influence our actions and their outcomes. How we view the world and our effect on it certainly relates to how we perceive and cope with stressors. Clearly, an internal locus of control is important for behavior change including stress management.

Like hostility, locus of control is unequivocally linked to the stress–health relationship. Knowledge about these dimensions of our personality can be revealing and instructive. Our responses to stress and our

---

**Locus of control** is a psychological concept referring to a person's beliefs about the underlying causes of events in his or her life.

People with an **internal control orientation** believe that outcomes are contingent on their actions; people with an **external control orientation** believe that outcomes are determined by events or forces outside their personal control.

coping methods are shaped by many factors, including personal experience, family background, social and societal influences, and the specific situational context. Some factors are within our control and others are beyond our control.

As suggested earlier, if you are concerned about a personality score or characteristic, or if the level of stress in your life is causing you problems with getting through the day, make an appointment with a counselor at the campus counseling center or student health center. You will find professionals whose job it is to help you cope with your experiences. They will be glad to talk with you and can provide guidance and resources.

## STRESS MANAGEMENT TECHNIQUES

Stress management is mostly about techniques to assist us in dealing with challenges that are surmountable. These approaches are effective *within limits*. The challenges faced by a refugee, a homeless person, a terminally ill person, or the victim of a violent crime are in a different realm from the more routine stressors that most people face in their everyday lives. Standard stress management techniques will not solve truly dire situations, nor were they developed with that in mind. Disastrous circumstances and traumatic experiences require different approaches, resources, and expertise. As a side note, a sincere effort to consider our personal crises in light of those faced by people who lack the most fundamental needs can add perspective. A further step would be to assist those with greater needs. Whether it's volunteering at a homeless shelter or aiding an elderly neighbor with a project, a simple act of service and kindness to others can provide a restorative break from our own personal struggles.

Most of us can benefit from stress management. As referred to earlier when discussing Lazarus and Folkman's transactional model of stress and coping, accurate appraisal of the stressor followed by effective coping is central to successful stress management. Initially, we make a judgment about the stressfulness of an event. How stressful is it? Is it manageable, positive, or irrelevant? Next is an appraisal of our coping options and resources. What options are available to me? Can I successfully apply the necessary steps to manage the stressor? Clearly, coping with modern-day stressors is not automatic. Fight-or-flight is rarely the appropriate response. Indeed, coping is a process that's always changing. It's a learned pattern that requires effort. And remember that coping is an effort to *manage* the situation—complete control and mastery are not necessary (or possible) in most cases. Successful coping is dependent on your overall health and energy, a positive belief, problem-solving skills, and social support.

To reinforce and complement the stress management suggestions from psychologists Lazarus and Folkman, we provide the following strategies from neuroscientist Robert Sapolsky, Ph.D.:

- *Learn to accurately recognize signs of stress.* This is the important first step. We must learn to recognize the signs and to identify the circumstances most responsible for the stress response. As noted earlier, it's important to "know thyself."
- *Find an enjoyable outlet and practice it regularly.* Take part in an activity or hobby that helps you release frustrations, and set aside time to do it regularly. The kind of activity is not critical as long as it's one you enjoy and is not stressful to others.
- *Seek control in the face of stress, but be realistic.* A can-do outlook is important. We generally have options to control stressors in a positive manner. Gather information, make a plan, and take action, but be realistic. We cannot control events that have already occurred, nor should we try to control future events that are uncontrollable.
- *Develop social support through strong relationships.* Nurture your social network. We are social creatures and long to be part of something larger than ourselves, whether it's a family unit or some other kind of group. This is true even for the most independent and individualistic among us. Remember, though, that strong relationships work both ways—they are reciprocal and dynamic. To have a good friend, you must be a good friend.

Article
6.4

Deep breathing or meditation can alleviate symptoms of stress.

In addition to these general strategies, specific stress management techniques are available. A few of the best known and accessible are described briefly below. The first four—deep breathing, progressive muscle relaxation, visualization, and meditation—are all based on inducing a relaxation response in which one consciously focuses on countering or reducing the natural physiological stress responses (e.g., increases in breathing rate and muscle tension). In contrast, physical activity dissipates stress by simulating the body's call to action inherent in the fight-or-flight response. All stress management techniques have been shown to be effective for some people, but no single technique works well for everyone. Consider these like choices on a menu. Depending on your personal characteristics, preferences, and experiences, some will appeal to you more than others. The key is to find an approach that meets your needs and fits your lifestyle.

The only way to find out which technique works for you is through trial and error. Nearly all college campuses provide a variety of courses and workshops on stress management techniques. Take a class. Experiment. Reading about the techniques is simply not enough. We learn by doing. Listen to your own reactions and trust your instincts. You will be able to tell which techniques really work for you.

### Deep Breathing

Deep breathing is a simple technique that is easily mastered and takes only a few minutes. Sit or lie down in a comfortable position with a straight spine. Begin by breathing deeply, using the full capacity of the lungs. Expand the chest and abdomen with each deep inhalation and then empty the lungs with a complete exhalation. Don't strain; this should be done comfortably. Allow the chest to rise and fall with each breath. The breathing rate should be slower than normal. Attempt to balance the time of the inhalation (a few seconds) with that of the exhalation. Deep breathing is most effective if practiced daily for 5 to 10 minutes.

### Progressive Muscle Relaxation

Progressive muscle relaxation is a technique in which one systematically contracts and relaxes different muscles in a sequential order coupled with deep breathing exercise. It can be performed in a seated or supine position. To try this technique, begin with the muscles of the right foot. Inhale deeply, contract the muscles, then exhale as you release the contraction and relax your foot completely. Notice how relaxation in this part of your body feels and enjoy the sensations. Next, go to the calf of your right leg, and proceed similarly through the major muscle groups in the rest of your body. The process takes

# Health & the Media Distress, Eustress, and Humor

"A clown is like an aspirin, only he works twice as fast."

—Groucho Marx

When we think of stress, our images are nearly always negative—conflict, sickness, grief, or sadness—reflecting the turmoil and angst of the human condition. These negative aspects have been captured in art through the ages. Yet, we know stress also can be positive. In a modern view with a twist, both eustress and distress are captured in Gary Larson's The Far Side® cartoon. Chuckling at this cartoon should remind us that humor is a most useful stress buster. As Bob Newhart once said, "Laughter gives us distance. It allows us to step back from an event, deal with it, and then move on." By poking fun at the absurdity or incongruity of life's situations, humor facilitates coping and healing. Hospitals now use clowns and humor intervention as a regular part of their care systems. So look for the mirth in those stressful situations, because your sense of humor is a valuable tool for maintaining positive mood and overall well-being.

## THE FAR SIDE® By GARY LARSON

only about 10 minutes and promotes relaxation by dissipating peripheral tension. Remain still and quietly enjoy the effects afterward.

### Visualization

Creative visualization, or the use of imagery, can be an effective stress reduction technique. This exercise is generally done in conjunction with deep breathing or progressive muscle relaxation, but it can be practiced by itself. Find a quiet place and make yourself comfortable—sit or lie down, with legs uncrossed and spine straight. Close your eyes and visualize a peaceful scene in nature—for example, a perfect, undisturbed place on a beach, an island, or a mountain or in a forest or a garden. It may be an actual place that you recall or a place that you are simply imagining. Immerse yourself in this beautiful and peaceful place by focusing on the details of the setting—see the colors and textures, hear the sounds, smell the fragrances, feel the breeze. With 5 to 10 minutes of visualization, you can create a mini-vacation and have a real break from the daily grind.

### Meditation

Meditation is a technique that has been used for centuries in Asian cultures. In the 1970s, Harvard cardiologist Herbert Benson studied people who practiced transcendental meditation and noted their remarkable ability to reduce their blood pressure and heart rate. Dr. Benson became a leading proponent of mind–body medicine and helped make the meditation technique accessible to Americans through his book *The Relaxation Response*. He distilled meditation down to its essential techniques, removing them from their Eastern religious context.

There are many types of meditation, but most involve adopting a passive attitude toward one's thoughts as they come and go. To try meditation, find a quiet environment and sit comfortably with your eyes closed. Pay attention to your breathing, or silently repeat a word or phrase with each exhalation. As your mind wanders (and it will), simply notice it and bring your attention back to your breathing. Practice for 15 to 20 minutes every day or at least three or four days a week. Like deep breathing, progressive muscle relaxation, and visualization, meditation induces the relaxation response.

### Physical Activity

Physical activity is one of the most natural ways to reduce stress, partly because it simulates the action of the classic fight-or-flight response. During exercise, we process (metabolize) stress chemicals and lessen the damaging effects associated with their accumulation. As discussed in Chapter 3 on fitness, regular physical activity imparts many health benefits, including an immediate reduction in tension

Regular exercise has many benefits—stress relief among them.

and anxiety. Physical activity is convenient and readily available—when you are really stressed out, just put on your sneakers and go for a walk or a jog. You might be surprised by how effective 20 to 30 minutes of exercise can be in helping you deal with even the most difficult situations. The type of exercise is not critical. Nearly all types of activity reduce stress. The key is to find an activity that you enjoy, can maintain, and will engage in regularly.

In this section, we have provided both overall strategies and specific techniques to assist you in managing stress. A central theme woven throughout this chapter is the importance of balance. That is, to effectively deal with stress, we must strive to balance our lifestyle behaviors (nutrition, exercise, sleep) with work, family, and social responsibilities. Simply put, strong lifestyle behaviors better equip us to face stressors of all kinds, from the unexpected or uncontrollable to the minor annoyances in our daily routine. Moreover, self-knowledge, along with a healthy lifestyle, provides the basis for the ongoing development of self-management skills that enable us to set and reach goals and overcome obstacles.

Article 6.5

The college years are an opportune time to hone these life skills. Be proactive, seek answers, and use campus resources. Stress is part of life, and to a great degree we have the ability to control stressors and our responses to them. Stress need not be dreaded—rather, it should be welcomed. Separate the wheat from the chaff—the daily hassles from more significant events—and realize that in most cases, stress can be a positive force in your life.

## ✓ NEED TO KNOW

The college years present different challenges for different people. For many, it's often a highly stressful time. To prevent unnecessary stress, use time management to reach goals. To manage excessive stress, understand how you perceive and respond to stress (locus of control). Based on self-knowledge and time-tested recommendations, develop a set of coping strategies. Find a stress management technique that works for you and practice it on a regular basis. Be aware that colleges provide many resources, from specific courses to professional counseling, to assist students in dealing with excessive stress. Be proactive—seek answers, use campus resources, and tailor your own approach to stress management.

## ARTICLES

6.1 "Poll Shows Stress Pains Many in College." *USA Today.* This poll conducted by the Associated Press and mtvU indicates that stress continues to be prominent among many college students.

6.2 "Strong Medicine Speaks: Recollections from the Matriarch of a Once Hidden Tribe." Smithsonian.com. Stress is not just an individual phenomenon; it can affect groups too, often as a function of race, ethnicity, or culture. In this article the matriarch of a Native American tribe reflects on the struggles for survival and identity.

6.3 "Professors' Guide: Top Ten Secrets to College Success." *U.S. News & World Report.* Tips from professors to incoming students on how to flourish in college.

6.4 "Change in Lifestyle Is the Best Kind of Cure." *Milwaukee-Wisconsin Journal Sentinel.* When counseling and medication do not do enough to improve anxiety and depression, science turns back toward the basics—diet, exercise, nature, and spirituality—to further improve patients' lives.

6.5 "Unraveling Beliefs." *Edge.* Understanding how personal beliefs are set and become familiar and how established beliefs can be changed are big steps toward understanding behavior and human nature.

## SELF-ASSESSMENTS

6.1 Recent Life Changes Questionnaire
6.2 Hostility Questionnaire
6.3 Locus-of-Control Questionnaire

## Website Resources

American Academy of Sleep Medicine
   **www.sleepeducation.com**
American Institute of Stress
   **www.stress.org**
American Psychological Association: Stress
   **www.apa.org/topics/stress/index.aspx**
Jed Foundation: College Stress
   **www.jedfoundation.org/students**

Medline Plus: Interactive Tutorial on Managing Stress
   **www.nlm.nih.gov/medlineplus/tutorials/managingstress/htm/
   index.htm**
National Institute of Mental Health
   **www.nimh.nih.gov**
National Sleep Foundation
   **www.sleepfoundation.org**
Stanford Prison Study
   **www.prisonexp.org**
University of Chicago Student Counseling & Resource Service:
   Time Management
   **http://counseling.uchicago.edu/services/asap/timemgmt**
University of Georgia Health Center: Managing Stress
   **www.uhs.uga.edu/stress/index.html**
U.S. News Professors' Guide
   **www.usnews.com/education/blogs/professors-guide**

## Knowing the Language

distress, 224
eustress, 224
external control orientation, 241
fight-or-flight response, 226
general adaptation syndrome, 225
hostility, 234
internal control orientation, 241
locus of control, 241

status syndrome, 236
stress, 224
stressor, 224
tend-and-befriend response, 236
time management, 239
transactional model of stress
   and coping, 228
type A behavior, 234

## Understanding the Content

1. Define and provide examples of common physical and psychological stressors.
2. Discuss both the general adaptation syndrome model and the transactional model of stress and coping and then contrast them.
3. Describe the signs and symptoms of excessive stress. What steps should a person take if he or she is experiencing these signs or symptoms?
4. Describe several stress management techniques and how they relieve stress.

1. How do modern-day stressors differ from those of our ancestors who lived several thousand years ago? Consider how our society is organized differently today and the impact of technology on our daily lives.
2. The stress–illness relationship is reciprocal. Excessive stress can lead to or worsen disease, and, conversely, dealing with an illness can compound a person's level of distress. Have you experienced this firsthand with family or friends? Describe circumstances that show how stress can be both a cause and a consequence of illness.
3. Explain the concept of locus of control. Using yourself or someone you know well, describe and discuss how a person's locus of control positively or negatively impacts his or her ability to assess and cope with stress. How can one move along the locus-of-control continuum from more external to more internal control?

## Selected References

Benson H. *The Relaxation Response*. New York: Morrow, 1975.

Colten HR, Altevogt BM (eds.). *Committee on Sleep Medicine and Research. Sleep Disorders and Sleep Deprivation: An Unmet Public Health Problem*. Washington, DC: National Academies Press, 2006.

Covey SR. *The 7 Habits of Highly Effective People*. New York: Simon & Schuster, 1989.

Curio G, Ferrara M, DeGennaro L. Sleep loss, learning capacity and academic performance. *Sleep Medicine Reviews* 10: 323–337, 2006.

Dallman MF, Pecoraro N, Akana SF, et al. Chronic stress and obesity: A new view of "comfort food." *Proceedings of the National Academy of Sciences* 100 (20): 11696–11701, 2003.

Diener E, Biswas-Diener R. *Happiness: Unlocking the Mysteries of Psychological Wealth*. Malden, MA: Blackwell, 2008.

Friedman M, Rosenman RH. *Type A Behavior and Your Heart*. New York: Knopf, 1974.

Holmes TH, Rahe RH. The social readjustment rating scale. *Journal of Psychosomatic Research* 11: 213–218, 1967.

Jacobs L, Hyman J. *The Secrets of College Success*. San Francisco: Jossey-Bass, 2010.

Lazarus RS, Folkman S. *Stress, Appraisal and Coping*. New York: Springer, 1984.

Lovallo WR. *Stress and Health: Biological and Psychological Interactions* (2nd ed.). Thousand Oaks, CA: Sage, 2005.

Marmot M. *The Status Syndrome: How Social Standing Affects Our Health and Longevity.* New York: Henry Holt, 2004.

McEwen BS. Effects of stress on the developing brain. *Report on Progress, Dana Foundation,* March 2011.
**www.dana.org/WorkArea/showcontent.aspx?id=31374**

McEwen BS, Lasley EN. *The End of Stress as We Know It.* Washington, DC: Joseph Henry Press, 2002.

Miller MA, Rahe RH. Life changes scaling for the 1990s. *Journal of Psychosomatic Research* 43 (3): 279–292, 1997.

Rotter JB. Generalized expectancies for internal versus external control of reinforcement. *Psychological Monographs* 80 (whole no. 609), 1966.

Ruark J. Positive psychology: An intellectual movement for the masses. *Chronicle of Higher Education,* August 3, 2009.
**http://chronicle.com/article/An-Intellectual-Movement-for/47500/**

Sapolsky RM. *Why Zebras Don't Get Ulcers* (3rd ed.). New York: Henry Holt, 2004.

Sellers FS. If Obama grows old before his time, stressed-out cell tips might be to blame. *Washington Post,* January 19, 2009.

Selye H. *Stress in Health and Disease.* Boston: Butterworth, 1976.

Selye H. *The Stress of Life.* New York: McGraw-Hill, 1956.

Society for Neuroscience. *Brain Facts: A Primer on the Brain and Nervous System.* Washington, DC: Society for Neuroscience, 2008.
**www.sfn.org/index.aspx?pagename=brainfacts**

Taylor SE. Tend and befriend: Biobehavioral bases of affiliation under stress. *Current Directions in Psychological Science* 15 (6): 273–277, 2006.

Williams R, Williams V. *In Control: No More Snapping at Your Family, Sulking at Work, Steaming in the Grocery Line, Seething in Meetings, Stuffing Your Frustration.* New York: Rodale, 2006.

Williams V, Williams R. *Lifeskills: 8 Simple Ways to Build Stronger Relationships, Communicate More Clearly, and Improve Your Health.* New York: Times Books, 1997.

Zimbardo PG. Stanford Prison Study: A Simulation Study of the Psychology of Imprisonment Conducted at Stanford University.
**www.prisonexp.org**

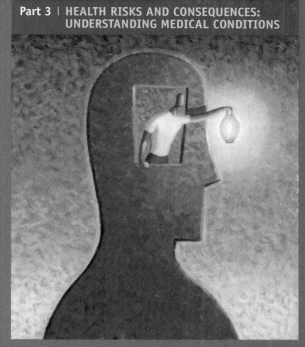

*You can handle depression in much the same way you handle a tiger.... If depression is creeping up and must be faced, learn something about the nature of the beast. You may escape without a mauling.*

— R. W. Shepherd

# Chapter 7

## MENTAL HEALTH AND DISORDERS

Until recently, mental illness was often kept secret. But today more people seek treatment openly, as anyone watching television will note upon seeing the frequent ads for anti-anxiety and antidepression drugs such as Paxil, Zoloft, and Cymbalta. This openness is fortunate, given that mental illness is fairly common. Twenty percent of the U.S. population is affected by it, according to the Centers for Disease Control and Prevention. Depression is the most common mental illness, and it is also the leading cause of disability and suicide. In Chapter 7 we explore the concept and characteristics of mental health and common problems related to mental health; we then discuss mental illness and options for seeking help.

# Mental Health

MIND, BODY, AND CULTURE

BASIC MENTAL HEALTH DEFINITIONS AND THEORIES

CHARACTERISTICS OF GOOD MENTAL HEALTH

# Personal and Social Problems Related to Mental Health

SUICIDE

DRUG ABUSE

VIOLENCE

EATING DISORDERS

# Mental and Personality Disorders

ANXIETY DISORDERS

MOOD DISORDERS: DEPRESSION AND MANIA

PERSONALITY DISORDERS

SCHIZOPHRENIA

# Treatment

**IN THE BOOK** *College of the Overwhelmed* (2005), Richard Kadison and Theresa Foy diGeronimo state that over the previous 13 years, college campuses saw depression double, thoughts of suicide triple, and sexual assaults quadruple among students. They report that 45 percent of college students say they are depressed, 10 percent claim they experience suicidal thoughts, and 44 percent report binge drinking. The American College Health Association's survey, based on an assessment of college students' mental state over the previous 12 months, reported the following for 2010:

- 19 percent had felt things were hopeless at some point
- 23 percent had felt overwhelmed by all they had to do
- 21 percent felt lonely
- 23 percent felt very sad
- 13 percent felt so depressed that it was difficult to function
- 17 percent felt overwhelming anxiety
- 17 percent felt overwhelming anger

The behaviors associated with depression, suicide, and related alcohol abuse can greatly affect a student's academic and personal life.

Knowing the signs and symptoms of mental disorders, as well as the available treatments, is important for any student today. Most people will experience anxiety, depression, and difficulty adjusting to life's circumstances at some point. For some people these are short and self-correcting problems, but for others they can be long-term and significantly interfere with daily life.

Article
7.1

Not that long ago there was little understanding of the physiology related to mental disorders, and there were not many treatments. But as the role of brain chemicals called *neurotransmitters* was unraveled, new drugs were developed in addition to the many counseling approaches already available. Further, since the underlying physical causes of disorders such as anxiety and depression are now better understood, people tend to view these illnesses as the physical diseases they are. The stigma of admitting to suffering from depression or anxiety has diminished greatly. There has never been more effective help available to those suffering with mental illness or disorders than there is today. Truly, there is no good reason for anyone to suffer in silence anymore.

Article
7.2

## ➤ Mental Health

Maintaining good mental health is as important to good quality of life as is maintaining good physical health. We gauge **mental health** by assessing several factors, including how fulfilling people's relationships are, how well they adapt or cope with adversity, the level of their communication skills, their resilience, and their self-esteem.

## FIGURE 7.1 INTERACTION OF BODY, MIND, AND ENVIRONMENT

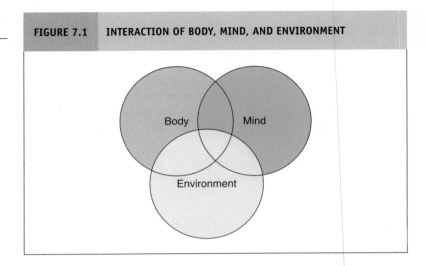

## MIND, BODY, AND CULTURE

The interdependence of the physical, mental, social, and spiritual dimensions of health are emphasized throughout *iHealth*. This notion remains true in regard to mental health. The word **psychosomatic** refers to the mind's influence on the body. In Chapter 6 the body's physical reaction to stress was discussed. Biology and emotions also influence each other, as shown in Figure 7.1.

When we are angry, our body responds by secreting certain types of chemical messengers called *hormones* that, in turn, influence neurotransmitters in the brain that relate to mood. When our body produces too little of certain neurotransmitters, depression can result. Just as the body has a fight-or-flight response to danger or stress (see Chapter 6), it also may respond to thoughts and feelings with back or chest pain, changes in appetite, constipation, high blood pressure, insomnia, upset stomach, weight loss, or weight gain.

Culture can also influence our mental health. When society emphasizes the importance of something an individual member of that culture can't attain, it causes conflict and potentially negative mind–body outcomes. Conversely, some institutions and organizations (such as religious or support groups) can greatly improve mental health and

**Mental health** is the successful performance of mental functions resulting in productive activities.

**Psychosomatic** refers to the influence of the mind (*psyche*) on the way the body (*soma*) functions.

one's sense of well-being. This influence of culture is hard to measure but is nonetheless an important factor that individuals must include in making decisions regarding mental health.

## BASIC MENTAL HEALTH DEFINITIONS AND THEORIES

When discussing mental health, there are a few basic terms you should know. *Behavior* is how someone acts. **Motivation** is something that leads to a behavior. **Self-concept** is a set of core beliefs and values that you feel describes yourself. **Self-esteem** is how you feel—either positively or negatively—about your core qualities and attributes. And finally, *assertiveness* is being very open and honest about declaring your rights, whereas *aggressiveness* is forceful behavior with the intent to dominate.

### Maslow's Hierarchy of Needs

Abraham Maslow's (1970) hierarchy of needs is a model that describes the motivation for behavior. As shown in Figure 7.2, Maslow's contention is that people display behaviors in order to meet needs. Further, he describes five levels of needs. The first level represents the most basic physiological needs—for food, water, and shelter.

Once our physiological needs are satisfied, we need to meet the psychological needs of feeling safe and secure. If these two basic levels of needs are met, then people tend to be motivated by needs higher in Maslow's hierarchy, such as the desire for love and belonging or for self-esteem. Successful people who seem to be living life to its fullest might be seen as reaching the level of self-actualization, though some say this level is questionable, since we can never really know what our full potential is.

### Simple Behavior Paradigm

Using Maslow's hierarchy of needs as a reference point, we can conclude that our behavior is either need-directed or goal-oriented. A simple paradigm to describe behavior is presented in Figure 7.3. The needs referred to in this figure can be the needs identified by Maslow (physiological needs, safety and security). Once the need is identified, people display an instrumental behavior to meet the need. If the behavior leads to achieving the goal, we get relief.

We discover early in life that the real world is rarely as simple as what Figure 7.3 describes. That is, our behaviors don't always result in

**Motivation** is the state of being energized to perform a task.

**Self-concept** is a stable set of beliefs about one's qualities and attributes.

**Self-esteem** is how one feels, good or bad, about one's qualities and attributes.

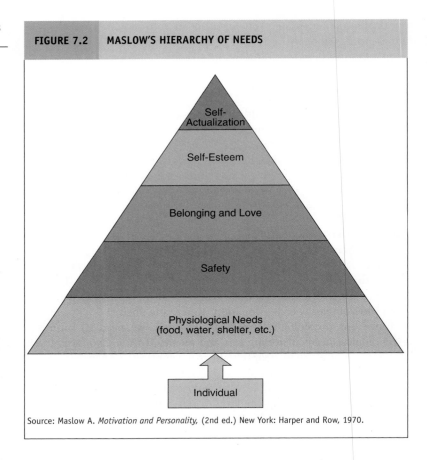

**FIGURE 7.2    MASLOW'S HIERARCHY OF NEEDS**

Self-Actualization

Self-Esteem

Belonging and Love

Safety

Physiological Needs
(food, water, shelter, etc.)

Individual

Source: Maslow A. *Motivation and Personality,* (2nd ed.) New York: Harper and Row, 1970.

a need being met. Often we display a behavior, and the need is not met; the goal is not reached. The result of a need not being met is displayed in Figure 7.4. Basically, we experience tension, frustration, and conflict, and then we respond. For example, we often interpret family expectations and personal expectations for success as needs or goals. When the expectations are not met or the goal is not reached, how we respond can result in relief or in no relief, in which case the tension, frustration, and conflict can either increase or lessen.

### Responding to Unmet Needs and Defense Mechanisms
When a need is not being met, the simplest response is anger. Another way to respond is to be assertive and challenge something (or someone) to try to get the need met. If anger and assertiveness do not work, then people often become aggressive, which involves either verbal or physical domination. It is not a good approach for resolving conflict

**FIGURE 7.3    SIMPLE BEHAVIOR PARADIGM**

Goal or Need

↓

Instrumental Behavior

↓

Goal Reached

↓

Relief

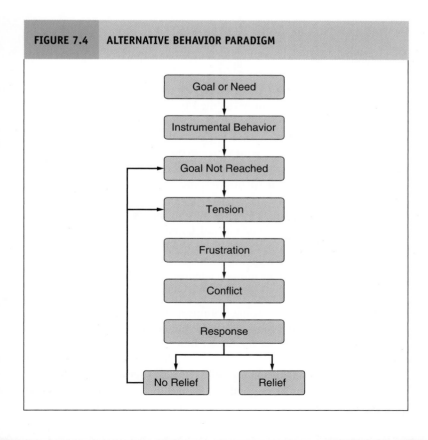

**FIGURE 7.4    ALTERNATIVE BEHAVIOR PARADIGM**

Goal or Need

↓

Instrumental Behavior

↓

Goal Not Reached

↓

Tension

↓

Frustration

↓

Conflict

↓

Response

No Relief          Relief

and often is counterproductive, especially if the aggressiveness is extreme or violent.

Another common way we respond to unmet needs is to protect or defend our ego, our conscious state of how we perceive ourself; hence, these responses are called *defense mechanisms.* One such mechanism is rationalization, or making excuses for our need not being met. Another defense mechanism is denial, or simply not acknowledging that there is any frustration or conflict. Displacement is expressing our frustration by attacking another target—for example, a person has a bad experience with a coworker but takes out her frustration on her spouse. Repression, or selective forgetting, is another defense mechanism—we refuse to think about the event that led to the frustration. Reaction formation is displaying behaviors that are the opposite of the ones that we are actually feeling. Finally, projection formation is accusing another person of the same unacceptable behaviors that we have displayed.

Use of defense mechanisms is normal. However, they can be harmful if they are overused to the point where the individual never deals directly with the problem.

## CHARACTERISTICS OF GOOD MENTAL HEALTH

The National Mental Health Association has identified 10 characteristics of people who are mentally healthy:

Self
Assessment
7.1

1. They feel good about themselves.
2. They do not become overwhelmed by emotions such as fear, anger, love, jealousy, guilt, or anxiety.
3. They have lasting and satisfying personal relationships.
4. They feel comfortable with other people.
5. They can laugh at themselves with others.
6. They have respect for themselves and for others even if there are differences.
7. They are able to accept life's disappointments.
8. They can meet life's demands and handle problems when they arise.
9. They make their own decisions.
10. They shape their environment whenever possible and adjust to it when necessary.

These characteristics have some common themes that are related to Maslow's hierarchy of needs, the behavior paradigm, and the use of defense mechanisms. These themes include a positive self-image, good communication skills, a sense of humor, a healthy response to unmet needs, and good problem-solving skills. It makes sense that people who display the characteristics of good mental health are well balanced, good problem solvers, and accept personal responsibility for their behavior.

✓ **NEED TO KNOW**

Good mental health allows people to cope with the stresses and challenges of life. People's behaviors are motivated by their physical and emotional needs. According to Maslow's hierarchy, the most basic needs are the body's needs for food and shelter. Once those needs are met, people attempt to fill the most basic emotional needs, including a need for feeling safe and secure. When a need remains unmet, frustration results. Often people cope with unmet needs by using defense mechanisms such as denial, displacement, repression, reaction formation, and projection formation.

# ➤ Personal and Social Problems Related to Mental Health

Since mental health involves judgment, coping, communication, relationships, biology, and feelings, it is easy to see how most personal and societal problems are related to mental health. Some examples of social and personal problems related to mental health include suicide, drug abuse, violence, and eating disorders.

### SUICIDE

Suicide is the eighth leading cause of death in the United States and the third leading cause of death among 15- to 24-year-olds. We know

Some places, such as the Golden Gate Bridge in San Francisco, attract people contemplating suicide. Suicide hotline phones have been installed on bridge walkways to help prevent people from jumping.

that depression is usually a precursor to suicide and that depression has a strong biological basis. So to say that suicide is "just" a mental health problem would be wrong.

Suicide can be examined in the context of the behavior paradigm discussed earlier. For example, when a need (food and shelter, safety and security, love and belonging, self-esteem) is not met, and tension, frustration, and conflict continue, then suicide can be the response. In the late 1800s sociologist Emile Durkheim identified three types of suicides. An egoistic suicide is ending one's life as a response to not being able to assimilate into a group or society—for example, a student taking his life after having severe difficulty fitting into the college environment. By contrast, an altruistic suicide is taking one's life to advance a cause or an ideal. Last, anomic suicides occur when the person or group that provided a sense of security no longer exists. The loss of a social network can cause such persistent frustration, conflict, and depression that a person may choose suicide. An example of an anomic suicide would be an elderly man who kills himself after his wife dies.

Notice in all of these descriptions that the person chooses suicide. Life becomes so difficult that the person perceives suicide as the only remedy. Suicide as a choice represents the ultimate personal defeat.

Unfortunately, most suicides are preceded by warning signs that may go unnoticed. Such warning signs include feelings of hopelessness, withdrawing from family and friends, sleeping too much or too little, feeling tired most of the time, acting compulsively, losing interest in most activities, giving away prized possessions, isolating oneself socially, feeling depressed, acting irrationally, being preoccupied with death, behaving recklessly, abusing alcohol or drugs, and being unable to concentrate. Many of the warning signs for suicide are also symptoms of depression, which is strongly related to suicide.

There are steps you can take to prevent suicide if you notice warning signs:

- Always take suicidal comments seriously.
- Try not to act shocked by what a suicidal person might say.
- Do not handle the situation by yourself—get assistance from a health professional.
- Listen attentively to everything that the person has to say.
- Comfort the person with words of encouragement.
- Let the person know that you are deeply concerned.
- If you perceive the person is at high risk of suicide, do not leave him or her alone.
- Talk openly about suicide.
- If the person talks about committing suicide with a firearm that he or she owns, call the police so that they may remove the firearm.

- Don't be judgmental.
- Be careful about statements you make.
- Listen; be gentle, kind, and understanding.
- Let the person express emotion in the way that he or she wants.

It takes time and patience, but you must understand that the suicidal person is in pain and sees few other options. With medical intervention, the crisis can end, and through therapy the person can recover.

## DRUG ABUSE

Much information regarding drug abuse is discussed in Chapter 4. Here it is important to note that attempting to modify one's mood is a common response to tension, frustration, and conflict. The extent to which one binge drinks can be directly related to coping problems. Also, stimulants, depressants, and hallucinogens can serve as chemical Band-Aids that exert a psychoactive effect to lessen the intensity of the response to tension, frustration, and conflict. However, this is a quick fix, and it is counterproductive to solving the problem because of the potential for a new problem: drug dependence.

In some ways it is understandable that drug misuse and abuse is such a common problem related to mental health. The effects are immediate and can be powerful enough so that one's problems just don't seem as bad—that is, until the effects of the drug wear off. When that happens, the problems are still there, and some people respond immediately by modifying their mood to feel better once again. It's not long before using drugs as a coping mechanism creates compound problems—first, not only having to cope with the initial problem, but second, now having to deal with a drug problem.

## VIOLENCE

According to a Centers for Disease Control and Prevention study, the cost in the United States of medical care, rehabilitation, and loss of productivity due to violence is estimated at more than $224 billion a year. In 2006 the CDC reported that homicide claimed the lives of over 18,000 Americans, whereas suicide was responsible for the deaths of over 33,000 Americans. Homicide is the second leading cause of death for people between 15 and 34, and it is the leading cause of death for African Americans in this age group. There were nearly 30,000 firearm-related deaths in 2004, and more than 2 million non-fatal violence-related injuries occurred in the United States.

Article
7.3

Violence is a serious mental health issue and is largely preventable. Violent behaviors and mental illness are not necessarily related—that is, only a small percentage of those who are diagnosed as mentally ill are violent. The causes of violence are related to larger social problems such as stress, dangerous environments, unemployment, drugs, and poverty. Like many other topics we will cover in this chapter, violence represents a choice, and this choice can be the response to tension, frustration, and conflict described in the earlier paradigm.

## Breaking It Down Predicting Violent Behavior

In April 2007, Seung-Hui Cho, a senior at Virginia Polytechnic Institute and State University, shot to death two students near their campus dormitory rooms. A short time later Cho chained the doors of a classroom building and systematically murdered 30 additional students and faculty before committing suicide as police approached him. The so-called Virginia Tech Massacre is the most deadly school shooting in U.S. history.

The biggest question is what motivated Cho to murder so many? A Governor's Task Force report could not find definitive explanations for Cho's actions. However, it uncovered many warning signs that indicated Cho might be a threat either to himself or to those around him.

Cho appears to have been a lonely young man with poor social skills. Students taunted and bullied him in high school, most likely because he was Korean and had poor English language skills. Not being able to express himself well, he internalized this rejection and became an introvert with an undisciplined fantasy life. He fantasized about committing violent acts. Cho sent a video manifesto to NBC News the morning of his attack at Virginia Tech. These actions reflected a stoic, determined, irrational man who wanted to make people pay the ultimate price for his problems. His victims were simply in the wrong place at the wrong time.

In the years leading up to the massacre, some people noticed that Cho needed help. He was referred and evaluated for psychological care, but sadly, he was never made to continue with therapy. Cho's violent fantasies and sense of alienation from people around him worsened. That, combined with the easy ability to buy weapons, resulted in the tragedy.

Several lessons can be learned from the Virginia Tech Massacre. A key point is that Cho fit the profile of a lonely, ostracized person who was capable of acting out violently. Unfortunately, the people around him were not networked in such a way that the full threat could become obvious before Cho acted out. When Cho was referred to counseling and didn't follow through, there was no mechanism to track what was happening with him. Strict privacy laws helped create a situation where Virginia Tech staff and faculty had no comprehensive record of the incidents that the faculty and staff at his high school had reported. If there had been such a record, perhaps when several female college students accused Cho of stalking them, charges might have been pressed, and Cho might have been forced to get help. Instead, Cho's brushes with mental health authorities and the criminal justice system remained slight, so he wasn't flagged in the gun dealers' database as a person who should not be allowed to purchase firearms. Without guns, the scope of whatever Cho chose to do would have been greatly diminished.

It should be noted that most people with Cho's apparent history of mental disorders and social problems do not resort to lashing out at others. If they act out, usually they turn their anger inward and take their own life. However, suicide has great cost not only to the person but also to the person's family and friends. Although stopping people from acting out violently on innocent bystanders is extremely important, preventing suicides is also an important goal, and it can be achieved with the same steps that can minimize the chance of another school massacre.

The Virginia Tech Massacre shows that individuals, both teachers and students, often have good instincts about pinpointing people who could benefit from counseling, psychiatric medications, and, in some cases, hospitalization to prevent violent acts. The challenge is to track at-risk individuals so that they don't fall through the cracks like Cho did. With a good tracking system, easing of the privacy laws in situations like these, and the right people involved in discussions about the behaviors they are observing and the appropriate interventions, horrible incidents like this one can be prevented.

## EATING DISORDERS

As discussed in Chapter 2, the eating disorders anorexia nervosa and bulimia nervosa cause people to starve themselves or engage in binge-and-purge eating behavior. Eating disorders can be a response to unmet needs relating to self-esteem or perception of body image. According to the National Eating Disorders Association, the causes of eating disorders are psychological, interpersonal, and social. Psychological factors include low self-esteem, feelings of inadequacy or lack of control in life, and depression, anxiety, anger, or loneliness. Interpersonal factors include troubled family and personal relationships, difficulty in expressing emotions and feelings, history of being teased or ridiculed based on size or weight, and history of physical or sexual abuse. Social factors include cultural preferences that glorify thinness and place value on obtaining the "perfect body," narrow definitions of beauty that include only specific body weights and shapes for women and men, and cultural norms that value people on the basis of physical appearance and not inner qualities and strengths. These psychological, social, and cultural factors are all related to the Maslow model and the behavior paradigm described earlier.

Clinically, according to the American Psychiatric Association, **anorexia nervosa** has the following symptoms:

- Fear of being fat when at or below normal weight
- Restricting eating so weight falls more than 15 percent below what is considered healthy
- Distorted body image that creates a sense of obesity even when overly thin
- In women, the absence of at least three consecutive menstrual cycles

**Bulimia nervosa,** according to the American Psychiatric Association, is characterized by binge eating and inappropriate compensatory methods to prevent weight gain, such as self-induced vomiting or misuse of laxatives and diuretics. Bulimia has the following symptoms:

- Recurrent episodes of binge eating (at least twice a week for three months)
- Complete loss of control during eating binges
- Persistent overconcern with body shape and size
- Regular self-induced vomiting or use of laxatives or diuretics to prevent weight gain
- Strict dieting, fasting, or exercising to prevent weight gain

**Binge eating disorder** is a relatively new classification of eating disorders. It is characterized by overeating as a response to frustration and conflict. Unlike bulimia, binge eating disorder does not involve purging after overeating.

Eating disorders have serious physical consequences. Anorexia nervosa can result in low blood pressure, reduction of bone density, muscle loss and weakness, and kidney failure. Bulimia nervosa can result in

**Anorexia nervosa** is an eating disorder characterized by self-starvation, excessive thinness, and a distorted body image.

**Bulimia nervosa** is an eating disorder characterized by binge eating and compensatory methods to rid the body of food.

**Binge eating disorder** is characterized by excessive overeating.

gastric rupture, inflammation of the esophagus, tooth decay, peptic ulcers, and pancreatitis. Eating disorders when extreme can result in death. No one knows how many deaths each year are related to eating disorders, primarily because official statistics of cause of death, such as kidney failure or suicide, do not show whether there is a link to an eating disorder. However, studies of anorexic patients have reported death rates from 4 to 25 percent.

✓ **NEED TO KNOW**

Many personal and social problems are related to mental health, including violence against others, suicide, binge drinking, drug use, and eating disorders. While each of these problems may have a biological component as a cause, they all also relate to the psychological, social, and cultural factors described by both the Maslow hierarchy of needs and the behavior paradigm model.

# ➤ Mental and Personality Disorders

Mental disorders are perhaps the most misunderstood kind of illness. We often use terms like *schizophrenic, bipolar,* and *obsessive-compulsive* to describe people, but in reality these are clinical terms that are used to identify profound disorders. Medical and psychodynamic perspectives are used in discussing abnormal behavior. The medical perspective is grounded in the physiological reasons for a condition, and the psychodynamic perspective contends that these disorders are a result of psychological conflicts and represent a means of coping with these conflicts. There is ample evidence supporting each perspective as well as a combination of perspectives—that is, both medical and psychodynamic factors interact—and the consequence is a condition that can be diagnosed.

## ANXIETY DISORDERS

**Anxiety** is excessive worry and concern that is extremely unpleasant and involves apprehension, fear, and panic. Symptoms of anxiety disorders include trembling, jumpiness, inability to relax, racing heart, irritability, hyperactivity, insomnia, and apprehension. There are several classifications of anxiety problems. **Generalized anxiety disorder (GAD)** is constant and uncontrollable worry and concern about

Self Assessment 7.2

**Anxiety** is excessive worry and concern.

**Generalized anxiety disorder (GAD)** is constant and uncontrollable worry or concern about everything.

everything. When anxiety comes on after a traumatic event—anything from a violent attack to an accident or the sudden death of a loved one—**posttraumatic stress disorder (PTSD),** where persistent frightening thoughts, feelings and memories interfere with one's life, may result. **Panic disorders** are sudden, overwhelming attacks of fear. Usually the attacks are short but frequent. A person experiencing a panic attack has uncontrolled thoughts of impending doom for themselves or someone else, experiences intense anxiety symptoms, and may even pass out.

**Phobias** are fears of specific events, objects, or situations. There are many different kinds of phobias. Examples are autophobia (fear of being alone), pharmacophobia (fear of taking medicine), musophobia (fear of mice), microphobia (fear of microbes), hydrophobia (fear of water), acrophobia (fear of heights), and claustrophobia (fear of being in closed spaces). The number of potential phobias is infinite. The response to a phobia can be intense anxiety symptoms like those in panic attacks. People who have claustrophobia and find themselves in an enclosed area such as an elevator or closet may experience panic attack symptoms.

Finally, **obsessive-compulsive disorder (OCD)** is a condition characterized by repetition of the same act over and over again (compulsion) as a response to persistent unwanted thoughts or images (obsession). The behavior is acted out in a ritualistic manner. Examples of OCD symptoms include constantly checking a door to make sure it is locked or constantly washing one's hands.

## MOOD DISORDERS: DEPRESSION AND MANIA

Mood disorders are serious and disabling instabilities in emotions. The extremes of mood disorders are depression and mania.

**Depression** is feelings of worthlessness, indecisiveness, guilt, sadness, and apprehension. We wouldn't be human if we didn't experience depression at points in our lives because of deaths, disappointments, and conflicts. Usually, however, the intensity of these feelings wanes,

---

**Posttraumatic stress disorder (PTSD)** is an anxiety disorder that can occur after experiencing a frightening event in which physical harm may have occurred.

**Panic disorders** are sudden, overwhelming attacks of fear.

**Phobias** are fears of specific objects or events.

**Obsessive-compulsive disorder (OCD)** is repetition of an act over and over again as a response to unwanted thoughts.

**Depression** is characterized by feelings of worthlessness, indecisiveness, guilt, sadness, and apprehension.

and the depression naturally lifts. But sometimes depression is a long-lasting state rather than a passing mood. In this case, depression can cause many personal, professional, and relationship problems. **Mania** is characterized by an elevated mood in which the person appears extremely excitable and hyperactive, makes grandiose and incomprehensible statements, and has rambling thoughts.

There are three types of depressive illness: major depression, dysthymia, and bipolar illness. According to the National Institute of Mental Health, symptoms of major depression include

- Sadness, irritability, excessive crying, anxiety, or hopeless feelings
- Decreased energy and feelings of fatigue
- Loss of interest or pleasure in usual activities
- Appetite and weight changes
- Sleep disturbances
- Thoughts of death or suicide attempts
- Difficulty concentrating, making decisions, remembering
- Chronic aches and pains not explained by any other physical condition

Article
7.4

**Dysthymia** is a form of depression that is long-term and less severe than major depression, but it still impairs functioning to some degree. **Bipolar disorder,** which sometimes is referred to as *manic-depressive illness,* includes two states: extreme elation (mania) followed by the extreme low of depression. If the symptoms of depression are experienced only during a specific season, such as winter, when the days are short, the diagnosis may be **seasonal affective disorder (SAD).**

Depression is a serious college health issue and certainly an impediment to academic success. It is important for anyone who experiences five or more of the symptoms of depression for two weeks or longer to seek some help from a health professional.

A person in a manic episode is hyperactive, believes he or she can do anything, and often talks in a rambling, incoherent manner. Although elation can be a symptom some people actually enjoy, a manic episode can make people delusional, and their actions can badly

---

**Mania** is characterized by an extremely elevated mood and subsequent hyperactive behaviors.

**Dysthymia** is a form of depression that has long-term but less severe effects than major depression.

**Bipolar disorder** (sometimes referred to as *manic-depressive illness*) involves swings between mania (extreme elation) and depression.

**Seasonal affective disorder (SAD)** is when symptoms of depression are experienced during a specific season of the year.

disrupt their life and relationships. Symptoms of mania include repeatedly starting new tasks, outbursts of inappropriate anger, grandiose sense of knowing more than others, extravagant spending, and energetic exercise. Hospitalization may be required to stabilize the person's mood in severe cases.

## PERSONALITY DISORDERS

Personality disorders are groups of persistent behaviors that impair social, academic, or professional functioning or cause personal distress. Common personality disorders include paranoid personality disorder, schizoid personality disorder, and schizotypal disorder.

A person suffering from **paranoid personality disorder** is excessively distrustful and suspicious of others, expects to be abused by others, doesn't confide in others, and may be extremely jealous. Schizoid personality disorder can result in extreme detachment from social situations and limited emotions in interpersonal relations. Finally, a person with a schizotypal disorder is usually socially isolated, exhibits bizarre behaviors and beliefs about the world, and is suspicious of others.

## SCHIZOPHRENIA

**Schizophrenia** is a severe personality disorder that involves distorted thoughts and perceptions, atypical communication, inappropriate emotion, abnormal motor behavior, and social withdrawal. There are five types of schizophrenia.

Paranoid schizophrenics experience delusions and auditory hallucinations. They trust no one and are constantly on guard because they are convinced that others are plotting against them. Catatonic schizophrenia is characterized by excessive inactivity. The person can retain the same posture for long periods of time and may alternate between violent behavior and being immobile and totally unresponsive to the outside world. Disorganized schizophrenics experience extreme delusions, hallucinations, and have inappropriate patterns of speech, mood, and movements. Extreme laughing and crying at unsuitable times are hallmark signs of disorganized schizophrenics.

**Paranoid personality disorder** is characterized by excessive distrust and suspicion of others.

**Schizophrenia** is a severe mental disorder that involves distorted thoughts and perceptions, atypical communications, inappropriate emotion, and abnormal motor behavior. Forms of schizophrenia include paranoid, catatonic, disorganized, undifferentiated, and residual.

A schizophrenic who experiences delusions, hallucinations, and disorganized behavior but lacks other specific symptoms is classified as an undifferentiated schizophrenic. Finally, residual schizophrenia is a condition in which at least one episode of schizophrenia has occurred, but there are currently no prominent psychotic symptoms.

✓ **NEED TO KNOW**

Mental disorders are some of the most misunderstood illnesses. When people's behavior appears different, often it is incorrectly interpreted as a disorder. Mental disorders, like physical disorders, have common sets of symptoms that are characteristic of those having the disorder. The symptoms can range from mood disorders to severe disorders such as anxiety disorders, mania, and schizophrenia.

# ➤ Treatment

Psychotherapy and biomedical therapy are two approaches used to treat many of the disorders described in this chapter. In most instances a combination of both psychotherapy and biomedical therapy is used.

Psychotherapy is performed by a psychotherapist. A psychotherapist can be a psychologist, psychiatrist, a psychiatric nurse, or a counselor. In all instances there are licensure and certification requirements for people performing psychotherapy. (See Chapter 12 for a more detailed explanation of the educational backgrounds of various health professionals.)

The psychological techniques employed in psychotherapy include such approaches as psychodynamic, humanistic, person-centered, gestalt therapy, existential therapy, and behavior therapies, systematic desensitization, implosive therapy, flooding, biofeedback, aversive conditioning, token economy, cognitive therapy, rational-emotive therapy, feminist therapy, and group therapy. See Figure 7.5 for a summary of the different techniques.

The biomedical approach involves the use of drug therapies to treat the disorder. In general the drugs used in treating these disorders include anti-anxiety drugs, antipsychotic drugs, antidepressant drugs, lithium, and electroconvulsive therapy. (Some of these drugs were discussed in Chapter 4.) Anti-anxiety drugs are minor tranquilizers such as Valium and Xanax. These drugs are designed to be used short-term. Anti-psychotic drugs are major tranquilizers that are used long-term and are capable of acting on the psychotic process itself. Antidepressant drugs such as Prozac, Zoloft, Paxil, and Cymbalta act on the neurotransmitters

## FIGURE 7.5 APPROACHES TO PSYCHOTHERAPY

**Aversive conditioning:** Client experiences unpleasant stimuli (shock, verbal insults) after behaving undesirably.

**Behavior therapy:** Principles of social learning are used to assist people in forming accurate perceptions of their feelings and themselves.

**Biofeedback:** Monitoring of body functioning provides feedback to the client.

**Cognitive therapy:** Client is taught to understand the irrationality of his or her thoughts or behaviors.

**Encounter groups:** Confrontational strategies are used to allow members to express true feelings.

**Existential therapy:** Emphasis is placed on free will and using the free will to develop insight and self-understanding.

**Family therapy:** This form of group therapy is directed at families.

**Feminist therapy:** Focuses on role of society and the role of discrimination in daily life.

**Flooding therapy:** Client is placed in a real situation that he or she fears, normally accompanied by the therapist.

**Gestalt therapy:** An approach that employs role-playing and confrontation.

**Group therapy:** Psychotherapeutic principles are applied to a group.

**Humanistic therapies:** The focus is on conscious thoughts and present times as opposed to psychodynamic (unconscious thoughts and past experiences).

**Implosive therapy:** Clients imagine and deal with their worst fears in a safe environment with a therapist.

**Marital therapy:** Husbands and wives receive therapy together to assist them in a more productive relationship.

**Modeling:** Client watches another person perform the feared behavior and with the help of the therapist copies that behavior.

**Person-centered therapy:** A warm, supportive environment is created where a person feels accepted and can reveal true feelings.

**Psychodrama:** Role-playing strategies are used including role reversal.

**Psychodynamic therapies:** Freudian insight therapies are used and involve free association and dream analysis; can be focused on the unconscious and past experiences.

**Self-help groups:** These support groups assist people in displaying behaviors to reduce risk of recidivism to a previous problem behavior (alcohol dependence).

**Sensitivity groups:** Strategies are used to promote self-awareness and trust of others.

**Systematic desensitization:** Principles of relaxation and visualization are used.

**Token economy:** Tokens are given as rewards for behavior in an effort to shape the behavior.

## Health & the Media *Advertising Antidepressants*

Zoloft is a selective serotonin reuptake inhibitor (SSRI), one of the most widely prescribed antidepressant among that category of drugs. Drugs like Zoloft have made a positive difference in many people's lives. However, in 2004 Zoloft advertisements contained a cartoon character that asked, "Are you sad or anxious? Tired all of the time? Not sleeping well? Losing interest in things and people you love? Do these feelings stop you from enjoying life? These could be the signs of depression. When the cause is unknown, Zoloft can help." The ads were deemed misleading by the Food and Drug Administration (FDA) and pulled because the possible risks and side effects from taking Zoloft were not adequately described. The issue of whether drug companies should advertise to consumers directly—in effect, asking them to go to their doctor to get a specific drug, rather than going to the doctor with a problem and allowing the physician to evaluate prescription needs—remains controversial today.

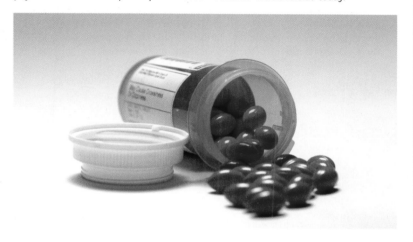

norepinephrine and/or serotonin. These medications have been very successful in treating depression and have made a major difference in people's lives. Lithium is used to control the swings in bipolar mood disorders.

Electroconvulsive therapy (ECT) is a procedure in which electrodes administer shocks to the patient, who experiences a seizure and then lapses into unconsciousness. When conscious, the patient feels better because the ECT has affected nerve cells and the root physiological causes of depression. Exactly what happens neurologically after ECT is unclear, but it provides relief for some people. Because it has some serious risks, ECT is normally used only when all other treatments have failed. ECT can speed or slow the heartbeat and cause memory loss. When psychotherapy and biomedical therapy are not effective in keeping a person functional, institutionalization may be the only remaining option, especially for people who are dangerous to themselves or others.

**NEED TO KNOW**

People who suffer from mental or emotional problems should be encouraged to know that interventions can help. After the condition is properly diagnosed, the appropriate treatment can be prescribed. Treatment can include counseling or medication or both. There have been tremendous advances in medications used to treat mental and emotional conditions. Medications such as anti-anxiety drugs and antidepressants have made a positive difference in many lives. Even people with profound mental problems might not need to be institutionalized as they were years ago. There are many options both in medications and counseling.

## ARTICLES

7.1 "A Nation of Wimps." *Psychology Today.* Parents are making wimps of their children, resulting in mental health problems when the child reaches college.

7.2 "Mental Health Service Utilization Among College Students in the United States." *Journal of Nervous and Mental Disease.* A comprehensive examination of service utilization and help-seeking behavior for mental health problems among college students in the United States.

7.3 "Conceptualizing the Engaging Bystander Approach to Sexual Violence Prevention on College Campuses." *Journal of College Student Development.* The "engaging bystander" is an approach to prevent sexual violence including rape and can be a viable intervention to decrease sexual violence on college campuses.

7.4 "Sleep Debt and Depression in Female College Students." *Psychiatry Research.* The relationship between sleep habits and depressive symptoms among female college students is examined in this study.

## SELF-ASSESSMENTS

7.1 Are You on the Correct Path to a Healthy Self Esteem?
7.2 Test Anxiety Questionnaire

## Website Resources

American Psychiatric Association. Healthy Minds. Healthy Lives **www.healthyminds.org**
Anxiety Disorders Association of America **www.adaa.org**
Centers for Disease Control and Prevention **www.cdc.gov**
Freedom From Fear **www.freedomfromfear.com**
Internet Mental Health **www.mentalhealth.com**
Jed Foundation **www.jedfoundation.org/students**
Mental Health America (formerly National Mental Health Association) **www.nmha.org**
National Eating Disorders Association **www.nationaleatingdisorders.org**
National Institute of Mental Health **www.nimh.nih.gov**
Obsessive-Compulsive Foundation **www.ocfoundation.org**

Substance Abuse and Mental Health Services Administration
**www.samhsa.gov**
Suicide.org: Suicide Awareness, Prevention, and Support
**www.suicide.org**

## Knowing the Language

anorexia nervosa, 266
anxiety, 267
binge eating disorder, 266
bipolar disorder, 269
bulimia nervosa, 266
depression, 268
dysthymia, 269
generalized anxiety disorder
  (GAD), 267
mania, 269
mental health, 256
motivation, 257
obsessive-compulsive disorder
  (OCD), 268

panic disorders, 268
paranoid personality
  disorder, 270
phobias, 268
posttraumatic stress disorder
  (PTSD), 268
psychosomatic, 256
schizophrenia, 270
seasonal affective disorder
  (SAD), 269
self-concept, 257
self-esteem, 257

## Understanding the Content

1. What is Maslow's hierarchy of needs and what does it have to do with mental health?
2. What can happen when needs are not met? What is the range of responses to tension, frustration, conflict?
3. What are the characteristics of good mental health?
4. What are the differences between mood disorders and personality disorders?
5. What are the common treatments used in treating mental disorders?

## Exploring Ideas

1. How does one know the difference between someone who is different and someone who is mentally ill?
2. How can a clear understanding of mental health lessen the personal and social problems related to mental health?

3. Why is it so hard for people to admit they are having mental health problems? What can be done to help create a better environment for people to seek help?

## Selected References

American College Health Association. *National College Health Assessment: Reference Group Summary.* Baltimore, MD: American College Health Association, 2010.

American Psychiatric Association. *Diagnostic and Statistical Manual of Mental Disorders* (4th ed.). Washington, DC: American Psychiatric Association, 2000.

American Psychiatric Association. *Let's Talk Facts About Eating Disorders.* American Psychiatric Association, 2005.

Centers for Disease Control and Prevention. *Violence Prevention.* January 27, 2009. **www.cdc.gov/violenceprevention**

Durkheim E. *Suicide: A Study in Sociology* (trans. Simpson G, Spaulding JA). New York: Free Press, 2000.

Glanze W. *Mosby's Medical and Nursing Dictionary* (5th ed.). St. Louis, MO: Mosby, 2002.

Kadison R, diGeronimo T. *College of the Overwhelmed.* San Francisco: Jossey-Bass, 2005.

Kitzrow M. The mental health needs of today's college students: Challenges and recommendations. *NASPA Journal* 41(1): 165–183, 2003.

Marano H. A nation of wimps. *Psychology Today* 40: 25–32, 2004.

Maslow A. *Motivation and Personality* (2nd ed.). New York: Harper & Row, 1970.

Narrow WE, Rae DS, Robins LN, Regier DA. Revised prevalence estimates of mental disorders in the United States. *Archives of General Psychiatry* 59(2): 131–145, 2002.

National Institute of Mental Health. *Eating Disorders.* Bethesda, MD: National Institute of Mental Health, 2002.

National Institute of Mental Health. *Facts about Anxiety Disorders.* Bethesda, MD: National Institute of Mental Health, 2003.

Nordenberg L. Dealing with the depths of depression. *FDA Consumer* 32 (4) July–August 1998. **www.fda.gov/fdac/features/1998/498. dep.html**

Shortell S, Kaluzny A. *Health Care Management: Organizational Design and Behavior.* Albany, NY: Delmar, 2000.

Sontag D. Who was responsible for Elizabeth Shin? *New York Times,* April 28, 2002.

Steers RM, Porter LW. *Motivation and Work Behavior.* New York: McGraw-Hill, 1987.

Taylor S. *Health Psychology* (5th ed.). New York: McGraw-Hill, 2003.

U.S. Department of Health and Human Services. *Healthy People 2010.* Washington, DC: U.S. DHHS, 2000.

U.S. Public Health Service. *Mental Health: A Report of the Surgeon General.* Washington, DC: U.S. PHS, 2002.

Wrobel G. Accessing Medicaid Funding for School Based Mental Health Programs. Presented at the National Association of School Psychologists, Washington, DC, February 10–12, 2001.

Cardiovascular disease is an equal opportunity affliction. In fact, more women than men die from heart disease, and the same is true for stroke.

— AMERICAN HEART ASSOCIATION

# Chapter 8

## HEART DISEASE AND STROKE

In this chapter, we focus on understanding coronary heart disease (CHD) and stroke, the two most common types of cardiovascular disease. We discuss the underlying disease process of atherosclerosis and review the signs, risk factors, and treatments for CHD and stroke. Prevention measures to reduce risk of CHD and stroke are highlighted.

## Cardiovascular Disease

CORONARY HEART DISEASE

STROKE

## Symptoms

HEART ATTACK ALERT—KNOW THE SIGNS

STROKE ALERT—KNOW THE SIGNS

ACT IN AN EMERGENCY

## Risk Factors

CIGARETTE SMOKING

HIGH BLOOD PRESSURE

HIGH BLOOD CHOLESTEROL

PHYSICAL INACTIVITY, OBESITY, AND DIABETES

OTHER RISK FACTORS

## Interventions

BEHAVIORAL APPROACH

PHARMACOLOGICAL APPROACH

SURGICAL APPROACH

## Prevention

**IN THE YEARS** following World War II, America was buzzing. Families reunited, new families began, suburban communities around cities mushroomed, and the economy boomed. Life was upbeat. Americans were optimistic about their health, too. In contrast to the hard times of the Great Depression and World War II, people living in the postwar period benefited from major advances in health and medicine. For example, public health systems ensured cleaner water and sanitary-waste disposal, while the advent of antibiotics brought major killers like tuberculosis and pneumonia under control. Yet, these good times were overshadowed by the rise in death and disability due to cardio-vascular disease.

Due to the growth in desk jobs and the popularity of labor-saving devices such as the washing machine and motorized lawn mower, people were getting much less physical activity than their parents had. In addition, the typical American diet changed to one where whole milk, butter, and red meats were commonplace rather than special occasion foods. Additionally, in 1950 the world was mostly unaware of the dangers of tobacco, which was especially unfortunate, given that about half of all American adults smoked.

Although heart disease rates in the United States had been increasing since the late 1930s, doctors had little advice for their patients on the control or prevention of heart conditions. Doctors thought that atherosclerosis was an inevitable part of the aging process and that blood pressure increased with age to enable the heart to pump blood through an older person's narrowed arteries. Similarly, the causal connections linking smoking, high-fat diet, and sedentary living to heart disease were not yet established. Doctors had scant evidence that modifying certain behaviors could help their patients prevent serious heart and vascular conditions. The standard treatment for people who survived a heart attack was four to six weeks of strict bed rest. Today people are encouraged to get up and walk as soon as they are medically stable, often within the first day following a heart attack or associated surgery.

In the 1950s, researchers began to investigate the potential roles of a high-fat diet and physical inactivity on the increased rates of cardio-vascular disease. By the 1970s a growing body of scientific studies provided strong evidence that both of those lifestyle habits contributed to the rise in cardiovascular disease. Today complex surgeries and powerful drugs are available to treat the many forms of cardiovascular disease. But an advancement at least as important as those sophisticated medical treatments is our understanding that cardiovascular disease can often be prevented. Staying active, not smoking, and making good dietary choices throughout life greatly reduces our risk of what remains the number one cause of death in the United States.

Article
8.1

This chapter focuses on understanding the two most common types of cardiovascular disease: coronary heart disease (CHD) and stroke. The underlying disease process of atherosclerosis is reviewed, followed by a synopsis of CHD and stroke, including their signs, risk factors, and treatments. The cardiovascular risk factors that are modifiable, along with preventive lifestyle behaviors, are emphasized throughout.

## ➤ Cardiovascular Disease

*Cardiovascular disease* is a general term that encompasses a broad array of diseases of the heart (*cardio-*) and blood vessels (*-vascular*). Cardiovascular disease has been the number one killer in the United States for many decades. In recent years, 4 of every 10 deaths among Americans are due to cardiovascular disease. Coronary heart disease (CHD) and stroke are the two most common types, together accounting for about 70 percent of all cardiovascular deaths. Other cardiovascular deaths are attributable primarily to congestive heart failure, a decline in the heart's pumping capacity (7 percent); high blood pressure, or hypertension (7 percent); and peripheral arterial disease (4 percent). The remaining cardiovascular deaths are caused by a variety of other less common heart and blood vessel disorders. Less than 1 percent of deaths are due to congenital cardiovascular defects.

A disease process called **atherosclerosis** causes both CHD and stroke. The term derives from the Greek words *athero,* meaning "gruel" or "paste," and *sclerosis,* meaning "hardness." Atherosclerosis involves a buildup of patchy deposits—primarily fatty substances, cholesterol, cellular waste products, and calcium—inside the arteries. These deposits are collectively referred to as *plaque.* As the plaque accumulates, the arteries thicken and harden, becoming less elastic.

The process of plaque deposition is not uniform or equally distributed within an artery, but rather it is irregular and scattered. As plaque accumulates within an artery, blood flow is increasingly restricted as the inner diameter of the vessel becomes rougher and smaller. The combination of less elasticity of vessel walls and increased pressure within vessels weakens arteries and makes them vulnerable to rupture. As atherosclerosis develops, it becomes more likely that a blood clot will

**Atherosclerosis** is the process in which the inner layers of arteries become irregular and thick due to accumulation of plaque (fatty deposits); over time, this process can lead to obstructive buildup within the arteries and weakening of the arterial walls.

form, blocking a narrowed artery. A clot can form within a narrowed artery (thrombus), or a clot can form in another part of the body and migrate to a narrowed artery (embolus). Complete obstruction of an artery or, less frequently, the bursting of an arterial wall can occur. If this occurs in the heart, we call it a *heart attack*. If it occurs in the brain, we call it a *stroke*.

Atherosclerosis may also occur in arteries far from the heart or brain—in the legs, pelvis, or arms, for example. This condition is known as *peripheral arterial disease*. It is much less common than heart attack or stroke as a cause of death, but it can be painful and limit one's activities. Cramping and fatigue in the legs while walking are early symptoms.

Atherosclerosis is a process that occurs throughout the body, although it may progress at different rates from one site to another. With that in mind, it's clear that a person at risk for any one of these three conditions—heart attack, stroke, or peripheral vascular disease—is also at risk for the other two. Moreover, atherosclerosis is often an underlying or contributing factor to hypertension and congestive heart failure.

Until the 1990s, atherosclerosis was chiefly considered a disease of middle age. It was viewed as a disease that could start in childhood but usually developed during midlife and beyond. New studies have significantly shifted this view. We now know that atherosclerosis can progress more rapidly and earlier in life, even in people in their 20s. At the other end of the age range, older people who have tightly controlled their cardiovascular risk factors have relatively low rates of heart disease and stroke. Such evidence indicates that age by itself is not as strong a determinant of atherosclerosis as was once believed; this evidence provides a powerful incentive to reduce one's risk factors regardless of age.

Atherosclerosis is initiated by inflammation with subsequent scarring and calcification of the innermost layer of the artery (endothelium). Substantial evidence demonstrates that premature onset or accelerated atherosclerosis is caused by tobacco smoke, high blood pressure, high cholesterol, physical inactivity, obesity, and diabetes—all of which are largely modifiable. These and other risk factors are discussed later in this chapter. In the next two sections, we will present the key terms and concepts about heart disease and stroke, respectively.

## CORONARY HEART DISEASE

Do you wonder what it feels like to have a heart attack? In the opening paragraphs of her book *Heartsounds,* Martha Weinman Lear tells the true story of her physician husband having a heart attack and the string of events that followed it:

> He awoke at 7 A.M. with pain in his chest. The sort of pain that might cause panic if one were not a doctor, as he was, and did not know, as he knew, that it was heartburn.
>
> He went into the kitchen to get some Coke, whose secret syrups often relieve heartburn. The refrigerator door seemed heavy, and he noted that he was having trouble unscrewing the bottle cap. Finally he wrenched it off, cursing the defective cap. He poured some liquid, took a sip. The pain did not go away. Another sip; still no relief.
>
> Now he grew more attentive. He stood motionless, observing symptoms. His breath was coming hard. He felt faint. He was sweating, though the August morning was still cool. He put fingers to his pulse. It was rapid and weak. A powerful burning sensation was beginning to spread through his chest, radiating upward into his throat. Into his arm? No. But the pain was growing worse. Now it was crushing—"crushing," just as it is always described. And worse even than the pain was the sensation of losing all power, a terrifying seepage of strength.
>
> On some level he stood aside and observed all this with a certain clinical detachment. Here, the preposterous spectacle of this naked man holding a tumbler of Coke and waiting to die in an orange Formica kitchen on a sunny summer morning in the 53rd year of his life.
>
> I'll be damned, he thought. I can't believe it.

**Coronary heart disease (CHD)**—also referred to as *coronary artery disease*—is a condition in which the blood supply to the heart muscle (myocardium) is partially or completely blocked due to atherosclerotic narrowing of one or more coronary arteries. CHD causes about one out of every six deaths in the United States. CHD was once widely thought to be a disease of men, and even today many people still believe this to be the case. But the statistics consistently show this to be false. CHD is the single largest killer of American males *and* females, with the total number of deaths about evenly split between the genders.

On average, men develop CHD about 10 years earlier than women because, until menopause, women are somewhat protected from the disease by their high levels of estrogen. Among women, heart disease is often perceived as an "older woman's disease," and it is the leading cause of death among women aged 65 years and older. However, heart disease is also the third leading cause of death among women aged 25–44 years and the second leading cause of death among women

---

**Coronary heart disease (CHD)** is a condition in which the coronary arteries are narrowed or blocked, usually because of atherosclerosis.

Cross section of a coronary artery reveals a large atherosclerotic plaque with a fibrous cap (arrow) and thick core (arrowhead).

aged 45–64 years. With regard to race/ethnicity, the prevalence of CHD for people aged 18 and older is similar for Whites (12 percent) and African Americans (10 percent) and lower for Hispanics (6 percent) and Asians (5 percent).

CHD is a chronic, progressive condition. As the plaque builds up in the coronary arteries, the blood flow channels become more and more restricted, with a likely outcome being chest pain or **heart attack** if the artery becomes completely blocked. The medical term for chest pain is *angina pectoris,* or more commonly just **angina.** Typical angina is uncomfortable pressure, squeezing, or pain in the chest, and it can vary widely in intensity. Angina often occurs when the heart needs more blood during physical exertion such as climbing a flight of stairs or running for a few seconds. Angina may also occur when experiencing strong emotions. Some people may have unstable angina in which chest pain occurs unexpectedly at rest. Nitroglycerin is the drug most

**Heart attack** is tissue death (infarction) to part of the heart muscle (myocardium) due to an insufficient blood supply when a coronary artery becomes blocked. The medical term for heart attack is *myocardial infarction.*

**Angina,** or *angina pectoris,* is the medical term for chest pain or discomfort caused by a restricted blood supply to the heart.

often used to treat angina. This drug is a coronary vasodilator. It causes the blood vessels to relax and thus allows the channels inside the vessels to open up and improve blood flow.

A heart attack, or myocardial infarction, occurs when one or more of the coronary arteries are blocked. This can happen when plaque tears or ruptures, creating a snag where a blood clot forms and completely blocks the artery. If the blood supply is cut off for more than a few minutes, the cardiac muscle cells suffer permanent damage and die. Depending upon the severity of the heart damage, the consequences can vary widely from a minor heart attack to sudden death. Fifty percent of men and 64 percent of women who died suddenly of CHD had *no previous symptoms* of the disease. This is a sobering statistic. Many of you may know of a person who died this way.

## STROKE

**Stroke** is a disorder in which an artery to the brain becomes blocked or ruptures, resulting in death of brain tissue. When counted separately from other cardiovascular diseases, stroke ranks third among all causes of death behind diseases of the heart and cancer. Stroke accounts for about 1 out of every 18 deaths in the United States. More women than men die from stroke. Stroke is also the second most common cause of disabling neurologic damage after Alzheimer's disease. Of those who survive a stroke, 15–30 percent suffer long-term disabilities. Over two-thirds of all strokes occur in people older than 65. In adults over 55, the lifetime risk for stroke is greater than one in six. Women have a higher risk than men, perhaps due to their longer lifespan. With regard to race/ethnicity, African Americans are more likely than Whites, Asians, or Hispanics to have a stroke and die from it. Although stroke is much more common in older people than in younger adults, they do sometimes occur in younger individuals, especially if there is uncontrolled high blood pressure.

Most strokes are due to atherosclerosis, the same underlying disease process that leads to heart attacks. In a stroke, the arteries supplying blood to the brain are affected. For this reason, strokes are sometimes referred to as *brain attacks.* The medical term for stroke is *cerebrovascular accident,* so called because the disorder affects the blood vessels (*-vascular*) to the brain (*cerebro-*). There are two types of stroke:

---

A **stroke** is brain-cell injury caused by a blockage or rupture of a blood vessel in the brain. Stroke is characterized by loss of muscle control, mental function, vision, sensation, and/or speech and other symptoms that vary with the extent and severity of brain damage. The medical term for stroke is *cerebrovascular accident.*

ischemic and hemorrhagic. The term *ischemic* refers to decreased blood flow due to constriction or obstruction of an artery. Most strokes (about 87 percent) are ischemic. In these cases, an artery to the brain has become blocked or occluded. Deprived of their blood supply and thus oxygen and nutrients, the affected brain cells can be permanently damaged.

A transient ischemic attack, sometimes called a *mini-stroke,* is a less serious variation of the ischemic stroke. In a transient ischemic attack, blood supply to part of the brain is compromised but only for a brief time. In this case, normal blood flow reestablishes quickly, and brain tissue does not die. However, a transient ischemic attack is a warning sign of an impending ischemic stroke.

Hemorrhagic strokes are less common (about 13 percent of all strokes) but are more dangerous than ischemic strokes. In this type of stroke, a blood vessel ruptures where the arterial wall has weakened. This not only prevents normal blood flow but also results in blood leaking into or around brain tissue, which in turn leads to life-threatening complications. Hemorrhagic strokes are more lethal than ischemic strokes.

When a stroke occurs, the resulting brain injury causes a loss of muscle control, mental function, vision, sensation, or speech, or a combination of these functions. Strokes usually damage only one side of the brain. Because nerves cross in the brain, symptoms appear on the side of the body opposite the injured side of the brain. Strokes affect people in different ways, depending on the type of stroke (ischemic vs. hemorrhagic), the specific area of the brain, and the extent of the brain injury.

✓ **NEED TO KNOW**

Cardiovascular disease includes all diseases of the heart and circulatory system. Coronary heart disease (CHD) and stroke are the two major types of cardiovascular disease and are the first and third leading causes of death in America, respectively. Atherosclerosis, a chronic progressive process of obstructive plaque buildup and weakening of the arterial walls, is the underlying cause of both CHD and stroke.

## ➤ Symptoms

Every adult in America should be able to recognize the symptoms of heart attacks and strokes and know the steps to take to activate the emergency medical system. Onset of symptoms should trigger an immediate response. You may be the only person available to provide assistance. Remember that emergency therapy for heart attack and stroke is critical for saving lives and reducing disabilities. The cardinal signs of a heart attack and of a stroke and the appropriate actions to take are presented in the next sections.

## HEART ATTACK ALERT—KNOW THE SIGNS

In the opening to this chapter's section on CHD, Dr. Lear struggles with disbelief and pain as he experiences a heart attack (described in the excerpt from *Heartsounds*). As a doctor, he knows the signs, yet he is trying to deny them. The thought that it must be something else— it *cannot* be a heart attack—is a typical initial response for many knowledgeable adults. Many people experiencing a heart attack are not sure what's wrong and wait too long before getting help. Know the signs of a heart attack, not only for your own sake but for the sake of others who may be indecisive about getting emergency care.

What are the classical signs of a heart attack? Many think a heart attack is sudden and intense, like the Hollywood portrayal where the character suddenly clutches his chest in anguish and falls over dead after an intense physical effort or emotionally charged event. A heart attack can occur this way, but the truth is that two out of three people who have heart attacks experience warning signs a few days or weeks beforehand. A person may notice only mild pain or discomfort from time to time. Or chest discomfort (angina) may become more frequent and occur with less and less physical exertion. Even those who have had a heart attack may not recognize their symptoms, because the next heart attack can have entirely different ones.

The most recognizable symptom of a heart attack is chest pain that may spread to the back, neck, jaw, left arm, both arms, or abdomen. The pain can range from slight discomfort or pressure to an unbearable squeezing or crushing sensation. It may persist or go away and return. The location of the pain can vary—it may occur in one or more of these sites and not in the chest at all. People who have a heart attack without chest pain are more likely to be over 75, have diabetes or heart failure, or have had a stroke. The chest pain of a heart attack is similar to the pain of angina but is generally more severe, lasts longer, and is not relieved by rest or nitroglycerin. Pain in the abdomen is sometimes mistaken for indigestion. Shortness of breath often accompanies chest discomfort, but it also can occur before chest discomfort. Other symptoms may include breaking out in a cold sweat, nausea, or light-headedness.

To summarize, *heart attack warning signs* are

- Chest discomfort or pain
- Discomfort in one or both arms, back, neck, jaw or stomach
- Shortness of breath
- Cold sweat, nausea, or light-headedness

It's worth repeating that women are as vulnerable to a heart attack as men. Heart disease is the number one killer of both women and men, and women account for just over half of all heart attack deaths. There is an average age difference, with women being about 10 years older than men when they have a heart attack. Please note that women are less likely than men to believe they're having a heart attack and more likely to delay seeking emergency treatment. As with men, women's most common heart attack symptom is chest pain or discomfort. But women are more likely than men to experience some of the other symptoms, particularly shortness of breath, nausea/vomiting, and back or jaw pain.

## STROKE ALERT—KNOW THE SIGNS

Strokes are most common in older people, but they are not rare among young adults. A stroke can occur in a young fit person if known risk factors are not being controlled, or occasionally they are caused by a hole in the heart—a patent foramen ovale. (All people are born with flap-like openings in their hearts, but for most the opening closes by itself shortly after birth.) It's important to be alert to the signs of both heart attack and stroke across the adult age range.

Unlike those of a heart attack, the signs of stroke are not widely recognized by the public. In a recent study by the Centers for Disease Control and Prevention, only 44 percent of American adults recognized the major warning signs. Admittedly, symptoms of a stroke can vary widely depending on the exact location of the blockage or bleeding in the brain. Each area of the brain is supplied by specific arteries. For example, if an artery supplying the area of the brain that controls the movement of the right arm is blocked, then the right arm becomes weak or paralyzed. Similarly, a loss of vision, sensation, speech, movement, or mental function can be the sign of a stroke, depending on the specific area of the brain affected.

The most common early symptoms of an ischemic stroke are sudden numbness, weakness, or paralysis of the face, arm, or leg on one side of the body; sudden confusion with difficulty speaking or understanding speech; sudden dimness or loss of vision, particularly in one eye; loss of balance or coordination, leading to falls; and sudden, severe headache. Symptoms of a transient ischemic stroke are the same but usually disappear within minutes. Symptoms of a hemorrhagic stroke are also largely the same as those of an ischemic stroke, but sudden severe headache may be more common along with nausea and vomiting, temporary or persistent loss of consciousness, and very high blood pressure.

To summarize, *stroke warning signs* are

- Sudden numbness or weakness of face, arm, or leg, especially on one side of the body
- Sudden confusion and trouble speaking or understanding

- Sudden trouble seeing in one or both eyes
- Sudden trouble walking, dizziness, loss of balance or coordination
- Sudden severe headache with no known cause

A person does not have to experience multiple symptoms to be having a stroke. Even if only one symptom is present, seek medical attention right away. Some people decide to ignore symptoms if they last only a few minutes. Yet, such a decision is a high-risk gamble with much to lose. Transient ischemic attacks often signal that a major stroke is on the way. People who have a transient ischemic attack should see a doctor immediately.

## ACT IN AN EMERGENCY

Starting medical treatment as soon as possible is critical when a person is experiencing a heart attack or stroke. The sooner emergency care is begun, the lower the risk of death or disability. There are clot-dissolving drugs and procedures that can open blocked arteries, but they must be delivered quickly—within the first one to three hours—to be effective.

It's critical to take action. Nearly everywhere throughout the country, a call to 9-1-1 will activate emergency medical service and ensure quick arrival by trained paramedics. Be sure to note as much of the following information as you can for the paramedics and emergency room team:

- What are the symptoms?
- What time did the symptoms begin?
- Does the person have any medical conditions?
- What drugs, if any, does the person take?

The paramedics will be able to start medical treatment, monitor the patient on the way to the hospital, call ahead to prepare the emergency team, and provide the quickest possible transport.

In the unusual instance where 9-1-1 is not available, drive the person to the nearest hospital emergency room. Call ahead if possible and alert them that you are coming. People who may have had a heart attack or stroke should not attempt to drive themselves, because an impaired driver is a hazard to everyone on the road.

Be aware that you may face obstacles in taking the appropriate action—primarily from the person you are trying to assist! Many reasons can surface to delay calling 9-1-1. People can't believe a heart attack or stroke is happening to them. Symptoms are not what they expected. People wait to see if the symptoms will go away. They want to try and treat the symptoms themselves. They call a family member for advice. They call the doctor and wait for a return call. They try to make arrangements for children or other dependent family members before seeking emergency care. They fear large medical bills. Although these are rational reasons, none of them are good enough to postpone *emergency* treatment. Although it may be tempting to wait, a delay in calling 9-1-1 can result in death or lifelong disability.

If the symptoms turn out to be related to some less serious problem, consider that as good news. The paramedics and emergency room team will not fault you for your quick and decisive actions to the known signs of a heart attack or stroke. Unfortunately, their dilemma is often just the opposite. They are sometimes unable to effectively treat people who waited too long before coming. In some cases, the time-sensitive window for using the most successful treatments may have closed.

## Breaking It Down Defibrillators—From the Emergency Room to the Shopping Mall

You may have seen automated external defibrillators (AEDs) conspicuously mounted in shopping malls, airports, fitness centers, and sports arenas. In the years ahead, you'll be seeing more of them—from work sites and churches to country clubs and casinos. They save lives. But how did the defibrillator come from the emergency room to the shopping mall?

We've seen the scene depicted on TV many times. The patient suddenly loses consciousness and has no pulse. It's a case of cardiac arrest, and a "Code Blue" is called for immediate response by a trained team of nurses and doctors. The resuscitating team continues advanced cardiac life support until the patient recovers or dies. The good news—on TV and in real life—is that cardiac arrest is often reversed by the electric discharge of a defibrillator.

Nearly a quarter of all deaths in the United States are attributed to sudden cardiac arrest, which results from disturbances in the electrical activity of the heart—most commonly, ventricular fibrillation. During this abnormal heart rhythm, the ventricles begin to quiver—visualize a bowl of writhing worms—rather than contracting in unison. This causes a sudden cessation of normal circulation of the blood due to failure of the heart's ventricles to contract effectively. Cerebral hypoxia, or lack of oxygen supply to the brain, causes victims to immediately lose consciousness and stop breathing. If left untreated, cardiac arrest invariably leads to death within minutes.

Most of these deaths are due to underlying CHD and are associated with a heart attack. Sudden cardiac arrest occurs primarily in middle-aged

*(Continued)*

and elderly people. Though the average age is about 65, some people are in their 30s or 40s. For many, there is no previous history of heart problems. Sudden cardiac arrest is often the first symptom and it can occur anytime, anywhere. By its very nature, sudden cardiac arrest is unpredictable.

The good news is that with the growing availability of AEDs in public places, successful treatment for cardiac arrest is much more likely. During ventricular fibrillation, electrical energy is present in the heart, but it is chaotic. If the heart can be shocked—called *defibrillation*—a normal heart rhythm may be restored. Due to advances in computer technology, AEDs are smart devices that automatically diagnose the abnormal heart rhythm and provide the necessary shock as appropriate. Learning to use an AED is highly intuitive and surprisingly simple. Many report that it's easier than learning CPR. AED courses last about three or four hours and include hands-on practice. AED training and related resources are offered through several organizations, including the American Heart Association and the American Red Cross.

*The key to successful treatment is to be quick.* The shorter the time from collapse to defibrillation, the better the chances of survival. If defibrillation is delayed for more than 10 minutes, survival rates drop to less than 5 percent. The challenge is to respond to every victim of sudden cardiac arrest within minutes. If the time from the 9-1-1 call to defibrillation is seven minutes or less, as many as one-third to one-half of sudden cardiac arrest victims found in ventricular fibrillation can be resuscitated.

To summarize, *cardiac arrest* warning signs are:

• Sudden loss of responsiveness (no response to tapping on shoulders)
• No normal breathing

If the signs of cardiac arrest are present, tell someone to call 9-1-1 and get an AED (if one is available), and begin CPR immediately. Use an AED as soon as it arrives. If you are alone with a person who has the signs of cardiac arrest, call 9-1-1 and get an AED if possible before you begin CPR.

Since 1960, cardiopulmonary resuscitation (CPR) has been taught to millions of people using the simple memory prompt of A-B-C for the steps of airway, breathing, and compressions. This changed in 2010 when the American Heart Association revised the guidelines and rearranged the three steps from A-B-C to C-A-B (Figure 8.1). The new first step is doing chest compressions, then establishing the airway, and

**FIGURE 8.1    NEW CPR GUIDELINES: C-A-B**

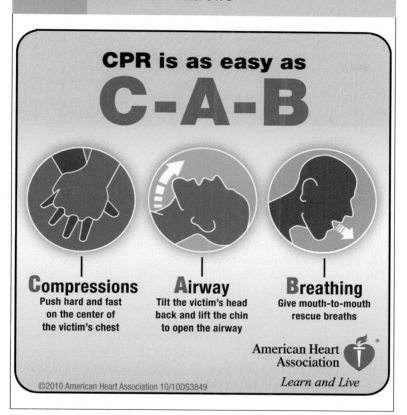

then performing rescue breathing. The new guidelines apply to adults, children, and infants. The AHA has found that chest compressions alone save many lives. The old approach caused delays in chest compressions (crucial for keeping the blood circulating).

The new guidelines may inspire more people to perform CPR—nearly everyone can do chest compressions whereas mouth-to-mouth breathing is difficult if you're not trained. The recommended rate of compressions is 100 times per minute (about the same beat as the 1970s pop classic "Stayin' Alive" by the Bee Gees). Remember, the new way is C-A-B for compressions, airway, and breathing. Better yet, take a course and learn (or renew) CPR and AED skills. If you needed help, you would hope that a bystander would know what to do. It may well be that we will be the bystander, not the victim. We need to be ready.

✓ **NEED TO KNOW**

You should know the warning signs of a heart attack and those of a stroke and how to activate the emergency medical system in your area. Time is of the essence. The sooner emergency care is begun, the lower the risk of death or disability. Learning CPR (cardiopulmonary resuscitation), knowing how to use an AED (automated external defibrillator), and keeping your certifications current are excellent ways to keep up-to-date and maintain practical—and potentially life-saving—skills.

## ➤ Risk Factors

With the rapid rise in cardiovascular disease during the first half of the 20th century, the U.S. Public Health Service decided to undertake a large-scale study to investigate why. Researchers wanted to learn which biologic and environmental factors were responsible. They agreed on an epidemiological study, a new approach at the time, to learn how and why those who developed heart disease differed from those who remained disease-free.

In 1948, the town of Framingham, Massachusetts, was selected as the study site, and 5,209 healthy residents (30–60 years of age, men and women) were enrolled. Each underwent a detailed medical history, physical examination, and comprehensive laboratory tests. Every two years, participants returned for similar exams. In 1971, another group was recruited for the "offspring study": 5,124 children (and spouses) of the original group. Currently, the "third generation" (children of the offspring group) are being enrolled and will be studied to further understand how genetic factors relate to cardiovascular disease.

Extensive longitudinal data from the Framingham Heart Study led to the identification of the major CHD risk factors. In fact, the Framingham researchers coined the term *risk factor* in 1961. The Framingham study has played a central role in influencing health care professionals to place greater emphasis on prevention and on detecting and treating cardiovascular disease risk factors in their earliest stages. In the years ahead, look for reports from the Framingham study as researchers continue to update and expand our knowledge about the causes, prevention, and control of cardiovascular disease.

Since the 1970s, risk factors for heart disease and stroke have been described as one of two types: nonmodifiable or modifiable. Risk factors that *cannot* be modified or changed are age, gender, and heredity. Increasing age is a risk factor. Men are at greater risk than women. And a family history of early heart disease—particularly in parents, grandparents, or siblings—is a risk factor. Early or premature heart disease is usually defined as occurring before age 65.

Risk factors that *can* be modified, treated, or controlled include six major factors and several other contributing factors. Most of you are aware of the three classic risk factors of smoking, high blood pressure, and elevated blood cholesterol. But you may not know that physical inactivity, obesity, and diabetes are also major risk factors. In the next few pages, we'll take a closer look at each of these six risk factors as they are the ones under our control. Dr. Paul Dudley White, the father of modern cardiology, once wrote that heart disease before age 80 is our fault, not God's or nature's will. That is, atherosclerosis is a largely preventable disease.

## CIGARETTE SMOKING

A smoker's risk is directly related to the number of cigarettes smoked daily. The nicotine and carbon monoxide in tobacco smoke reduce the amount of oxygen carried in the blood. These and other substances in tobacco smoke reduce HDL ("good") cholesterol, damage blood vessel walls causing plaque to buildup, and may trigger the formation of blood clots. In addition to increasing one's chances of having a heart attack or stroke, smoking causes cancer and lung disease, is the strongest risk factor for peripheral arterial disease and sudden cardiac death, and harms the fetus during pregnancy. Moreover, constant exposure to the tobacco smoke of others (secondhand smoke) can be as harmful as smoking.

Cigarette smoking is the single most preventable cause of disease and death in the United States. Despite the multiple harmful effects of tobacco and large-scale efforts to curb its use, tens of thousands of Americans still smoke. The latest figures indicate nearly one in four Americans over the age of 16 smokes. On average, smokers have twice the risk of heart attack and stroke as nonsmokers. Yet, remarkably, a large portion of a smoker's risk disappears two years after stopping; by 10 years, a former smoker's risk is similar to a nonsmoker's. If you smoke, the single best thing you can do for your health is to stop. All physicians agree on this point. Also, think of family and friends who smoke and what you can do to help them quit. (For suggestions, see You Can Quit Smoking Now! at **www.smokefree.gov.**)

## HIGH BLOOD PRESSURE

**High blood pressure,** or **hypertension,** is a condition in which blood pressure is consistently elevated over repeated readings on different

**High blood pressure** or **hypertension** is a chronic elevation of blood pressure, defined as a systolic pressure of 140 mm Hg or higher and/or a diastolic pressure of 90 mm Hg or higher.

days. Blood pressure is the force with which the blood pushes against the walls of the arteries. If blood pressure is continuously high, the heart is working harder than it should, and over time this will damage both the heart and the blood vessels.

When blood pressure is measured, two values are recorded. The higher value, or systolic pressure, reflects the highest pressure in the arteries when the heart contracts. The lower value, or diastolic pressure, reflects the lowest pressure in the arteries during the relaxation phase following a contraction. Blood pressure is written as systolic pressure/diastolic pressure; for example, 120/80 mm Hg (millimeters of mercury). This reading is referred to as "120 over 80." Although blood pressure today is increasingly measured with automated monitors, it's useful to understand the standard method on which it's based.

Conventionally, blood pressure is measured with a sphygmomanometer—an inflatable cuff with a gauge that measures the pressure of blood flowing through the main artery in the arm. Listening with a stethoscope placed over the artery below the cuff, a doctor or nurse inflates the cuff until it compresses the artery tightly enough to temporarily stop blood flow. Then the cuff is gradually deflated. When the pressure in the cuff equals the maximum pressure in the artery, the artery opens, and the sound of blood rushing through is amplified by the stethoscope. This is the systolic pressure. As the cuff pressure is reduced further, the sound suddenly becomes faint. This is the diastolic pressure—the pressure exerted when the heart relaxes between beats.

A sphygmomanometer measures blood pressure.

*Hypertension* is defined as a systolic pressure at rest that averages 140 mm Hg or higher, a diastolic pressure at rest that averages 90 mm Hg or higher, or both. As shown in Table 8.1, the higher the blood pressure, the greater the risks. In most people with hypertension, both systolic and diastolic pressures are high. Although hypertension can be successfully controlled, in most cases (over 90 percent of the time) its actual cause remains a medical mystery. This condition is formally known as *essential* or *primary hypertension.*

Hypertension is widespread in the U.S. population, affecting nearly one in three adults. Of those with hypertension, about 30 percent don't

**TABLE 8.1    CLASSIFICATION OF BLOOD PRESSURE**

| CATEGORY | SYSTOLIC (mm Hg) | | DIASTOLIC (mm Hg) |
|---|---|---|---|
| Normal | <120 | and | <80 |
| Prehypertension | 120–139 | or | 80–89 |
| Hypertension Stage 1 | 140–159 | or | 90–99 |
| Hypertension Stage 2 | ≥160 | or | ≥100 |

Note: High blood pressure is not diagnosed based on a single reading. If an initial reading is high, a second reading should be taken a few minutes later. Elevated readings should then be confirmed in the other arm.

Source: *Seventh Report of the Joint National Committee on Prevention, Detection, Evaluation and Treatment of High Blood Pressure,* 2003 **(www.nhlbi.nih.gov/guidelines/hypertension).**

know that they have it. There is a popular myth that people can "sense or feel" when their blood pressure is high. This is a false belief. Some folks think that if they don't feel ill, they must be OK. The truth is that hypertension typically has no symptoms for many years. This is why hypertension is known as the silent killer.

Compared to people with normal blood pressure, those with uncontrolled hypertension have a two- to threefold greater risk of heart attack and a three- to fourfold greater risk of stroke. Other prominent risks include kidney damage and heart failure. Hypertension is significantly more common in African Americans, adults over age 75, and people who are obese.

If you don't already know your blood pressure or if it's been more than a year since you had it checked, get a reading and record it. Everyone should know their blood pressure. If you have hypertension, work out a plan with your doctor to control it. There are a variety of approaches using combinations of weight reduction, dietary changes, aerobic exercise, stress management, and drug therapy.

## HIGH BLOOD CHOLESTEROL

A **high blood cholesterol** level, technically known as *hypercholesterolemia,* is another important modifiable risk factor. A total cholesterol value equal to or greater than 240 mg/dL (milligrams per deciliter of blood) is defined as high, putting a person at increased risk of atherosclerosis and thus heart attack, stroke, and peripheral arterial disease. Elevated cholesterol values can be due to many factors: a diet high

**High blood cholesterol,** or hypercholesterolemia, is an abnormally elevated total cholesterol level as measured from a blood sample.

in saturated fats, smoking, obesity, physical inactivity, and diabetes. Like hypertension, high cholesterol has no symptoms, and many people are unaware that they have the risk factor. About one of five American adults has high blood cholesterol.

The National Institutes of Health recommends that everyone aged 20 and older should have their cholesterol levels measured. The preferred blood test is a fasting lipoprotein profile that measures not only total blood cholesterol but also its components: low-density lipoprotein (LDL) cholesterol, high-density lipoprotein (HDL) cholesterol, and triglycerides.

Cholesterol is transported throughout the circulatory system by combining with lipoprotein carriers that vary in size and weight (e.g., LDL, HDL). The LDL-cholesterol combination is readily deposited on arterial walls and is a major constituent of plaque. LDL cholesterol—a.k.a. the "bad" cholesterol—is the largest component of total cholesterol and the primary target for cholesterol-lowering treatment. Conversely, the HDL-cholesterol combination functions in just the opposite manner and prevents plaque buildup in the arteries. Thus, HDL cholesterol is dubbed the "good" cholesterol. It is the only blood lipid in which higher levels are better.

The classification system for total, LDL, and HDL cholesterol is presented in Table 8.2. Notice the target values: total cholesterol under

| TABLE 8.2 | CLASSIFICATION OF BLOOD LIPIDS |
|---|---|
| **TOTAL CHOLESTEROL (mg/dL)** | |
| <200 | Desirable |
| 200–239 | Borderline high |
| ≥240 | High |
| **LDL CHOLESTEROL (mg/dL)—PRIMARY TARGET OF THERAPY** | |
| <100 | Optimal |
| 100–129 | Near optimal |
| 130–159 | Borderline high |
| 160–189 | High |
| >190 | Very high |
| **HDL CHOLESTEROL (mg/dL)** | |
| <40 | Low |
| ≥60 | High |

Note: Exclusive of the LDL cholesterol, a low HDL cholesterol (<40) is a major risk factor. Conversely, a high HDL cholesterol (≥60) is cardioprotective.

Source: *Third Report of the Expert Panel on Detection, Evaluation, and Treatment of High Blood Cholesterol in Adults*, 2004 (**www.nhlbi.nih.gov/guidelines/cholesterol**).

200 mg/dL, LDL cholesterol under 100, and HDL cholesterol equal to or greater than 60. An overall index of CHD risk is determined from the ratio of total cholesterol to HDL cholesterol. Ratios range from 3 or less (e.g., 180/60), which would be low risk and highly desirable, to 10 or higher (e.g., 250/25), which would be high risk and require medical follow-up. An ideal target is to keep the total cholesterol well below 200, with the HDL cholesterol accounting for 30 percent or more.

Average ratios (total cholesterol/HDL cholesterol) are 3.3 to 3.8 for young adult men and 3.0 to 3.5 for young adult women. The more favorable ratio in women is due to their higher levels of HDL cholesterol, which is associated with the female hormone estrogen. This is one reason why women are at lower risk for CHD and stroke through midlife. After menopause (as estrogen levels diminish), women lose this HDL cholesterol advantage, and the incidence of atherosclerotic diseases increases. For both genders, total cholesterol and thus LDL cholesterol levels increase with age.

How do we decrease LDL cholesterol and increase HDL cholesterol? For most people with borderline values, a prudent low-fat diet and aerobic exercise, respectively, are effective approaches to improving the blood lipid profile. If your LDL level is high, it's important to meet with your doctor. Effective cholesterol-lowering (LDL) drug therapy is available as an additional treatment if needed.

Article 8.2

As you now see, understanding your lipid profile as a risk factor is not just a matter of knowing total cholesterol. Years ago, this was the case. But that was prior to the discovery of the lipid subcomponents and an understanding of their roles. Although the term *high blood cholesterol* (or hypercholesterolemia) continues to be widely used, it's now known to be an oversimplification. The more accurate term is **abnormal blood lipids** (or dyslipidemia, *dys-* means "abnormal"), which refers to elevations of total cholesterol, LDL cholesterol, and triglycerides and/or low HDL cholesterol. In the years ahead, the term *abnormal blood lipids* will eventually replace *high blood cholesterol*.

Everyone should know his or her blood lipid values. Only about half of young adults aged 20–44 undergo cholesterol screening, even though about 25 percent have abnormal lipid profiles. Moreover, the CDC recently reported that 20 percent of youths aged 12–19 have abnormal lipid levels. If you have not had a lipoprotein profile performed within the past several years, get one. You should be as familiar

---

**Abnormal blood lipids,** or dyslipidemia, is elevated levels of total cholesterol, LDL cholesterol, and triglycerides and/or low HDL cholesterol as measured from a blood sample.

## Health & the Media Health Messages That Strike a Chord

The American Heart Association (AHA) has long been a leader in communicating health messages to the public. In recent years, these messages have broadened from straightforward ads to raise awareness of risk factors and signs of a heart attack or stroke to more complex messages to motivate and enable behavior change. This new emphasis is captured in the "You're the Cure" campaign and encompasses not just individual behavior change but also advocacy for children, families, and communities. This print ad certainly strikes a chord. How can we not want to improve the health of children? It also makes us reflect on our responsibility as role models. The action points—advocating for daily PE and healthy food choices in school—clearly link the prevention of childhood obesity to reducing risk for heart disease and stroke. Highlighting the multiple benefits of healthy lifestyle behaviors is a key message that underlies chronic disease prevention. AHA is an excellent resource for up-to-date information on how to improve diet, exercise regularly, and manage risk factors.

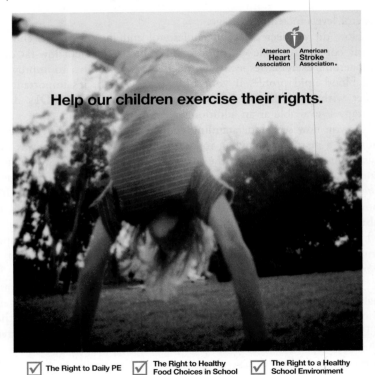

American Heart Association | American Stroke Association.

### Help our children exercise their rights.

☑ **The Right to Daily PE**   ☑ **The Right to Healthy Food Choices in School**   ☑ **The Right to a Healthy School Environment**

Childhood obesity is a growing epidemic that increases the risk of death and disability from heart disease and stroke. Don't miss your chance to shape a whole new generation of Americans and stop the nation's No. 1 and No. 3 killers — heart disease and stroke.

**Heart Disease and Stroke. You're the Cure.**
yourethecure.org

with your cholesterol levels as you are with your height, weight, BMI, and blood pressure.

## PHYSICAL INACTIVITY, OBESITY, AND DIABETES

Until the 1990s, the American Heart Association identified only three *major* risk factors that could be changed: cigarette smoking, high blood pressure, and high blood cholesterol. Other modifiable risk factors, described as *secondary* or *contributing* risk factors, were associated with an increased risk for cardiovascular disease, but their significance and prevalence had not yet been precisely determined. However, as the research evidence continued to mount, it became clear that several of the secondary risk factors were of similar importance as the first three. Accordingly, physical inactivity in 1992 and then obesity and diabetes in 1998 were upgraded to *major* risk factors.

### Physical Inactivity

Physical inactivity is an independent risk for heart attack and stroke. When inactivity is combined with overeating, obesity and diabetes can result. All contribute to the development of atherosclerosis. Conversely, regular moderate-to-vigorous exercise reduces the risk of heart and blood vessel diseases. Exercise can also favorably modify other risk factors by controlling blood cholesterol, obesity, and diabetes as well as lowering high blood pressure. Yet, only 3 in 10 adults are active enough to achieve these health benefits. Or put another way, 7 in 10 are not engaging in sufficient levels of physical activity. Although any increase in physical activity among the sedentary may impart some benefit, regularly engaging in moderate activities (e.g., 30 minutes of brisk walking 5 days a week) is known to improve cardiorespiratory function and lower the risk of cardiovascular disease. In general, physical activity follows a dose-response curve—the more active you are, the better. Refer to Chapter 3 for more information on physical activity and exercise guidelines.

Article 8.3

### Obesity

People with excess body fat—particularly if the fat is in the waist/trunk area (abdominal obesity)—are at higher risk of CHD. Obesity also contributes to the development of other risk factors for atherosclerosis: high blood pressure, high blood cholesterol, and diabetes. However, obesity puts people at higher risk of cardiovascular disease even if they don't have other risk factors. One in three American adults is obese (BMI of 30 or more; e.g., 5'5"/180 lb or 6'0"/221 lb = BMI of 30). Losing excess body fat reduces a person's risk for atherosclerosis as well as other associated disorders. In many cases, even modest weight loss

(5 to 10 percent of body weight) can help significantly. Refer to the section on healthy weight in Chapter 2 for information on safe and effective weight-loss and maintenance strategies.

## Diabetes

People who have diabetes have a two- to sixfold higher risk for developing atherosclerosis than those without diabetes. Diabetes—defined as a high blood glucose level (fasting value of 126 mg/dL or higher)—is a disease in which the body does not produce or respond properly to insulin. The most common form of diabetes is type 2, which usually develops in adults during middle age. In recent years though, onset of diabetes is occurring at younger ages. Among Americans aged 20 and older, 1 in every 11 persons has diabetes. Even when glucose levels are controlled, diabetics still have an increased risk of heart attack and stroke. Most diabetics die from cardiovascular disease. Diabetes damages the blood vessels and is linked with low HDL ("good") cholesterol, high triglycerides, and high blood pressure. Women who have diabetes are not protected from atherosclerosis before menopause. Also, physical inactivity and weight (fat) gain contribute to the development of diabetes. This dangerous combination of risk factors—elevated blood glucose, high blood fats, high blood pressure, and obesity—is called the *metabolic syndrome* (discussed in Chapter 10). For those with diabetes, regular medical checkups are essential. For everyone else, remember that diabetes is largely a preventable disease. Refer to Chapter 10 for an expanded discussion on diabetes.

## OTHER RISK FACTORS

Although not considered major risk factors, other factors are known to contribute to heart disease and stroke risk. Some people have particularly intense cardiovascular responses (e.g., sharp spikes in heart rate and blood pressure) to stressful conditions. Under conditions of continual stress, this high physiological reactivity can contribute to the development of cardiovascular disease. People who score high on personality traits of anger and hostility are also at higher risk. Such individuals, primarily men, typically display an explosive temper or expect the worst from people. This is damaging to their own health as well as unpleasant for those around them. Third, drinking too much alcohol can raise blood pressure and triglycerides and cause other cardiac problems as well as contributing to obesity, alcoholism, suicide, and accidents. As a side note, moderate alcohol consumption has been shown to reduce CHD risk by elevating HDL cholesterol. However, the evidence is not strong enough to recommend that teetotalers should begin drinking to improve their cardiovascular health!

Scientists continue to search for new clues that will lead to earlier diagnosis and a more complete understanding of cardiovascular disease. Promising variables of interest include homocysteine, which is an amino acid that appears to be associated with atherosclerosis and clot formation; lipoprotein (a), which may be harmful due to its role in preventing the breakup of clots; and viruses and other infectious agents that may damage blood vessel walls and start the atherosclerotic process. As research progresses, specific biochemical markers for these and other risk factors may eventually lead to additional or better methods for predicting or diagnosing cardiovascular disease.

To estimate your risk for CHD and stroke, see the Self-Assessment in Connect Resources. It may be eye opening to calculate risk profiles for a few relatives (siblings, parents, grandparents) as well. To get a sense of what your cardiovascular health status might be like in another 25 or 30 years, simply take a hard look at your parents. If you are concerned with what lies ahead, think about preventive approaches and be proactive. Today we know that heart disease is largely a consequence of lifestyle and everyday choices.

**303**

CHAPTER 8 HEART DISEASE AND STROKE

Self
Assessment
8.1 & 8.2

✓ **NEED TO KNOW**

Major risk factors for CHD and stroke are categorized as nonmodifiable and modifiable. The three nonmodifiable risk factors are increasing age, being male, and having a family history of CHD. The six modifiable risk factors are cigarette smoking, high blood pressure, abnormal blood lipids, physical inactivity, obesity, and diabetes. CHD and stroke are largely preventable diseases. Good nutrition, regular exercise, and a healthy weight are key elements to cardiovascular health.

# ➤ Interventions

The aim of this section is to provide a brief overview of the most common behavioral, pharmacological, and surgical approaches to reduce risk of heart attack and stroke and to treat atherosclerosis.

## BEHAVIORAL APPROACH

If you have one or more of the six modifiable risk factors, the first step should be to consider lifestyle modification to reduce risk. Your primary care doctor will be glad to hear of your willingness to make healthful changes and will help you develop an appropriate plan. Practical, science-based, online resources are cited throughout *iHealth* to help you break the smoking habit, improve eating and exercise patterns, and reach and maintain a healthy weight. If you plan these risk-lowering behavior

Article
8.4

changes on your own, it would be smart to consult with your physician before starting. It is important to have your doctor's support. Depending on your overall health status and risk profile, your doctor may feel it necessary to prescribe medications immediately along with your steps to improve lifestyle behaviors.

Occasionally a doctor may not support a person's desire to improve health habits and may recommend relying solely on medications to control risk factors. This approach is not common, but it does occur. If the doctor's rationale is unclear, then get a second opinion. A time-honored principle in the practice of medicine is to do the patient no harm. This reminds us that—even in the 21st century, when drugs are available for nearly every known malady—medications should be used only as needed. If nondrug alternatives such as lifestyle changes are available and feasible, they should be tried first or at least in combination with medications.

## PHARMACOLOGICAL APPROACH

This overview focuses on the use of medicines and the importance of patient–doctor communication to break tobacco dependence or treat and control high blood pressure and abnormal blood lipids. Dozens of other cardiovascular drugs are available to treat a multitude of related conditions. While discussion of these is beyond the scope of *iHealth,* an excellent resource to learn about specific prescription and over-the-counter drugs is the *Physicians' Desk Reference* website (**www.pdrhealth. com/drug_info/index.html**).

Nicotine replacement treatments via gum, inhaler, nasal spray, or patch are often prescribed for tobacco users who want to stop smoking, chewing, or dipping. Consult with your doctor about using nicotine or other drugs to help break the habit of tobacco dependence. He or she will gladly discuss drug treatment as well as counseling and behavioral options. Some doctors record history of tobacco use (i.e., current, former, never) as a vital sign along with their patients' pulse, blood pressure, temperature, and respiratory rate.

A nicotine patch can help a smoker quit by easing withdrawal symptoms.

If you use tobacco and value your

Drugs to treat and control high blood pressure and high blood cholesterol are two of the most common types of drugs prescribed in the United States. There are a variety of both anti-hypertensive drugs and LDL-cholesterol-lowering drugs available. Doctors have many choices regarding specific drugs and dosages. Yet, a major challenge to doctors is noncompliance, or patients not taking their medications. During initial drug treatments, many people abruptly stop taking the medication due to unpleasant side effects and *do not follow up* with their doctor. It's critical for people to report side effects to their doctor so that adjustments can be made. Successful treatment depends on the patient and doctor working in partnership, with the patient taking an active role in his or her own health.

In a sense, noncompliance is a natural response. Most people with high blood pressure or high cholesterol feel fine; they don't have symptoms of sickness. Yet, they are told they have high blood pressure or abnormal blood lipids, and it must be treated. In turn, the prescribed medicines may make them feel odd or ill or disrupt their normal patterns in some way—for example, they begin experiencing sluggishness, achiness, frequent trips to the toilet, difficulty sleeping, or a host of other side effects.

What is the solution? First, realize that high blood pressure and abnormal blood lipids need to be treated. The damage caused by either of these conditions is cumulative and permanent. If your doctor recommends drug therapy, side effects may occur. Be aware from the beginning that it may take several calls or office visits to find the right drug-dose combination. You need to be an active partner with your doctor to find a treatment that is satisfactory to both of you. Share this insight. If you know others who are having difficulty staying on their medicines, strongly encourage them to go back to their doctors.

## SURGICAL APPROACH

Since the 1960s, coronary angiography, also known as *cardiac catherization,* has been the gold standard for determining the degree of blockage in the coronary arteries. After a series of initial diagnostic tests, angiography is typically performed when CHD is suspected. In this procedure, a tiny hollow tube or catheter is inserted into an artery in the arm or leg and guided to the heart, where a contrast dye is released and X-rays are taken. From the resulting images, the degree of atherosclerosis—the narrowing of the coronary arteries—can be measured. If severe blockage is present in one or more coronary arteries, the options are usually coronary angioplasty (Figure 8.2) or

Interventions

## FIGURE 8.2 CORONARY ANGIOPLASTY

(A)          (B)          (C)

(A) From an artery in the leg or arm, a catheter (thin tube) is positioned in the narrow part of the coronary artery. A very thin wire tipped with an expandable balloon is threaded across the blocked area. (B) The balloon is inflated and deflated several times to compress the surrounding plaque and open the artery. The balloon is then deflated and the catheter removed. (C) The artery is now wider and blood can flow more easily.

Source: Reprinted with permission **www.americanheart.org.** Copyright © 2007, American Heart Association, Inc.

coronary artery bypass surgery. Multiple factors are considered in determining whether a patient is a candidate for either surgical procedure.

Both types of surgery are amazingly common, remarkably safe, and in the vast majority of cases, successful in restoring functional capacity and relieving symptoms such as chest pain (angina). However, if patients don't follow prescribed lifestyle changes and drug treatments after surgery, the surgical benefits may be relatively short-term. Some people find themselves back on the operating table a few years later for a second surgery. Over the past decade, on average about 1.2 million angioplasty procedures and 450,000 bypass surgeries are performed every year in the United States. That's about 3,300 angioplasties and 1,200 bypass surgeries per day, every day throughout the year, year after year!

### Coronary Angioplasty

**Coronary angioplasty,** or balloon angioplasty, is technically known as *percutaneous coronary intervention (PCI)* (*percutaneous* means "through the skin"). This catheter-based procedure is performed to open up a blocked coronary artery and restore blood flow to the heart muscle. Generally,

**Coronary angioplasty** is a surgical procedure in which a balloon-tipped catheter is inserted into a diseased, narrowed coronary artery; inflation of the balloon stretches the vessel opening, improving blood flow through it. Also called *balloon angioplasty,* and technically known as *percutaneous coronary intervention.*

coronary angioplasty is preferred to bypass surgery because it is less invasive and faster. During the procedure, the patient remains awake and conscious. The procedure involves guiding a catheter (thin tube) through a large peripheral artery (usually the femoral artery) into the aorta and eventually into the narrowed artery. A small inflatable balloon at the end of a wire is then threaded into position and inflated. This compresses the plaque that narrows the artery. In most cases, a drug-coated stent (a tiny wire mesh tube) is positioned in this newly opened artery and left permanently in place to help keep the artery open. After one or two days in the hospital, the patient usually returns home (see Figure 8.2).

### Coronary Artery Bypass Graft

**Coronary artery bypass graft,** commonly called *bypass surgery,* consists of grafting vessels taken from another part of the body (e.g., vein from leg or artery from chest wall) to a coronary artery and the aorta. Blood flow is thus rerouted, skipping over (bypassing) the narrowed or blocked area. In the traditional surgery, an incision is made down the center of the chest from the neck to the top of the stomach, and the breastbone is parted. The patient is on a heart-lung machine, which adds oxygen to the blood and circulates blood to other parts of the body during the surgery. This open-heart surgery can take four to six hours depending on the number of blood vessels to be grafted. The modifier before *bypass*—for example, *triple* or *quadruple*—refers to the number of arteries that are bypassed. The hospital recovery stay is typically five to seven days (Figure 8.3).

Other surgical techniques and technologies are being used more frequently. One increasingly popular method, called *off-pump coronary artery bypass,* avoids use of the heart-lung machine. This operation allows the bypass to be created while the heart is still beating. Another less-invasive alternative is the use of smaller incisions that avoid splitting the breastbone. Last, some bypass procedures are being performed using surgeon-directed robotics.

### Carotid Endarterectomy

**Carotid endarterectomy** is a surgical procedure done to prevent strokes by removing plaque from the carotid arteries. The carotid arteries are

**Coronary artery bypass graft,** or bypass surgery, creates a new route around a significantly narrowed coronary artery or multiple diseased arteries using a vein from the leg or an inner chest-wall artery, permitting increased blood flow to deliver oxygen and nutrients to the heart muscle. Bypass surgery is one of the most commonly performed major operations.

**Carotid endarterectomy** is a surgical procedure in which a narrowed carotid artery is opened and the plaque is removed to restore adequate blood flow to the brain.

## FIGURE 8.3    CORONARY ARTERY BYPASS GRAFT

Coronary bypass using the internal mammary artery

Internal mammary artery (from chest)

Aorta

Blocked coronary artery

Saphenous vein (from leg)

Blocked coronary artery

Coronary bypass using the saphenous vein

The cardiac surgeon will use a vein removed from the leg or an artery from inside the chest wall to provide a new path for blood flow from the aorta to the heart muscle.

located on each side of the neck and extend from the aorta to the base of the skull. Narrowed carotid arteries are diagnosed using a variety of medical imaging techniques. Although less well known and less frequently performed than angioplasty or bypass surgery, carotid endarterectomy is a common operation (over 90,000 per year) and a safe and long-lasting treatment.

The patient may be given a general anesthesia or, alternately, only the neck area may be numbed to allow the patient to communicate with the surgeon during the operation. The surgery involves making an incision to expose the narrowed carotid artery. The artery is temporarily clamped or bypassed, and another incision is made directly into the blocked section of the artery. The surgeon removes the plaque deposits, stitches the artery, removes the clamps or the bypass, and closes the neck incision. The procedure lasts about two hours. Following surgery, the average hospital stay is one or two days (Figure 8.4).

**FIGURE 8.4    CAROTID ENDARTERECTOMY**

2. Plaque is removed from the artery

Blocked section of carotid artery

1. Artery is opened at the blocked section, revealing plaque

3. Clean artery is sutured shut

The sequence illustrates the surgical removal of plaque from a carotid artery.

Source: Reprinted with permission **www.americanheart.org.** Copyright © 2007, American Heart Association, Inc.

We have reviewed three of the most common cardiovascular surgeries. Surgical techniques are continually being modified and improved. Moreover, applications of new technologies are providing new options for removing arterial plaque—for example, miniaturized devices and tools using the latest laser, mechanical, and chemical technology.

All three cardiac procedures can be viewed in tutorials with animation graphics at **www.nlm.nih.gov/medlineplus/tutorial.html.**

### Heart Transplants

As an endnote to this section on surgical approaches, we'll take a look at the ultimate cardiovascular surgery—heart transplantation. For a few patients with advanced heart disease, it may represent the only option left. The first heart transplant was performed in 1967 in Groote Schuur Hospital, Cape Town, South Africa, by Professor Christiaan Barnard and his surgical team. It was a milestone in medicine. The patient only lived for 18 days, succumbing in the end to pneumonia. But his new heart beat strongly to the end. Dr. Barnard showed the world that a human heart transplant was possible. The science of organ transplantation is now highly refined, and recipient outcomes are remarkably successful. Since 1990, there has been an average of over 2,100 heart transplants per year in the United States. Nationwide, over 240 medical centers perform heart transplants. Survival rates are 87 percent for one year and 71 percent for five years. As expected, the costs are enormous—surgery and treatments for the first year are estimated to be about $500,000.

> **NEED TO KNOW**
>
> Interventions to treat known risk factors for CHD and stroke can be categorized as behavioral, pharmacological, and surgical. Modifying lifestyle habits is a powerful approach to reducing risk factors. Motivation and perseverance are needed, but the cost and the side effects are minimal. Drugs are available to help people stop smoking and to control high blood pressure and abnormal blood lipids. Standard surgical procedures include angioplasty and bypass procedures to treat CHD and carotid endarterectomy to prevent stroke. Effective interventions often use combinations of behavioral, pharmacological, and surgical approaches.

## ➤ Prevention

Humans are intrigued with scientific and medical achievements. We are particularly dazzled by medical advances. The discovery of new drugs and the refinement of surgical techniques to treat cardiovascular disease are shining examples. With the constant highlighting of medical breakthroughs, we tend to minimize or overlook the enormous human pain and financial costs that come with heart disease and stroke—that is, until it strikes close to home.

No one purposely chooses a path that leads to disease and surgery, with the emotional and physical toll of the incisions, the tubes, and the pills. But by default, this is the path many follow. And more often than not, it leads to a life with limitations and loss of independence. In retrospect, many heart disease survivors encourage young people to pay attention to their health *now*. Don't wait until you're 40 or have a heart attack before you take stock of your lifestyle.

To gain insight into the emotional dimension and impact on quality of life, you should discuss the process of heart surgery with someone who has gone through it. A family member or a neighbor may be willing to share a firsthand account of the disease progression, surgery, and rehabilitation. Surgical options can indeed be life-saving treatments. Yet, if one can prevent the need for surgery by following a healthy lifestyle, then the choice seems clear.

Over 90 percent of people who develop atherosclerosis or experience a heart attack or stroke have one or more of the major risk factors. Science-based guidelines are available for all six of the modifiable risk factors. To keep your risk low, don't smoke, eat a prudent diet, exercise regularly, and maintain a healthy weight. Monitor your blood pressure, blood lipid profile, and blood glucose level and intervene as necessary to keep them in a healthy range. The central message is simple: cardiovascular disease is largely preventable through our own actions. The lifestyle habits you establish now will have a bearing on whether or when you will face drug therapy and surgery in the years ahead.

If the public were to adopt preventive measures, premature death and disability across all ages would decline markedly. A few notable scientists assert that cardiovascular disease need not influence one's quality of life until the age of 80 or later. Esteemed cardiologist Dr. Paul Dudley White stated that "a high, even 100 percent, mortality from cardiovascular disease nor sudden death itself are to be regretted, provided they take place at an advanced age after a healthy, happy, and useful life right up to the last minute."

**connect** Resources

## ARTICLES

8.1 "Paul Dudley White, MD, Preventive Cardiologist and Exercise Advocate." Author Phil Sparling writes a profile on the father of American cardiology.

8.2 "Lowering LDL Cholesterol Without Drugs." *U.S. News & World Report.* The challenges of how to treat high LDL cholesterol are discussed.

8.3 "Sedentary Behavior: Emerging Evidence for a New Health Risk." *Mayo Clinic Proceedings.* Prolonged sitting may have dire long-term health consequences distinct from those due to lack of regular exercise.

8.4 "Americans Confused about Effects of Wine, Sea Salt on Health. *Medical News Today.* Survey shows that many are confused when it comes to dietary recommendations regarding salt and wine.

 **SELF-ASSESSMENTS**

8.1 Disease Risk Questionnaire for Heart Disease
8.2 Disease Risk Questionnaire for Stroke

## Website Resources

### Specific Topics

American Red Cross: CPR and AED Courses
   **www.redcross.org/services/hss/courses/aed.html**
How Healthy Is Your Heart? (Texas Heart Institute)
   **http://hht.texasheartinstitute.org**
National Cholesterol Education Program
   **www.nhlbi.nih.gov/about/ncep/index.htm**
National Heart Attack Alert Program
   **www.nhlbi.nih.gov/about/nhaap**
National High Blood Pressure Education Program
   **www.nhlbi.nih.gov/about/nhbpep/index.htm**
Sudden Cardiac Arrest Association
   **www.suddencardiacarrest.org**
Tobacco Cessation
   **www.surgeongeneral.gov/tobacco**
Quit Smoking Today!
   **www.smokefree.gov**

American Heart Association (AHA)
**www.americanheart.org**
American Stroke Association
**www.strokeassociation.org**
CDC's Division for Heart Disease & Stroke Prevention
**www.cdc.gov/dhdsp**
MedlinePlus Tutorials on Diagnostic and Surgical Procedures
**www.nlm.nih.gov/medlineplus/tutorial.html**
*Physicians' Desk Reference*
**www.pdrhealth.com/drugs/drugs-index.aspx**

## Knowing the Language

abnormal blood lipids, 299
angina, 285
atherosclerosis, 282
carotid endarterectomy, 307
coronary angioplasty, 306
coronary artery bypass graft, 307
coronary heart disease
    (CHD), 284

heart attack, 285
high blood cholesterol, 297
high blood pressure
    (hypertension), 295
stroke, 286

## Understanding the Content

1. Define *atherosclerosis, coronary heart disease,* and *stroke.*
2. How do the signs of a heart attack differ from those of a stroke?
3. What is the difference between a modifiable and a nonmodifiable risk factor? Provide examples of each.
4. Give an example of a behavioral, a pharmacological, and a surgical intervention to reduce risk for cardiovascular disease.

## Exploring Ideas

1. Assume you are walking across campus early one morning, and you see a person lying on the ground who appears to have passed out. What would you do?
2. Prescription drugs are available to control high blood pressure and abnormal blood lipids, yet many people stop taking their

medicines. What are possible explanations for this situation? What are possible solutions?

3. What lifestyle behaviors will lower the likelihood that we develop atherosclerosis? Within the context of the modifiable risk factors, describe the key cardioprotective behaviors.

## Selected References

American Heart Association (AHA). Warning Signs of Heart Attack, Stroke and Cardiac Arrest.
**www.heart.org/HEARTORG/Conditions/Conditions_ UCM_305346_SubHomePage.jsp**

AHA. Cardiac Procedures and Surgeries
**www.heart.org/HEARTORG/Conditions/HeartAttack/Prevention TreatmentofHeartAttack/Cardiac-Procedures-and-Surgeries_ UCM_303939_Article.jsp**

Appel LJ, Frohlich ED, Hall JE, et al. The importance of population-wide sodium reduction as a means to prevent cardio-vascular disease and stroke: A call to action from the American Heart Association. *Circulation* 123: 1138–1143, 2011.

Archer E, Blair SN. Physical activity and the prevention of cardio-vascular disease: From evolution to epidemiology. *Progress in Cardiovascular Diseases* 53 (6): 387–396, 2011.

Artinian NT, Fletcher GF, Mozaffarian D, et al. Interventions to promote physical activity and dietary lifestyle changes for cardiovascular risk factor reduction in adults: A scientific statement from the American Heart Association. *Circulation* 122: 406–441, 2010.

Centers for Disease Control and Prevention (CDC). Awareness of Stroke Warning Symptoms—13 States and the District of Columbia, 2005. *MMWR* 57 (18): 481–485, 2008.

CDC. Prevalence of abnormal lipid levels among youths—United States, 1999–2006. *MMWR* 59 (2): 29–33, 2010.

Fiore MC, Jaen CR, Baker TB, et al. Treating Tobacco Use and Dependence: 2008 Update. Quick Reference Guide for Clinicians. Rockville, MD: U.S. DHHS. April 2009.
**www.gov/clinic/tobacco/tobaqrg.htm**

Framingham Heart Study: A Project of the National Heart, Lung and Blood Institute and Boston University.
**www.framinghamheartstudy.org**

Hurst JW. Meaningful quotations from Paul Dudley White. *Clinical Cardiology* 21: 617–618, 1998.

Kuklina EV, Yoon PW, Keenan NL. Prevalence of coronary heart disease risk factors and screening for high cholesterol levels among young adults, United States, 1999–2006. *Annals of Family Medicine* 8: 327–333, 2010.

Lear MW. *Heartsounds.* Pp. 11–12. New York: Simon & Schuster, 1980.

Mosca L, Benjamin EJ, Berra K, et al. Effectiveness-based guidelines for the prevention of cardiovascular disease in women—2011 update: A guideline from the American Heart Association. *Circulation* 123: 1243–1262, 2011.

National Heart, Lung, and Blood Institute (NHLBI), NIH. Heart and Vascular Diseases.
**www.nhlbi.nih.gov/health/public/heart/index.htm**

NHLBI, NIH. Seventh Report of the Joint National Committee on Prevention, Detection, Evaluation and Treatment of High Blood Pressure, 2003.
**www.nhlbi.nih.gov/guidelines/hypertension**

NHLBI, NIH. Third Report of the Expert Panel on Detection, Evaluation, and Treatment of High Blood Cholesterol in Adults, 2004.
**www.nhlbi.nih.gov/guidelines/cholesterol**

Piscatella JC, Franklin BA. *Prevent, Halt, and Reverse Heart Disease: 109 Things You Can Do.* New York: Workman Publishing, 2011.

Roger VL, Go AS, Lloyd-Jones DM, et al. Heart disease and stroke statistics—2011 update: A report from the American Heart Association. *Circulation* 123: e18–e209, 2011.
**http://circ.ahajournals.org/cgi/content/full/123/4/e18**

Shiroma EJ, Lee IM. Physical activity and cardiovascular health: Lessons learned from epidemiological studies across age, gender, and race/ethnicity. *Circulation* 122: 743–752, 2010.

U.S. Department of Health and Human Services. *How Tobacco Smoke Causes Disease: The Biology and Behavioral Basis for Smoking-Attributable Disease: A Report of the Surgeon General.* Atlanta, GA: CDC, 2010.
**www.cdc.gov/tobacco/**

World Health Organization (WHO) and CDC. *The Atlas of Heart Disease and Stroke.*
**www.who.int/cardiovascular_diseases/resources/atlas/en/**

The truth is, if you asked me to choose between winning the Tour de France and cancer, I would choose cancer. Odd as it sounds, I would rather have the title of cancer survivor than winner of the Tour, because of what it has done for me as a human being, a man, a husband, a son, and a father.

— LANCE ARMSTRONG

# Chapter 9

## CANCERS

In Chapter 9 we try to defuse the perception that cancer is synonymous with death. While people do die from cancer, there have been phenomenal advances in diagnosis and treatment. There is now hope where there was once none. This chapter discusses the basic disease process of cancer and also explains risks, prevention-oriented behaviors, early detection strategies, and treatment options.

# Chapter 9 | CANCERS

*BATTLE* **AND** *LOST* are two words often used by the media to describe people who have been diagnosed with cancer. Recently movie stars Patrick Swayze, Farrah Fawcett, and Dennis Hopper all lost their battles with cancer: Patrick Swayze of pancreatic cancer at age 57; Farrah Fawcett of anal cancer at age 62; and Dennis Hopper of prostate cancer at age 74.

The word *win* is not usually used in describing surviving cancer; instead, the words *cancer-free* or *cancer survivor* are favored. The reason for this can be summarized by another well-known saying: You don't know you're cured until you die of something else. That's because there is always a chance for recurrence with cancer. So while celebrities such as Sheryl Crow, Melissa Etheridge, Kylie Minogue, and Lance Armstrong have not necessarily "won" their battles with cancer yet, they have remained cancer-free and healthy since their treatments.

Reducing the impact of cancer is difficult because it requires proactive efforts on two fronts. People need to engage in healthy diet and behaviors throughout life to limit risk of developing cancer in the first place. Additionally, people should have regular screenings so in the event cancer does occur, it can be detected early and treated effectively. There are still many unknowns about why cancer strikes certain people and not others, and why some people respond better to treatment than others. But science continues to unravel these puzzles over time. Although the disease in Patrick Swayze, Farrah Fawcett, and Dennis Hopper followed the "traditional" pattern of late detection and a subsequently quick death, the good news is that more and more people are diagnosed with cancer early and respond favorably to treatments. Many become cancer-free after initial therapies and stay that way for the rest of their lives. And for others, cancer is not cured outright but is managed like a chronic disease, so that many people with cancer continue living productive lives despite being ill.

## ➤ Cancer

This year approximately 1,596,670 new cases of cancer will be diagnosed, and over 571,000 Americans will die from the disease. One in four deaths in the United States is attributable to cancer. The good news is that, according to the American Cancer Society, the 5-year survival rate for all cancers increased from 50 percent in 1975–1977 to 68 percent in 2006. More people are surviving cancer because of education, early detection methods, and sophisticated treatment.

**Cancer** is a broad term that refers to the growth and spread of abnormal cells in the body. The cell is the basic unit of life. Cells that are alike group together and form tissue. Tissue makes organs, and organs make up body systems. There are nine major body systems: cardiovascular, respiratory, digestive, endocrine, skeletal, muscular, nervous, reproductive, and excretory.

Human cells have two major characteristics. They "survive" by dividing into new cells, and each type of cell has a specific function. For example, cells in the digestive system may secrete digestive enzymes, while those on the tongue may allow you to taste.

Normally cells divide and create the same types of tissues that they came from. But sometimes, something goes wrong in the division process. Two unhealthy cells derive from a normal one, and then those two cells continue creating more abnormal cells. The abnormal tissue created can make an organ unhealthy. Unhealthy organs will make a body system malfunction. Figure 9.1 represents the progression of cancer. If the process goes on unchecked, death can result.

## CANCER TERMINOLOGY

A multitude of terms describe cancer and the disease process. The most basic ones are fairly simple. When a healthy cell becomes abnormal, it is said to mutate. Some **mutations** lead to cancers, but not all do. An abnormal cell that is not cancerous is referred to as **dysplasia.**

Chemicals from outside the body that influence cells to grow in abnormal ways are known as *carcinogens.* On the other hand, within the body, some people have genes in their DNA that are known to be correlated with increased chance for certain types of cancers. These are referred to as **oncogenes.**

Finally, when cancer spreads from its point of origin to another area, the process is known as **metastasis.** For example, one might hear that the cancer has metastasized from the lungs to the bone, meaning that

---

**Cancer** is the growth and spread of abnormal cells.

**Mutation** is the process by which a normal cell becomes abnormal.

**Dysplasia** is an abnormal cell that is not cancer.

An **oncogene** is a gene that increases the risk of cancer in a person who carries it.

**Metastasis** is the spread of cancer from its place of origin to somewhere else in the body.

## FIGURE 9.1  BODY STRUCTURE AND CANCER GROWTH

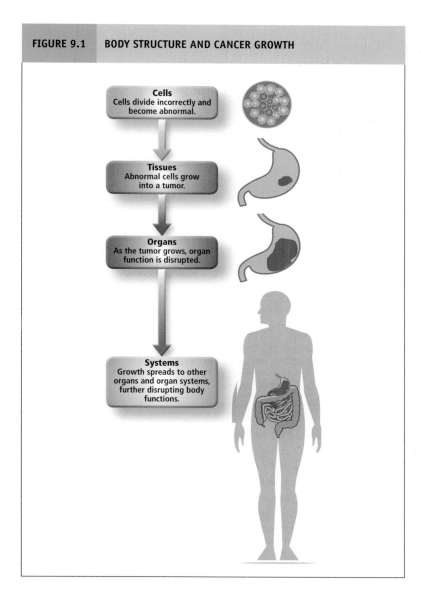

**Cells**
Cells divide incorrectly and become abnormal.

**Tissues**
Abnormal cells grow into a tumor.

**Organs**
As the tumor grows, organ function is disrupted.

**Systems**
Growth spreads to other organs and organ systems, further disrupting body functions.

the cancer has spread from the lungs to the skeleton. Figures 9.2 and 9.3 show diagrammatic representations of all of these terms.

When abnormal cells divide, they normally form a structure referred to as a *tumor*. A tumor is a stacking of cells, sometimes also called a *growth*. Tumors do not have to contain cancer cells—a benign tumor is a growth of normal cells, and a malignant tumor is a growth of

## FIGURE 9.2 LOSS OF CONTROL OF NORMAL CELL GROWTH

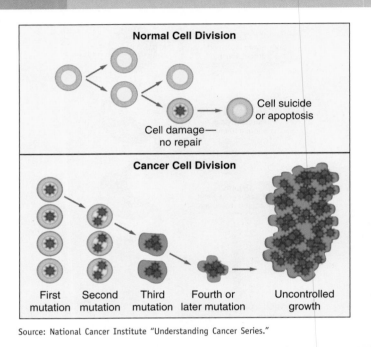

Source: National Cancer Institute "Understanding Cancer Series."

cancer cells. It should be noted that just because something is referred to as *benign* doesn't necessarily mean it is not dangerous. Some benign tumors can significantly interfere with the function of an organ and body system and, as a result, can be life-threatening.

Often the terms *tumor* and *cyst* are used interchangeably, but this is incorrect. Cysts are a mass of cells with fluid in the center. Tumors have solid centers. Both, however, are growths. Another difference is that cysts are usually benign.

Tumors normally arise from certain types of body tissues and are named in a way that defines their origin. Tumor names also end with the suffix *-oma*. **Sarcomas** are tumors that arise from bone, cartilage, or muscle. **Lymphomas** originate in lymphatic tissue, and **carcinomas**

**sarcoma** is a tumor that arises in bone, cartilage, or muscle.

**lymphoma** is a tumor that originates in lymphatic tissue.

**carcinoma** is a tumor that arises from epithelial tissue.

## FIGURE 9.3 METASTASIS

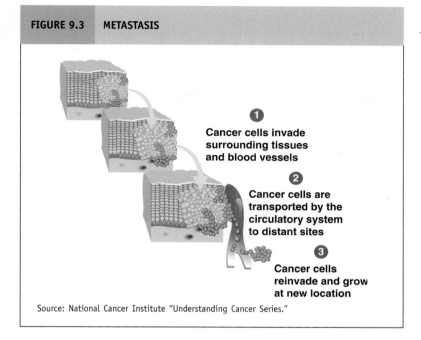

**1** Cancer cells invade surrounding tissues and blood vessels

**2** Cancer cells are transported by the circulatory system to distant sites

**3** Cancer cells reinvade and grow at new location

Source: National Cancer Institute "Understanding Cancer Series."

arise from epithelial tissue, such as that in the skin, nose, and mouth. From a clinical perspective, the specific location of the tumor is often referred to when discussing the tumor. For example, the term *basal cell carcinoma* describes a tumor that is made up of basal cells found in skin.

### ✓ NEED TO KNOW

Any cell in the body has the potential to mutate into an abnormal cell. Some cells are more susceptible than others, especially cells in the bone, muscle, cartilage, lymphatic, and epithelial tissue. When cells mutate into abnormal cells, there is a possibility that these abnormal cells will cause abnormalities in tissue or organs and that the cancer may metastasize to other areas of the body.

## ➤ Causes of Cancer

Many factors influence cellular change over time. Like many diseases, cancer generally has more than one cause.

There are 23 pairs of chromosomes in the nucleus of every cell in our body (except for red blood cells, sperm, and ova). **Deoxyribonucleic acid (DNA)** is the cellular molecule containing the genetic code that organisms need to function, and genes are made of DNA. Genes lie on the chromosomes and influence all sorts of body traits, from height and eye color to the propensity to develop certain types of cancers. If a person has a gene sequence that is linked with cancer, it usually means that at a certain point in a person's life, specific cells are more likely to grow abnormally than they would in a person without that oncogene.

In recent years health researchers have focused on decoding human DNA by mapping what different gene expressions do. Mapping the human genome is not a small task, because there are an estimated 20,000–25,000 genes in human DNA, with 3 billion chemical base pairs involved.

The alignment of the chemical base pairs spells out the genetic code, including disease. The Human Genome Project has estimated that there are about 1.4 million locations where single-base DNA differences occur in humans that seem to correlate with cancer and other diseases. The genetic sequences that are linked to a disease are sometimes referred to as "markers." In the case of cancer, having a marker does not mean the person will inevitably develop cancer. But it indicates that the person is at a much higher risk for developing a form of the disease if certain environmental variables are present. For example, people who have a marker for lung cancer but do not smoke have a low risk of lung cancer. If they do smoke, then their risk of lung cancer is very high— bigger than the risk of a smoker who doesn't have the lung cancer marker. Again, it is the marker combined with the unfavorable environ- ment (via smoking) that greatly increases the overall chance for cancer.

Although it sounds like science fiction, someday we may be able to alter a problematic line of code in a person's DNA and eradicate hereditary-linked cancers. Until then, the best way to deal with what we may be genetically predisposed to is to be aware of the kinds of cancer that run in our family, to try to live a healthy lifestyle, and to get early and regular screenings to minimize risks.

## ENVIRONMENT

Some chemicals in our environment can cause cancer. These substances are called **carcinogens.** Some of the more common ones include sulfur

> **Deoxyribonucleic acid (DNA)** is the genetic code inside nearly all cells that gives instructions on how the cells will divide, grow, and function.
>
> A **carcinogen** is a chemical or substance in the environment that can cause cancer in someone who is exposed to it.

dioxide, arsenic, asbestos, benzene, chromium, radon, soot, tar, vinyl
chloride, wood dust, and ultraviolet light.

Sulfur dioxide is a product of combustion engines and is a component in air pollution. Exposure to sulfur dioxide over time can cause cell mutations that contribute to the development of lung cancer. Arsenic is found in pesticides and has been linked to lung, skin, and liver cancer. Asbestos, a risk factor for lung cancer, was once a key chemical in glues, home insulation, and tile products. As a result, many construction workers who worked before asbestos was outlawed in the late 20th century were put at risk for cancer. Similarly, petroleum workers are often exposed to benzene, which has been linked to leukemia, and metal workers must deal with exposure to chromium, a chemical that increases the risk of lung cancer.

Radon is an underground gas found in geological pockets in many parts of the United States. It can leak through the foundation of homes unnoticed because it has no odor. Prolonged exposure to radon can increase the risk of lung cancer. Excessive soot and tar exposure, such as that experienced by industrial workers, has been linked to lung, skin, and liver cancers. Frequent exposure to wood dust has been associated with nasal cancer. Finally, exposure to ultraviolet light from the sun is strongly related to the development of skin cancer.

Again, it is important to note that exposure doesn't automatically mean disease. But people who have high levels of exposure to carcinogens run greater than average risks for developing certain cancers, and the longer the duration of exposure, the higher the probability of getting cancer. Environmental health specialists are very skilled at implementing ways to reduce exposure, so although an occupation may be risky, certain precautions like protective masks, sunscreen, or special clothing can help minimize harmful exposures.

## VIRUSES

Viruses are microorganisms that invade other organisms and use their cellular materials to replicate itself. (A more detailed explanation of viruses is in Chapter 11.) Since cancer involves abnormal replication of body cells, it makes sense that if viruses are capable of disrupting the genetic mechanisms in cells, their process might be a contributing factor to cancer. Fortunately, only a few viruses are thought to actually cause cancer.

Herpes virus 2, the most common form of genital herpes, can affect cervical cells and increase a woman's risk of cervical cancer. The same holds true for women infected with human papillomavirus (HPV). Hepatitis B affects liver cells and may increase the risk of liver cancer. Epstein-Barr virus (EBV), the cause of mononucleosis, increases the

The human papillomavirus (HPV) is a leading cause of cervical cancer in women. Pap smear tests are important screening tools in finding abnormal cells early.

risk of lymphoma, and human T-cell lymphotrophic virus is related to leukemia.

People who have been infected with cancer-linked viruses should be monitored closely. For example, a woman with a herpes 2 infection should have Pap smears more frequently than a woman who isn't infected with herpes 2. Understanding the early signs of related cancers is important so people can seek medical help early, if necessary. A more thorough discussion about herpes and HPV, including the issues surrounding Gardasil, the vaccine for HPV, can be found in Chapter 11.

## LIFESTYLE

As with so many diseases, the everyday choices we make can influence our risk for cancer. Lifestyles are a key factor in the etiology of many common cancers. Tobacco use is strongly implicated in the development of lung cancer. People who smoke 30 cigarettes or more each day have a 15 times greater risk of developing lung cancer than nonsmokers. Even smoke that nonsmokers inhale—secondhand smoke—can increase the risk of lung cancer. Additionally, combining cigarettes and alcohol increases the risk of cancer of the esophagus. People who drink more than four drinks a day and smoke have a 40 times greater chance

Self
Assessment
9.1

of developing cancer of the esophagus than people who don't combine heavy alcohol consumption with smoking.

Meat consumption and colon cancer are also related. The higher the consumption of red meat, the greater the risk of colon cancer. The population of the United States consumes large amounts of red meat and has one of the highest incidences of cancer of the colon. Specific information regarding reducing one's risk will be discussed later in the chapter.

> ✓ **NEED TO KNOW**
>
> Cancer is multicausal. There are both hereditary and environmental components to cancer. Depending upon the type of cancer, the hereditary influence might be stronger than the environmental or vice versa. It is critical that people know the kinds of cancers that run in their families and learn which environmental variables are related to the development of the cancer so that they can limit their exposure to those variables. If a certain type of cancer is present in their family, people need to assume they have a genetic predisposition and limit their risk.

# ➤ Diagnosing Cancer

Diagnosing cancer requires an examination of cells to determine if they are normal or malignant (cancerous). The protocol for diagnosis involves the same steps used for identifying any disease. It begins when people explain their medical history, describe their symptoms, and are examined by a medical professional.

### EXAMINATIONS AND BIOPSIES

When people have physical symptoms that are of concern, they usually visit a physician who asks about the severity of symptoms and the length of time they have been occurring. The physician performs physical examinations to determine health status, such as listening to the heart and lungs and measuring blood pressure. This examination may reveal suspicious findings that require further testing.

In the case of cancer, further testing can include examinations with imaging technologies such as X-rays, CT scans, or MRIs (see Chapter 12 for more explanation of some of these technologies). Some cancers leave traces in the blood, so tests may also be conducted on blood samples. For example, if a man has prostate cancer, his blood might have high levels of prostate specific antigen (PSA).

Mammograms are X-rays used to detect breast cancer.

If something looks abnormal in blood work or a scan image, a biopsy is performed. A **biopsy** is the removal and examination of a segment of the abnormal tissue or tumor. The cells are examined in order to determine if they are benign or malignant. Biopsies can be performed in a range of ways. The least invasive type is with a needle inserted into the tumor, which draws out cells for study. Other times, surgery may be needed to obtain a tissue sample. Most biopsies are uncomfortable but not usually highly painful.

## STAGING OF CANCER

Once cells are determined to be malignant, the next step is to determine how serious and advanced the malignancy is. In other words, how deep is the cancer and has it metastasized? **Staging** is the term used to determine how invasive the cancer is. There are three types of staging: tumors $(T)$, nodes $(N)$, and metastasis $(M)$. $T$, $N$, and $M$ values are assigned after the diagnosis of cancer.

If a tumor cannot be measured or found, then it is called $TX$. When there is no evidence of a primary tumor, a $TO$ is noted, which means that cancer has been diagnosed, but the tumor has not been found. If the tumor has not started to grow into the surrounding tissues, then

**Biopsy** is the removal and testing of a sample of cells or tissue to look for abnormalities.

**Staging** is a description of the size and spread of a cancer.

it is staged as *Tis*. Finally, *T1–T4* are used to describe the size and invasiveness of the tumor, with *T4* being the largest and most invasive.

*N* staging is also important because if the cancer has spread from the tumor to the lymph nodes, it very possibly has spread to other parts of the body, too. The notations in *N* staging include *NX, NO, N1, N2,* and *N3. NX* means that nearby lymph nodes cannot be measured. When the nearby lymph nodes don't contain cancer, an *NO* is assigned. *N1, N2,* and *N3* refer to the size, location, and number of lymph nodes involved. The higher the *N* value, the more lymph nodes involved and the more dangerous the cancer is.

*M* staging is used to describe the extent of metastasis of the cancer. Only three stages are used: *MX, MO,* and *M1. MX* means metastasis cannot be measured or found. *MO* means that there is no known distant metastases, and *M1* means metastases are present.

The evaluation of *TNM* will determine the course of treatment. As a general rule, the worse the *TNM* staging, the more intense the treatment. For people who are diagnosed with cancer, the staging they want to hear or see on their medical chart is *TX, NX, MX.*

### ✓ NEED TO KNOW

Diagnosing cancer is a complex and sophisticated process. Depending on the type of suspected cancer, a diagnosis may involve physical exams, X-rays, blood evaluation, and biopsy. Cancer must be staged, or rated, for an effective treatment plan to be devised. Staging describes three factors: whether a tumor has been found, if the original cancer has been discovered in lymph nodes as well, and if metastasized cancer can be found outside the original cancer site. Cancer tumors that are small and have not spread are the easiest to treat successfully.

## ➤ Common Cancer Sites

Any cell in the body has the potential to become cancerous. Figures 9.4 and 9.5 show the estimated cancer incidences and deaths by gender for 2011. It will be quickly noticed that the more common sites for cancer to develop include the breast, lung, colon, prostate, cervix, testicles, blood, and skin. We will examine these kinds of cancers with respect to signs and symptoms, risk factors, early detection, and treatment.

### BREAST CANCER

Of the estimated 230,000 new cases of breast cancer each year, 99 percent are found in women and less than 1 percent are in men. Breast cancer

### FIGURE 9.4 ESTIMATED CANCER BY GENDER

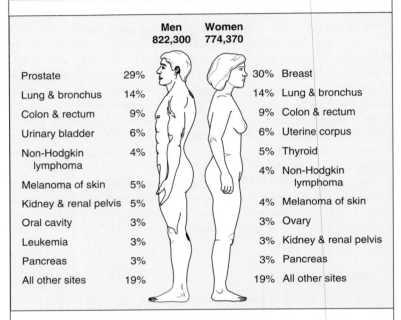

| | Men 822,300 | | Women 774,370 | |
|---|---|---|---|---|
| Prostate | 29% | | 30% | Breast |
| Lung & bronchus | 14% | | 14% | Lung & bronchus |
| Colon & rectum | 9% | | 9% | Colon & rectum |
| Urinary bladder | 6% | | 6% | Uterine corpus |
| Non-Hodgkin lymphoma | 4% | | 5% | Thyroid |
| | | | 4% | Non-Hodgkin lymphoma |
| Melanoma of skin | 5% | | | |
| Kidney & renal pelvis | 5% | | 4% | Melanoma of skin |
| Oral cavity | 3% | | 3% | Ovary |
| Leukemia | 3% | | 3% | Kidney & renal pelvis |
| Pancreas | 3% | | 3% | Pancreas |
| All other sites | 19% | | 19% | All other sites |

Excludes basal and squamous cell skin cancers except urinary bladder.

Source: Reprinted with permission from American Cancer Society. *Cancer Facts & Figures 2011.* Atlanta: American Cancer Society, Inc.

is the most common form of cancer diagnosed among women and the second most common site for cancer deaths in women. The most common symptoms of breast cancer are a lump in the breast or changes in the nipple. Although most lumps are benign, lumps still remain the most common symptom of breast cancer. Other symptoms include breast swelling, tenderness, nipple pain and/or dimpling, and nipple discharge. Any of these symptoms warrant immediate medical evaluation.

Like most cancers, the causes are unknown. Risk factors include a family history, a long menstrual history including periods that started early and ended late in life, obesity after menopause, postmenopausal hormone therapy, never bearing children, and having a first child after age 30. None of these events are strongly enough correlated with cancer to conclude cause and effect, but they are factors that increase one's relative risk.

Early detection of breast cancer is key to survival. The simplest early detection method is breast self-examination performed once a month.

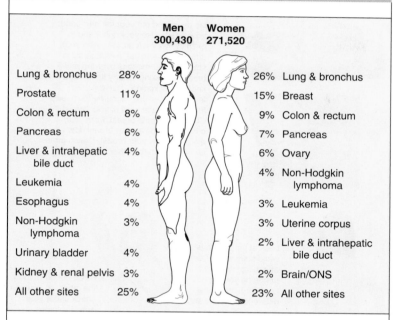

**FIGURE 9.5    ESTIMATED CANCER DEATHS BY GENDER**

|  | **Men**<br>**300,430** | **Women**<br>**271,520** |  |
|---|---|---|---|
| Lung & bronchus | 28% | 26% | Lung & bronchus |
| Prostate | 11% | 15% | Breast |
| Colon & rectum | 8% | 9% | Colon & rectum |
| Pancreas | 6% | 7% | Pancreas |
| Liver & intrahepatic bile duct | 4% | 6% | Ovary |
| Leukemia | 4% | 4% | Non-Hodgkin lymphoma |
| Esophagus | 4% | 3% | Leukemia |
| Non-Hodgkin lymphoma | 3% | 3% | Uterine corpus |
| Urinary bladder | 4% | 2% | Liver & intrahepatic bile duct |
| Kidney & renal pelvis | 3% | 2% | Brain/ONS |
| All other sites | 25% | 23% | All other sites |

ONS = Other nervous system.

Source: Reprinted with permission from American Cancer Society. *Cancer Facts & Figures 2011.* Atlanta: American Cancer Society, Inc.

Women who properly practice self-examinations have a higher probability of identifying a lump or tumor so that less invasive procedures can be used to remove the lump. Figure 9.6 shows the proper procedures for examinations.

Mammography is a type of X-ray examination of the breast. If a lump or mass is seen in the X-ray image, it will be biopsied. Unless directed by a physician, the general medical consensus is that all women should begin yearly mammograms at age 40. The earlier the breast cancer is detected, the less intense the treatment. If the cancer hasn't invaded other tissue or the lymph nodes, then all that may be necessary is a lumpectomy (removal of the growth). If the cancer is more advanced, then removal of the affected breast, called *mastectomy,* might be necessary. In addition to surgery, there may be a need for follow-up chemotherapy and/or radiation, both of which will be discussed in the section on cancer treatment.

**FIGURE 9.6    BREAST SELF-EXAMINATION**

1. Lie down and put your left arm under your head. Use your right hand to examine your left breast. With your 3 middle fingers flat, move gently in small circular motions over the entire breast, checking for any lump, hard knot, or thickening. Use different levels of pressure - light, medium, and firm - over each area of your breast. Check the whole breast, from your collarbone above your breast down to the ribs below your breast. Switch arms and repeat on the other breast.

2. Look at your breasts while standing in front of a mirror with your hands on your hips. Look for lumps, new differences in size and shape, and swelling or dimpling of the skin.

3. Raise one arm, then the other, so you can check under your arms for lumps.

4. Squeeze the nipple of each breast gently between your thumb and index finger. Report to your healthcare provider right away any discharge or fluid from the nipples or any lumps or changes in your breast.

Lung cancer accounts for approximately 14 percent of the new cases of cancer, or about 221,000 cases annually. It is the second most commonly diagnosed cancer among both men and women, and it is also the most typical site for cancer deaths among both genders. The most frequent symptoms for lung cancer include persistent cough, sputum streaked with blood, chest pain, and recurring bouts with respiratory infections, such as pneumonia and bronchitis.

Lung cancer tumors can grow and spread without symptoms. Unfortunately, lung cancer has a lower rate of survival than other cancers, mostly because it is usually discovered late. By the time a tumor is visible on an X-ray, it is well advanced.

Article 9.1

The most important risk factor for lung cancer is cigarette smoking. Other risk factors include exposure to secondhand smoke and to carcinogenic environmental chemicals. Although family history is always an important variable in the development of cancer, lung cancer is clearly more related to environmental exposure.

Chest X-rays, analysis of cells in sputum, and fiber-optic examination of the bronchial passages are detection methods. Unfortunately, they are not very effective for early detection. Treatment options include surgery, chemotherapy, and radiation.

## COLON CANCER

Approximately 141,000 cases of colon cancer are diagnosed each year in the United States. It is the third most common cancer, in both incidence and mortality, for both men and women. The most typical symptoms are rectal bleeding, blood in the stool, change in bowel habits, and cramping pain in the lower abdomen. Unfortunately, there are no early signs of the disease.

The major risk factors for colon cancer include family history, colon polyps, inflammatory bowel disease, low fiber diet, obesity, and a diet high in saturated fat and red meats.

Because there are no early signs of colon cancer, the emphasis is on early detection. Early detection can be done through a number of procedures. The simplest is a noninvasive procedure to determine if there is blood in the stool. Another procedure is an endoscopic exam called a *colonoscopy*; the person is given a sedative, and a scope is inserted deep into the bowel so that the bowel wall can be examined for cancer. An endoscopic exam is recommended for all adults over 50 years of age.

Treatment for colon cancer can range from removal of the tumor to removal of sections of the colon. It depends on how advanced the cancer is. Follow-up with chemotherapy and radiation may also be necessary.

## PROSTATE CANCER

Prostate cancer is the most commonly diagnosed cancer among men and typically affects men over 50 years of age. Many experts say that, like women's risk of breast cancer, if men live long enough, they will eventually develop prostate cancer. Approximately 240,000 new cases of prostate cancer are diagnosed each year.

Like many other of the cancers discussed, symptoms usually occur in the advanced stages. The common symptoms include weak or interrupted urine flow, inability to urinate, need to urinate frequently, blood in the urine, pain or burning with urination, and pain in the lower back, pelvis, or upper thighs. Symptoms usually mean the cancer has spread.

Risk factors for prostate cancer are age, ethnicity, and family history. The older a man is, the greater the risk. More than 70 percent of all prostate cancer cases are diagnosed in men older than 65. African American men have the highest prostate cancer rates in the United States.

Treatment options for prostate cancer usually include surgery, chemotherapy, and radiation. In early stage prostate cancer, radioactive seed implants can be inserted into the prostate to shrink the tumor. However, some prostate cancers are slow growing, and if a man is quite old, the cancer may be monitored and not removed because it might not present a threat to life and health.

## CERVICAL CANCER

The cells of the cervix are susceptible to mutation especially with the presence of certain viruses such as HPV. Cervical cells can change and over time mutate into cancer cells without a woman experiencing other symptoms. Approximately 12,700 new cases of cervical cancer are diagnosed each year.

Symptoms of cervical cancer don't usually occur until the abnormal cervical cells invade surrounding vaginal and cervical tissue. Then, the symptoms are usually abnormal vaginal bleeding and vaginal discharge. The main risk factor for cervical cancer is infection with HPV. Also, women who had sexual intercourse at an early age or who have had multiple partners are also at higher risk.

The Pap test is the most common early detection measure used to determine the health of the cervical cells and the first indication of cancer. A Pap test consists of a swab of cervical cells that are examined under a microscope. A trained lab technician can distinguish between healthy cells and cancer cells. Sometimes a Pap test will be reported as dysplasia. This term describes cells that aren't normal yet aren't cancer either. Women with dysplasia are monitored more closely and have Pap tests more often. If cervical cancer is diagnosed, then surgery, chemotherapy, and radiation are most likely to follow.

Testicular cancer is called a young man's cancer because the majority of the almost 8,200 diagnosed cases each year occur in men 20–40 years of age. Like other cancers, testicular cancer in the early stages has no specific symptoms. A common symptom is a lump in the testicle. The lump may or may not be painful. Testicular swelling, hardness, and a feeling of heaviness or aching in the scrotum or lower abdomen are other possible symptoms of testicular cancer.

Risk factors for testicular cancer are not clearly understood. Undescended testicles are the major risk factor. In the absence of risk factor information, the key is early detection. The American Cancer Society recommends that men, especially between the ages of 20 and 40, practice testicular self-examination (TSE) once each month. Figure 9.7 highlights the simple TSE procedures.

Article 9.2

Treatment for testicular cancer can range from chemotherapy to removal of the testicular lump to removal of the testicle or both testes.

## LEUKEMIA

When blood cells mutate and become cancerous, leukemia can result. Approximately 44,000 new cases of acute and chronic leukemia are diagnosed each year. Acute leukemia is the major form affecting children, and its symptoms appear quickly. Chronic leukemia is the major form affecting adults and is characterized by a slow progression of symptoms.

The major signs of leukemia are fatigue, paleness, weight loss, repeated infections, fever, bruising easily, nosebleeds, and other hemorrhages. Some of these symptoms are common to other conditions as well, making the diagnosing of leukemia difficult. The major risk factors for leukemia include exposure to environmental carcinogens, radiation, and specific types of viruses.

Other than paying close attention to ongoing fatigue, weight loss, and other symptoms with a follow-up diagnosis, there is no early detection method. Blood tests in suspect patients can indicate leukemia, and sometimes a bone marrow biopsy might be needed to examine bone marrow for cancer cells.

## SKIN CANCER

Skin cancer is an epidemic. There are over 2 million cases of skin cancer diagnosed in the United States each year. The good news is that most skin cancer is curable if detected early. Symptoms of skin cancer are more ambiguous than other forms of cancer discussed because the symptoms are mostly changes on the skin, so one has to notice those changes.

## FIGURE 9.7    TESTICULAR SELF-EXAMINATION

Spermatic cord

Epididymis

Testicle

**Self-Exam**

It's best to do a TSE during or right after a hot shower or bath. The scrotum (skin that covers the testicles) is most relaxed then, which makes it easier to examine the testicles.

1. Use both hands to gently roll each testicle (with slight pressure) between your fingers. Place your thumbs over the top of the testicle, with the index and middle fingers of each hand behind the testicle, and then roll it between your fingers.
2. You should be able to feel the epididymis (the sperm-carrying tube), which feels soft and ropelike and is slightly tender to pressure; it is located at the top of the back part of each testicle. This is a normal lump.
3. Remember that one testicle (usually the right one) is slightly larger than the other for most men—this is also normal.
4. When examining each testicle, feel for any lumps or bumps along the front or sides. Lumps may be as small as a grain of rice or a pea.
5. If you notice any swelling, lumps, or changes in the size or color of a testicle, or if you have any pain or achy areas in your groin, let your doctor know right away.

Lumps or swelling may not be cancer, but they should be checked by your doctor as soon as possible. Testicular cancer is almost always curable if it is caught and treated early.

Source: "How to Perform a Testicular Self-Exam" from TeensHealth.org. This information was reprinted with permission from KidsHealth, one of the largest resources online for medically reviewed health information written for parents, kids, and teens. For more articles like this one, visit **www.KidsHealth.org** or **www.TeensHealth.org.** Copyright: 1995–2011. The Nemours Foundation/KidsHealth.

There are three major types of skin cancer. **Basal cell carcinoma** usually appears as flat, firm, pale areas of the skin or as small, raised,

**Basal cell carcinoma** is a flat, firm, pale area of the skin or a small, raised, pink or red shiny area.

pink or red shiny areas. **Squamous cell carcinoma** appears as growing lumps with a rough surface or as flat, red patches that grow slowly. **Malignant melanoma** represents approximately 3 percent of skin cancers diagnosed but causes more than 75 percent of deaths, so it is considered the most dangerous of the skin cancers.

Malignant melanoma, the fifth and seventh most common form of cancer diagnosed in males and females, respectively, is very aggressive, and the incidence is rising faster than any other cancer in the United States. Malignant melanoma appears as an unusual mole, and if untreated it will grow deep into the body and metastasize. Melanomas appear asymmetrical—that is, one side doesn't match the other. They also tend to have irregular borders and wide variation in colors including yellow, green, and red tinges. Finally, the size of melanomas tends to be more than 6 mm (¼ in.), or about the size of a pencil eraser.

Article
9.3

The chief risk factor for malignant melanoma is exposure to the sun. It is estimated that 65 percent of melanomas are related to ultraviolet (UV) exposure. There are three major forms of UV rays, called UV-A, UV-B, and UV-C. All forms of ultraviolet light are found in the sun's rays, and when the rays reach the skin, they traumatize it. The skin responds by secreting pigment, which is what causes a suntan. So a suntan is not a sign of health but rather a sign of the skin trying to protect itself from damage. Tanning booths are also a source of UV rays (see "Breaking It Down" on the safety of tanning booths).

Self
Assessment
9.2

Early detection for malignant melanoma uses an *A, B, C,* and *D* screening. *A* stands for "asymmetrical." Symmetrical moles are usually not melanoma, which have irregular edges. Likewise, the borders (*B*) of the moles observed should be round, not irregular. The color (*C*) of a malignant melanoma is not brown, but might be brownish, red, yellow, or green. It does not look like a typical, common brown mole. Finally, a malignant melanoma will have a diameter (*D*) more than 6 mm or the size of a pencil eraser. If any mole on the body has abnormal characteristics of *A, B, C,* and *D*, a follow-up evaluation is necessary. Figure 9.8 shows the *A, B, C, D* of identifying malignant melanoma.

Treatment for malignant melanoma is like that for other cancers: surgery, chemotherapy, and radiation. Generally speaking, the earlier a melanoma is diagnosed, the better the outcome. If found in the early stages, then all that may be necessary for treatment is the removal of the mole.

---

**Squamous cell carcinoma** appears as a growing lump with a rough surface or as a flat, red patch that grows slowly.

**Malignant melanoma** is the most dangerous form of skin cancer because it is fast growing and can metastasize quickly.

**FIGURE 9.8    IDENTIFYING MALIGNANT MELANOMA**

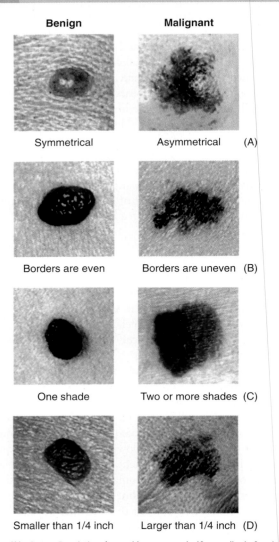

Source: The Skin Cancer Foundation (www.skincancer.org/self_exam/look_for.php).

Studies show that more than 2 million new cases of skin cancer will be diagnosed in the United States this year and that over 10,000 deaths will be traced to skin cancer in the same time period. Exposure to the sun is the major risk factor associated with the development of skin cancer, especially the deadliest skin cancer, melanoma. Approximately 28 million Americans visit tanning booths each year, and many assume that tanning booths are safer than regular sun exposure. Is this a correct assumption?

In fact, tanning booths are not safer than the sun. Booth equipment doesn't emit much UV-B light, which is what causes surface damage and sunburns. Instead, booths emit mostly UV-A light, which penetrates deeper into the skin and can damage internal organs or a person's DNA. UV-A exposure can increase the risk of melanoma.

A case in point. Anna Tremblay was a student at James Madison University in Virginia. She used tanning booths frequently, feeling it was a "social thing to do." Just before her senior year, she noticed a mole on her lower hip. After a trip to the dermatologist and a biopsy, she was diagnosed with melanoma.

Anna then had surgery to remove a large section of tissue from the area around the melanoma as well as other suspicious areas on the waist. According to Anna, her whole midsection "was just completely cut up. It was horrible." In the next four years she had two other melanomas diagnosed and treated. The good news is that Anna is a cancer survivor—however, because of her overuse of tanning booths, she now has to visit a dermatologist every six months for the rest of her life.

According to the Skin Cancer Foundation,

- UV light is a proven human carcinogen.
- Exposure to tanning beds before age 35 increases melanoma risk by 75 percent.
- People who use tanning beds are 2.5 times more likely to develop squamous cell carcinoma.
- Occasional use of tanning beds almost triples the chances of developing melanoma.

Yes, tanning booths can be found anywhere—spas, shopping malls, hotels. Just because they are abundant doesn't mean they are safe. For years the American Cancer Society and other groups have been very vocal regarding the dangers of tanning booths. Finally, there has been a response. President Bush signed the Tanning Accountability and Notification Act (TAN Act), which gives the Food and Drug Administration the authority to regulate tanning equipment including language used on warning labels. Expect to see the public's view of the safety of tanning booths change to regarding them as a high-risk behavior in the next few years.

In Spring–Summer 2011 the Food and Drug Administration (FDA) released new sunscreen regulations that will be implemented by Summer 2012. The aim of the new regulations is to educate the consumer on the benefits or lack of benefits in using a particular sunscreen. The following are among the new regulations:

- Broad-spectrum labeled sunscreens must provide protection from both UV-A and UV-B radiation.
- Those products with an SPF (sun protection factor) of 15 or higher can make the claim that they protect against skin cancer if used as directed with other sun protection measures.
- Sunscreens with an SPF of 2–14 are required to have a warning stating that the product has not been shown to help prevent skin cancer or early aging.
- The terms *sunblock, sweatproof,* and *waterproof* can no longer be included on sunscreen labels.
- A sunscreen can claim to be water resistant, but the product must specify it offers 40 or 80 minutes of protection while swimming or sweating. Sunscreens that are not water resistant must include a direction instructing consumers to use a water-resistant sunscreen if swimming or sweating.
- Sunscreens cannot claim to provide sun protection for more than 2 hours without reapplication.
- The FDA emphasized that sunscreen alone is not enough and should be used in conjunction with a complete sun protection regimen, including finding shade and wearing long pants, long-sleeved shirts, hats, and sunglasses.

Protecting against skin cancer is simple. In addition to consistently using a broad-spectrum, water-resistant sunscreen (SPF of 15 or higher) and applying 1 ounce to your entire body 30 minutes before going outside and reapplying every 2 hours or immediately after swimming or excessive sweating, the following should be observed:

- Limit exposure to the sun between 10 a.m. and 2 p.m.
- Do not burn.

### ✓ NEED TO KNOW

There are signs and symptoms for the common sites for cancer. Through an understanding of the signs and symptoms and the early detection methods, you can reduce your risk of being a cancer-mortality number and increase the probability of a successful outcome with the cancer. Many cancers are a result of choices people make—diet, smoking, sun exposure, and use of certain medications. Knowing the long-term effect of your health choices and acting appropriately can significantly reduce your risk.

- Avoid tanning and UV tanning booths.
- Cover up with clothing, including a broad-brimmed hat and UV-blocking sunglasses.
- Examine your skin head-to-toe every month to check for suspicious moles (*A, B, C, D* evaluation).
- See your physician for a professional skin exam each year.

## ➤ Cancer Treatment

Cancerous tissue must be removed in some manner. Surgery is the chief option for excising both the cancer and surrounding tissue. Once the cancer is removed, then a radiation and/or chemotherapy regime is instituted in order to prevent it from growing back.

Article 9.4

**Chemotherapy** simply means "chemical therapy," or the use of a variety of anticancer drugs. Some cancers do not require surgery and can be cured with just chemotherapy, whereas other cancers require both surgery and "chemo." There are many categories of anticancer drugs, some of which are quite toxic and have a very narrow margin of safety. The whole emphasis of chemotherapy is to kill new cancer cells before the cancer reoccurs.

Chemotherapy is hard on the body. Although drugs are becoming more precisely targeted, they often kill all fast-growing cells in a body, not just the cancerous ones. (People on chemotherapy sometimes lose their hair, because scalp cells are fast growing.) Chemotherapy also can suppress the immune system and leave a person open to infection. Further, it can cause nausea and weakness.

**Radiation therapy** is the last component of cancer treatment. Similar to chemo, the goal of radiation treatment is to destroy both cancer cells and cells that divide rapidly, which could be cancer cells. This treatment increases the likelihood that cancer cells remaining after surgery will be destroyed along with any cells that might become cancerous. In addition to killing cancer cells, radiation can help reduce symptoms if a cancer cure is not possible.

Although there have been many remarkable advances in cancer treatment, there is no guarantee that surgery, chemotherapy, and radiation will be effective with everyone. What has been described is the conventional approach, and the implementation of this treatment protocol requires the clinical judgment of physicians and the decision of

**Chemotherapy** is the use of numerous drugs to kill cancer cells.

**Radiation therapy** exposes cancer-ridden body areas to radiation doses to kill cancerous cells.

## Health & the Media Quack Cancer Treatments

Amigdalina (amygdalin) has often been referred to as vitamin $B_{17}$. However, it is not really a vitamin but a chemical found in the pits of apricots and other fruits. *Laetrile* is the common term for the drug form of the chemical. Because laetrile produces cyanide, which is a poison that kills cells, it has been marketed (particularly in Mexico) as a cancer cure. Amygdalin was first used as a cancer treatment in Russia in the 1840s. But modern studies show no scientific or clinical evidence that laetrile cures cancer. Nonetheless, some people diagnosed with cancer are tempted to try laetrile despite the numerous studies indicating it won't work.

Why are people susceptible to this quack drug? Some people do not research treatments before embracing them, so they remain ignorant of the science and evidence. This makes them easy prey for those who continue to market laetrile therapy. Others may have tried traditional cancer therapies but remain uncured. People who are desperate to extend their life may try almost any treatment if they think it gives them even the tiniest chance for improvement. Still others are drawn to the idea that "natural" or "simple" cures like laetrile, a drug derived from plants, must be better than invasive surgery or the arduous regimens of radiation or chemotherapy. So for a variety of reasons, quack drugs like laetrile continue as cancer treatments.

the patient. Cancer is such a serious condition that there is wisdom in getting a second opinion—not just about the diagnosis but also before committing to an aggressive treatment protocol. Finally, and most importantly, early detection is critical to increase the options for less intense treatment and survival.

More people are surviving cancer. Effective treatment modalities are the key to survival—surgery, chemotherapy, and radiation. Although these therapies are not pleasant, they are effective. There is much more hope for surviving cancer today than there was just a few years ago.

## EARLY DETECTION AND PREVENTION

Each type of cancer discussed has implications for early detection. Unfortunately, some kinds of cancer do not have symptoms until the cancer is advanced. Further, pain is a symptom of advanced cancer, so pain is not an early warning sign and should not be considered one. Figure 9.9 shows the array of cancer screenings available, when they should be done, and the appropriate age group.

To make cancer symptoms easy to remember, the American Cancer Society created the acronym CAUTION. If any of the symptoms below are noticed for at least two weeks, then a follow-up medical evaluation should be undertaken. CAUTION stands for

**C**hanges in bowel or bladder habits, like bloody stool/urine, or painful elimination

**A** sore that doesn't heal—a sign of skin cancer

**U**nusual bleeding or discharge—possibly a symptom of cervical or bladder cancer

**T**hickening or lump in the breast or elsewhere

**I**ndigestion or difficulty in swallowing—digestive-tract cancer symptoms

**O**bvious change in color of a wart or mole—a key sign of skin cancer

**N**agging cough or hoarseness—symptoms of lung or throat cancer

Increasing the options to prevent cancer focus mainly on the choices people make that affect risk. These choices are related to tobacco use, diet, and exposure to environmental carcinogens.

Tobacco is related to most cases of lung, mouth, and throat cancer, so abstaining from tobacco would be a significant effort in reducing the risk of respiratory cancers. Diets high in saturated fat and red meat

✓ **NEED TO KNOW**

There is not always a clear way to prevent cancer because we do not know with confidence what is related to the development of certain cancers. Just as important as prevention is early detection. CAUTION provides a simple framework for a basic set of symptoms that might indicate cancer. Learn and apply them. They may save your life.

**FIGURE 9.9** **RECOMMENDED CANCER SCREENINGS**

## Site & Recommendation

### Breast

◆ Yearly mammograms are recommended starting at age 40. The age at which screening should be stopped should be individualized by considering the potential risks and benefits of screening in the context of overall health status and longevity.

◆ Clinical breast exam should be part of a periodic health exam about every 3 years for women in their 20s and 30s and every year for women 40 and older.

◆ Women should know how their breasts normally feel and report any breast change promptly to their health care providers. Breast self-exam is an option for women starting in their 20s.

◆ Screening MRI is recommended for women with an approximately 20%–25% or greater lifetime risk of breast cancer, including women with a strong family history of breast or ovarian cancer and women who were treated for Hodgkin disease.

### Colon & Rectum

Beginning at age 50, men and women should begin screening with 1 of the examination schedules below:

◆ A fecal occult blood test (FOBT) or fecal immunochemical test (FIT) every year

◆ A flexible sigmoidoscopy (FSIG) every 5 years

◆ A double-contrast barium enema every 5 years

◆ A colonoscopy every 10 years

### Prostate

◆ The PSA test and the digital rectal examination should be offered annually, beginning at age 50, to men who have a life expectancy of at least 10 years. Men at high risk (African American men and men with a strong family history of 1 or more first-degree relatives diagnosed with prostate cancer at an early age) should begin testing at age 45. For both men at average risk and high risk, information should be provided about what is known and what is uncertain about the benefits and limitations of early detection and treatment of prostate cancer so that they can make an informed decision about testing.

increase the risk of cancer of the colon, so moderation in intake of saturated fats and red meat will reduce one's risk of cancer of the colon. Environmental carcinogens range from ultraviolet light to industrial chemicals, and reducing exposure will reduce risk.

## FIGURE 9.9    RECOMMENDED CANCER SCREENINGS (*continued*)

### Uterus

◆ **Cervix:** Screening should begin approximately 3 years after a woman begins having vaginal intercourse, but no later than 21 years of age. Screening should be done every year with regular Pap tests or every 2 years using liquid-based tests. At or after age 30, women who have had 3 normal test results in a row may get screened every 2 to 3 years. Alternatively, cervical cancer screening with HPV DNA testing and conventional or liquid-based cytology could be performed every 3 years. However, doctors may suggest a woman get screened more often if she has certain risk factors, such as HIV infection or a weak immune system. Women aged 70 and older who have had 3 or more consecutive normal Pap tests in the last 10 years may choose to stop cervical cancer screening. Screening after total hysterectomy (with removal of the cervix) is not necessary unless the surgery was done as a treatment for cervical cancer or precancer.

◆ **Endometrium:** The American Cancer Society recommends that at the time of menopause all women should be informed about the risks and symptoms of endometrial cancer and strongly encouraged to report any unexpected bleeding or spotting to their physicians. Annual screening for endometrial cancer with endometrial biopsy beginning at age 35 should be offered to women with or at risk for hereditary nonpolyposis colon cancer (HNPCC).

### Cancer-related Checkup

◆ For individuals aged 20 or older undergoing periodic health examinations, a cancer-related checkup should include health counseling and, depending on a person's age and gender, might include examinations for cancers of the thyroid, oral cavity, skin, lymph nodes, testes, and ovaries, as well as for some nonmalignant diseases.

◆ American Cancer Society guidelines for early cancer detection are assessed annually in order to identify whether there is new scientific evidence sufficient to warrant a reevaluation of current recommendations. If evidence is sufficiently compelling to consider a change or clarification in a current guideline or the development of a new guideline, a formal procedure is initiated. Guidelines are formally evaluated every 5 years regardless of whether new evidence suggests a change in the existing recommendations. There are 9 steps in this procedure, and these "guidelines for guideline development" were formally established to provide a specific methodology for science and expert judgment to form the underpinnings of specific statements and recommendations from the Society. These procedures constitute a deliberate process to ensure that all Society recommendations have the same methodological and evidence-based process at their core. This process also employs a system for rating strength and consistency of evidence that is similar to that employed by the Agency for Health Care Research and Quality (AHCRQ) and the US Preventive Services Task Force (USPSTF).

Source: American Cancer Society, *Cancer Facts and Figures,* 2008. Atlanta: American Cancer Society, Inc.

Knowing the Language

 **connect** Resources

 **ARTICLES**

9.1 "The Deadliest Cancer." *Newsweek.* This article highlights why lung cancer is considered the deadliest cancer.

9.2 "Getting to the Root of Testicular Cancer." *ED Insider.* Epididymitis and testicular torsion are two conditions affecting young males. This article highlights the diagnosis and treatment of both.

9.3 "The Sunscreen Myth: How Sunscreen Products Actually Promote Cancer." *Natural News.com.* This controversial article's premise is that sunscreens might not protect one from skin cancer.

9.4 "Conquering Cancer in the 21st Century: Leading a Movement to Save More Lives Worldwide." *Health Education and Behavior.* The executive director of the American Cancer Society writes about the current state of the global fight against cancer.

 **SELF-ASSESSMENTS**

9.1 Cancer Risk Factors
9.2 Skin Cancer Prevention

## Website Resources

Alliance for Cervical Cancer Prevention **http://alliance-cxca.org**
American Cancer Society **www.cancer.org**
American Institute for Cancer Research **www.aicr.org**
American Medical Association **www.ama-assn.org**
American Public Health Association **www.apha.org**
Centers for Disease Control and Prevention **www.cdc.gov**
Harvard Center for Cancer Prevention **www.diseaseriskindex. harvard.edu**
MedlinePlus Cancer Information **www.nlm.nih.gov/medlineplus/ cancers.html**
National Comprehensive Cancer Network **www.nccn.org**
Skin Cancer Organization **www.skincancer.org**

## Knowing the Language

## Understanding the Content

1. What is meant by *cancer* and *metastasis*?
2. Where are the most common sites where cancer occurs, and what are the major risk factors for each site?
3. What are the major methods used to treat cancer? Are they successful?
4. How can cancer be prevented?
5. What does the acronym CAUTION mean?

## Exploring Ideas

1. Why is it that when people hear the word *cancer*, they think immediately of death?
2. At which sites are college-age students at risk for cancer? What can be done to reduce risk?
3. What steps should be taken after a person is diagnosed with cancer?
4. Is there a role for complementary and alternative medicine in cancer treatment, and if so when?
5. Do you think the statement is true that if a person lives long enough he or she will most likely develop cancer? If so, why would this be true?

## Selected References

American Academy of Dermatology. The Darker Side of Tanning. 2004.
 **www.aad.org/public/publications/pamphlets/sun_darker.html**
American Cancer Society (ACS). *Cancer Facts and Figures.* Atlanta, GA: American Cancer Society, 2011.
ACS. *Cancer: What Causes It. What Doesn't.* Atlanta, GA: American Cancer Society, 2006.

Callee EE, et al. Overweight, obesity, and mortality from cancer in a prospectively studied cohort of U.S. adults. *New England Journal of Medicine* 348: 1625–1638, 2003.

Chao A, et al. Meat consumption and risk of colorectal cancer. *Journal of the American Medical Association* 293 (2): 172–182, 2005.

Christenson LJ, Borrowman TA, Vachon CM, Tollefson MM, Otley CC, Weaver AL, Roenigk RK. Incidence of basal cell and squamous cell carcinomas in a population younger than 40 years. *Journal of the American Medical Association* 294 (6), 2005.

Curry SJ, Byers T, Hewitt M, eds. *Fulfilling the Potential of Cancer Prevention and Early Detection.* Washington, DC: National Academic Press, 2003.

Elmore JG, et al. Screening for breast cancer. *Journal of the American Medical Association* 293 (10): 1245–1256, 2005.

Fung T, et al. Major dietary patterns and the risk of colorectal cancer in women. *Archives of Internal Medicine* 163 (3): 309–314, 2005.

Kapp J, Yankaskas BC, LeFevre ML. Are mammography recommendations in women younger than 40 related to increased risk? *Breast Cancer Research and Treatment* 119: 485–490, January 2009.

Matias KP. Studies of the viral origins of some cancers lead to new prevention, treatment strategies. *OncoLog* 39 (1), 2004.

Paules RS, Aubrecht J, Corvi R, Bernward G, Kleinjans JC. *Moving Forward in Human Cancer Assessment.* Bethesda, MD: National Institutes of Environmental Health Sciences, December 2010.

Raloff J. Sun struck: Data suggest skin cancer epidemic looms. *Science News Online* 168 (7), Aug. 13, 2005.

Ruckington C, Straus JJ. *The Encyclopedia of Cancer.* New York: Facts on File, 2005.

U.S. Food and Drug Administration. FDA Sheds Light on Sunscreens, June 2011. **www.fed.gov/ForConsumers/ConsumerUpdates/ucm258416.htm**

Good health is a
serious business. Like
life itself, it has to be
worked at and it takes
on added meaning
with effort.

— Norman Cousins

# Chapter 10

## DIABETES

In this chapter, we focus on what public health experts
describe as the fastest-growing chronic disease among
Americans today—diabetes. Metabolic syndrome (associated
with diabetes, heart disease, and obesity) is also discussed.
The interrelatedness of these chronic conditions highlights
the importance of establishing a balanced lifestyle at an
early age.

**DIABETES IS DISABLING,** deadly, and on the rise. New evidence indicates that one in three Americans born in 2000 will develop diabetes. Due to the rapid rise in prevalence—a tripling over the past three decades—and the dire prediction for further increases, an expanded look at this disease called *diabetes* is warranted. An understanding of diabetes is important because it may well affect our personal health or the health of those close to us. Moreover, facing the challenges of diabetes today provides a striking example of how lifestyle, medicine, and technology converge in 21st-century American society.

The Greeks described the disease as a "melting down of the flesh and limbs into urine." Indeed, the symptoms of diabetes have been recognized for centuries. Early records describe a puzzling and deadly condition that caused intense thirst, excessive urine production, and a wasting away of the body. And, oddly, the urine of those afflicted was sweet. Thus, the full medical term, *diabetes mellitus,* comes from the Latin words meaning "siphon" (in reference to excessive urine output) and "sweet like honey," respectively.

Little was understood about the cause of diabetes until the late 19th century, when the pancreas, a little-known organ, was discovered to play a central role. Experiments involving the removal of the pancreas from dogs resulted in diabetes, confirming the relationship between the organ and the disease. The focus then shifted toward identifying a substance in the pancreas that could be the key to solving the diabetes puzzle. This led to the discovery of insulin in 1921. For this remarkable scientific achievement, Canadian researchers Frederick G. Banting and John Macleod were awarded the 1923 Nobel Prize in Medicine.

Subsequent events continued to advance our understanding and treatment of diabetes. Soon after the discovery of insulin, Eli Lilly and Company started commercial production of insulin from the pancreases of animals. Concurrently, home testing kits for sugar (glucose) in the urine were developed. Yet, it would be the 1950s before it was fully realized that diabetes could be caused in two ways. This finding spurred the discovery of (noninsulin) drugs to lower blood glucose levels. In the 1970s, treatment innovations included blood glucose meters and insulin pumps. They were followed in the early 1980s by the commercial production of bioengineered "human" insulin.

Despite these major advances in treating the disease, diabetes among Americans has skyrocketed. Researchers agree that these rising numbers are due to the widespread combination of overeating and physical inactivity among a large proportion of the population. This "fattening of America" is clearly triggering the onset of diabetes along with increasing risk for heart disease and stroke. Related to these changes, a pattern of chronic disease risk factors has been recognized and in recent years has come to be known as *metabolic syndrome.*

In large part, diabetes, like atherosclerosis, is an unintended consequence of our technologically advanced, affluent society where food is plentiful, and daily physical demands are nearly nonexistent. For those with diabetes, the disease is not reversible or curable. Thankfully though, it is highly treatable. And for those without diabetes, the key concept is prevention. Let's learn about diabetes and see what we can do to turn the tide, both for ourselves and for society.

## ➤ Diabetes

**Diabetes** is the seventh leading cause of death in the United States, behind heart disease, cancer, stroke, lower-respiratory-tract disease (primarily tobacco-related emphysema), unintentional accidents (primarily motor vehicle accidents) and Alzheimer's disease. Over 8 percent of the population has diabetes (26 million people), with about the same number of males and females being affected. Of these, about 27 out of 100 are undiagnosed. That translates into nearly 7 million people who have the disease but are unaware of it. The risk for early death among people with diabetes is at least two times that of people without diabetes.

Among Americans aged 20 or older, 11.3 percent have diabetes. As shown in Figure 10.1, the prevalence of diabetes increases with age. For those 65 and older, the prevalence is nearly 27 percent. Risk of diabetes is also associated with race/ethnicity, as illustrated in Figure 10.2. Native Americans, Mexican Americans, and Blacks are about one and a half to two times more likely to have diabetes than Asian Americans and Whites of similar age.

Just what is diabetes? Diabetes is a group of disorders in which there is a defect in the transfer of glucose (sugar) from the bloodstream into cells. This leads to abnormally high levels of blood glucose, which is known as **hyperglycemia** (*hyper-* means "high" or "elevated"; *glycemia* refers to glucose in the blood). Blood glucose levels are controlled by **insulin,** a

---

**Diabetes**—or technically *diabetes mellitus*—is a group of disorders characterized by hyperglycemia resulting from defects in insulin production, insulin action, or both. **Hyperglycemia** is high blood glucose levels and is the hallmark of uncontrolled diabetes. **Insulin** is a hormone produced in the pancreas that helps glucose pass into the cells where it can be used for energy.

**FIGURE 10.1** **PREVALENCE OF DIABETES BY AGE GROUP**

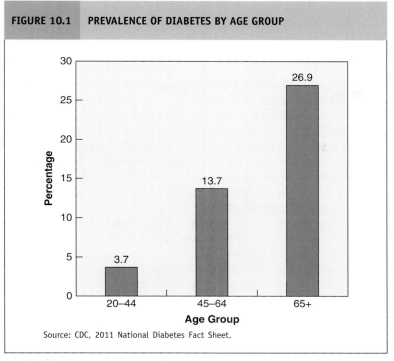

Source: CDC, 2011 National Diabetes Fact Sheet.

**FIGURE 10.2** **PREVALENCE OF DIABETES BY RACE/ETHNICITY (AGED 20 AND OLDER)**

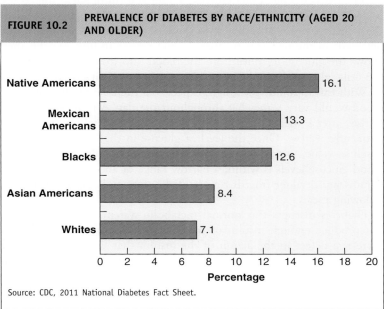

Source: CDC, 2011 National Diabetes Fact Sheet.

hormone produced by the pancreas that helps move glucose from the blood into the cells of muscles and other tissues.

## PANCREAS, METABOLISM, AND DIABETES

The pancreas, sandwiched between the stomach and the spine, is an oblong gland about the size and shape of a flattened banana. Part of it lies behind the stomach, and the other part is nestled in the curve of the small intestine (duodenum). The pancreas makes hormones and enzymes that help the body digest and use food. Throughout the pancreas are clusters of cells called the *islets of Langerhans.* These islets are made up of two types of cells: alpha cells, which make glucagon, a hormone that raises the level of glucose in the blood, and beta cells, which make the hormone insulin.

Balancing the release of glucagon and the release of insulin into the bloodstream to regulate glucose needs of the body is normally an efficient physiological system. However, if the beta cells do not produce enough insulin, diabetes will develop. Diabetes can also result if the body does not respond properly to the insulin that is made. Last, diabetes can occur by a combination of both defects—insulin deficiency and insulin resistance.

To better understand diabetes, let's consider what happens when a person eats. Once in the gastrointestinal tract, food is broken down into constituents including glucose, a simple form of sugar that is the body's primary source of energy. Glucose passes through the wall of the intestine and is absorbed into the bloodstream and stimulates the beta cells in the pancreas to produce and release insulin. Insulin then allows the glucose to move from the blood into the cells. Once inside the cells, glucose is used for energy or stored until it's needed.

With this in mind, you might expect that the level of glucose in the blood would vary somewhat throughout the day. And indeed it does. It rises after a meal and returns to a baseline level within about two hours after eating. Once the level of glucose in the blood returns to a baseline value, insulin production decreases. Standard variation in blood glucose levels is within a narrow range of about 70 to 110 milligrams per deciliter (mg/dL) most of the time and up to 140 mg/dL following meals.

Diabetes disrupts this normal metabolic system. If the body does not produce enough insulin to move the glucose into the cells or if there is a defect in the action of the insulin that limits its effect, the resulting high level of glucose in the blood and the inadequate amount of glucose in the cells together produce the symptoms and complications of diabetes. There are three main types of diabetes: type 1, type 2, and gestational diabetes.

Type 1 diabetes is diagnosed in children, teenagers, and young adults. The incidence of type 1 diabetes peaks at puberty. In this form of diabetes, the beta cells, the insulin-producing cells of the pancreas, are destroyed by the body's immune system. This abnormal autoimmune response—a targeted attack and destruction of the body's own cells—is linked to genetic predisposition, but it may also be associated with environmental factors. Although pieces of the puzzle are coming together, the actual causes are not yet well understood. The eventual permanent destruction of all or nearly all of the beta cells typically leads to absolute insulin deficiency—that is, a complete inability to produce insulin. Most people who have type 1 diabetes develop it before age 25 and must take insulin for the rest of their lives. Due to the acute onset of symptoms (e.g., increased urination, increased thirst, unexplained weight loss), type 1 diabetes is nearly always diagnosed soon after symptoms appear. Although the preferred term is *type 1 diabetes,* this condition is also referred to as *insulin-dependent diabetes* or *juvenile diabetes.* From a public health perspective, it's important to note that only 5 to 10 percent of people with diabetes have this form of the disease.

## TYPE 2 DIABETES

Type 2 diabetes usually develops in people older than 40 and becomes more common with age. It is by far the most prevalent type of diabetes—over 90 percent of all people with diabetes have type 2. In this type of diabetes, the pancreas continues to produce insulin, but the body develops what is known as *insulin resistance.* This is a condition in which the body's cells do not use insulin properly. Initially, the pancreas compensates by producing more insulin at higher than normal levels. Over time, however, the pancreas cannot supply enough insulin in response to meals. Excess body fat (adipose tissue) is the primary cause of insulin resistance and the chief risk factor for type 2 diabetes. It's estimated that 80–90 percent of people with type 2 diabetes are obese. This type of diabetes, like type 1, is also associated with a complex genetic predisposition and tends to run in families. In contrast to type 1 though, type 2 develops gradually. People can have high blood glucose levels for years—with ongoing damage to tissues—yet

Article
10.1

---

Type 1 diabetes develops during childhood or young adulthood due to pancreatic beta cell destruction. This form includes cases of diabetes caused by an autoimmune process and those with unknown etiology.

Type 2 diabetes, the most common form of diabetes, encompasses cases that range from an inability to make enough insulin (secretory defect) to an inability to use the insulin that is made (insulin resistance).

have no outward symptoms. The only way to tell is with regular screening for diabetes. Type 2 is also referred to as *noninsulin-dependent diabetes* because insulin is usually not needed to treat the condition, at least initially.

For many decades, type 2 diabetes was considered solely a disease of middle age and commonly referred to as *adult-onset diabetes.* From the 1930s until the 1990s, if a child or young adult had diabetes, it was known that they had type 1 (juvenile diabetes). Type 2 diabetes was simply not seen in children or young adults. But then in the 1990s, a few unusual cases were reported. Physicians began to diagnose type 2 diabetes in individuals in their 30s, 20s, and even occasionally in their teens. This was both surprising and puzzling. What could cause premature development of type 2 diabetes? Were these cases rare occurrences, or were they early indications of a troubling trend?

Twenty years later, we know the answer: Development of type 2 diabetes in children and young people is primarily a consequence of excess body weight (an obesity epidemic), which in turn is largely ascribed to unhealthy eating and sedentary lifestyle. The prevalence of American children and adolescents who are overweight has tripled over the past three decades. Since about 90 percent of type 2 diabetes is attributed to weight gain, it's easy to see why type 2 diabetes is rising among our youth. There is also evidence that exposure to diabetes *in utero* (gestational diabetes) may be a major contributor. Although the epidemiology of type 2 diabetes in children and teenagers is limited, clinical reports and regional studies indicate type 2 diabetes is being diagnosed more frequently, particularly in Native Americans, Mexican Americans, and African Americans. The International Diabetes Federation states that type 2 diabetes in the young is a global phenomenon affecting children in both developed and developing countries.

## GESTATIONAL DIABETES

**Gestational diabetes** develops in about 6 out of 100 women during the late stages of pregnancy. It is more common among obese women, certain ethnic/racial groups (African American, Hispanic, Native American), and those with a family history. This form of diabetes is typically caused by the development of insulin resistance late in pregnancy. Gestational diabetes requires treatment to normalize the maternal blood glucose levels to avoid complications in the infant. Treatment usually consists of dietary changes and avoiding excess weight gain.

**Gestational diabetes** is diabetes that first appears during pregnancy; it affects about 6 percent of pregnant women.

Although gestational diabetes usually resolves after the baby is born, women who develop it are more likely to develop type 2 diabetes later in life. Following pregnancy, a small proportion of women with gestational diabetes (5–10 percent) are found to have type 2 diabetes, and a larger proportion (40–60 percent) are at risk for developing type 2 diabetes within the next 5 to 10 years. For additional information on gestational diabetes, go to the American Diabetes Association's website (**www.diabetes.org/gestational-diabetes.jsp**).

## PRE-DIABETES

**Pre-diabetes** is a condition that causes blood glucose levels to be higher than normal but not high enough for a diagnosis of diabetes. People with pre-diabetes are at increased risk for developing diabetes. This borderline condition is similar to the pre-hypertension category for blood pressure. Among those 20 and older, CDC estimates that there are three times as many Americans with pre-diabetes as those with diabetes. Before people develop type 2 diabetes, they almost always have pre-diabetes. Recent evidence indicates that initial damage to the body, especially the heart and circulatory system, starts during pre-diabetes. However, not all individuals with pre-diabetes inevitably progress to diabetes. Interventions work. Improving diet, increasing physical activity, and losing weight can reverse pre-diabetes and delay or prevent diabetes. Being diagnosed with pre-diabetes represents an important crossroad at which a choice must be made. It is a last window of opportunity for true prevention, because once diabetes is developed, it doesn't go away.

✓ **NEED TO KNOW**

Diabetes is a group of metabolic diseases characterized by hyperglycemia resulting from defects in insulin secretion, insulin action, or both. Type 1 diabetes develops during childhood due to destruction of the beta cells of the pancreas. Lifelong insulin therapy is required. Type 1 accounts for 5–10 percent of all cases of diabetes. Type 2 diabetes generally appears during adulthood and is associated with weight gain and insulin resistance. It is by far the most common (over 90 percent of all cases). Pre-diabetes is a transitional condition in which the blood glucose level is higher than normal but not high enough for a diagnosis of diabetes. People with pre-diabetes are at high risk for developing type 2 diabetes. For these people, several lifestyle strategies are available to prevent or delay the onset of the disease.

**Pre-diabetes** is a borderline condition in which the blood glucose level is between normal and diabetic levels.

# ➤ Complications

We all know individuals with diabetes. Yet, unless we live with a person who has diabetes or have it ourselves, it's difficult to fully appreciate the disease. People with diabetes may experience many serious, long-term complications. Some complications begin within months of the onset of diabetes, although most develop over a period of years. Nearly all complications are progressive. If not managed, diabetes can be extremely disabling in a number of ways.

## DAMAGE TO BLOOD VESSELS

Uncontrolled diabetes damages both the small blood vessels (such as arterioles, capillaries, and venules) and the large ones (arteries and veins). Compounds accumulate within the tiny vessels that compromise the microvascular systems, causing them to thicken and leak. Blood flow is restricted, especially to the skin and nerves. High glucose levels also cause the levels of fats in the blood to rise, hastening atherosclerosis in the larger blood vessels. As a result, atherosclerosis occurs at younger ages and is at least twice as common in people with diabetes as in those without diabetes.

## HEART ATTACK AND STROKE

Over time, elevated blood glucose levels and compromised circulation harm multiple organs, including the heart and brain. Angina, heart attack, stroke, and heart failure can result. Heart disease and stroke cause about two out of three deaths among people with diabetes.

## EYE DISEASE AND BLINDNESS

Diabetic eye disease is the leading cause of blindness in adults. Complications from diabetes primarily result in damage to the retina (retinopathy) but also include cataracts and glaucoma. Diabetic retinopathy is caused by a breakdown of the small blood vessels in the retina. All three diabetic complications of the eye can result in loss of vision and eventual blindness.

## KIDNEY DISEASE

Over 40 percent of all new cases of kidney disease are in people with diabetes. Diabetic kidney disease develops as the tiny blood vessels in the kidney are damaged, and the system to filter the blood is slowly degraded. Eventually, this can lead to kidney failure requiring dialysis or kidney transplantation.

Diabetes is a leading cause of blindness in the United States.

## NERVE DAMAGE

In 60–70 percent of people with diabetes, high blood sugar and related metabolic factors lead to nerve damage (neuropathy). Although nerve problems can occur in every organ system, the most common is peripheral neuropathy, which causes pain, tingling, or numbness (loss of feeling) in the toes, feet, legs, hands, and arms. Blisters and sores may appear on numb areas of the foot because pressure or injury goes unnoticed. Peripheral neuropathy may also cause muscle weakness and loss of balance and coordination.

## AMPUTATIONS

Poor circulation and nerve damage can lead to ulcers, infections, and poor wound healing. People with diabetes are especially likely to have skin breakdown and infections of the feet and legs. Such wounds typically heal slowly or not at all. More than half of all lower-limb amputations in the United States occur in people with diabetes.

The complications just highlighted are only the major ones. There are other outcomes, less vivid but still debilitating. Diabetes can also compromise immune function; flu- and pneumonia-related deaths are three times more likely among people with diabetes than those without diabetes. And there are gender-specific concerns such as pregnancy complications affecting women and their babies and the risk of impotence among men.

Although diabetes-related complications can be severe, they don't have to be. The more tightly a person with diabetes controls his or her blood glucose level (glycemic control), the less likely it is that these complications will develop or worsen. Early detection, comprehensive medical care, and vigilant self-management are proven strategies in preventing or minimizing complications. Regular medical exams should include careful screening for heart disease and stroke, eye disease, kidney disease, skin and foot infections, and nerve damage.

✓ **NEED TO KNOW**

Early diagnosis of diabetes is extremely important because medical complications from untreated diabetes are extensive. Over time high glucose levels in the bloodstream and insufficient levels in the cells cause irreversible damage. Both microvascular and macrovascular systems are affected. Serious complications include heart disease, stroke, blindness, kidney damage, nerve damage, and lower-limb amputations. The key to preventing or minimizing complications is to control blood glucose levels and associated risk factors such as hypertension, abnormal blood lipids, and overweight/obesity. Moreover, people with diabetes should follow preventive care practices for their eyes, kidneys, and feet.

## ➤ Diagnosis and Control

As previously mentioned, undiagnosed diabetes is common; up to 27 percent of people with type 2 diabetes are unaware of their condition. Similar to high blood pressure or abnormal lipid levels, type 2 diabetes can be present for years before a person has symptoms. And when symptoms develop, they may be subtle. Increased urination and thirst are mild at first and gradually worsen over weeks or months. Eventually, the person experiences extreme fatigue, is likely to develop blurred vision, and may become chronically dehydrated. Sadly, even during the early stages of type 2 diabetes—before the symptoms arise—uncontrolled high blood glucose (hyperglycemia) causes microvascular disease (e.g., damage to the retinas and kidneys) and may cause or contribute to macrovascular disease (e.g., heart disease, stroke, peripheral vascular disease). Undiagnosed diabetes is a serious condition.

For apparently healthy adults, testing for diabetes is recommended for everyone age 45 and older, particularly if overweight (i.e., a BMI equal to or greater than 25). If results are normal, testing should be repeated every three years. However, for individuals with known risk

factors for the development of diabetes, screening should begin earlier.
Targeted testing is suggested for adults and children who are overweight and have one or more of the following risk factors:

- Habitual physically inactivity
- Parent or sibling with diabetes
- Previous diagnosis of pre-diabetes
- Member of high-risk ethnic/racial group—Asian American, Black, Hispanic, Native American, Pacific Islander
- High blood pressure
- Abnormal blood fats—HDL-cholesterol less than 35 mg/dL and/or triglycerides greater than 250 mg/dL
- Women who have been diagnosed with gestational diabetes or delivered a baby weighing more than 9 pounds

Awareness and appropriate action are critical. In a study from Oregon, two out of three adults at high risk for developing diabetes reported being unconcerned about their risk for developing the disease, and only one out of five had discussed their risk of diabetes with a health professional. These surprising findings indicate the need for increased recognition of future diabetes risk by high-risk individuals *and* health professionals.

To prevent or effectively treat diabetes, people must first be screened. The tests used to diagnose diabetes and pre-diabetes and the standard treatments for controlling the disease are reviewed in the next section.

## TESTING AND DIAGNOSIS

Diabetes and pre-diabetes can be diagnosed by measuring blood glu-
cose in one of four ways: a fasting plasma glucose test, an A1c test, an oral glucose tolerance test, or a random plasma glucose test. Each test has advantages and disadvantages.

The *fasting plasma glucose (FPG)* test is the most common measure. (Plasma is the fluid portion of blood after the cells are removed.) Fasting is defined as no caloric intake for at least 8 hours. Typically a blood sample is drawn in the morning after an overnight fast. Normal fasting glucose levels range from about 70–99 mg/dL. Pre-diabetes is defined as 100–125 mg/dL, while diabetes is diagnosed as a value of 126 mg/dL or above.

A second approach is the *A1c* test. No fasting is required for this blood test. The A1c test indicates a person's average blood sugar level for the past two to three months. An A1c level between 5.7 and 6.4 percent indicates pre-diabetes, while a level of 6.5 percent or higher indicates diabetes. This test is not for everyone, though, and should not be used for pregnant women, people who have had recent severe bleeding or blood transfusions, those with kidney or liver disease, and people with blood disorders. (More on the A1c test in the upcoming section on managing diabetes.)

A third method is the *oral glucose tolerance test (OGTT)*. The OGTT requires a fasting plasma glucose test, followed by drinking a standard glucose solution (75 grams dissolved in water) to "challenge" one's system, and then 2 hours later another blood draw. Pre-diabetes is indicated if the 2-hour value is between 140 and 199 mg/dL, and diabetes is indicated if the value is 200 mg/dL or higher. The OGTT is not widely used, as it's more burdensome on patients (requires fasting, multiple blood draws), more time-consuming, and more costly. In certain cases though, it may be the best choice. (Figure 10.3 summarizes the diagnostic values for the first three methods.)

The fourth and least common approach is to measure the *random plasma glucose*. In this test, the blood sample can be taken at any time of day without regard to when the last meal was eaten. A diagnosis of diabetes is indicated if the glucose level is 200 mg/dL or above *and* the person has the classic symptoms of diabetes (i.e., increased urination, increased thirst, unexplained weight loss).

Regardless of the method used, if diabetes is diagnosed, it must be confirmed with a subsequent test on a separate day. Any one of the four tests can be used to confirm an initial positive diagnosis. Of the four, the fasting plasma glucose test (FPG) is the preferred method and most widely accepted. It's a routine measurement made on blood samples during annual physical exams. The test is easy to perform, relatively convenient for patients, and low cost.

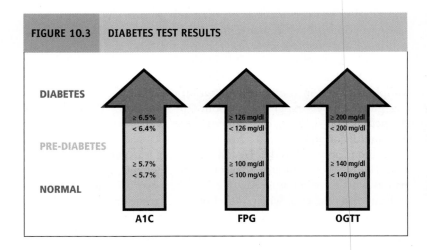

**FIGURE 10.3   DIABETES TEST RESULTS**

DIABETES

| | ≥ 6.5% | ≥ 126 mg/dl | ≥ 200 mg/dl |
| | < 6.4% | < 126 mg/dl | < 200 mg/dl |

PRE-DIABETES

| | ≥ 5.7% | ≥ 100 mg/dl | ≥ 140 mg/dl |
| | < 5.7% | < 100 mg/dl | < 140 mg/dl |

NORMAL

| A1C | FPG | OGTT |

The goal for successfully treating diabetes is to do what the body does naturally for most people—to maintain the proper balance between glucose and insulin. In diabetes the glucose–insulin synergy is impaired, either due to a lack of insulin being produced (insulin deficiency), an inability to effectively use the insulin (insulin resistance), or a combination of the two. Even with these limitations, the overall physiological processes remain operational. Food still makes the blood glucose level rise. Insulin and exercise make it fall. But the normal responsiveness and sensitivity to these variables are lacking.

Consequently, treatment of diabetes involves carefully controlling the type and amount, sequencing, and interaction among diet, exercise, and, for most people, drugs. Among adults with diagnosed diabetes, 12 percent take insulin only, 14 percent take both insulin and oral medication, 58 percent take oral medication only, and 16 percent are treated without drugs (Figure 10.4). With multiple factors to coordinate, it is easy to understand why diabetes self-management education is an integral part of medical care. The goal of diabetes treatment never stops. It is to keep blood glucose levels within the normal range as much as possible. If blood glucose levels are carefully controlled, complications are less likely to develop.

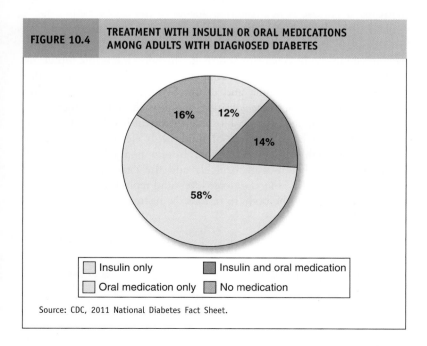

**FIGURE 10.4** TREATMENT WITH INSULIN OR ORAL MEDICATIONS AMONG ADULTS WITH DIAGNOSED DIABETES

16% 12%
14%
58%

☐ Insulin only   ■ Insulin and oral medication
☐ Oral medication only   ■ No medication

Source: CDC, 2011 National Diabetes Fact Sheet.

Keeping blood glucose levels from getting too high—hyperglycemia—is the primary challenge. But the problem with tightly controlling levels to prevent high blood glucose is that low blood glucose, or **hypoglycemia,** may occur. Most cases of low blood glucose—generally considered lower than 70 mg/dL—are caused by an "overshoot" or excessive effect of the insulin or oral medications taken to lower the blood glucose levels. Hypoglycemia is uncommon among people without diabetes.

Symptoms of hypoglycemia can begin slowly or suddenly and progress from mild discomfort to severe confusion to fainting or coma. Hypoglycemia should be treated immediately because prolonged hypoglycemia can cause brain damage. Symptoms are relieved within minutes of consuming sugar in any form such as a few ounces of fruit juice or a regular (not diet) soft drink or a few pieces of candy. Many people with diabetes carry these quick-fix foods, glucose tablets, or foil packets of a glucose-containing liquid. Milk is actually better than juice or glucose because it has lactose, fat, and protein, and this combination not only raises blood sugar but also keeps it more stable over time. However, milk is not easily carried or always readily available. A doctor may prescribe a glucagon kit for those prone to hypoglycemia, as an injection will quickly raise one's blood glucose. Family, friends, and coworkers can be taught how to inject glucagon in an emergency.

Less frequent but even more dangerous is a condition called **ketoacidosis.** If glucose is not readily available to the body's tissues, fat is broken down as a source of energy, and ketones are produced as a byproduct. If the body burns too much fat too quickly, ketones will accumulate in the bloodstream and make the body too acidic, upsetting normal chemical balance and leading to ketoacidosis. Untreated, this condition can lead to coma and death. Symptoms include excessive thirst and urination; nausea; vomiting; rapid, shallow breathing; stomach and chest pain; and fatigue. Hospital treatment involves intravenous administration of large amounts of fluids with electrolytes to replace those lost through excessive urination. Insulin is also generally given intravenously so that it works quickly and the dose can be adjusted frequently. Controlling blood glucose levels and replacing fluid and electrolytes usually allow the body to restore the normal acid–base balance.

**Hypoglycemia** is low blood glucose levels and can occur as a side effect of diabetes treatment.

**Ketoacidosis** is a life-threatening condition requiring immediate treatment; it is associated with uncontrolled diabetes and characterized by accumulation of ketones in the blood and increased acidity of the blood.

Diabetes is a complex disease and best treated with a team approach. Two key elements for optimally managing diabetes are patient education and a specialized medical team. People with diabetes benefit greatly from learning as much as possible about the disease—particularly, the practical, everyday steps that must be taken to control it. For example, self-testing of blood glucose is a daily routine. People with diabetes check their blood glucose level several times throughout the day using a drop of blood from a finger prick and a small, easy-to-use glucose monitor. Each test indicates the blood glucose level at that particular time and can guide the person's subsequent actions regarding eating, exercise, and medications.

A specialized medical team provides patient education along with medical care. If the person's primary care doctor does not have expertise and experience in treating diabetes, the person is typically referred to an endocrinologist, a physician specializing in the treatment of hormonal and metabolic diseases. Other members of a diabetes-care medical team often include a nurse practitioner or a physician assistant, a dietitian, an exercise specialist, a pharmacist, and a mental health professional such as a social worker, a psychologist, or a counselor. Many are certified as diabetes educators by the American Association of Diabetes Educators (**www.aadenet.org**), a multidisciplinary professional organization that ensures the delivery of quality self-management training to diabetic patients.

An important marker of blood glucose management (glycemic control) is the A1c test because it indicates how well blood glucose has been controlled over the past several months. As glucose circulates in the blood, some of it spontaneously binds to hemoglobin A (the primary form of hemoglobin). Hemoglobin is the protein that carries oxygen in the red blood cells. Once the glucose is bound to the hemoglobin A, it remains there for the life of the red blood cell (about 120 days). The more glucose there is in the blood, the more it binds to hemoglobin A. This combination of glucose and hemoglobin A is called *A1c* or *hemoglobin A1c* (see the earlier discussion of the A1c test). Measuring this compound reflects the overall blood glucose level over the previous two to three months. The A1c test helps the patient and doctor know if the treatment plan to control the diabetes is working or needs to be adjusted. A1c should be measured two to four times a year, and the goal is to have a reading that is less than 7 percent.

People with diabetes should let friends and coworkers know about their diabetes so that they are aware of the needs associated with diabetes management—such as dietary control, medications, and for some people, injections. Those with diabetes should also carry or wear

Individuals with diabetes may wear a medical alert bracelet to ensure quick medical intervention in an emergency.

a medical identification bracelet or tag to alert emergency workers and other health care professionals to the presence of diabetes. This information allows medical professionals to start life-saving procedures quickly and appropriately, whether treating a diabetes-related emergency or an injury or accident unrelated to the disease.

To deal with the complexities of diabetes, treatment and management should be individualized and address medical, psychosocial, and lifestyle issues. Acceptance of the disease and compliance with a management plan are not trivial issues. A team approach works only if the patient takes an *active role* in his or her care. In most cases, a person with diabetes is master of his or her fate. The actions a person chooses will determine how full a life he or she leads and to what degree disability is prevented.

### Management of Type 1 Diabetes

Due to the lack of insulin production, type 1 diabetes is the most difficult form of diabetes to control. Type 1 is treated with insulin replacement along with a structured diet and physical activity regimen. Eating times, types and amounts of foods and beverages, and physical activity patterns should be consistent from day to day. Blood glucose is measured several times a day, and multiple insulin injections are necessary. Insulin can't be taken by mouth because the digestive juices destroy it. Most people find giving the injections to be simple and relatively painless because the needle is very small. Insulin is given at regular intervals, usually two to four times a day. Each injection may contain one type or a combination of different types

Article
10.3

## Health & the Media Ratcheting Up PSAs from Risk Awareness to Disease Management

Diabetes is now so widespread in the United States that PSAs such as this are designed for a broad audience—not just for people with diabetes but also their families and friends. Perhaps more than any other chronic disease, diabetes requires the individual's daily vigilance and appropriate actions to manage the disease. Using cartoonlike characters to catch the eye, this PSA is an example of how an information-dense message can be conveyed in a creative and engaging manner. The highlighted A, B, Cs combine the diabetes-specific measurement of A1c with measurements of blood pressure and cholesterol (discussed in Chapter 8), reinforcing the interrelatedness of the major cardiovascular and metabolic diseases.

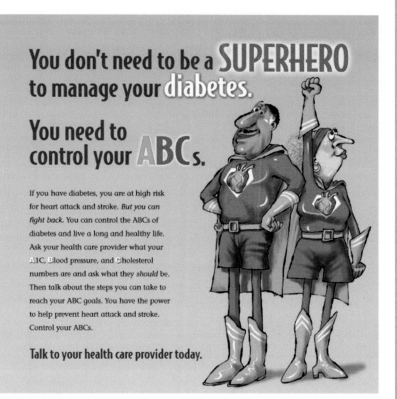

Source: National Diabetes Education Program.

of insulin—short-acting, intermediate-acting, or long-acting. As an alternative to injections, insulin pumps are increasingly being used. These pumps are small, computerized devices—about the size of a compact cell phone—worn outside the body (in a pocket, pouch, or on a belt). They provide continuous insulin delivery through a small, soft tube. Future prospects for treatment include the possibility of delivering insulin through an inhaler.

## Breaking It Down "Human" Insulin— A First in Genetic Engineering

Since the discovery of insulin in 1921, a variety of insulins have been developed to meet the needs of people with diabetes. Harvesting human pancreases from corpses was not practical commercially, so the pancreases of cows and pigs were used instead. Both have "insulin activity" in humans because they are nearly identical to human insulin, differing in only one or a few amino acids (protein building blocks). However, even a slight difference is enough to elicit an allergic response in some people.

To overcome this problem, researchers looked for ways to make better insulin. Since the early 1980s, two methods have been used to make human insulin from nonhuman sources. One method involves the use of enzymes to convert insulin from pigs into human insulin by altering the one amino acid that is different. The second and more widely used method comes from genetic engineering, or recombinant DNA technology. Eli Lilly and Company marketed the first biogenetically engineered synthetic human insulin in 1982.

Genetic engineering is the manipulation of the genetic material of cells in the laboratory to change hereditary traits or produce biological products. Techniques include isolating, copying, and multiplying DNA (genetic material); recombining DNA from different species; and transferring DNA from one species to another, bypassing the reproductive process. In this instance, bacteria are genetically altered to produce human insulin in large amounts. To provide a reliable source of human insulin, researchers obtain from human cells the DNA carrying the gene with the information for making human insulin. They then make a copy of this DNA and move it into a bacterium. As the bacterium grows in the lab, the microbe splits from one cell into two cells, and both cells get a copy of the insulin gene. As these two microbes grow, they divide into four, those four into eight, and so forth. And, remarkably, because the cells have a copy of the genetic "recipe card" for insulin, they produce insulin.

This synthesized human insulin is identical to the insulin naturally produced in healthy humans. The recombinant DNA technology put to rest the fear that insulin production from animals would not be able to meet the need of the ever-increasing diabetic population. It had been forecast as early as 1976 that by the early 1990s demand would outstrip supply. Today, insulin from cows is no longer available, and insulin from pigs is being phased out. The additional good news is that the cost of "human" insulin has remained similar to that of animal-derived insulin.

Genetic engineering is a controversial issue. And it should be. After all, genetic engineering provides the means to alter the normal biology of living organisms by increasing the yield of a crop species, introducing a novel trait, or producing a new protein. As such, it brings on a host of legal, regulatory, and ethical challenges. In the case of "human" insulin, there has been little debate. A major medical need was met, and no major side effects or long-lasting adverse events have been identified.

Currently, biotechnology products are regulated by the U.S. Department of Agriculture, the Environmental Protection Agency, and the Food and Drug Administration. Together, these agencies are empowered by law to use three criteria when assessing new products: safety, efficacy, and quality. Is the product sufficiently safe for humans and the environment? Does the product work as intended? Can the quality of the product be assured? Other considerations include the potential or probable social and economic impacts of the product. Clearly, the more we know about biotechnology, the better prepared we are to make personal choices and provide input on policies about the use of new technologies and their products.

### Management of Type 2 Diabetes

In the past, type 2 diabetes was sometimes considered the milder form of diabetes. This is no longer the case. Although most people with type 2 do not require insulin, the consequences of not controlling high blood glucose can lead to the same serious metabolic and tissue damage complications as type 1. Generally, type 2 can be controlled with diet and exercise, especially if detected early. When lifestyle measures don't provide adequate blood glucose control, then medication in tablet form is used. The different types of medicine work in one of several ways: helping the beta cells of the pancreas make more insulin, increasing the use of glucose and decreasing glucose production, slowing the absorption of glucose from the intestine, or stimulating insulin release from the pancreas. Over time, even a careful diabetes management

Blood glucose monitors help those with diabetes manage the disease.

plan (i.e., optimal diet, exercise, oral medication therapies) may not be sufficient to keep type 2 diabetes under control. If this occurs, then insulin injections may become necessary.

✓ **NEED TO KNOW**

The most widely used criterion measure for diagnosing diabetes is a fasting blood glucose level equal to or greater than 126 mg/dL. Pre-diabetes is indicated when the fasting blood glucose level is in the borderline range of 100–125 mg/dL. Since one out of four people with type 2 diabetes are undiagnosed, it's important to know the risk factors and be screened as appropriate. The goal of diabetes treatment is to keep blood glucose levels within the normal range. Hypoglycemia and ketoacidosis are related conditions that may occur with poor glycemic control. With the help of a diabetes health care team, a management plan addressing life-style, medical, and psychosocial issues is tailored to each individual. The key then becomes successful implementation and maintenance. In the final analysis, diabetes is about self-care.

## ➤ Prevention of Type 2 Diabetes

To date, there is no known method to prevent type 1 diabetes, although pancreatic islet transplantation shows promise and may become a viable option for selected patients within the next decade. In marked contrast to type 1, type 2 diabetes is largely a preventable disease. This is an important point to emphasize because the projected rise in type 2 diabetes is ominous. Unless population-wide lifestyle changes occur, public health experts forecast that approximately one out of three people born in the year 2000 will develop diabetes.

Responsibility to take action rests squarely on the shoulders of individuals and families. They need to avoid health-compromising habits and take the initiative to establish health-promoting practices. Once a person has diabetes, the decision to make smart choices seems so clear *in retrospect*. Humans, unlike other animals, have the capacity to plan and then accordingly take a course of action. We should apply this capacity to our health and the prevention of disease just as we do in other aspects of our lives.

Be aware of the risk factors for diabetes and pre-diabetes, and be screened as appropriate. Remember that approximately one-fourth of all people with diabetes may be undiagnosed and that diabetes is occurring at earlier ages. Being overweight and having a family history of diabetes are the two most apparent risk factors. The relative risk for diabetes increases with increasing BMI. For the extended list of risk factors and guidelines for screening, refer to the earlier section "Diagnosis and Control."

Self Assessment 10.1

## FINDINGS FROM THE DIABETES PREVENTION PROGRAM

For those who already have been diagnosed with pre-diabetes, the potential to prevent the onset of diabetes with diet and exercise is promising. In a major three-year clinical trial known as the Diabetes Prevention Program, high-risk participants randomly assigned to a lifestyle intervention group reduced their risk of getting diabetes by 58 percent. The lifestyle intervention focused on healthful changes in diet and physical activity. For example, participants reduced intake of saturated fats and increased intake of whole-grain foods. They also built up to and maintained physical activity at 30 minutes per day—through brisk walking or similar moderate-intensity exercise. In a second group, participants were treated with standard diabetes oral medication. They reduced their risk of getting diabetes by 31 percent—a nice reduction, but not as great as the reduction for those in the lifestyle intervention. Those in the lifestyle intervention group lost about 6 percent of their body weight compared to no weight loss among those in the medication group.

This large study was conducted at 27 centers nationwide and involved over 3,000 people with pre-diabetes. Participants ranged in age from 25 to 85 with an average age of 51, and nearly half were from minority groups that disproportionately develop type 2 diabetes. All were overweight, with an average BMI of 34. The structured lifestyle intervention worked as well in men as women, in all ethnic groups, and across the age range. The study ended a year early because the data clearly answered the main research question regarding the effectiveness of a lifestyle intervention to delay the development of type 2 diabetes. Ending a clinical trial study early due to excellent results is highly unusual. While both the lifestyle and oral medication treatments were found to be effective, the lifestyle intervention (diet and exercise) was found to be better.

The best strategy for preventing pre-diabetes and type 2 diabetes is to eat properly, exercise regularly, and maintain a healthy weight. The overall health benefits of positive diet and exercise behaviors are truly astounding. Conversely, the detrimental health effects of chronically poor lifestyle habits are extensive as well. The multifactorial and global aspects of diet and physical activity on health are further illustrated in the next section on metabolic syndrome.

### NEED TO KNOW

Type 2 diabetes is a largely preventable disease, yet its prevalence among Americans has been climbing steadily since the 1980s. Prevention depends primarily on awareness and proactive steps by individuals and families. If you know someone with advanced diabetes, your incentive to prevent diabetes may be particularly meaningful. The tools for prevention are readily available by incorporating a healthy diet and physical activity and maintaining a healthy weight. Even for those who are overweight and/or prediabetic, the potential to prevent or slow the progression to diabetes through lifestyle intervention is a real option. Research has convincingly shown that a reasonable program of proper diet and exercise substantially reduces the risk of getting diabetes.

## ➤ Metabolic Syndrome

Metabolic syndrome is a cluster of interrelated metabolic and cardiovascular risk factors that appear to directly promote type 2 diabetes and atherosclerosis. Over the last few years, leading health organizations including the National Heart Lung and Blood Institute (NHLBI), American Heart Association (AHA), World Health Organization (WHO), and International Diabetes Association have issued official scientific statements to define and describe metabolic syndrome and to provide up-to-date guidance on diagnosis and treatment.

**TABLE 10.1    DEFINITION AND CRITERIA OF METABOLIC SYNDROME**

Metabolic syndrome is defined as having three or more of the following five criteria:

| RISK FACTORS | CRITERIA |
| --- | --- |
| Abdominal obesity (waist girth) | > 40 inches for men, > 35 inches for women |
| Triglycerides | ≥ 150 mg/dL |
| HDL cholesterol | < 40 mg/dL for men, < 50 mg/dL for women |
| Blood pressure | ≥ 130/85 mm Hg |
| Fasting blood glucose | ≥ 110 mg/dL |

Source: SM Grundy et al. *Circulation* 112: 2735–2752, 2005.

## WHAT IS METABOLIC SYNDROME?

Although it remains unclear whether **metabolic syndrome** has a single cause, it appears that it can be precipitated by multiple underlying risk factors. The most important of these are abdominal obesity and insulin resistance. Other associated conditions include physical inactivity, hormonal imbalance, aging, and genetic or ethnic predisposition. Population studies show that metabolic syndrome confers a twofold increase for heart disease and stroke, and in individuals without established type 2 diabetes, an approximate fivefold increase in risk for developing diabetes as compared with people without the syndrome.

Several different sets of criteria have been proposed over the past decade for diagnosis of metabolic syndrome. The criteria most widely accepted are those adopted by the AHA and the NHLBI. As presented in Table 10.1, these include five common clinical measurements: waist circumference, triglycerides, HDL cholesterol, blood pressure, and fasting blood glucose. The presence of abnormalities in any three of these five measures constitutes a diagnosis of the syndrome.

Since the 1980s, substantial research has shown that accumulation of upper body fat (on the trunk)—also known as abdominal or visceral fat—is more highly associated with both type 2 diabetes and atherosclerosis than lower body fat (on the hips and thighs). For this reason, large waist circumference (i.e., greater than 35 inches for women and 40 inches for men) is used in lieu of a high BMI as a criterion for metabolic syndrome.

**Metabolic syndrome** is a cluster of conditions—excess abdominal fat, abnormal cholesterol levels, high blood pressure, and elevated blood glucose—that occur together and increase risk for coronary heart disease, stroke, and type 2 diabetes.

FIGURE 10.5 SCHEMATIC DEPICTING INTERRELATIONSHIPS AMONG LIFESTYLE BEHAVIORS, PHYSIOLOGICAL RESPONSES, AND DISEASE OUTCOMES

The summary schematic in Figure 10.5 presents a simple depiction of a complex web of interactions and likely causal links among lifestyle factors, human physiology, and metabolic syndrome. The middle box reflects a biological "mixing pot"—still a scientific black box in many respects—where multiple physiological systems are attempting to adapt to health-compromising factors as well as to one another. Behaviors can be viewed as input; the biological "pot" is where compensatory interplay among systems and disease processes occurs; and the resulting related diseases that constitute metabolic syndrome are presented as output. Over time, cascading and wide-ranging effects toward disease (or health) can result from basic lifestyle choices.

## TREATMENT GOALS AND STRATEGIES

The primary goal in treating metabolic syndrome is to reduce risk for atherosclerosis—namely, heart disease and stroke—and to decrease the risk for type 2 diabetes in people who do not yet have the disease. As in managing the diseases separately, the first-line approach is to reduce the major risk factors: reduce LDL cholesterol, blood pressure, and blood glucose levels to the recommended goals, and if a smoker, to stop.

At age 27, Mike acknowledged that he was overweight but gave little thought to his overall health. After all, he was simply a big person, still relatively young, and busy with work and home activities. Then he volunteered to give blood during a blood drive at work and was turned away because of high blood pressure. Surprised by this, he saw his doctor, who confirmed his hypertension and told him that his blood lipids were off the chart, too. His doctor was direct and to the point: "You need to lose 70 pounds. It's time to get serious about your health." Mike suddenly realized that his poor eating habits and his sedentary lifestyle had caught up with him, and he was at risk for heart disease and diabetes as well as many other diseases.

Whenever possible, initial treatments for metabolic syndrome should begin with lifestyle interventions—weight loss in overweight and obese people, a change in dietary patterns toward a prudent diet (low in saturated fats and refined sugars; high in whole grains, fruits, vegetables), and an increase in regular physical activity. Such changes will produce a reduction in all metabolic syndrome risk factors simultaneously. The greatest benefit will be derived from consistent and lasting lifestyle intervention. As a second tier of treatment, an array of drug therapies are available for individual risk factors and are often used in combination with positive lifestyle modifications.

Mike decided to do something about his deteriorating medical condition and the inattention he had shown to his health. He made a promise to himself to turn his situation around. He started going to the gym regularly and made consistent adjustments in his diet, eating less processed foods and more fruits and vegetables. He relates, "I didn't cut out all the fun stuff; rather I just began to make better choices." These days, Mike feels healthier than he has in a long time. He is glad he finally recognized the need to take action and now would not have it any other way.

## ONGOING PROFESSIONAL DEBATE

The definition of *metabolic syndrome* and the concept itself are still evolving. A consensus among the major professional societies has yet to be achieved. In a joint scientific review and position statement, the American Diabetes Association and the European Association for the Study of Diabetes report that too much essential information is missing to warrant the designation of "metabolic syndrome" as a new syndrome and question the value of doing so. As an interesting aside, the American Diabetes Association recently proposed a similar concept of cardiometabolic health as a measure of a person's risk for diabetes and heart disease.

In contrast to the doubts of the American and European diabetes associations about the usefulness of metabolic syndrome, the International Diabetes Federation, the American Heart Association, and the National Heart Blood Lung Institute are aligned in support of the concept. Their shared view is that early detection and intensive management of metabolic syndrome are warranted. They contend that while no single treatment for metabolic syndrome is yet available, lifestyle changes—such as improving diet and increasing physical activity—provide a solid basis for treatment. In addition, new drug treatments that would reduce several risk factors concurrently are under development and may have a significant impact on reducing both cardiovascular disease and diabetes in the years ahead.

These professional differences of opinion appear to be more about the interpretation and use of the concept than about its scientific basis. Regardless, further research will continue to shed light on our understanding and application of metabolic syndrome to both personal and public health. In closing, the term *metabolic syndrome* describes a condition in which metabolic and atherogenic risk factors cluster in the same people more often than would be expected by chance. This provides a practical means for early detection of individuals at high risk for type 2 diabetes and cardiovascular disease and indicates an interaction among diseases once thought to be separate conditions.

In related initiatives, the American Cancer Society, American Diabetes Association, and American Heart Association have joined together to promote clinical and public health interventions that reduce prevalence of tobacco use, poor diet, and insufficient physical activity—the major risk factors for cardiovascular disease, diabetes, and cancer. Perhaps over the next decade, as research progresses and we learn more about metabolic syndrome, professional organizations will reach consensus. Stay tuned. In the meantime, all are united in supporting prevention and early detection of chronic disease.

### ✓ NEED TO KNOW

Metabolic syndrome is a clustering of risk factors associated with diabetes and cardiovascular disease. Metabolic syndrome provides a striking example of the continuous interaction among circulatory, metabolic, endocrine, and immune systems in their adaptations to lifestyle behaviors. Our body's physiological systems do not operate separately. Rather, complex collective and compensatory influences are at work among them. Likewise, our health behaviors affect more than a single system or disease. Indeed, lifestyle habits have overall effects—for better or worse.

## ARTICLES

10.1 "How and Where Fat Is Stored Predicts Disease Risk Better Than Weight." University of Texas Southwestern Medical Center. A leader in diabetes research explains an important point in understanding the cause of diabetes and metabolic syndrome.

10.2 "Type 2 Diabetes Surges in People Younger Than 20." *Washington Post.* A disease formerly associated with adults is now occurring in children and teens.

10.3 "Creating a Family Culture of Healthy Eating One Step at a Time." *Diabetes Health.* A mother provides insights and practical tips on making dietary changes for the whole family when her son is diagnosed with type 1 diabetes.

## SELF-ASSESSMENT

10.1 Disease Risk Questionnaire for Type 2 Diabetes

## Website Resources

### DIABETES

American Association of Diabetes Educators
  **www.aadenet.org**
American Diabetes Association
  **www.diabetes.org**
GlaxoSmithKline's Diabetes.com
  **www.diabetes.com**
International Diabetes Federation **www.idf.org**
Joslin Diabetes Center **www.joslin.harvard.edu**
National Diabetes Education Program
  **http://ndep.nih.gov**

### METABOLIC SYNDROME

American Heart Association
  **www.heart.org/HEARTORG/Conditions/More/
  MetabolicSyndrome/Metabolic-Syndrome_UCM_002080_
  SubHomePage.jsp**
National Heart, Lung, and Blood Institute, NIH
  **www.nhlbi.nih.gov/health/dci/Diseases/ms/ms_whatis.html**

## Knowing the Language

diabetes, 352
gestational diabetes, 356
hyperglycemia, 352
hypoglycemia, 364
insulin, 352

ketoacidosis, 364
metabolic syndrome, 373
pre-diabetes, 357
type 1 diabetes, 355
type 2 diabetes, 355

## Understanding the Content

1. Where is insulin produced, and what is its role in the body?
2. Explain the differences among type 1 diabetes, type 2 diabetes, and pre-diabetes.
3. What are the risk factors for diabetes?
4. Define *metabolic syndrome* and the criteria for diagnosis.

## Exploring Ideas

1. Type 2 diabetes is by far the most common form of the disease, yet it's largely preventable. Its prevalence in the population is at an all-time high and projected to rise even higher. Why is this happening, and what needs to be done to turn the tide?
2. Just as with high blood pressure and abnormal blood lipids, we should know the numbers that define the condition. What fasting blood glucose levels define pre-diabetes and diabetes? What is the A1c measurement, and when is it used?
3. Explain how eating a healthy diet and exercising regularly lowers a person's risk for developing type 2 diabetes and metabolic syndrome.

## Selected References

Alberti KG, Eckel RH, Grundy SM, et al. Harmonizing the metabolic syndrome: A joint interim statement of the International Diabetes Federation Task Force on Epidemiology and Prevention; National Heart, Lung, and Blood Institute; American Heart Association; World Heart Federation; International Atherosclerosis Society; and International Association for the Study of Obesity. *Circulation* 120: 1640–1645, 2009.

American Diabetes Association. The Cardiometabolic Risk Initiative, 2006. **http://professional.diabetes.org/ ResourcesForProfessionals.aspx?cid=60379**

American Diabetes Association. Standards of medical care in diabetes. *Diabetes Care* 34: Supplement 1, S11–S62, 2011.

Blaha M, Elasy TA. Clinical use of the metabolic syndrome: Why the confusion? *Clinical Diabetes* 24: 125–131, 2006.

Centers for Disease Control and Prevention (CDC). Children and Diabetes. **www.cdc.gov/diabetes/projects/cda2.htm**

CDC. Childhood Overweight and Obesity. **www.cdc.gov/obesity/childhood/**

CDC. National Diabetes Fact Sheet, 2011. **www.cdc.gov/diabetes/pubs/factsheet11.htm**

Danaei G, Finucane MM, Lu Y, et al. National, regional, and global trends in fasting plasma glucose and diabetes prevalence since 1980: Systematic analysis of health examination surveys and epidemiological studies with 370 country-years and 2.7 million participants. *Lancet* 378: 31–40, 2011.

Diabetes Prevention Program Research Group. Reduction in the incidence of type 2 diabetes with lifestyle intervention or metformin. *New England Journal of Medicine* 346: 393–403, 2002. **http://content.nejm.org/cgi/content/full/346/6/393**

Eckel RH, Alberti KG, Grundy SM, et al. The metabolic syndrome. *Lancet* 375: 181–183, 2010.

Eckel RH, Kahn R, Robertson RM, et al. Preventing cardiovascular disease and diabetes: A call to action from the American Diabetes Association and the American Heart Association. *Diabetes Care* 29:1697–1699, 2006. **http://care.diabetesjournals.org/cgi/content/short/29/7/1697**

Eyre H, Kahn R, Robertson RM, et al. Preventing cancer, cardiovascular disease, and diabetes: A common agenda for the American Cancer Society, the American Diabetes Association, and the American Heart Association. *CA: A Cancer Journal for Clinicians* 54: 190–207, 2004. **http://caonline.amcancersoc.org/cgi/content/full/54/4/190**

Grundy SM, Cleeman JI, Daniels SR, et al. AHA/NHLBI scientific statement: Diagnosis and management of the metabolic syndrome. *Circulation* 112: 2735–2752, 2005. **http://circ.ahajournals.org/cgi/content/full/112/17/2735**

International Diabetes Association. *Diabetes Atlas.* **www.eatlas.idf.org**

International Diabetes Association. The IDF consensus worldwide definition of the metabolic syndrome, 2005. **www.idf.org/home/index.cfm?node=1429**

Kahn R, Buse J, Ferrannini E, et al. The metabolic syndrome: Time for a critical appraisal: Joint statement from the American Diabetes Association and the European Association for the Study of Diabetes. *Diabetes Care* 28: 2289–2304, 2005.

Kemple AM, Zlot AI, Leman RF. Perceived likelihood of developing diabetes among high-risk Oregonians. *Preventing Chronic Disease* [serial online], November 2005.
**www.cdc.gov/pcd/issues/2005/nov/05_0067.htm**

Marwick TH, Hordern MD, Miller T, et al. Scientific statement: Exercise training for type 2 diabetes mellitus. *Circulation* 119: 3244–3262, 2009.
**http://circ.ahajournals.org/cgi/content/full/119/25/3244**

Nobel Prize in Physiology or Medicine, 1923.
**http://nobelprize.org/medicine/laureates/1923**

Public Health Agency of Canada. The Many Faces of Diabetes—Mike's Story.

Sanders LJ. *The philatelic history of diabetes: In search of a cure.* Alexandria, VA: American Diabetes Association, 2001.

Steinberger J, Daniels SR. AHA Scientific statement: Progress and challenges in metabolic syndrome in children and adolescents. *Circulation* 119: 628–647, 2009.
**http://circ.ahajournals.org/cgi/content/full/119/4/628**

Epidemics have often
been more influential
than statesmen and
soldiers in shaping
the course of political
history, and diseases
may also color the
moods of civilizations.

— René Dubos

# Chapter 11

## INFECTIONS

The relationship between people and microbes has in part
defined our world. Who hasn't heard of the plague? The
great influenza epidemic? HIV/AIDS? In Chapter 11 we examine all facets of the infectious disease process including signs,
symptoms, treatment, risk factors, and risk reduction. At the
end of the chapter we explore emerging issues, from new
diseases to bioterrorism.

## Communicable Disease Process
PATHOGENS
MODE OF TRANSMISSION
PORTALS OF ENTRY AND EXIT
STAGES OF RESPONSE

## Fighting Disease
IMMUNE SYSTEM
VACCINES
ANTIBIOTICS
ANTIVIRALS
PREVENTION

## Common Bacterial Infections
STAPH INFECTIONS
STREP INFECTIONS

## Common Viral Infections
COMMON COLD
INFLUENZA
MONONUCLEOSIS
HERPES 1 (ORAL HERPES)
HEPATITIS

## Common Fungal Infections

## Sexually Transmitted Infections
CHLAMYDIA
GONORRHEA
PELVIC INFLAMMATORY DISEASE
SYPHILIS
HERPES 2 (GENITAL HERPES)
HUMAN PAPILLOMAVIRUS
PREVENTION OF SEXUALLY TRANSMITTED INFECTIONS
HIV AND AIDS

## Bioterrorism

> The fate of most microbes that invade us is quick death. Sometimes,
> though, a microbe finds in humans an ideal environment, with plenty of
> nourishment and mere Maginot resistance. And it has its own weapon;
> it can attack or elude white blood cells, produce toxins, and kill and
> feed on tissues anywhere from the toes to the depths of the brain. If it
> multiplies unhindered, it may kill the host. But should that happen
> before the germ finds transport to another home, the meeting becomes a
> dead end for host and parasite alike.

As the quote from Karlen's book describes, the world is filled with
microbes that infect and sicken humans. Some cause illnesses that are
easy to transmit but prove more annoying than serious. Others are
life-threatening but hard to catch. A few are unfortunately both deadly
and easy to spread. An example of the last type of infection is the one
that was responsible for the influenza pandemic of 1918, which is
estimated to have killed tens of millions of people—more than died
in World War I.

In the second half of the 20th century, the development of antibiotics greatly reduced the number of deaths from bacteria infections.
But microbes have mutated and adapted defenses against many antibiotics in the past few decades. Each year approximately 18,000 Americans die from MRSA (methicillin-resistant *Staphylococcus aureus*), a
common bacteria that has become resistant to antibiotics. Because of
this resistance, the bacteria can multiply unhindered and may kill the
host.

In this chapter we will discuss the communicable disease process
and the human immune response that protects us. We will also describe
some of the more common infections that affect people today.

## ➤ Communicable Disease Process

The common link shared by all communicable diseases is that they are
caused by microorganisms called **pathogens,** *germs,* or *microbes.* Thousands of communicable diseases have been identified. The American
Public Health Association publishes the *Control of Communicable Diseases in Man,* the definitive resource that describes all communicable
diseases and all facets of the communicable disease process including
transmission, prevention, and treatment.

---

**Pathogens** are microorganisms that cause communicable disease.

Any communicable disease is defined by not only the pathogen responsible for the disease but also the process by which the pathogen can infect people. The communicable disease process involves pathogens, reservoir, modes of transmission, hosts, and stages of response (incubation, prodromal, acute, and recovery). Communicable diseases follow the process shown in Figure 11.1.

## PATHOGENS

Six major groups of pathogens cause communicable diseases. These include bacteria, viruses, fungi, rickettsia, metazoa, and protozoa. Most common diseases are caused by bacteria, viruses, and fungi. Pathogens are living organisms and, as such, must have a place where they can live and reproduce in their natural environment. This place is termed a *reservoir*. Not surprisingly, the reservoir for the most common diseases that affect people is the human body.

## MODE OF TRANSMISSION

Infection occurs when a pathogen leaves the reservoir (that is, an infected person) and enters another person. This process is referred to as the *mode of transmission*. **Direct modes of transmission** are person to person via coughing, sneezing, or sexual contact. **Indirect modes of transmission** include vectors and vehicles. Vectors can be insects, such as mosquitoes or ticks, that carry a pathogen. An insect that carries a pathogen bites a person in order to feed and as a result gives the person the pathogen that causes disease. Vehicles are substances like water and food. If a pathogen exists in the vehicle, it is consumed. Inanimate objects such as drinking glasses and eating utensils are also considered vehicles, since people can pick up pathogens from their contaminated surfaces.

## PORTALS OF ENTRY AND EXIT

Pathogens require portals of entry and exit in order to infect a person and for that person to pass the infection to others. Portals include the nose, mouth, and reproductive system. The skin normally protects against infection, but when its surface is broken by a cut, scrape, or insect bite, then it too becomes a possible portal of entry. Finally, during sexual activity, pathogens can be transmitted from mucous membrane to mucous membrane.

---

**Direct mode of transmission** is disease transmission through person-to-person contact. **Indirect mode of transmission** is disease transmission via food or insects.

## FIGURE 11.1    CHAIN OF INFECTION

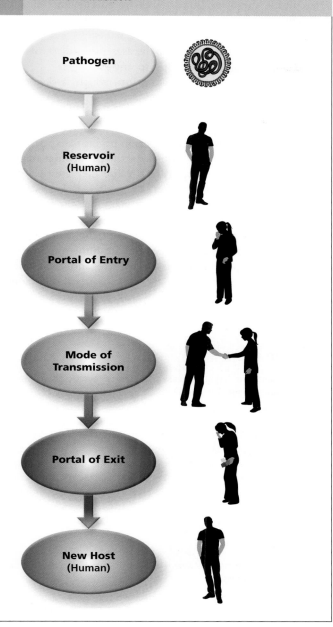

## STAGES OF RESPONSE

Once inside the body, pathogens have specific mechanisms of action on body cells. There are many variations within pathogen groups that result in differences in infection mechanisms. Some of these will be noted when discussing selected diseases. Regardless of the variations, there are four stages of response to any pathogen.

The first stage is called **incubation,** which is defined as the time between exposure to the pathogen and the onset of clinical symptoms. It is the time when the pathogen is reproducing in the system and doing whatever it uniquely does to take over the body.

After incubation, the infected person begins to experience early symptoms of the disease, called *prodrome* or the **prodromal stage.** During the prodromal stage, most people don't realize they are sick, and they tend to attribute the symptoms to something else—lack of sleep, allergies, or general tiredness. As the symptoms get more intense and the person begins to feel sick, the infection enters the **acute,** or peak **stage.**

One of three things can happen after the acute stage: death (the pathogen wins), **recovery** (the person's immune response system wins), or relapse (the person begins to recover and then goes back into another acute stage). Relapse normally occurs if a person doesn't get the right amount of rest or stops taking prescribed medication too soon, allowing the pathogen to once again gain the upper hand.

### ✓ NEED TO KNOW

Most common infectious diseases are caused by bacteria, viruses, and fungi. Direct modes of transmission are person to person via coughing, sneezing, or sexual contact. Indirect modes of transmission include vectors (such as insects) and vehicles (such as food, utensils, or other objects). Stages of infection are incubation, when symptoms have not yet appeared; prodromal, when symptoms first begin to emerge; and acute, when the full-blown infection is obvious. The acute stage is followed by recovery if the host successfully conquers the infection, or by death if the pathogen completely overwhelms the host. In long-term infectious diseases, the acute stage may sometimes be followed by a series of partial recoveries and relapses to the acute stage.

**Incubation** is the time between exposure to a pathogen and the onset of the infection's symptoms.

In the **prodromal stage** the person experiences the early symptoms of a disease. The **acute stage** is the period when a person is the sickest with an infection.

**Recovery** is overcoming the infection and getting better.

# ➤ Fighting Disease

Our body interprets infection with a pathogen as an invasion and tries to fight. A war of sorts ensues, with the pathogen trying to multiply on one side, and the body trying to kill off the pathogens on the other. The most effective method of fighting infections is our own immune system. Other methods include drugs such as vaccines, antibiotics, and antivirals.

## IMMUNE SYSTEM

The immune system continually guards against foreign substances called **antigens.** Pathogens are considered antigens. White blood cells called **leukocytes** are the most basic unit of the immune system. Phagocytes and lymphocytes are the two main types of leukocytes. **Phagocytes** will surround, engulf, and digest pathogens or other material that is recognized as being foreign to the body. Phagocytes can also be specialized. For example, neutrophils are a type of phagocyte that primarily targets bacteria. A clinical application of this knowledge about different kinds of white blood cells is a blood test ordered by a physician to determine neutrophil count. If the count is higher than normal, it indicates a bacterial infection, which then has implications for the physician's recommendations about treatment.

**Lymphocytes** originate in the bone marrow, and they can stay in the bone marrow and develop into B lymphocytes, often referred to as **B cells.** T lymphocytes, or **T cells,** are those that leave the bone marrow and mature in the thymus gland. T cells and B cells work in partnership. If a pathogen invades the body, it is detected by the B cells, which produce antigen-specific **antibodies,** specialized proteins capable of destroying antigens. The T cells then destroy the pathogens.

---

An **antigen** is a foreign substance in the body that triggers the production of antibodies.

**Leukocytes** are white blood cells.

**Phagocytes** are white blood cells that surround and destroy foreign substances in the body.

**Lymphocytes** are a type of white blood cell and are the most basic unit of immunity. **B cells** are lymphocytes that produce antibodies. **T cells** are small circulating lymphocytes that mediate immune response.

**Antibodies** are proteins that are produced to destroy antigens, including pathogens.

The process of immunity is defined by lymphocytes and antibodies, but the broader types of immunity include activity immunity and passive immunity. In active immunity, the protection develops after direct exposure to the pathogen. Cells in our immune response recognize the pathogen if we are subsequently exposed, and that increases our body's capability to fight that particular type of infection. Passive immunity is a process by which people get antibodies from another source, such as when infants ingest them in breast milk. Passive immunity is short-lived.

## VACCINES

**Vaccines** can be an effective way to prevent an infection. When people are vaccinated, they are given a weakened or dead form of the pathogen, and they develop an immunity to it through their body's formation of antibodies. Figure 11.2 shows the diseases for which vaccinations are available.

## ANTIBIOTICS

As their name implies, **antibiotics** fight bacterial infections. They are antibodies that, once administered, either destroy the bacteria directly or block bacterial biological processes, causing the pathogens to self-destruct. Antibiotics are specific to certain types of bacteria, so a diagnosis must be made in order to prescribe the correct drug. It is also important that once an antibiotic is prescribed, the person takes the whole prescription in the course of treatment. If not, resistant strains of the bacteria can result. Resistance to antibiotics is becoming a serious problem because the altered bacteria cause infections that can become very virulent, difficult to treat, and deadly.

Some individuals are allergic to antibiotics, and their reaction to them can be life-threatening. Physicians should ask any patient about known antibiotic allergies before prescribing an appropriate drug.

## ANTIVIRALS

**Antivirals** are drugs that block the reproductive ability of viruses; they can be effective in treating certain viral conditions such as influenza.

**Vaccines** are a treatment made from weakened or dead pathogens that allow the body to build up immunity against specific diseases.

**Antibiotics** are antibodies given as a drug that disrupt bacterial processes and stop an infection from growing.

**Antivirals** are drugs that treat viral infections.

## FIGURE 11.2 ADULT IMMUNIZATION SCHEDULE

| VACCINE ▼ / AGE GROUP ▶ | 19–49 Years | 50–64 Years | ≥ 65 Years |
|---|---|---|---|
| Tetanus, Diphtheria, Pertussis (Td/Tdap)[1],* | 1 dose Td booster every 10 yrs | | |
| | Substitute 1 dose of Tdap for Td | | |
| Human papillomavirus (HPV)[2],* | 3 doses females (0, 2, 6 mos) | | |
| Measles, Mumps, Rubella (MMR)[3],* | 1 or 2 doses | 1 dose | |
| Varicella[4],* | 2 doses (0, 4–8 wks) | | |
| Influenza[5],* | | 1 dose annually | |
| Pneumococcal (polysaccharide)[6,7] | | 1–2 doses | 1 dose |
| Hepatitis A[8],* | 2 doses (0, 6–12 mos or 0, 6–18 mos) | | |
| Hepatitis B[9],* | 3 doses (0, 1–2, 4–6 mos) | | |
| Meningococcal[10],* | 1 or more doses | | |
| Zoster[11] | | | 1 dose |

For all persons in this category who meet the age requirements and who lack evidence of immunity (e.g., lack documentation of vaccination or have no evidence of prior infection).

Recommended if some other risk factor is present (e.g., on the basis of medical, occupational, lifestyle, or other indications).

*Covered by the Vaccine Injury Compensation Program.

(Continued)

**FIGURE 11.2  ADULT IMMUNIZATION SCHEDULE (*continued*)**

| INDICATION ▶<br><br>VACCINE ▼ | Pregnancy | Immuno-compromising conditions (excluding human immunodeficiency virus [HIV]), medications[13], radiation[13] | HIV infection[3,12,13] CD4+ T lymphocyte count <200 cells/L | HIV infection[3,12,13] CD4+ T lymphocyte count ≥200 cells/L | Diabetes, heart disease, chronic pulmonary disease, chronic alcoholism | Asplenia[12] (including elective splenectomy and terminal complement component deficiencies) | Chronic liver disease | Kidney failure, end-stage renal disease, receipt of hemodialysis | Health care personnel |
|---|---|---|---|---|---|---|---|---|---|
| Tetanus, Diphtheria, Pertussis (Td/Tdap)[1,*] | 1 dose Td booster every 10 yrs ― Substitute 1 dose of Tdap for Td ||||||||
| Human papillomavirus (HPV)[2,*] | 3 doses for females through age 26 yrs (0, 2, 6 mos) ||||||||
| Measles, Mumps, Rubella (MMR)[3,*] | Contraindicated | Contraindicated | Contraindicated | 1 or 2 doses ||||||
| Varicella[4,*] | Contraindicated | Contraindicated | Contraindicated | 2 doses (0, 4–8 wks) ||||||
| Influenza[5,*] | 1 dose TIV annually ||||||| | 1 dose TIV or LAIV annually |
| Pneumococcal (polysaccharide)[6,7] | | 1–2 doses ||||||||
| Hepatitis A[8,*] | 2 doses (0, 6–12 mos or 0, 6–18 mos) ||||||||
| Hepatitis B[9,*] | 3 doses (0, 1–2, 4–6 mos) ||||||||
| Meningococcal[10,*] | 1 or more doses ||||||||
| Zoster[11] | Contraindicated ||| 1 dose |||||

■ For all persons in this category who meet the age requirements and who lack evidence of immunity (e.g., lack documentation of vaccination or have no evidence of prior infection).

■ Recommended if some other risk factor is present (e.g., on the basis of medical, occupational, lifestyle, or other indications).

*Covered by the Vaccine Injury Compensation Program.

Report all clinically significant postvaccination reactions to the Vaccine Adverse Event Reporting System (VAERS). Reporting forms and instructions on filing a VAERS report are available at **www.vaers.hhs.gov**. Additional information about the vaccines in this schedule is available at **www.cdc.gov/vaccines**

Source: CDC.

## Health & the Media Hand Sanitizer Dangers

Can the alcohol in hand sanitizers cause poisoning? You may have heard a story about a little girl who was rushed to the emergency room after becoming lethargic and unable to focus her eyes. Tests failed to discover the problem until a preschool teacher reported that children witnessed the child licking hand sanitizer before falling ill. Blood alcohol tests then showed the girl had dangerously high levels of alcohol in her system. The story ends with strict cautions about how deadly hand sanitizer can be.

Although this tale was widely distributed via e-mail with enough factual errors (such as an impossibly high blood alcohol level) that led it to be classified as an urban myth, the basic premise behind the story is true. Hand sanitizers contain up to 65 percent alcohol, and if ingested in sufficient amounts, they can cause alcohol poisoning. Although this isn't an issue for adults, who understand that sanitizer is for washing and not drinking, accidental poisoning could occur with small children.

Although nonalcoholic versions of hand sanitizers are available, some doctors and health policy administrators caution strongly against using this type. In this case, the worry is that widespread use of these alternative sanitizers may help build drug-resistant "superbugs." (See "Breaking It Down" for more information on drug-resistant infections.) Alcohol-based sanitizers are believed to kill more types of bacteria than other types, and the mechanism by which they work does not create drug-resistant pathogens.

Given their ability to reduce the spread of gastrointestinal and respiratory illness and the fact their use doesn't increase drug-resistant microbes, getting rid of alcohol-based hand sanitizers entirely is probably too strong a reaction. They have their place in the fight against infections. However, keeping them out of reach of children and allowing children to use them only with adult supervision are wise practices.

Tamiflu is an example of an antiviral. Use of antiviral drugs is tricky because in many instances there is a narrow therapeutic window for effectiveness at the very beginning of the infection. Most people don't visit their physician until they are very ill, when the use of antivirals is less effective, if not contraindicated.

## PREVENTION

Vaccines, antibiotics, and antivirals are all valuable ways to prevent infections or lessen their intensity and duration. Good hygiene is also important in the prevention of infections. Perhaps the most important behavior one can perform to prevent disease is to wash hands frequently. Many of the more common pathogens are found on hands and thus are capable of being transmitted to other people. Additionally, maintaining a good lifestyle (such as exercising regularly, eating healthy foods, and getting enough sleep routinely) also helps keep the immune system in good shape, which in turn helps the body fight off infections.

### ✓ NEED TO KNOW

The human immune system is by far the most effective tool for fighting off infections. White blood cells, called B cells, target antigens by creating antibodies, while other white blood cells (T cells) then destroy the pathogens. Vaccines are drugs that are administered to prevent infections. Antibiotics are drugs that kill bacteria, and antiviral drugs fight viruses. People who maintain good health habits and are well rested will usually have a better immune response against infections than people who are stressed or have unhealthy habits. All people can decrease the chance of infections by frequently washing their hands.

## ➤ Common Bacterial Infections

Bacteria are very simple pathogens. It should be noted that many bacteria do not cause disease and can even be beneficial to human health. Bacteria are single-celled plants that, after entering a body, divide until they reach sufficient numbers to cause symptoms. One cell becomes two, two cells become four, four cells become eight, and so on until they reach billions and trillions. It is only after huge numbers of bacteria are present that a person becomes aware of the infection, because that is the point at which symptoms arise.

There are many common bacterial infections. Some will be covered in this section and some will be covered in the section "Sexually

Transmitted Infections." Because most foodborne diseases (food poisoning) are bacterial, those diseases are discussed in Chapter 2.

## STAPH INFECTIONS

Staph (staphylococcal) bacteria are common bacteria found on the skin and the membranes that line the nose and throat. In most instances the bacteria are harmless, but if conditions are right, the bacteria can invade the body, secrete a toxin, and result in disease. Common **staph infections** include impetigo, boils, and cellulitis.

Impetigo is a contagious skin infection that can result when the staph bacteria invades the skin through a crack or broken area. During an impetigo infection, blisters can appear, and the affected skin can become red. When the blisters burst, the infection can spread, and the area where the blister fluid dries can have a crusty appearance. Antibiotics can clear up the infection quickly.

Boils are inflamed, pus-filled lumps on the skin that are also caused by staph bacteria. Normally these lumps are infected hair follicles. To avoid spreading the infection, it is important that the boil not be burst. A hot compress can shrink the boil and facilitate drainage. In some instances antibiotics are prescribed to facilitate ending the infection.

Cellulitis is a staph infection of the skin and the tissues beneath. Usually the infection results from a wound. Cellulitis normally affects the neck, face, and legs. In addition to redness of the affected skin, fever and chills can result. Again, antibiotics are used to treat the infection.

Toxic shock syndrome is an uncommon staph infection, but because it is largely preventable and the people with the highest risk are young menstruating women, it warrants discussion. In rare instances, toxic shock syndrome results when a woman inserts a tampon without first washing her hands. Staph bacteria on the hands is transmitted to the vagina via the tampon. If the staph grows in sufficient numbers, it can secrete a toxin that causes a sudden drop in blood pressure, high fever, skin rash, dizziness, disorientation, and possibly shock. The mortality rate is about 3 percent. Treatment is the same antibiotics used for other staph infections.

## STREP INFECTIONS

**Streptococcal** (strep) **infections** are common, with the most common being strep throat. One of the least common yet most highly publicized

**Staphylococcal infections** include cellulitis, impetigo, skin boils, and the much-feared, drug-resistant MRSA.

**Streptococcal infections** include strep throat and flesh-eating bacteria.

Pathogens capable of surviving antibiotics and other medications designed to kill them are called *superbugs.* Such pathogens, the most common of which is methicillin-resistant *Staphylococcus aureus* (MRSA), have the potential to become a significant medical and public health problem.

MRSA is colonized in approximately 1 percent of the population. The bacterium itself is not harmful unless it invades the skin or body organs and causes infection. There are about 90,000 reported infections each year. These bacteria are a real danger, because infection has a 20 percent mortality rate.

Until recently MRSA was a problem mostly found in hospitals and nursing homes, where approximately 85 percent of the reported cases originate. These settings are ideal for transmission because elderly and/ or sick people tend to be more susceptible to infections. In the case of hospitals, invasive procedures such as surgery also provide an easy way for these bacteria to find their way into the body.

Although medical facilities are the riskiest locations for coming into contact with MRSA, infection can occur in any setting, especially where towels, soap, or equipment are shared by many. This is why we have seen outbreaks of MRSA in students at the same school, among U.S. soldiers returning from Afghanistan and Iraq, and even within the ranks of the St. Louis Rams football team.

MRSA is not the only superbug. Other strains of *Staphylococcus aureus* are becoming antibiotic resistant. *Enterococcus,* which is responsible for infections that range from the urinary tract to heart valves, and *Streptococcus pneumonia,* which can cause pneumonia and meningitis, are also developing tolerance to drugs that formerly killed them easily. There is also some evidence that the pathogens responsible for gonorrhea, salmonella, and *E. coli* disease are also becoming antibiotic resistant.

If more superbugs emerge, we could potentially see a new era where the leading causes of death will be communicable diseases, much as it was during the centuries before modern advances in medical care. In that event, medical efforts would shift to emphasizing the prevention of communicable diseases instead of chronic illnesses such as diabetes and heart disease. Further, if this scenario does play out, we could see decrease in both lifespan and life expectancy.

A hopeful point is the fact that superbugs were created through unintended consequences and sloppy practices that people can avoid, once they are aware of the dangers. This is a case where everyday actions by many will be a better defense than relying on science to create ever-stronger drugs to fight resistant, ever-stronger bacteria. Not sharing towels, washing hands frequently, taking the entire antibiotic prescription, and not insisting on antibiotics when the doctor says they are unnecessary are all ways that each of us can help prevent the emergence of new superbugs.

is flesh-eating bacteria. Strep throat usually starts one to five days after exposure, and its chief symptoms include fever, sore throat, and swollen neck glands. A simple throat culture can confirm the diagnosis, and antibiotics can be effective in treating the condition. In extreme or untreated cases, the initial strep infection can develop into a body rash known as scarlet fever, or turn into rheumatic fever, which causes heart problems.

Invasive Group A *Streptococcus* gets a lot of publicity because of its devastating and potentially disfiguring results. This kind of strep bacteria destroys fatty tissue and muscle, thereby gaining the nickname "flesh-eating bacteria." Usually the mode of transmission is an untreated skin wound. The wound becomes infected with strep, and tissue death occurs. Antibiotics can stop the infection, but any tissue that died will not grow back.

One in ten people carry the bacteria responsible for meningococcal meningitis or **bacterial meningitis.** The bacteria are transmitted by close contact between people, which is why outbreaks are known to happen in places such as college dorms. Some people have enough of an immune deficiency that the bacteria get into the bloodstream, affect the brain, and produce the symptoms associated with bacterial meningitis. These symptoms include severe headache, stiff neck, fever, frequent vomiting, and a rash. Fewer than 5 percent of victims will die. If the infection spreads, a condition called *septicemia* results, and the death rate can rise to around 20 percent or higher.

Bacterial meningitis and septicemia are very serious. When young people move into a college dorm or other setting where they come into close contact with a large number of people, they are at higher risk of exposure to the bacteria. Vaccination is the best method of prevention. In addition, it is important to be aware of the symptoms so that medical attention can be sought before the symptoms get worse. Early medical attention with antibiotics can mean the difference between life and death.

Article 11.1

**Bacterial meningitis** is an infection that can affect the brain and is potentially fatal.

# ➤ Common Viral Infections

Viruses are mysterious organisms. They are very simple—a strand of RNA or DNA wrapped in a protein coat. Viruses have the capability of invading the body and using the person's own cells as genetic material to replicate. This process baffles scientists, and because of its complexity, it has been difficult to medically intervene and rid the body of viruses in the way that antibiotics rid the body of bacteria. So the quality of the individual's immune response system, which can destroy the virus, is usually the key to dealing with viral infections. Examples of viral infections are the common cold, influenza, mononucleosis, herpes, and hepatitis. (Sexually transmitted viral infections will be covered later in the chapter.)

A virus as seen through a high-powered microscope.

Over 100 different viruses can cause what we term the *common cold*. Over 50 percent of colds are caused by rhinoviruses, which are viruses that are in the nose. It makes sense that the symptoms of a cold are a runny nose, nasal congestion, a sore throat, and sometimes a headache and fever.

Most adults have two to three colds each year. There is no cure for the common cold, and since a healthy immune response system is very effective in eliminating the virus, the symptoms last about a week and tend to be self-limiting. Because most cold viruses are transmitted by the hands, the most effective way to prevent the spread of colds is to wash one's hands frequently and cover the mouth when sneezing or coughing.

## INFLUENZA

Influenza, or the flu, spreads from person to person through coughing or sneezing. Shaking hands with an infected person is also a common mode of transmission; if people cough into their hand or wipe their nose, they can easily pass the virus on when they touch someone else. Influenza is similar to the common cold, but the symptoms are usually more severe. The incubation period for influenza is usually one to three days, and the symptoms include headache, tiredness, body aches, fever, and chills. There is no cure for the flu. A person's natural immune response will be helped if the flu sufferer gets plenty of rest and drinks lots of fluids.

There are three types of influenza: type A, type B, and type C. The most widespread is type A.

A sense of seriousness regarding influenza reached a fever pitch in spring 2009 when novel Influenza A, a subtype called H1N1 virus, was detected in humans. Mexico reported the first cluster of infections, followed soon after by the United States. H1N1 spread rapidly throughout the rest of the globe. Within a few months of its first detection, the World Health Organization officially classified H1N1 as a pandemic. With approximately 17,000 deaths attributed to H1N1, the pandemic did not turn out to be

This electron-microscope view shows an influenza virus (yellow) budding from a host cell. The host cell nucleus is black.

as serious as originally feared. In August 2010 the H1N1 pandemic was declared officially over.

The *H* and *N* in the virus's name refer to two different kinds of proteins: hemagglutinin (allows the virus to attach to cells) and neuraminidase (in part responsible for releasing new viruses from cells). There are 16 types of hemagglutinin and 9 types of neuraminidase, and we can identify viruses by their specific protein makeup. For instance, the H3N2 virus was responsible for the Hong Kong flu epidemic in the late 1960s. Some but not all of these protein combinations are capable of causing human influenza.

Influenza A spreads from person to person. Symptoms of Influenza A are typical of other human flus: fever, cough, runny nose, aches, fatigue, and chills. Typically infected persons are contagious from one day before symptoms arise to about a week after symptoms subside. The best way to prevent Influenza A infection is the same protocol for preventing other forms of influenza: Cover the nose and mouth when sneezing or coughing, wash hands often, and avoid contact with sick people when possible.

If you do become infected with Influenza A, it is important to do your part to help prevent passing it on to others. The CDC advises that people with influenza-like symptoms stay home from work or school until at least 24 hours after they are free of fever or signs of a fever (such as chills or fatigue) without using fever-reducing medications like acetaminophen or ibuprofen.

Flu vaccinations are an effective way to prevent the flu. The best time to get the vaccine is between October to mid-November because it takes about two weeks for the vaccination to develop protection against influenza. Influenza should be taken seriously because complications can result, including pneumonia and, in rare cases, paralysis.

## MONONUCLEOSIS

Mononucleosis is a common viral infection that as many as 95 percent of adults in the United States will contract by the time they are 40 years old. Epstein-Barr virus is the pathogen that causes mononucleosis. It is found in the saliva of the infected person and may be spread through direct contact, which is why it is nicknamed the "kissing disease."

Mononucleosis has a long incubation period. Approximately 30–50 days after exposure, the person can experience a fever, sore throat, swollen glands in the back of the neck, and fatigue. Symptoms can last anywhere from a week or two to several months. Although most people experience mono only once, it is possible for the virus to lie dormant and reactivate later, resulting in another episode of symptoms. As with influenza, treatment includes rest to help the immune system.

## HERPES 1 (ORAL HERPES)

The most common types of this virus are **herpes simplex virus 1 (HSV 1)** and herpes simplex virus 2 (HSV 2). HSV 1, or oral herpes, will be discussed here, and HSV 2, or genital herpes, will be discussed in the section "Sexually Transmitted Infections."

The classic HSV 1 symptom is a cold-sore lesion on or near the mouth. The sores will appear for a week or two and then subside. The virus will the lie dormant and can reactivate at almost any time. The first outbreak of cold sores is usually the worst and most painful. HSV 1 is not dangerous unless one has a compromised immune system, and the infection spreads and affects the nervous system. Medications are available to reduce the severity of the symptoms, but no medications exist that actually rid the body of the virus. To prevent the spread of herpes, limit saliva contact with an infected person, cover cold sores if possible, and wash hands often.

## HEPATITIS

**Hepatitis** is a generic term meaning "inflammation of the liver." There are several types of the disease, categorized as A, B, or C, depending in part on the mode of transmission. Hepatitis A can be present in the feces and is normally contracted through eating food prepared by someone who is infected and did not wash his or her hands after using the bathroom. Hepatitis B and C are contracted through contact with infected blood via transfusions, dirty needles, or sexual intercourse.

Since hepatitis affects the liver, a key symptom is a yellowing of the skin and eyes called *jaundice*. Other symptoms include brown urine, diarrhea or light-colored stool, fever, loss of appetite, stomach pain, nausea, and fatigue. These symptoms usually begin about four weeks after exposure, can last for a long time, may be quite intense, and are not usually self-limiting but do impair functioning. Hepatitis C victims can carry the virus the rest of their lives. Hepatitis is largely preventable. If restaurant workers wash their hands before touching food, risk of hepatitis A for customers is extremely low.

---

**Herpes simplex virus 1 (HSV 1)** infections are common incurable oral infections, and cold sores around the mouth and lips are the most typical symptom.

**Hepatitis** is a generic term for an infection that causes inflammation of the liver.

**FIGURE 11.3    UNIVERSAL PRECAUTIONS**

1. *Using gloves* to provide a barrier between the hands and potentially infectious body fluids or items contaminated with body fluids. Wash hands immediately after removing gloves.

2. *Wearing* face protection such as masks to prevent droplets of potentially infectious body fluids from being inhaled.

3. *Wearing* protective body clothing such as disposable laboratory coats when there is potential for body fluids to be splashed onto the body.

4. *Washing hands* thoroughly if there is contact with body fluids.

5. *Washing surfaces* that have been exposed to body fluids.

6. *Avoiding injuries* caused by potentially contaminated needles and any other sharp instruments.

7. *Placing* all used gloves and disposable items exposed to body fluids in a specially designated hazardous-materials container.

Bloodborne diseases such as hepatitis B or HIV are best prevented by limiting exposure to potentially infectious body fluids, including blood, through following universal precautions. These precautions include three main practices: wearing a barrier between exposed skin and body fluids; washing hands; and placing exposed materials in a specially designated hazardous-materials receptacle.

Drugs are available to treat hepatitis, and vaccinations are available for hepatitis A and B. Also, the FDA recently approved a new drug, Incivek, which shows much promise in curing liver disease caused by hepatitis C.

Hepatitis B and C, which are the bloodborne forms of hepatitis, can be successfully prevented by using what are termed "universal precautions." All health care workers and many other workers are required to learn these precautions.

Figure 11.3 lists the universal precautions. After reviewing the list, you can easily see that the main effort is to protect the portal of entrance—the skin and nose—from contact with blood products or body fluids. Adhering to universal precautions reduces risk by blocking the portal of entrance through use of masks, gloves, and protective clothing. If implemented correctly, these precautions will significantly limit one's risk of bloodborne diseases.

✓ **NEED TO KNOW**

Options for treating viral diseases are limited. A healthy immune system and frequent hand washing are the best defenses against viruses such as influenza. Avoiding contact with herpes sores is perhaps the best low-risk behavior to prevent a herpes 1 infection. Mononucleosis has been referred to as the kissing disease and the risk of getting it is increased by deep kissing with an infected person. However, many people get mononucleosis just through close person-to-person contact. Symptoms include sore throat, swollen glands, and extreme fatigue. Finally, to avoid contracting bloodborne diseases such as HIV and hepatitis, one should follow universal precautions. Universal precautions are based on three main practices: wearing a barrier between exposed skin and body fluids; washing hands; and placing exposed materials in a specially designed hazardous-materials receptacle.

## ➤ Common Fungal Infections

Fungi are pathogens capable of a wide range of infections, from minor annoyances like athlete's foot and ringworm to serious, life-threatening lung infections such as histoplasmosis.

Athlete's foot is caused by coming into contact with fungal spores commonly found on locker-room floors (hence *athlete's foot*). Skin from an infected person is shed, and a barefoot person stepping on the infected skin runs a risk of also becoming infected. The key symptoms of athlete's foot are redness, itching, and cracking of skin, usually between the toes. Normally, applying a topical antifungal medication will clear up the infection quickly. Prevention efforts include wearing flip-flops when walking on floors used by many barefooted people, especially in locker rooms, and keeping the feet dry.

Ringworm is a fungal infection normally confined to the scalp. The infection appears as a red circle on the scalp, and because it is raised, it looks like a worm. Direct physical contact with an infected person or animal is the chief method of developing the infection. Ringworm is highly contagious and can affect both children and adults. Once diagnosed, ringworm can be successfully treated with topical antifungal medications.

Self
Assessment
11.2

## ➤ Sexually Transmitted Infections

Sexually transmitted infections (STIs) are common diseases caused by bacteria or viruses. Pathogens can be transmitted through sexual activities such as vaginal intercourse, anal intercourse, or oral sex. The common STIs include chlamydia, gonorrhea, syphilis, herpes 2, and human papillomavirus (HPV).

## CHLAMYDIA

*Chlamydia* is a type of bacteria found in infected body fluids from the penis or vagina. The bacteria is transmitted during sexual contact. Symptoms typically appear 7–30 days after exposure. They usually include a discharge from the penis, vagina, or rectum; cramps or pain in the lower abdomen in women; burning or itching around the opening of the penis; pain in the testicles; and painful urination. Many people with chlamydia do not have symptoms, but they can still spread the disease. Women who are asymptomatic might not be aware of the chlamydia infection until they experience pelvic inflammatory disease (PID). However, vaginal discharge with odor or bleeding between cycles can indicate infection, and medical attention is required. Antibiotics can successfully treat chlamydia.

## GONORRHEA

Gonorrhea, another sexually transmitted bacterial infection, is similar to chlamydia. The symptoms are virtually the same. However, symptoms usually appear sooner than chlamydia, 2–7 days after exposure. Untreated gonorrhea in women can lead to pelvic inflammatory disease. Vaginal discharge with odor or bleeding between cycles could indicate infection, and medical attention is required. Gonorrhea can be successfully treated with antibiotics.

## PELVIC INFLAMMATORY DISEASE

**Pelvic inflammatory disease (PID)** is a serious complication of untreated chlamydia and gonorrhea. When the disease is not treated, the bacteria can find their way to the cervix, uterus, fallopian tubes, and eventually the lower pelvic cavity. The symptoms of PID include lower abdominal pain and abnormal vaginal discharge, fever, pain in the right upper abdomen, painful intercourse, and irregular menstrual bleeding. PID causes more than 100,000 women per year to become infertile. Another possible complication of PID is ectopic pregnancy, where the fertilized egg implants in the fallopian tube or the ovary (see Chapter 5).

**Pelvic inflammatory disease (PID)** is a serious, painful condition often related to untreated chlamydia or gonorrhea.

PID can be difficult to diagnose because the symptoms can be similar to those of many other diseases. Antibiotics can be used to treat PID, but any damage to pelvic structures will remain.

## SYPHILIS

Syphilis is another sexually transmitted infection. Unlike chlamydia and gonorrhea, the signs and symptoms are dependent on which stage of syphilis the person is experiencing.

The first stage of syphilis is called the *primary stage*. An infectious, painless lesion or sore called a *chancre* appears at the point of sexual contact. The chancre will most likely appear 10–90 days after exposure and remain for an average of 21 days, after which it will disappear naturally. Unfortunately, the disappearance of the chancre doesn't mean the person is cured. It indicates he or she is moving into the *secondary stage* of the disease.

During the secondary stage, the bacteria spreads, and a rash appears all over the body. This rash can look like a sunburn or take the form of wartlike bumps and white patches in the mouth. In addition to the rash, an infected person might also have a fever, swollen glands, sore throat, patchy hair loss, headaches, weight loss, and malaise. The rash and other symptoms can last 2–6 weeks and will disappear.

If untreated during the primary and secondary stages, the bacteria will become even more disseminated and will damage body organs. This state is termed the *latent stage*, and most often it has no symptoms. A person can be in the latent stage for years before there are symptoms of organ damage, such as paralysis, blindness, and heart damage. This damage marks the last stage of syphilis, termed the *tertiary stage*.

The bacteria can be eliminated with antibiotics. At any stage in the infection, a person can receive the antibiotics and be cured. However, if organ damage occurs, it will not be reversed by antibiotic treatment.

## HERPES 2 (GENITAL HERPES)

**Herpes simplex virus 2 (HSV 2)** is the sexually transmitted form of herpes. Approximately 2–12 days after exposure, a person develops small sores or lesions around either the external reproductive organs or the mouth, depending on the point of sexual contact and infection.

Article 11.2

> **Herpes simplex virus 2 (HSV 2)** is an incurable viral infection; it is usually sexually transmitted, and lesions around the point of sexual contact are the most common symptom.

These sores can be quite painful and will normally last for a week or two before disappearing. However, like herpes 1, when the sores disappear, it doesn't mean that the person is cured; rather, the virus has gone into dormancy and can reactivate at any time. There are medications that can limit the intensity or severity of the symptoms, but there is no cure—once infected, always infected. About 16 percent of Americans between the ages of 14–49 are infected with herpes 2. Women with herpes 2 infections have a higher risk of cervical cancer and run the risk of not being able to vaginally deliver a baby, especially if there are active sores.

## HUMAN PAPILLOMAVIRUS

Human papillomavirus (HPV) is responsible for a condition commonly called *genital warts*. HPV is transmitted sexually, and the warts appear either externally or internally on the genitals between six weeks and eight months after exposure. In some instances people have the infection but never develop warts, leaving them unaware they have an STI. Approximately 50 percent of sexually active women will be infected with HPV at some point in their lives and as a result are at higher risk of cervical cancer. As with herpes 2, they may have difficulty with a vaginal delivery of a baby, depending on whether the warts are in the vagina. Genital warts are treated by applying medications to the warts (causing the warts to fall off), freezing the warts with liquid nitrogen, using electrical heat (cauterizing), or laser therapy.

Article 11.3

A new vaccine is available to protect against HPV. Gardasil provides protection against four types of HPV, including two that are responsible for the majority of cases of cervical cancer. It is believed that most of the HPV infections that lead to cervical cancer are acquired shortly after women become sexually active. The Centers for Disease Control and Prevention (CDC) recommends that all 11- and 12-year-old girls be vaccinated with Gardasil. The objective is to reduce cervical cancer, and if vaccination begins early, then the incidence of cervical cancer could be significantly reduced in the next 20–30 years.

Two controversies arise from the CDC recommendation of Gardasil. First, the vaccine must be administered in three separate injections with a cost of around $350. Second, many ethical issues are raised in administering the vaccine to 11- and 12-year-olds. Some parents believe the vaccine is too new to recommend widespread use, because not all its side effects may yet be known. And some parents believe administering the vaccine may somehow encourage girls to have sex earlier than they would otherwise, because they feel it is safer. Despite these issues, since HPV can lead to more serious conditions, the vaccination is becoming common practice for girls and women.

## PREVENTION OF SEXUALLY TRANSMITTED INFECTIONS

Sexually transmitted infections can be prevented in a number of ways. First, abstinence is the lowest-risk preventive behavior. Second, use of condoms greatly reduces rates of transmission. Condoms are not 100 percent protection against STIs, but they do provide a barrier that blocks the portals of entry and exit.

✓ **NEED TO KNOW**

Sexually transmitted infections (STIs) are preventable. High-risk sexual choices can result in high risk for an STI. Condoms offer some protection. Pain upon urination, urethral or vaginal discharge, sores around the genital area, and pelvic pain all can be signs of an STI and require medical attention. Infertility can result from untreated STIs. A new vaccine offers some protection against the HPV virus, which is a leading cause of cervical cancer.

### HIV AND AIDS

**HIV** and **AIDS** represent two ends of the same viral infection. Because this disease has such important life-and-death dynamics and is such a politically charged issue, we will discuss it independently of the common sexually transmitted infections.

The human immunodeficiency virus (HIV) is both the cause of acquired immunodeficiency syndrome (AIDS) and an infection itself. The term **HIV positive** is used for a person who has been shown to carry the virus but appears to have no symptoms; people whose infections have progressed to the point where they show symptoms are said to have AIDS. If the disease progresses, the person begins to experience fever, weight loss, swollen lymph glands, and white patches in the mouth.

Article
11.4

HIV is transmitted through body fluids such as blood, semen, vaginal secretions, and breast milk of HIV-infected women. Once in the body, HIV attacks the immune system's T cells (described in the "Immune System" section earlier in this chapter). HIV changes the way T cells function so that over time, the T cells stop sending messages to B cells to produce antibodies to fight infections. As the immune system becomes increasingly deficient because of a lack of

Self
Assessment
11.3

**HIV** is the human immunodeficiency virus. **AIDS** is the end-stage disease caused by HIV.

**HIV positive** is the term for a person who has the HIV infection but doesn't exhibit any symptoms yet.

antibodies, the infected person is susceptible to what are termed *opportunistic diseases* such as Kaposi's sarcoma (a skin lesion) and PCP (pneumocystis pneumonia).

The most common modes of transmission of HIV are dirty needles, anal intercourse, and high-risk sexual practices where tissue is torn, allowing contaminated blood to enter another person's body. It can take between six weeks and six months after exposure for someone to test positive for HIV. People who feel fine despite being HIV positive can still pass the virus on to others.

Through medical interventions, people can live productive lives despite HIV infection. There are medications available that, if used at the appropriate time, can limit the reproductive capability of HIV and greatly prolong an infected person's life. If these drugs are not used, then most likely the infection will progress to AIDS.

---

**NEED TO KNOW**

HIV is a relatively difficult disease to get. It breaks down the human immune system over time. Most HIV infections are a result of sexual relations with an infected person or from sharing needles when using drugs. Fortunately, being infected with HIV is not the death sentence it was years ago—but still, to take advantage of the life-saving medical interventions, a person should be diagnosed early.

---

## ➤ Bioterrorism

*Bioterrorism* was once a term used primarily in science-fiction movies. In recent years, with highly publicized "weapons of mass destruction" and the anthrax deaths after September 11, 2001, bioterrorism has become a concept that is now well integrated into our consciousness. It refers to the use of lethal pathogens in terrorism. The diseases of most concern in a bioterrorist context are anthrax, botulism, pneumonic plague, and smallpox. Figure 11.4 provides a clinical overview of the bioterrorist agents responsible for those diseases.

Anthrax is a bacterial disease most associated with cows. When humans are infected by inhaling anthrax spores, they experience flu-like symptoms, and after a brief time period when they think they are recovering, they lapse into respiratory failure and shock. Unless there is medical intervention with high-powered antibiotics, death is likely.

Botulism is a bacterial foodborne disease. Because we have such strict food preparation standards, botulism has not been a serious

# FIGURE 11.4 BIOTERRORIST AGENTS: WATCH FOR THESE SYMPTOMS

| Disease | Signs & Symptoms | Incubation Time (Range) | Person-to-Person Transmission | Isolation | Diagnosis | Postexposure Prophylaxis for Adults | Treatment for Adults |
|---|---|---|---|---|---|---|---|
| **Anthrax** *Bacillus anthracis* A. Inhalation | Flu-like symptoms (fever, fatigue, muscle aches, dyspnea, nonproductive cough, headache), chest pain; possible 1–2 day improvement then rapid respiratory failure and shock. Meningitis may develop. | 1 to 6 days (up to 6 wks) | None | Standard Precautions | Chest x-ray evidence of widening mediastinum; obtain sputum and blood culture. Sensitivity and specificity of nasal swabs unknown—do not rely on for diagnosis. | Prophylaxis for 60 days: Ciprofloxacin* 500 mg PO q 12h Or Doxycycline 100 mg PO q 12h Alternative (if strain susceptible and above contraindicated): Amoxicillin 500 mg PO q 8h *In vitro studies suggest that Levofloxacin 500 mg PO q 24h Or Gatifloxacin 400 mg PO q 24h Or Moxifloxacin 400 mg PO q 24h could be substituted | Inhalation anthrax Combined IV/PO therapy for 60d Ciprofloxacin 500 mg q 12h Or Doxycycline 100 mg q 12h, AND 1 or 2 additional drugs (vancomycin, rifampin, imipenem clindamycin, chloramphenicol, clarithromycin, and if susceptible penicillin or ampicillin) |
| B. Cutaneous | Intense itching followed by painless papular lesions, then vesicular lesions, developing into eschar surrounded by edema. | 1 to 12 days | Direct contact with skin lesions may result in cutaneous infection. | Contact Precautions | Peripheral blood smear may demonstrate gram positive bacilli on unspun smear with sepsis. | | Cutaneous anthrax Ciprofloxacin 500 mg PO q 12h Or Doxycycline 100 mg PO q 12h Recommendations same for pregnant women and immunocompromised persons |
| C. Gastrointestinal (GI) | Abdominal pain, nausea and vomiting, severe diarrhea, GI bleeding, and fever. | 1 to 7 days | None | Standard Precautions | Culture blood and stool. | Recommendations same for pregnant women and immunocompromised persons | |
| **Botulism** botulinum toxin | Afebrile, excess mucus in throat, dysphagia, dry mouth and throat, dizziness, then difficulty moving eyes, mild pupillary dilation and nystagmus, intermittent ptosis, indistinct speech, unsteady gait, extreme symmetric descending weakness, flaccid paralysis; generally normal mental status. | Inhalation: 12–80 hours Foodborne: 12–72 hours (2–8 days) | None | Standard Precautions | Laboratory tests available from CDC or Public Health Dept; obtain serum, stool, gastric aspirate and suspect foods prior to administering antitoxin. Differential diagnosis includes polio, Guillain Barre, myasthenia, tick paralysis, CVA, meningococcal meningitis. | Pentavalent toxoid (types A, B, C, D, E) 0.5 ml SQ may be available as investigational product from USAMRIID. | Botulism antitoxins available from public health authorities. Supportive care and ventilatory support. Avoid clindamycin and aminoglycosides. |
| **Pneumonic Plague** *Yersinia pestis* | High fever, cough, hemoptysis, chest pain, nausea and vomiting, headache. Advanced disease: purpuric skin lesions, copious watery or purulent sputum production; respiratory failure in 1 to 6 days. | 2–3 days (2–6 days) | Yes, droplet aerosols | Droplet Precautions until 48 hrs of effective antibiotic therapy | A presumptive diagnosis may be made by Gram, Wayson or Wright stain of lymph node aspirates, sputum, or cerebrospinal fluid with gram negative bacilli with bipolar (safety pin) staining. | Doxycycline 100 mg PO q 12 Or Ciprofloxacin 500 mg PO q 12h | Streptomycin 1 gm IM q 12h; Or Gentamicin 2 mg/kg, then 1.0 to 1.7 mg/kg IV q 8h Alternatives: Doxycycline 200 mg PO load, then 100 PO mg q 12h Or Ciprofloxacin 400 mg IV q 12h |
| **Smallpox** variola virus | Prodromal period: malaise, fever, rigors, vomiting, headache, and backache. After 2–4 days, skin lesions appear and progress uniformly from macules to papules to vesicles and pustules, mostly on face, neck, palms, soles, and subsequently progress to trunk. | 12–14 days (7–17 days) | Yes, airborne droplet nuclei or direct contact with skin lesions and secretions until all scabs separate and fall off (3 to 4 weeks) | Airborne (includes N95 mask) and Contact Precautions | Swab culture of vesicular fluid or scab, send to BL-4 laboratory. All lesions similar in appearance and develop synchronously as opposed to chickenpox. Electron microscopy can differentiate variola virus from varicella. | Early vaccine critical (in less than 4 days). Call CDC for vaccinia. Vaccinia immune globulin in special cases—call USAMRIID 301-619-2833. | Supportive care. Previous vaccination against smallpox does not confer lifelong immunity. Potential role for Cidofovir. |

Source: Adapted with permission from Bioterrorism Wallchart developed by North Carolina Statewide Program for Infection Control and Epidemiology (SPICE). Copyright 2003 by University of North Carolina at Chapel Hill.

407

problem. As a terrorist weapon, the organism would infect a person, and after incubation, dizziness, weakness, and paralysis would result. Unless botulism antitoxins are administered, the disease can be lethal.

Pneumonic plague is also caused by bacteria. A few days after exposure, the victim can spike a high fever and have a cough, chest pain, nausea, and vomiting. In the advanced form, skin sores will appear. Unless antibiotics are administered, respiratory failure and death can result.

Smallpox was once thought to be eradicated—meaning that enough of the total world population had been immunized to stamp out all infections. But in a bioterrorist context, the smallpox virus can be disseminated through the air. If people breathe in the smallpox virus, they can develop it. Symptoms include fever, vomiting, headache, and skin sores. Unlike the bacterial diseases, there is no cure for smallpox. The quality of the individual's immune response is the key to surviving smallpox. There is a smallpox vaccine that is derived from the virus, but because the disease was thought to have been eradicated, only a small supply of the vaccine is available.

Experts disagree on the extent of the threat of bioterrorism. Many of the diseases discussed here are caused by organisms that are hard to deliver to infect large numbers of people. But that doesn't mean that the organisms can't be manipulated to become easier to deliver and even more lethal. Bioterrorism should be considered a real threat.

Dealing with bioterrorism requires a comprehensive plan with involvement from every segment of American society. In an October 2007 Homeland Security Presidential Directive (HSPD-21), a national strategy for preparedness was presented. This strategy includes four major components: biosurveillance, countermeasure stockpiling and distribution, mass casualty care, and community resilience.

Biosurveillance measures include focused national and international activities to monitor disease occurrence and distribution for those diseases that are likely to be a part of bioterrorism in both animal and human populations. Countermeasure stockpiling and distribution involves ensuring that appropriate vaccines and drugs are available in the case of a real or potential bioterrorism event. Mass casualty care is the mobilization of public health and medical systems to treat those affected by a bioterrorism disease outbreak. Finally, community resilience is activities that communities and social networks can undertake to lessen the risk and damage done in such outbreaks.

HSPD-21 is key to both prevention and intervention activities to both protect citizens from effects of bioterrorist activities and to mobilize public health and medical sectors to deal with a bioterrorist event. The odds are something will eventually happen, and the impact of that event will be directly related to the degree of preparedness of the affected nation, with the United States being a key target. The need for a comprehensive plan that addresses the four major components is paramount and requires cooperation from institutions and individuals.

## ✓ NEED TO KNOW

Manipulating lethal organisms for the purpose of bioterrorism is a real threat. Although there is very little that individuals can do to physically protect themselves, paying attention to Homeland Security warnings and threat levels are key to identifying people or groups who may be involved in harming others through biology. A bioterrorism event is likely to happen at some point. The severity of such an event will be directly related to how well the critical components of HSPD-21 are implemented. Bioterrorism is a real threat, and we all have a role in prevention, especially in helping our respective communities be resilient.

**connect** Resources

 ## ARTICLES

11.1 "Adolescents at Risk: The Case for Meningococcal Vaccine." *Journal of Adolescent Health.* Challenges associated with early diagnosis of meningococcal disease are discussed.

11.2 "Genital Herpes: A Hidden Epidemic." *FDA Consumer.* An examination of the infection rate of genital herpes and why it is considered a hidden epidemic.

11.3 "Getting to Know Human Papillomavirus (HPV) and the HPV Vaccines." *Journal of the American Osteopathic Association.* A practical article on the spread of HPV and availability of HPV vaccines.

11.4 "A Way Forward: The National HIV/AIDS Strategy and Reducing HIV Incidence in the United States." *Journal of Acquired Immune Deficiency Syndrome.* The plan to deal with HIV/AIDS in the United States is the focus of this article.

## SELF-ASSESSMENTS

11.1 Do You Know How to Wash Your Hands?
11.2 Personal Infectious Disease Record
11.3 Sexually Transmitted Infections Quiz

## Website Resources

American Medical Association **www.ama-assn.org/ama**
American Public Health Association **www.apha.org**
Centers for Disease Control and Prevention **www.cdc.gov**
Healthology **www.healthology.com**
Infectious Disease Society of America
    **www.idsociety.org**
MedlinePlus (NIH)
    **www.nlm.nih.gov/medlineplus/infectiousdiseases.html**
Medscape (WebMD)
    **www.medscape.com/infectiousdiseaseshome**
National Foundation for Infectious Diseases
    **www.nfid.org**
National Institute of Infectious Diseases
    **www.nih.go.jp/niid**
World Health Organization
    **www.who.int/topics/en**

## Understanding the Content

1. Describe the communicable disease process using the following terminology: *pathogen, reservoir, mode of transmission, portal of entry, portal of exit, incubation, prodromal stage, acute stage,* and *recovery.*
2. What are the main mechanisms for fighting disease?
3. What is MRSA and why are most people at risk for it?
4. Why can PID be a problem associated with chlamydia and gonorrhea?
5. What is HPV and why should women be concerned about it?
6. What is the difference between HIV, HIV positive, and full-blown AIDS?
7. What are the main bioterrorism agents of concern?

## Exploring Ideas

1. Why should we be so concerned about superbugs, and whose role is it to prevent the spread of these pathogens?
2. Should Gardasil be required for all girls beginning at ages 11 or 12? If so, why? If not, why not?
3. Should there be mandatory HIV testing to determine the extent of HIV infection? Why or why not?
4. What has been done since September 11, 2001, to prevent a bioterrorism event? Is America ready?

American Public Health Association. *Control of Communicable Disease in Man* (17th ed.). Washington, DC: American Public Health Association, 2000.

Brown J. *Don't Touch That Doorknob.* New York: Warner Books, 2001.

Centers for Disease Control and Prevention. *Healthy People 2010,* 2010.

Fauci AS. Emerging infectious diseases: A clear and present danger to humanity. *Journal of the American Medical Association* 292 (15): 1887–1888, 2004.

Garrett L. The lessons of HIV/AIDS. *Foreign Affairs* 84 (4): 51–65, July/August 2005.

Garrett L. Probable cause. *Foreign Affairs* 84 (4): 3–23, July/August 2005.

Harrison LH, Dwyer DM, Maples CT, Billmann L. Risk of meningococcal infection in college students. *Journal of the American Medical Association* 281 (20): 1906–1910, May 26, 1999.

Karlen A. *Man and Microbes.* New York: Putnam, 1995.

Miller J, Engelberg S, Broad W. *Germs.* New York: Simon & Schuster, 2001.

Preston, R. *The Hot Zone.* New York: Random House, 1994.

The White House. Homeland Security Presidential Directive/HSPD-21. Released October 18, 2007. **www.whitehouse.gov/news/releases/2007/10/print/20071018-10.html**

When it comes to your
health, I recommend
frequent doses of that
rare commodity—
common sense.

— VINCENT ASKEY, M.D., PRESIDENT,
AMERICAN MEDICAL ASSOCIATION

# Chapter 12

## THE U.S. HEALTH CARE SYSTEM

In this chapter, we describe the U.S. health care system and
its components. Because of the growing interest in health
care options beyond those of mainstream medicine, a review
of complementary and alternative medicine in addition to
conventional Western medicine is included. We finish with an
overview on the emerging concept of integrative medicine.

# Chapter 12 | THE U.S. HEALTH CARE SYSTEM

## Organization of Our Health Care System

COMPONENTS AND LEVELS OF CARE

MAJOR CHALLENGES: CONTROLLING COSTS AND REDUCING ERRORS

## Western Medicine

PHYSICIANS: M.D.'s AND D.O.'s

DENTISTS

PODIATRISTS

OPTOMETRISTS

CLINICAL PSYCHOLOGISTS

ALLIED HEALTH CARE PROFESSIONALS

## Complementary and Alternative Medicine (CAM)

COMPARISON WITH WESTERN MEDICINE

NATIONAL CENTER FOR COMPLEMENTARY AND ALTERNATIVE MEDICINE

ALTERNATIVE MEDICAL SYSTEMS

MIND–BODY INTERVENTIONS

BIOLOGICALLY BASED THERAPIES

MANIPULATIVE AND BODY-BASED METHODS

ENERGY THERAPIES

BEING A CRITICAL CONSUMER OF CAM

## Integrative Medicine

**EACH OF US** has some familiarity with the U.S. health care system because we've all been patients. Most of you also have a family member or friend who works in health care. Yet, basic information on how our medical system works and the impact of health care reform are only background noise for many of you, as your parents or family watch over your medical needs. You have no compelling reason to understand the health care system. But the time is coming when you will. In contrast, some of you already face responsibility for your own health care. Perhaps you are a returning adult student, or you lost your coverage as a dependent on a parent's health insurance plan when you turned 18 or 21.

As the current or soon-to-be decision maker for your own health care, you need a working knowledge of the U.S. system to use it effectively. Our health care system is complex and continually changing. For the uninformed, it can be confusing and downright overwhelming. In this chapter we present the fundamentals of the health care system to help prepare you to be your own advocate. We provide an overview of 21st-century medicine, explain the key players in conventional Western medicine, review the realm of complementary and alternative medicine (CAM), and end with a profile of a future, blended system known as *integrative medicine.*

As a side note, we also provide a glimpse into potential occupations that may be appealing. Many of you may in fact eventually work in health care—either directly as a health care professional or indirectly in a health-related business. Among all jobs in the U.S. economy, those in the health care sector are expected to be among the fastest growing over the next decade.

## ➤ Organization of Our Health Care System

### COMPONENTS AND LEVELS OF CARE

The U.S. health care system is a multilevel, market-based network of individuals and organizations that provide and underwrite medical services. Our current system began as a simple two-party arrangement between a family doctor and a patient. The patient would either go to the doctor's office for care, or the doctor would make a "house call" (go to the patient's home). Patients paid doctors directly, and those payments were sometimes bartered—goods or services (for instance, food from a farmer) instead of money. Over the decades, this straightforward practice of medicine evolved into a complex health care system. Today in addition to the general practitioner or family doctor, there are a myriad of physician specialists and allied health professionals, a multitude of high-tech instruments and specialized facilities for medical tests and procedures, and a wide array of third-party health care insurers that help patients pay for all those services.

In today's system, health care is described as being at one of three levels: primary, secondary, or tertiary. **Primary health care** involves diagnosis and treatment of common illnesses such as acne, influenza, high blood pressure, or depression. A family practice physician usually provides primary care; thus, he or she is known as the *primary care provider.* Your primary care provider orders standard tests such as urinalysis, blood tests, and X-rays to aid in diagnosis and treatment.

Health problems that are less common, more complex, or persistent may require **secondary health care.** This is the realm of the specialist. There are several approaches to finding a specialist, but the typical route is a referral from your primary care provider. For example, a patient may visit his or her primary care physician to treat migraine headaches. If the migraines persist despite the primary care physician's best efforts, then the physician will likely refer the patient to a neurologist, a doctor who specializes in treating nervous system disorders.

The tests and therapies provided by secondary care may solve the health problem. But if they do not, then **tertiary health care** can come into play. Tertiary care is the most complex set of medical services, involving many types of health care specialists and taking place at a medical center or specialized clinic. If, for instance, a neurologist is unsuccessful in helping the migraine sufferer, then he or she might consult with yet another specialist, such as an endocrinologist, and more complex tests might be ordered, such as an MRI (magnetic resonance imaging) to assess brain function.

## MAJOR CHALLENGES: CONTROLLING COSTS AND REDUCING ERRORS

In terms of highly trained health professionals and cutting-edge medical technology, the United States is one of the top countries in the world. Yet, despite recognized excellence in medical resources, significant weaknesses exist in our health care system. First, the American approach to health care is the most expensive in the world. Medical economists predict that continuation of spiraling costs will have dire consequences and that policy changes are needed sooner rather than later. Second, the rate of preventable medical errors that result in illness,

---

**Primary health care** is the diagnosis and treatment of simple, routine illnessess.

**Secondary health care** is the use of specialists for more complex or unusual conditions.

**Tertiary health care** is the utilization of complex medical services and networks in order to diagnose and treat the most challenging medical conditions.

disability, or death is unacceptably high. What's being done to reduce medical mistakes? As consumers and citizens, these two major challenges warrant our attention.

### Health Care Costs

The major cost categories for health care are hospitals, physician and related clinical services, prescription drugs, and nursing home care. Predictably, hospital care and physician/clinical services account for over half of annual health care costs. Highly trained medical professionals justifiably earn high salaries, and state-of-the-art specialty equipment is extremely expensive to develop, manufacture, and maintain. The main concern is the *rate of rise* in the cost of health care. Health care spending has exceeded overall growth in the U.S economy in recent decades. Put another way, for individuals and families, increases in the cost of health insurance and out-of-pocket medical expenses have consistently outpaced inflation and growth in workers' earnings.

Factors such as medical litigation, the aging population, and treatment for those without insurance contribute significantly to increasing health care costs. Today, physicians routinely carry malpractice insurance; high-risk specialists like obstetricians and surgeons pay malpractice premiums of over $100,000 per year. The costs that physicians must bear to practice medicine are ultimately passed on in patient fees. A second factor pushing health care costs higher is the "graying" of America—the fastest-growing segment of our population is people over age 60. Elderly individuals require more health care services simply due to their age; consequently, as this proportion of the population increases, so do the total expenditures for medical care.

A third factor contributing to rising health care costs is the large number of uninsured people: in 2009, approximately 50 million Americans, about one out of six, had no health care insurance. Uninsured individuals do not seek medical care unless it is absolutely necessary, so most are treated at emergency rooms, and the costs are underwritten with tax dollars. Currently, the availability of low-cost or free care to treat routine medical problems or conduct preventive screening is minimal. Limited services are provided through state, county, and city public health departments and benevolence organizations. Finding a solution to the uninsured problem is a major national challenge.

Article
12.1

Health care reform legislation passed by Congress in 2010 is a major step toward addressing rising health care costs and providing coverage to the uninsured. However, it will take years to fully implement and a decade before we know the impact on controlling costs (see Chapter 13's section on health care reform). In the foreseeable future, we should continue to view health insurance as a necessity, not an option. Without it, medical care is not affordable. Information on how to select a health insurance plan is presented in the next chapter (see Chapter 13's section on understanding health insurance).

### Medical Errors

We've read about the tragic cases. A woman dies from an overdose during chemotherapy. A man has the wrong leg amputated. An 8-year-old dies during "minor" surgery due to a drug mix-up. A comprehensive national study by the prestigious Institute of Medicine of the National Academy of Sciences found that medical errors were a leading cause of death and injury. Researchers estimated that between 44,000 and 98,000 Americans die in hospitals each year as a result of medical errors. Even with the lower estimate, deaths due to preventable medical errors exceeded deaths due to motor vehicle accidents (43,000), breast cancer (42,000), or AIDS (16,000).

Indeed, the problem is probably much larger. Hospital patients represent only a small proportion of the total number of people at risk. More medical care and increasingly complex care is provided in outpatient surgical centers, medical clinics, physicians' offices, and nursing homes. Retail pharmacies and home care are also settings for medical errors. Clearly, health care is not as safe as it should be. In stark terms, this landmark study demonstrated the need for initiating a comprehensive approach to improving patient safety.

As a result of national attention, significant steps have been taken to create safety systems within health care organizations from top to bottom. For example, many hospitals have gone to electronic patient

Article 12.2

records in which all medications are recorded and noted when administered; this minimizes errors due to illegible handwriting, paper records, and different personnel across shifts. Yet, despite reforms to improve health care services, progress has been slow. Fundamental change takes time and commitment by all stakeholders. Knowing that preventable medical errors are *not* a rare occurrence should reinforce our commitment to being active, engaged partners in our own treatment and medical management. Tips on preventing medical errors, especially those related to medicines and hospital stays, are presented in the next chapter (see

Receiving the wrong drug or the correct medication at the wrong dose are examples of preventable medical errors.

Chapter 13's sections "Prescription and OTC Medicines" and "Medical Tests and Procedures").

With regard to the U.S. health care system, there are two clear messages for the individual consumer: (1) have adequate health insurance, and (2) be vigilant for medical errors. At the societal level, Americans should support policies to provide health care that is cost effective, safe, and available to everyone.

✓ **NEED TO KNOW**

The U.S. health care system is a complex, market-based network of individuals and organizations. Medical care is provided at three levels: primary, secondary, and tertiary. Controlling health care costs and reducing medical errors are major challenges. In the American system both health insurance and vigilance are fundamental to receiving quality health care.

# ➤ Western Medicine

Health care in the United States is predominantly in the form of Western medicine—that is, science-based medicine that was largely developed in Europe and North America (the Western world). *Western medicine,* also known as *conventional medicine* or *biomedicine,* can be defined as medicine practiced by mainstream medical doctors and allied health professionals. To maintain a high standard of care, these health care professionals adhere to strict educational and licensing criteria. As consumers of health care, we need to have some familiarity with how doctors and allied health care workers are trained and credentialed.

When the call goes out over the plane's intercom, "Is there a doctor on board?" you can be sure the attendant is calling for a physician, not a college professor. Yet, general knowledge about health care doctors other than physicians and dentists—such as podiatrists, optometrists and clinical psychologists—is fairly limited. In each case, these doctors can function as independent health care practitioners and must be licensed to practice. A brief review of the training, specializations, and overlap among these mainstream health care doctors is provided next.

### PHYSICIANS: M.D.'s AND D.O.'s

There are two types of **physicians:** the M.D. (doctor of medicine) and the D.O. (doctor of osteopathic medicine). Both M.D.'s and D.O.'s

A **physician** is either a doctor of medicine (M.D.) or a doctor of osteopathy (D.O.). Nearly all physicians trained and licensed in the United States have three or more years of residency training following graduation from medical school.

are trained to use all the tools of modern health care including a vast array of medical tests, drugs, and surgery to diagnose and treat illnesses and injuries. In 2010, there were an estimated 900,000 active physicians (about 7% are D.O.'s) in America. About one-third are women.

M.D.'s and D.O.'s are much more similar than different. The main distinction is that osteopathic medicine places special emphasis on the body's musculoskeletal system, preventive medicine, and holistic care. As a result, D.O.'s are more likely than M.D.'s to be primary care doctors and practice family medicine, internal medicine, pediatrics, or obstetrics/gynecology. D.O.'s are often referred to as *osteopaths*, which is a shortened term for *osteopathic physician*.

### Physician Education

Medical education typically extends 7–11 years beyond the under-graduate degree. This is divided between four years of medical school and three to seven years of postgraduate medical education (referred to as *residency*). Most of the first two years of medical school is spent in laboratories and classrooms taking core science courses such as anatomy, biochemistry, physiology, microbiology, pathology, and pharmacology as well as courses in human behavior, medical ethics, and medical law. During years three and four, students learn to take medical histories, examine patients, and diagnose illnesses under the supervision of physicians in hospitals and clinics. Students learn acute, chronic, rehabilitative, and preventive care in broad areas of medicine such as internal medicine, surgery, psychiatry, obstetrics/gynecology, pediatrics, and geriatrics.

### Physician Specialties and Board Certifications

Following medical school, almost all physicians enter a residency in a major hospital or medical center. A residency is graduate medical education in a specialty that takes the form of paid on-the-job training. Residencies and additional training commonly last from three to seven years. This advanced training prepares doctors for board certification in a specialty. This process is overseen by the American Board of Medical Specialists, which comprises 24 specialty boards, ranging from anesthesiology to radiology.

Board certification is not just a topic of interest among physicians—it's also relevant to consumers who want quality health care. Simply put, it's best to select a doctor who is board certified whenever possible. Board certification attests to the highest level of training in a specialty area. A few familiar medical specialties are highlighted in Table 12.1. These can be broadly grouped as primary care specialties, medical specialties, and surgical specialties. In most cases, we are referred to medical and surgical specialists by our primary care doctor.

**TABLE 12.1     EXAMPLES OF PHYSICIAN SPECIALTIES**

| PRIMARY CARE | MEDICAL SPECIALTIES | SURGICAL SPECIALTIES |
|---|---|---|
| Family Medicine | Dermatology | Colon & Rectal Surgery |
| Internal Medicine* | Emergency Medicine | Neurological Surgery |
| Pediatrics* | Ophthalmology | Orthopedic Surgery |
| Obstetrics & Gynecology | Otolaryngology (ear/nose/throat) | Plastic Surgery |
| | Psychiatry | Thoracic Surgery |
| | Urology | Vascular Surgery |

*Within both internal medicine and pediatrics, physicians can pursue additional training in subspecialties such as cardiovascular disease, pulmonary disease, oncology, infectious disease, and endocrinology.

Source: American Board of Medical Specialties **(www.abms.org/Who_We_Help/Physicians/ specialties.aspx).**

The eye specialist (ophthalmologist) and skin specialist (dermatologist) are two whom many of us have already visited. And, we may have been seen by an emergency medicine physician when we went to the ER (emergency room/department) after an accident or for a severe sudden-onset illness. You can determine if a physician is board certified via the medical specialty websites (see Website Resources at the end of the chapter).

### Primary Care Physicians

The **primary care physicians** are our family or personal doctors. Most specialize in family medicine, internal medicine, pediatrics, or obstetrics/gynecology. They are skilled at diagnosing and treating common medical problems. Equally important, they know when to refer us to a medical or surgical specialist. In this role, they serve as gatekeepers and guides to a vast array of medical specialists and resources. In fact, some insurance plans require that people always see their primary care physician first (except for emergencies) before seeking other care.

Article 12.3

Even if you can go directly to a specialist, there are good reasons to have a primary care physician. People without medical training have

A **primary care physician** is the front-line doctor (an M.D. or D.O.) who spends most of his or her time diagnosing and treating common and routine illnesses and diseases. Most specialize in family medicine, internal medicine, pediatrics, or obstetrics/gynecology.

limited skills in diagnosis and knowing when to see which specialist. We should recognize our limitations and rely on our primary care doctors for their expertise (see Chapter 13's section "Caring for Yourself"). Plus, if a serious problem requires seeing several doctors, being able to rely on a primary care doctor to coordinate care and integrate findings is invaluable.

The aim is to have a primary care physician with whom you've established a relationship over a period of years—a doctor who knows you well, provides ongoing medical care, refers you to specialists as needed, interprets results, and generally advises you on medical matters. In addition to being board certified, it's important to select a primary care doctor who is a good communicator and with whom you feel comfortable. A solid patient–doctor relationship is based on confidence and trust.

Doctors specializing in internal medicine (internists) focus on the primary care of adults, particularly the diagnosis and (nonsurgical) treatment of diseases of the internal organs. They are trained to solve diagnostic problems in which multiple illnesses and diseases may be occurring at the same time. They also are trained to advise people on disease prevention, women's health, substance abuse, and mental health, as well as common problems of the eyes, ears, skin, nervous system, and reproductive organs. Although their focus is on the internal organs, they do treat the whole person. (Do not confuse *internists* with *interns*, who are doctors in their first year of residency training.)

Just as internists specialize in adult medicine, pediatricians are the primary care specialists in the medical care of infants, children, and adolescents. Obstetricians and gynecologists are trained in the medical and surgical care of the female reproductive system and associated disorders. They are also trained and often serve as primary care physicians for women.

## ✓ NEED TO KNOW

Most 21st-century physicians (M.D.'s or D.O.'s) are highly trained specialists with three or more years of training beyond medical school. Adults should have a primary care physician who is a family medicine specialist or an internist. Women may elect to rely on their obstetrician/gynecologist as their primary doctor. Infants, children, and adolescents should be seen by a pediatrician or family medicine specialist. To receive the best medical care, consumers should seek out physicians who are board certified. Finally, it's important to select a primary care doctor who is a good communicator and with whom you feel comfortable.

**Breaking It Down** Doctors and Drug Companies: Who's in Control?

423

CHAPTER 12 THE U.S. HEALTH CARE SYSTEM

An anonymous woman tries to disentangle a shopping cart from an interlocked row of carts outside a suburban store. She is frustrated and angry. She becomes even more exasperated when another shopper enters the frame, calmly unhooks a cart, and glides smoothly on her way. Watching this TV advertisement unfold, it might look like the woman is experiencing little more than a normal bout of tension or stress. But the folks at the drug company Lilly know better. This woman may need a powerful antidepressant because she is suffering from a severe form of mental illness known as PMDD. "Think it's PMS? It could be PMDD," intones the voiceover.

Not everyone agrees with the drug company's assessment. This example was taken from the book *Selling Sickness: How the World's Biggest Pharmaceutical Companies Are Turning Us All into Patients*. Authors Roy Moynihan and Alan Cassels argue that the pharmaceutical industry is no longer focused on selling cures for disease, but rather on marketing drugs to the masses. They provide persuasive evidence that the big drug companies now influence all facets of medication use—research, approval, marketing, and the doctors and their patients.

*Selling Sickness* is just one of many books to delve into this remarkable entanglement of capitalism, medicine, and culture. When the arthritis pain drugs Celebrex and Vioxx were recalled from the market because of reports that they increased the risk of heart disease, troubling questions arose. Were these drugs prematurely pushed through the approval process in the rush to get them to market? The intrusion of drug companies into the practice of medicine has been described as scandalous and fraudulent. Even those who are sympathetic to the drug companies recognize that the situation is—at the very least—troubling and problematic. Consumers should be alert and concerned.

A few statements of fact: Many prescription drugs are truly lifesaving and life-sustaining in their ability to help cure or manage specific diseases and illnesses. For some medical conditions, compelling evidence from years of careful research has shown that specific drug therapies are effective and safe. Examples include statin drugs to manage high cholesterol and synthetic insulin for type 1 diabetes. Drugs are also often expensive, and all have side effects.

So what's the problem? Through strategic and systematic corporate sponsorship, drug companies have undue influence in the promotion

*(Continued)*

and sales of prescription drugs. To begin with, a large proportion of research at medical schools is funded by drug companies. Less noticeable because it's omnipresent is the benefactor role of drug companies in the lives of physicians from medical school till retirement. Such support pervades both medical education (medical school, residency training, and continuing education) and clinical practice. Drug companies sponsor all sorts of educational and social events from luncheons for medical students to lavish seminars for physician specialists. Drug company representatives who regularly visit physicians to present new products have an array of thank-you gifts and favors to bestow.

But of all the inroads to influence forged by the drug companies, perhaps the most far-reaching is direct marketing to the public. Through slick "awareness-raising" campaigns, the drug industry has capitalized on the American illusion that we can have it all—eternal youth, beauty, sexual desire, enhanced intellect, and continual happiness—by taking a pill. This has led to the creation or exaggeration of medical conditions such as PMDD (premenstrual dysphoric disorder, a severe form of premenstrual syndrome), motivational deficiency disorder, adult attention-deficit disorder, social anxiety disorder, female sexual dysfunction, and erectile dysfunction. Doctors are no longer just subliminally conditioned to prescribe drugs. They are now confronted by patients who saw an advertisement and subsequently ask for, and sometimes demand, the new drug.

The goal of for-profit companies is to increase sales, often aggressively within the limits of the law. In their ambition, drug companies have steadily pushed the envelope to broaden the base of potential clients beyond those who are sick to the healthy too. This has required new corporate strategies aimed at creating markets for their products. Moynihan asks, "Is the goal of pharma [the drug industry] a disease for every pill?"

In today's world, many factors influence how doctors prescribe drugs to their patients. We must remember that doctors are human just like the rest of us. They are not immune from influences inherent in the system of medical training and practice. The influence of drug companies is another compelling reason to select your doctor with care. Find one who accepts you as not just a patient, but as a partner in your own health care. And before asking your doctor for that new medicine you saw advertised, do your homework on the drug and its targeted medical condition. You may be just fine without it.

# DENTISTS

Nearly every reader has visited a dentist within the last year or two. In America, we are fortunate to have regular access to dentists to help ensure good oral health. **Dentists** prevent, diagnose, and treat problems with teeth and with mouth tissue. They commonly remove tooth decay, fill cavities, interpret X-rays, straighten teeth, and repair or replace damaged or diseased teeth. They also perform corrective surgery on gums and supporting bones to treat gum diseases. They provide instruction on oral hygiene including diet, brushing, flossing, and the use of fluorides, as well as administer anesthetics and write prescriptions. In 2010, there were about 200,000 active dentists in the United States.

As with medical school students, most students who are admitted to dental school hold an undergraduate degree. Dental school is typically four academic years. During the last two years, students treat patients in dental clinics, under the supervision of licensed dentists. Most dental schools award the degree of doctor of dental surgery (D.D.S.). The rest award an equivalent degree, doctor of dental medicine (D.M.D.). A major difference between the education of a physician and a dentist is the extent of postgraduate education. For medical school graduates, a three-year residency is standard. In contrast, most dental school graduates go straight into practice after graduation. Most become general practitioners, handling a variety of dental needs. Only about one in eight new graduates enroll in postgraduate programs to prepare for a dental specialty. Orthodontists who straighten teeth with braces or retainers constitute the largest group of specialists. Oral and maxillofacial surgeons, who operate on the mouth and jaws, and periodontists, who treat gums and bone supporting the teeth, are two other types of specialists.

## PODIATRISTS

A **podiatrist** is to the foot what a dentist is to the mouth. The podiatrist—or doctor of podiatric medicine (D.P.M.)—specializes in the prevention, diagnosis, and treatment of foot and ankle disorders. A podiatrist makes independent judgments, prescribes medications, and performs surgery. The foot may be the first area to show signs

---

A **dentist** is a doctor of dental surgery (D.D.S.) or dental medicine (D.M.D.), whose practice includes problems with teeth and gums and other aspects of oral health.

A **podiatrist** is a doctor who holds a doctor of podiatric medicine (D.P.M.) degree and whose practice focuses on medical problems of the foot and lower leg.

of serious conditions such as diabetes or heart disease. In this role, podiatrists often become a vital link in the patient's health care team.

Although podiatry has been a recognized medical practice for nearly a century, the profession remains poorly understood. Most foot and ankle problems are treated by primary care physicians or orthopedic surgeons (M.D.'s/D.O.'s). Although podiatrists are foot and ankle specialists, there is substantial overlap in medical care of foot injuries by physicians and podiatrists. Because there are only about 15,000 podiatrists nationwide, many Americans simply do not have access to podiatric care.

The medical training to become a podiatrist is similar to that for an M.D. or D.O. The curriculum leading to a D.P.M. is four years long. The first two years are classroom instruction and laboratory work; they are followed by two years of supervised clinical rotations. Graduation from podiatric medical school is followed by a two-year residency in a hospital-based program.

## OPTOMETRISTS

Doctors of optometry (O.D.'s) are health care professionals for the eye. The primary function of **optometrists** is correcting what are known as *refractive errors*. A refractive error is due to the eye not bending light correctly, resulting in a blurred image. Refractive errors are the most common eye disorders, and they include nearsightedness, farsightedness, and astigmatism. Optometrists prescribe corrective lenses both in the form of glasses and contact lenses. In addition they counsel people regarding their visual needs and associated surgical and nonsurgical options related to their occupations, avocations, and lifestyle.

### Optometric Education
A four-year curriculum leads to the O.D. degree. Nearly all O.D.'s enter the workforce immediately following graduation. A small percentage complete an optional one-year residency in a specific area of practice.

### Optometrist Versus Ophthalmologist
Both optometrists and ophthalmologists are referred to as "eye doctors." Indeed, there is overlap in the services they perform. But there are differences as well. An ophthalmologist is a physician, with eight or more years of education beyond college (medical school, and at least four years of specialty training), who performs a full range of eye-related

An **optometrist** holds an O.D. degree and is primarily trained to evaluate refractive errors and prescribe corrective glasses or contacts.

Optometrists use glasses or contact lenses to correct refractive errors of the eye.

medical care, including surgery. In comparison, an optometrist has four years of education beyond college (4-year professional degree in optometry) and mainly examines eyes, prescribes corrective lenses, and advises on nonsurgical management of certain eye problems. As a final note, let's consider the optician. An optician is a technician licensed to fit and dispense eyeglasses and contact lenses according to a written prescription from an ophthalmologist or optometrist. The training and certification of opticians vary from state to state.

## CLINICAL PSYCHOLOGISTS

**Clinical psychologists** are mental health practitioners. They work closely with physicians, often referring patients to each other. Clinical psychologists constitute the largest specialty group within the broad field of psychology. Clinical psychologists help people with mental/emotional illness adjust to life. They also assist medical and surgical patients in dealing with illnesses or injuries. For example, in physical rehabilitation centers, clinical psychologists can be found treating patients with spinal cord injuries, chronic pain or illness, stroke, and neurological conditions.

A **clinical psychologist** holds a Ph.D. or Psy.D. in clinical psychology and provides psycho-socio-behavioral therapies to help people adjust to or overcome emotional problems or mental illnesses.

Clinical psychologists work with individuals of all ages from infants to older adults, as well as families, groups, and organizations. They use a wide range of assessments and interventions to promote mental health and to alleviate discomfort and maladjustment. Interventions are directed at preventing and treating emotional conflicts, personality disturbances, and psychopathology. Common interventions include psychotherapy, psychoanalysis, behavior therapy, marital and family therapy, group therapy, biofeedback, cognitive retraining, social learning approaches, and environmental consultation and design. Many clinical psychologists are also involved in research, teaching and supervision, program development and evaluation, and public policy.

### Doctoral Education in Clinical Psychology

A doctoral program in clinical psychology—leading to either a Ph.D. or Psy.D. degree—takes five to seven years and requires substantial coursework in personality and psychopathology and a one-year internship. The American Psychological Association accredits clinical psychology doctoral programs. All states require a license to practice clinical psychology.

### Clinical Psychologist Versus Psychiatrist

As between optometrists and ophthalmologists, overlap exists between clinical psychologists and psychiatrists. The main difference is that psychiatrists are physicians who can order medical tests to assist in diagnoses and prescribe medications for treatment. Although the clinical psychologist's training is firmly rooted in psychology and the psychiatrist's in medicine, both are experts in mental health and, in fact, often work together in complementary fashion on health care teams in hospitals and clinics.

### ✓ NEED TO KNOW

Along with the familiar physician (M.D., D.O.), a number of other doctors provide health care services. In addition to the dentist (D.D.S., D.M.D.), there are the doctoral-level professions of podiatrist (D.P.M.), optometrist (O.D.), and clinical psychologist (Ph.D., Psy.D.). Understanding the similarities and differences among these three professions versus the physician specialists of orthopedist, ophthalmologist, and psychiatrist, respectively, is important in making decisions about health care needs related to the foot, eye, and the mind.

## ALLIED HEALTH CARE PROFESSIONALS

In conventional Western medicine, complex illnesses are treated and managed by medical teams led by physicians. The health care team contains a mix of allied health care professionals depending on the patient's particular medical condition. There are over 50 recognized allied health professions. They range from audiologists (hearing) and prosthetists (artificial limbs) to technologists trained in specialized medical services from medical imaging to surgery. As mentioned in the chapter introduction, many of you will eventually work in health care—as doctors, allied health care professionals, or employees in a health-related business. Knowing that job growth in the health care sector is projected to remain strong, you may wish to investigate related educational programs and career paths. Four allied health professionals with which you—as a patient—are likely to interact are the registered nurse, physician assistant, physical therapist, and registered dietitian.

### Registered Nurses

**Registered nurses (R.N.'s)** constitute the largest health care profession, with 2.6 million jobs in the United States. Most R.N.'s work as staff nurses, providing health care services to patients under the direction of physicians and other health care practitioners. Round the clock, nurses are the true front-line caregivers. In the hospital or clinic, when a doctor orders a treatment or test, it's the nurse who typically administers or supervises the procedure. Basic duties include checking vital signs, dressing wounds, administering treatment and medications, educating and reassuring patients, and providing support to patients' family members. Additionally, R.N.'s record medical histories and symptoms, help perform diagnostic tests and analyze results, and assist with patient follow-up and discharge. In some cases, R.N.'s direct health screenings, immunization clinics, blood drives, and public seminars on various medical conditions.

There are three main paths to becoming an R.N.: a bachelor of science degree in nursing (B.S.N.), an associate degree in nursing, and a diploma. In 2006, over 700 colleges offered the bachelor's degree (typically a four-year program), about 850 community and junior colleges offered the associate degree (two to three years), and only about 70 hospital-based programs offered the diploma (about three years). Generally, licensed graduates of any of the three types of educational programs qualify for entry-level positions as staff nurses. Accelerated B.S.N. programs also are available for people who have a bachelor's or higher degree in another field. In 2006, about 200 of these programs were available.

A **registered nurse (R.N.)** is a graduate of a nursing school (diploma, associate degree, or undergraduate degree) who has passed the licensing exam for the R.N. credential.

Some R.N.'s choose to become advanced practice nurses by obtaining a master's degree in one of four areas—as a nurse practitioner, clinical nurse specialist, nurse anesthetist, or nurse midwife. Nurse practitioners provide basic preventive health care to patients and increasingly are serving as primary and specialty care providers in medically underserved areas. Clinical nurse specialists provide direct patient care and expert consultations in a particular nursing specialty (related to a disease, a body organ or system, or a patient population). Nurse anesthetists administer anesthesia, monitor the patient's vital signs during surgery, and provide postoperative care. Nurse midwives provide primary care to women, including gynecological exams, family planning advice, prenatal care, assistance in labor and delivery, and neonatal care.

### Physician Assistants

**Physician assistants (P.A.'s)** are health professionals licensed to practice medicine with a physician's supervision. Within the physician–P.A. relationship, P.A.'s can have significant autonomy in medical decision making and provide a broad range of diagnostic and therapeutic services. P.A.'s can take medical histories, perform physical exams, order and interpret laboratory tests, diagnose and treat illnesses, counsel patients, assist in surgery, and set fractures. In nearly all states they can prescribe medicines under the supervision of an M.D. or D.O.

Most P.A. programs consist of a two-year master's program. All programs emphasize primary care. Nearly all successful applicants already have a bachelor's degree. P.A.'s often have prior experience as registered nurses, while others come from varied backgrounds, including the military corps/medics and allied health occupations such as respiratory therapists, physical therapists, and paramedics. Many P.A.'s obtain additional training in a primary care specialty—family medicine, internal medicine, pediatrics, or obstetrics and gynecology. Others may opt for specialty fields, such as cardiovascular surgery, orthopedics, or emergency medicine.

### Physical Therapists

Under the guidance of a physician, **physical therapists (P.T.'s)** provide treatments that help restore function, improve mobility, relieve pain, and prevent or limit permanent physical disabilities of people suffering from injuries or disease. Their patients range from accident victims with fractures and injuries to the spine and head to people with disabling

A **physician assistant (P.A.)** is a health care professional trained to provide routine primary care to patients under the supervision of a physician.

A **physical therapist (P.T.)** is a health care professional who holds a degree in physical therapy and generally works in rehabilitation medicine helping patients restore musculoskeletal function.

conditions such as low back pain, arthritis, stroke, and cerebral palsy. P.T.'s most commonly provide care in hospitals, clinics, and private offices. There are over 100,000 P.T.'s working in the United States. Throughout most of the rest of the world, physical therapists are known as *physiotherapists*.

There are about 200 U.S. programs awarding the doctor of physical therapy (D.P.T.). The degree transitioned from a master's (M.P.T.) to a doctorate over a 10-year period starting in the late 1990s. Nearly all programs require applicants to have an undergraduate degree with a core set of science courses. D.P.T. programs are three to four years with clinical internships interspersed throughout. P.T.'s can enter the workforce as generalists and treat patients with a wide range of conditions, or they can specialize in areas such as pediatrics, geriatrics, orthopedics, sports medicine, neurology, and cardiopulmonary rehabilitation.

## Registered Dietitians

**Registered dietitians (R.D.'s)** are food and nutrition experts who typically work in one of four areas: clinical, community, management, or consultant dietetics. Clinical dietitians provide nutritional services for patients in institutions such as hospitals and nursing care facilities.

They confer with doctors and other health care professionals to coordinate medical and nutritional needs for patients. Over half of all full-time R.D.'s work as clinical dietitians. Community dietitians work in public health clinics, home health agencies, and HMOs, where they counsel individuals and groups on nutritional practices to prevent disease and promote health. Management dietitians oversee large-scale meal planning and preparation in places such as school and company cafeterias. Consultant dietitians work on a contract basis for individual clients or organizations such as wellness programs, sports teams, supermarkets, and nutrition-related businesses.

Many registered dieticians work for hospitals and nursing care facilities to ensure that the nutritional needs of patients are met.

A **registered dietitian (R.D.)** is a food and nutrition expert who holds a degree in dietetics and has passed the national R.D. exam.

To be eligible for the R.D. exam, the standard route is to complete an accredited bachelor's degree in nutrition/dietetics. There are over 200 bachelor's and master's degree programs in the United States. The curriculum includes course and laboratory work in all four dietetics practice areas as well as an approved internship. R.D.'s are trained to translate the science of nutrition into practical solutions across the lifespan and for a variety of diseases and conditions. There are over 50,000 practicing full-time R.D.'s. Many pursue additional graduate training to prepare for advanced clinical positions, to work in public health, or to go into research. Given the current diet-related health problems faced by Americans, the value of a dietitian in advising patients and working with other health care professionals to coordinate medical care has never been greater.

For additional information on these and other types of allied health care professions, see the websites listed at the end of the chapter. Related to both consumer information and career prospects, it should be noted that competition is keen, and educational standards are continually increasing for allied health care professional preparation programs. As with health care doctors, the job opportunities in allied health careers are excellent, and future demand is projected to remain high.

✓ **NEED TO KNOW**

A patient's needs may require the expertise of a health care team that includes one or more physicians and a mix of allied health care professionals. The team approach is particularly important in diagnosing, treating, and managing complex illnesses. As a consumer, it's important to understand how these supporting professionals contribute to patient care. The training and roles of allied health care professionals—such as nurse, physician's assistant, physical therapist, and dietitian—are varied and multifaceted and continue to evolve over time.

## ➤ Complementary and Alternative Medicine (CAM)

In addition to conventional or Western medicine, to which most of us are accustomed, there is a wide variety of other approaches to health care collectively referred to as **complementary and alternative medicine (CAM).** Chiropractic and acupuncture are two well-known examples.

**Complementary and alternative medicine (CAM)** is a group of diverse medical and health care systems, practices, and products that are not currently considered to be part of Western or conventional medicine.

| TABLE 12.2 | COMPARISON OF BASIC PRINCIPLES: WESTERN MEDICINE VERSUS ALTERNATIVE MEDICINE |
|---|---|
| **PRINCIPLES OF WESTERN MEDICINE** | **PRINCIPLES OF ALTERNATIVE MEDICINE** |
| Rooted in the scientific method and guided by empirical evidence from research | Often rooted in traditional medicine based on ancestral practices |
| Illness has a physical cause due to pathogens, environment, lifestyle, genetic factors, aging | Illness is due to an imbalance in the person or between the individual and others |
| Diagnosis of illness is based on established signs and symptoms that occur across patients | Illness is different in each person; evidence is case-based |
| Focus is to heal via outside intervention as with drugs and/or surgery | Focus is on helping the body's capacity for self-repair |
| Use of specialists and advanced technology to diagnose and treat illness | Based on metaphysical premises that may not be testable |

CAM practices are based on principles quite different from those of mainstream Western medicine. For this reason, CAM is also known as *nonconventional medicine. Complementary medicine* specifically refers to practices used at the same time but not necessarily in conjunction with conventional medical practices, whereas *alternative medicine* refers to practices used instead of conventional treatments.

## COMPARISON WITH WESTERN MEDICINE

The fundamental differences between Western medicine and CAM are summarized in Table 12.2. The foundation of Western medicine is science, the scientific method is the discovery and accumulation of knowledge through systematic and rigorous research. In contrast, CAM practices are often rooted in culture-specific traditions and medical customs passed down across generations. CAM practices, also referred to as *traditional medicine*, are still widely used in parts of Asia, Africa, and Latin America.

The Western medicine approach involves the diagnosis and treatment of illness within a biomedical framework using highly trained specialists and advanced technology. Western medicine focuses on curing illness and disease through drugs and surgery, based on objective scientific evidence. In contrast, CAM is generally case-based rather than research-based and often has spiritual or metaphysical underpinnings that are not readily testable by the scientific method. For most forms of CAM, illness is thought to be caused by an imbalance within the individual or between the individual and others, and treatment is directed toward assisting the body's innate capacity for self-repair and restoration of balance.

Thus, the very nature of CAM—where interpretation of similar symptoms, diagnosis of illness, and prescribed treatments may vary widely from one patient to the next—makes CAM practices difficult if not impossible to study using the scientific method. Standard research methods typically involve studying hundreds of subjects with the same illness to test the effectiveness of a given treatment.

Western medicine is evidence-based and the bedrock for health care in the 21st century. However, CAM is routinely used by significant segments of our population, and some CAM practices may provide healing benefits for certain patients. A recent government survey found that about 40 percent of American adults reported using some form of CAM on a regular basis. Patients' perceptions about limitations in Western medical care are reflected in their increasing expenditures for alternative treatments. About half of these costs are paid out of pocket because insurance companies do not authorize payment for most CAM therapies.

As strong as Western medicine is, it cannot answer all our questions about health and disease. Even the foremost medical researchers agree on this point. And, conversely, as unproven as CAM appears to those who understand the world through science, the fact remains that some alternative therapies help people get better. The difficulty is in reconciling our inability to prove cause and effect between certain CAM practices and what appears to be a potent benefit.

With that in mind, we should remain open to the possibility that CAM offers beneficial treatments, yet always examine specific practices based on their own merits and evidence. As consumers of health care, our challenge is to do our homework on the effectiveness and safety of a CAM practice and to investigate the practitioner's qualifications and experience *before* making a decision about treatment.

## NATIONAL CENTER FOR COMPLEMENTARY AND ALTERNATIVE MEDICINE

In 1998 the National Institutes of Health (NIH) created the National Center for Complementary and Alternative Medicine (NCCAM) in response to the growing interest in alternative medicine and the need for an objective resource for information and guidance on these diverse practices. The primary objectives of the NCCAM are twofold: to investigate alternative healing practices in the context of rigorous science and to disseminate authoritative information to the public and professionals.

The NCCAM has developed a category system to organize the large number of assorted practices and treatments within alternative medicine. We will follow this system and provide examples of common therapies within each category. The NCCAM organizes alternative medicine into five major categories: alternative medical systems, mind–body interventions, biologically based therapies, manipulative and body-based methods, and energy therapies. From the onset, it should be recognized that these are broad domains and that overlap exists.

For the most popular forms of alternative medicine, we will also describe educational and licensing requirements. In contrast to Western medicine, professional preparation programs for practitioners of alternative medicine are generally much less rigorous and systematic. Practice standards and credentialing are often lacking or not uniform.

## ALTERNATIVE MEDICAL SYSTEMS

Alternative medical systems are integrated systems of medical care that are separate from the Western medical system. Traditional Chinese medicine and homeopathic medicine are two examples. Alternative medical systems vary widely from each other because each is based on its own unified body of thought and practice that reflects unique historical origins and underlying philosophies. As illustrated in Figure 12.1, the domain of alternative medical systems can cut across the other four categories. To illustrate, traditional Chinese medicine utilizes specific treatments based on *qi* (pronounced *chee* and roughly translated as "life" or "vital energy"), herbs, and Chinese massage that are also considered modalities within energy therapies, biologically based therapies, and manipulative therapies, respectively.

**FIGURE 12.1    ORGANIZATION OF ALTERNATIVE PRACTICES**

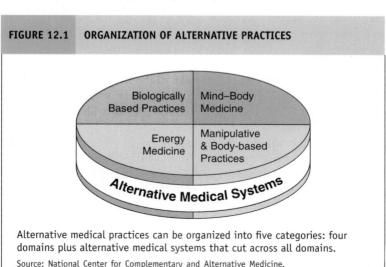

Alternative medical practices can be organized into five categories: four domains plus alternative medical systems that cut across all domains.

Source: National Center for Complementary and Alternative Medicine.

An acupuncturist carefully places needles in the body.

### Traditional Chinese Medicine and Acupuncture

Traditional Chinese medicine is a system of medicine that has been practiced in China for over 3,000 years. A fundamental principle is that to remain healthy, harmony must be maintained within the body and between the body and nature. This view is represented in the distinctive yin-yang theory that encompasses the concepts of opposites, interdependence, and change. This theory and its many associated concepts (beyond the scope of this brief overview) reflects a coherent, well-developed medical system and a wide variety of therapeutic methods. Traditional Chinese medicine continues to be widely practiced in China today alongside Western medicine.

In the Western world, **acupuncture** is the best known of the traditional Chinese medicine treatments. Acupuncture is the practice of inserting small needles into carefully selected points along the body's energy pathways. Needles are positioned just under the skin or deeper into the muscle and then either manually rotated or electrically stimulated.

**Acupuncture** is an alternative medicine procedure used in or adapted from traditional Chinese medicine in which specific body areas are pierced with fine needles to treat a variety of illnesses.

Acupuncture treatment is based on the belief that by adjusting the body's *qi*, or vital energy, healing can occur.

Acupuncture has been most thoroughly studied as a potential treatment for two conditions: low back pain and nausea/vomiting. Systematic reviews of multiple studies indicate acupuncture is more effective for relief of low back pain than no treatment or sham (pretended) treatment. Moreover, when acupuncture is added to conventional therapies, it relieves pain and improves function better than conventional therapies alone. Yet, all effects are small. Multiple studies have also assessed whether acupuncture can be used to reduce nausea and vomiting (typically postoperative or following chemotherapy). Overall results indicate that acupuncture can be effective, particularly on the first day.

Practitioners of acupuncture are known as *acupuncturists*. The National Certification Commission for Acupuncture and Oriental Medicine has been providing bona fide certification in acupuncture since 1985. These certificates are accepted for licensure in about 40 states. Refer to the Commission's website to find a certified acupuncturist and for information on state licensure (**www.nccaom.org**).

### Homeopathy

Homeopathy is another example of an alternative medical system. Homeopathy is based on the *law of similars.* This refers to the observation that medicines can produce in healthy people the same symptoms they cure in the sick. This concept—also known as *like cures like*—was derived from simple trial and error or empirical observations. Homeopathic treatment involves giving extremely dilute medicines to trigger the patient's innate ability to heal. Homeopathic medicines are natural remedies derived from animal, plant, and mineral sources and are sold as over-the-counter products.

Homeopathy was developed over 200 years ago in Europe by Samuel Hahnemann, a German physician. His followers immigrated to the United States in the mid-1800s and established the American homeopathic movement, which flourished for several decades. However, the tide turned in the first half of the 20th century. As medical science (Western medicine) grew, and more and more modern drugs were discovered, homeopathy lost its appeal.

Even though all formal degree programs were disbanded by 1950, homeopathy has persevered over the decades and still has its advocates. Seminars and courses continue to be offered by homeopathic interest groups. A resurgence of interest in homeopathy has occurred in recent years as part of the broader interest in self-care and alternative medicine. Because there is no federal licensure exam, the current practice of homeopathy is generally limited to medically licensed physicians

(M.D.'s, D.O.'s) who use selected homeopathic remedies along with conventional medical treatments.

The scientific basis and medical effectiveness of homeopathy remain dubious. Although there may be instances in which like cures like the concept does not qualify as a universal principle. A limited number of studies have evaluated homeopathic treatments. Few carefully controlled randomized studies have been conducted due to the lack of positive findings from smaller studies. Systematic reviews of homeopathic treatments find no conclusive evidence of effectiveness for any specific medical condition. Although the risk of serious side effects from using highly diluted homeopathic remedies appears low, there is no compelling theory or solid evidence to support their use.

## MIND–BODY INTERVENTIONS

The overarching premise of mind–body treatments is that a potent connection exists between our mind and our physical health. This view is readily acceptable to many people. As discussed in Chapters 6 and 7, the reciprocal mind–body link is well established and is a reflection of our holistic nature. Our thoughts and emotions can affect our physical health, just as physical illness can affect our thinking and feelings. Several mind–body interventions such as psychotherapy, biofeedback, and hypnosis have been carefully studied and systematically developed and are now recognized by many experts as mainstream Western medicine practices.

Most mind–body interventions, however, are still placed under the umbrella of CAM practices. Movement therapies are a grouping that includes tai chi and yoga as well as less familiar movement pattern/ postural awareness regimens like the Alexander technique and the Feldenkrais method. They are used to reduce stress and treat a variety of disorders from asthma to osteoporosis. Creative therapies are another grouping; these interventions typically use art, dance, or music as a means to treat people with communication or psychological disorders. Spiritual healing is a third grouping in which practitioners and in some cases laypeople use purposeful focused intention to help cure another person; faith healing and intercessory prayer are examples, respectively.

Meditation is one of the oldest and most widely practiced mind–body therapies. Meditation and its different forms evolved from Eastern religions. During meditation one focuses on breathing or on a mantra (a single word or syllable) and is taught to disregard other thoughts and emotions. Meditation is a self-administered tool for mental and physical relaxation that gives a sense of control and autonomy. It should be practiced daily to fully accrue its benefits.

Although anecdotal reports are persuasive and meditation appears to be safe and poses little risk, systematic reviews show that the scientific evidence is weak or insufficient to demonstrate therapeutic effectiveness for any specific health condition. Many people practice meditation simply as a lifestyle choice—not to treat a specific medical condition but rather because meditation imparts a sense of relaxation and self-awareness. Aspects of meditation are closely related to other mind–body therapies including deep breathing, progressive muscle relaxation, and yoga.

## BIOLOGICALLY BASED THERAPIES

A biologically based therapy uses specific compounds, foods, or special diets—typically derived from natural sources—to treat an illness or disease. Examples include using aloe to treat a burn or consuming ginger to alleviate nausea. These therapies are referred to as biologically based because the use of the compound or food is believed to have a positive physiological effect in treating a given medical condition. Of all the CAM categories, biologically based therapies may be the broadest, with several hundred treatments including but not limited to the use of plant-based products (herbals or botanicals), animal-based products, vitamins, and minerals. The vast majority of therapies involve the ingestion of a specific compound.

A recent survey by the NCCAM reported that about one in five American adults use natural products. Echinacea, ginseng, ginkgo, garlic, and glucosamine were the most popular. The top 10 natural medicines, their typical uses, and level of evidence are summarized in Table 12.3. Note that for half of the natural remedies, evidence of effectiveness is mixed or uncertain; that is, some studies have found positive effects while others show no benefit. For ginger, glucosamine, and soy, the level of evidence to treat specific conditions is promising, but more research is needed. Finally, there is good evidence that fish oils lower cardiovascular risk and St. John's wort is effective in treating mild to moderate depression. However, not a single natural medicine among the 10 most popular has compelling evidence to support its use.

Several key points are important to keep in mind when thinking about using a biologically based therapy. These CAM products are chemically active and can interact with other compounds, foods, and drugs. For this reason, you would be wise to first discuss the pros and cons of any natural product with your doctor, especially if you are on medications, including birth control pills, or have a chronic health condition. Also, be aware that nearly all natural products are classified as dietary supplements, not as drugs (see the section on dietary supplements in Chapter 2). Consequently, the purity, effectiveness, and safety of the compound must always be questioned. As a reminder,

**TABLE 12.3   POPULAR NATURAL MEDICINES USED BY AMERICANS**

| NATURAL PRODUCT | COMMON CONDITION TREATED | EVIDENCE |
|---|---|---|
| Echinacea | prevent/treat colds, flu, infections | mixed |
| Garlic supplements | prevent/treat infections | mixed |
| Ginger supplements | prevent/treat nausea & vomiting | promising |
| Ginkgo | memory loss, variety of illnesses | mixed |
| Ginseng | reduce susceptibility to illness | mixed |
| Glucosamine | joint pain, osteoarthritis | promising |
| Fish oils (omega-3 fatty acids) | circulatory disorders | good |
| Peppermint | digestive disorders | mixed |
| Soy supplements | menopause hot flashes, high cholesterol | promising |
| St. John's wort | depression | good |

Source: Based on information from MedlinePlus (www.nlm.nih.gov/medlineplus/druginformation.html); and the National Center for Complementary and Alternative Medicine (http://nccam.nih.gov/health/herbsataglance.htm).

conventional medicines—both over-the-counter and prescription—go through a rigorous drug approval process by the FDA before they go to market, but this is *not* the case for dietary supplements, so it is buyer beware.

In the United States, herbalists and practitioners of other biologically based therapies have no standardized training or certification, and most are not medically qualified. Hundreds of natural products have been studied. For nearly all, evidence of effectiveness is negative or insufficient; for a few, evidence is mixed or promising. General contraindications are pregnancy and lactation. Additional precautions should be taken by people on medications or with chronic health conditions. Individual biologically based therapies should be thoroughly investigated for proof of effectiveness and safety.

## MANIPULATIVE AND BODY-BASED METHODS

In the United States, the three most common types of manipulative and body-based methods (manual therapies) are osteopathic manipulation, chiropractic adjustment, and therapeutic massage. In manual therapy, practitioners use their hands to manipulate the patient's soft tissues (primarily muscle and adipose tissue) and musculoskeletal joints, including the spine. The techniques and uses of these three manual therapies vary somewhat with the type of practitioner—osteopath, chiropractor, or massage therapist.

As described earlier in this chapter, the osteopath or D.O. goes through training similar to the M.D.—both are physicians (Western medicine). A notable difference though is that osteopathic medicine emphasizes manipulative techniques as a key part of medical training and an important clinical skill, particularly in the diagnosis and treatment of musculoskeletal problems. In general, osteopathic manipulative treatment is broadly accepted as part of conventional Western medicine. In contrast, chiropractic adjustment and therapeutic massage are still considered alternative practices.

### Chiropractic

The health care philosophy of chiropractic is centered on the body's inherent recuperative abilities and embraces a holistic view of the patient's well-being. A **chiropractor,** also known as a doctor of chiropractic **(D.C.),** primarily works with people whose health problems are related to the body's muscular, nervous, and skeletal systems, especially the spine. Chiropractors believe that interference with these systems impairs normal functions, lowers resistance to disease, and can cause pain. Chiropractic was established in 1895 by D. D. Palmer and is now practiced worldwide.

Chiropractors take medical histories, conduct clinical exams, and often use X-rays. The most common treatment procedure is known as *chiropractic adjustment,* also called *spinal manipulation.* Chiropractic adjustment—manipulating the patient's joints, particularly the spine— is used to reduce pain and restore joint function. This procedure seldom causes discomfort, and people often report improvements in their symptoms immediately following treatment. Chiropractors do not perform surgery or prescribe drugs but often recommend changes in lifestyle—in eating, exercise, and sleeping habits. As needed, chiropractors refer patients to mainstream physicians (M.D.'s or D.O.'s).

In the United States, a standardized curriculum must be followed to become a chiropractor. The D.C. degree is awarded after completion of a 4-year course of study at one of the 15 accredited chiropractic programs in the country. At least two years of undergraduate education is required for entry, although many applicants enter with an undergraduate degree. During the first two years, students complete classroom and laboratory work in basic sciences, while the last

---

A **chiropractor (D.C.)** typically works with people whose health problems are associated with the muscular, nervous, and skeletal systems, especially the spine. Chiropractic adjustment is a common treatment to relieve neck and back pain. The effectiveness of such treatment holds promise, but conclusive evidence is lacking.

Complementary and Alternative Medicine (CAM)

two years provide clinical training with emphasis in manipulation and spinal adjustment. All states have licensing boards for chiropractic, and many health insurance companies provide coverage for chiropractic care.

There are over 50,000 chiropractors across the United States. The majority are solo practitioners. Seeing a chiropractor—particularly for a back, neck, or pain-related problem—is not an unusual event. It's estimated that 1 in 10 American adults visited a chiropractor within the last year. Chiropractic is also gaining acceptance among Western medicine practitioners, and some physicians refer patients to chiropractors for treatment of back pain.

Many studies have been done on chiropractic and back pain. Findings are mixed—some researchers report positive effects, and others found no benefit. As is common in research on alternative practices, many of these studies are not well designed, which limits the interpretation of findings. Moreover, back pain is difficult to study because the cause is often never known, and in most cases the condition resolves within several weeks regardless of the treatment. Overall the evidence to support the use of chiropractic adjustment as an effective treatment for back pain is not convincing; spinal manipulation is no more or no less effective than conventional treatments. Use of chiropractic for other conditions is even less compelling.

Several precautions should be noted. Due to high-speed manipulations of some adjustment techniques, people with osteoporosis should not undergo chiropractic treatments. Also, damage to the arteries that run along the vertebrae is a potential serious risk during spinal adjustment, but this appears to be a rare risk for healthy people.

### Therapeutic Massage

Therapeutic massage, or massage therapy, is one of the most popular forms of CAM. The central principle of therapeutic massage is that the body's soft tissues will function optimally when the circulatory and lymphatic systems are unimpeded. There are different types of therapeutic massage (for example, Swedish, shiatsu, neuromuscular). Most involve similar manual techniques such as stroking, kneading, and stretching, and these are often combined during a treatment session. Therapeutic massage is generally used to treat joint and muscle pain and to reduce high stress levels.

A client usually sees a therapist with a diagnosis—and often a referral—from a physician or with a self-diagnosis or symptom. Therapists take a brief medical history to rule out contraindications such as skin infections, acute inflammations, or recent injuries and may ask questions to better understand the diagnosis or health complaint.

During the session, the therapist requests feedback as to how much pressure is preferred. Palpation, or touch, is fundamental to therapeutic massage and allows the therapist to identify areas of muscle tension or fluid accumulation with appropriate amounts of pressure for each individual, while also conveying a sense of caring.

In the United States, considerable variability still exists from school to school regarding the length and amount of training and from state to state regarding licensing. However, the National Certification Board for Therapeutic Massage, established in 1992, has become the leading organization in setting professional standards and administering written competency exams—over 90,000 people have been certified. When provided by a qualified therapist, therapeutic massage appears to be beneficial for musculoskeletal pain and for anxiety and depression. The evidence is promising but not unequivocal. Direct risks are minimal.

## ENERGY THERAPIES

Energy therapies include a variety of alternative treatments based on the use, modification, or manipulation of energy fields. This category is the most controversial of the five NCCAM categories due largely to the untestable premises upon which many of the therapies are based. Most energy therapies assume that matter and energy are similar and that matter is simply a denser form of energy; matter is readily perceived whereas energy is not, yet it is present. Some energy therapies are associated with traditional Asian medicine; others draw upon modern physics-based principles of energy.

Energy therapies can be divided into two groups. Veritable (or bioelectromagnetic) energy therapies use electromagnetic or mechanical forces in unconventional ways to treat patients. They are referred to as *veritable* (meaning "real") because they involve specific, measurable wavelengths and frequencies. Examples include magnetic therapy, light therapy, and sound energy therapy. In comparison, putative energy (or biofield) therapies are based on theorized energy or life forces emanating from the body. These energies are known as *putative* (meaning "reputed" or "supposed") because they are unmeasurable; biofields are simply assumed to exist. Examples are qigong from China, reiki from Japan, and therapeutic touch (laying-on of hands).

Qualifications of practitioners or healers vary widely. Some practices have credentialing or training programs; others do not. Some practitioners of energy therapy believe that all people have the capacity to be healers; others regard the ability to use healing energies as a gift given only to people who are unusually spiritual.

Based on systematic reviews of research, none of the energy therapies have been found to be effective in treating medical conditions. Extra precautions should be taken to carefully assess potential risk and benefit for any of the energy therapies.

## BEING A CRITICAL CONSUMER OF CAM

If you are considering using a nonconventional medical treatment, it's especially important to know how to get reliable and credible information. Compared to Western medicine, alternative medicine is generally unregulated. Thus, misinformation, misleading claims, and outright hoaxes abound. The key is to sort the honest and credible practitioners from the modern-day quacks. Use the following tips to assess information on alternative medicine practices and products found on the Internet:

1. Who runs the web page? Is it a credible professional (.org), educational (.edu), or governmental group (.gov)? Or a business set up to market a product (.com)? Generally, the .edu, .gov, and .org sites are more trustworthy than the .com sites.
2. Be wary of sites that diagnose illnesses or suggest an individual course of treatment. These services should be provided only by a medical professional who knows the patient's medical history and has performed a proper examination.
3. Be suspicious of quasi-scientific statements that go against common sense or known health principles. Discount any treatments or products that make claims about miracle cures.
4. Don't rely on a single website for the final word. Always cross-check your information on multiple independent websites known to be reputable. For example, use the following websites as a starting point or to verify information from other sources:

   NCCAM: **http://nccam.nih.gov**
   Quackwatch: **www.quackwatch.org**
   Office of Dietary Supplements: **http://ods.od.nih.gov**
   Food and Drug Administration: **www.fda.gov**

Remember, to find bona fide treatment options to a troubling health problem, seek solid information. Advertisements are sometimes disguised as health columns or news reports. Some are easy to spot, but others are more sophisticated and subtle. Convincing claims or personal success stories are not a substitute for scientific evidence. It is fair and appropriate to approach CAM practices with a healthy dose of skepticism. While some CAM approaches may be beneficial, you must take the time to separate the credible from the suspect. As always, your best guide to optimizing your health is accurate and trustworthy information.

## Health & the Media *Patent Medicines*

So-called patent medicines (protected by a patent or trademark and available without a doctor's prescription) were common following the Civil War. The illustration here is an example of a patent medicine trade card—an early form of advertising that extended the reach of peddlers and medicine shows. At county fairs and frontier settlements, doctors and druggists—often with suspect credentials—engaged in aggressive selling. Many were talented entertainers capable of wowing audiences with enthralling oratory and theatrics. Ayer's Sarsaparilla could "improve the complexion, purify the blood, and make the weak strong." Quackery continues today. Many ads, across all media—print, radio, TV, and the Internet—still use unsubstantiated claims of healing and generalized health benefits. Satisfaction "guaranteed," of course.

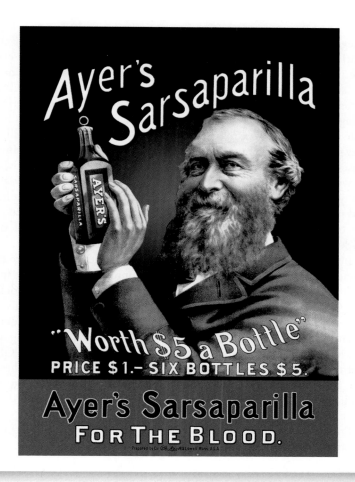

✓ **NEED TO KNOW**

Complementary and alternative medicine (CAM) encompasses a multitude of diverse treatments and approaches to healing that are outside conventional medicine. The National Center for Complementary and Alternative Medicine organizes CAM into five categories: alternative medical systems, mind–body interventions, biologically based therapies, manipulative and body-based methods, and energy therapies. Even though many Americans regularly use CAM, fundamental questions about the risks and benefits of many CAM therapies are yet to be answered. Continued research on CAM practices is needed. The bottom line is be a careful consumer and use due diligence.

## ➤ Integrative Medicine

Integrative medicine is the blending or combining of aspects of conventional Western medicine with those of complementary and alternative medicine (CAM). It's based on an awareness and appreciation of the strengths and weaknesses of both Western medicine and CAM. For example, in conventional medicine, the system of medical referral—being passed from specialist to specialist and having to undergo multiple tests—can be extremely frustrating for patients, especially if they're not getting better. People can begin to feel that they are simply "cases" or "specific conditions" rather than living, breathing individuals with their own unique histories and complex lives. Understandably, many people turn to CAM practitioners, who are known for holistic and patient-centered approaches. CAM practitioners tend to listen and get to know their patients better than mainstream physicians who work within a more regimented, time-constrained system.

Integrative medicine is a growing movement within health care that carefully selects and combines the most appropriate treatments from both realms of medicine, recognizing that neither Western medicine nor CAM has all the answers. Medical schools used to dismiss or ignore CAM, but now that has changed. The Consortium of Academic Health Centers for Integrative Medicine includes over 40 leading academic medical centers in the country such as Harvard, Duke, UCLA, and the Mayo Clinic. The Consortium's mission is to advance health care by educating medical students and physicians about integrative medicine and conducting research on CAM practices to better determine which treatments are effective or hold promise.

Prominent physicians Ralph Snyderman and Andrew Weil succinctly describe the appeal of integrative medicine for patients:

> Most Americans who consult alternative providers would probably jump at the chance to consult a physician who is well trained in scientifically

based medicine and who is also open-minded and knowledgeable about the body's innate mechanisms of healing, the role of lifestyle factors in influencing health, and the appropriate uses of dietary supplements, herbs, and other forms of treatment, from osteopathic manipulation to Chinese and Ayurvedic medicine. In other words, they want competent help in navigating the confusing maze of therapeutic options that are available today, especially in those cases in which conventional approaches are relatively ineffective or harmful.

As an example, low back pain is a widespread health problem, affecting up to one out of three adults in a given month. Conventional medicine is important in identifying serious, underlying problems such as a herniated disc, rheumatoid arthritis, infection, fracture, or cancer. If no underlying cause can be determined—which occurs in a large percentage of cases—conventional medicine has little to offer the patient. Yet, there is promising evidence that acupuncture can relieve pain and improve function. In a clinic that practices integrative medicine, the doctor would discuss acupuncture as a possible treatment and arrange for treatments if requested.

Self Assessment 12.1

Integrative medicine reaffirms the importance of the doctor–patient relationship, focuses on the whole person—not just a specific condition or disease—and makes use of all appropriate curative *and* preventive approaches. The bottom line is that physicians practicing integrative medicine are not restricted to a particular dogma, Western or Eastern, but rather guided by a "get the patient better" philosophy. Integrative medicine considers all factors that influence health and disease. This includes the individual's body, mind, and spirit as well as family, community, and society. This broad perspective recognizes that cultural expectations and public policies play significant roles in shaping a person's lifestyle and health behaviors and accordingly are considered in treating patients.

Article 12.4

## ✓ NEED TO KNOW

Integrative medicine is based on a holistic view of patient care and the promotion of optimal health. Integrative medicine neither accepts Western medicine nor rejects CAM uncritically; instead it brings together practices from both, based on good science and the needs of the patient. Integrative medicine is a powerful movement in modern medicine and is being promoted as a new model at leading academic medical centers across the country. Integrative medicine may become the mainstream medicine of the future.

## connect Resources

### ARTICLES

12.1 "Yes, Prevention Is Cheaper Than Treatment." *Newsweek.*
Dr. Dean Ornish makes the case for moving preventive medicine to the forefront of the American health care system.

12.2 "Improving Health Care Quality." *Permanente Journal.*
Fundamental strategies to improve health care are presented.

12.3 "Treat the Patient, Not the CT Scan." *New York Times.*
Technology can not replace a doctor's clinical skills.

12.4 "Alternative Medicine Is Mainstream." *Wall Street Journal.* The evidence is mounting that diet and exercise are the best cures for some of our worst ailments.

### SELF-ASSESSMENT

12.1 Understanding U.S. Health Care Services

## Website Resources

### MEDICINE—M.D.'S AND D.O.'S

American Medical Association **www.ama-assn.org**
Association of American Medical Colleges **www.aamc.org**
American Board of Medical Specialties **www.abms.org**
American Osteopathic Association **www.osteopathic.org**
American Association of Colleges of Osteopathic Medicine
   **www.aacom.org**

### DENTISTRY

American Dental Association **www.ada.org**
American Dental Education Association **www.adea.org**

### PODIATRY

American Podiatric Medical Association
   **www.apma.org**
American Association of Colleges of Podiatric Medicine
   **www.aacpm.org**

## OPTOMETRY

American Optometric Association **www.aoa.org**
Association of Schools and Colleges of Optometry
**www.opted.org**

## CLINICAL PSYCHOLOGY

Society of Clinical Psychology **www.div12.org**
National Register of Health Service Providers in Psychology
**www.nationalregister.org**

## NURSING

American Nurses Association **www.nursingworld.org**
Guide to Nursing Education and Careers
**www.allnursingschools.com/faqs**
Accredited Nursing Programs
**www.nlnac.org/Forms/directory_search.htm**

## PHYSICIAN ASSISTANT

American Academy of Physician Assistants **www.aapa.org**
Physician Assistant Education Association **www.paeaonline.org**

## PHYSICAL THERAPY

American Physical Therapy Association **www.apta.org**
Physical Therapist Education **www.apta.org/PTEducation/**

## DIETETICS

American Dietetic Association **www.eatright.org**
Commission on Dietetic Registration **www.cdrnet.org**

## COMPLEMENTARY AND ALTERNATIVE MEDICINE

National Center for Complementary and Alternative Medicine
(NCCAM) **http://nccam.nih.gov**
American Chiropractic Association **www.acatoday.org**
Council on Chiropractic Education **www.cce-usa.org**
American Massage Therapy Association **www.amtamassage.org**
National Certification Board for Therapeutic Massage and Bodywork
**www.ncbtmb.com**
National Certification Commission for Acupuncture and Oriental
Medicine **www.nccaom.org**

NCCAM: Herbs at a Glance
**http://nccam.nih.gov/health/herbsataglance.htm**
Quackwatch **www.quackwatch.org**
MedlinePlus: Herbs and Supplements
**www.nlm.nih.gov/medlineplus/druginfo/herb_All.html**

### GENERAL

Agency for Healthcare Research and Quality **www.ahrq.gov**
Health Care Careers, American Medical Association **www.ama-assn**
   **.org/ama/pub/education-careers/careers-health-care/directory**
   **.page**
Explore Health Careers **http://explorehealthcareers.org**
Consortium of Academic Health Centers for Integrative Medicine
   **www.imconsortium.org**

## Knowing the Language

acupuncture, 436
chiropractor (D.C.), 441
clinical psychologist, 427
complementary and alternative
   medicine (CAM), 432
dentist, 425
integrative medicine, 415
optometrist, 426
physical therapist, (P.T.), 430

physician, 419
physician assistant, (P.A.), 430
podiatrist, 425
primary care physician, 421
primary health care, 416
registered dietitian (R.D.), 431
registered nurse (R.N.), 429
secondary health care, 416
tertiary health care, 416

## Understanding the Content

1. Define and provide examples of primary, secondary, and tertiary health care.
2. Identify and discuss two of the major challenges facing our current health care system.
3. Define and contrast Western medicine with complementary and alternative medicine (CAM).

## Exploring Ideas

1. Western medicine is often referred to as evidence-based medicine. Explain what is meant by this statement. For example, consider the centrality of the scientific method, how physicians and allied health

professionals are trained in comparison with CAM practitioners, and the role of clinical trials in advancing medical knowledge.

2. Assume one of your parents has a recurring medical problem, and the doctors have been unable to effectively treat it. Your parent now wants to try a CAM approach that was recommended by a neighbor. What advice would you give? List and explain the steps you would take to check out this CAM practice or product.

3. Explain the concept of integrative medicine. How does it differ from Western medicine? What changes need to occur if integrative medicine is to become widely accepted?

## Selected References

Agency for Healthcare Research and Quality (AHRQ). Evidence Reports for Complementary and Alternative Care and Dietary Supplements.
**www.ahrq.gov/clinic/epcindex.htm#complementary**

AHRQ. Medical Expenditure Panel Survey.
**www.meps.ahrq.gov/mepsweb**

AHRQ. Patient Safety: One Decade After *To Err Is Human*. September/October 2009.
**www.psqh.com/septemberoctober-2009/234-september-october-2009-ahrq.html**

Cochrane Reviews. Complementary Medicine.
**www.cochrane.org/reviews/en/topics/22_reviews.html**

Commonwealth Fund. New Health Insurance Survey: 9 Million Adults Joined Ranks of Uninsured Due to Job Loss in 2010. March 2011.
**www.commonwealthfund.org/Content/News/News-Releases/2011/Mar/New-Health-Insurance-Survey.aspx**

Ernst E, Pittler M, Wider B. *Desktop Guide to Complementary and Alternative Medicine: An Evidence-based Approach* (2nd ed.). Philadelphia: Mosby, 2006.

Food and Drug Administration (FDA). How to Spot Health Fraud. February 2010.
**www.fda.gov/Drugs/EmergencyPreparedness/BioterrorismandDrugPreparedness/ucm137284.htm**

Helfand WH. *Quack, Quack, Quack: The Sellers of Nostrums in Prints, Posters, Ephemera, & Books.* Falls Village, CT: Winterhouse Editions, 2002.

Institute of Medicine. *Complementary and Alternative Medicine in the United States.* Washington, DC: National Academies Press, 2005.

Institute of Medicine. Summit in Integrative Medicine and the Health of the Public Agenda, February 2009.

Kaiser Family Foundation. Health Care Costs: A Primer, March 2009. **www.kff.org/insurance/7670.cfm**

Kohn L, Corrigan J, Donaldson M (eds.). *To Err Is Human: Building a Safer Health System.* Washington, DC: Institute of Medicine, National Academies Press, 2000.

Leape LL, Berwick DM. Five years after *To Err Is Human.* What have we learned? *Journal of the American Medical Association* 293: 2384–2390, 2005.

MedlinePlus: Herbs & Supplements. **www.nlm.nih.gov/medlineplus/druginfo/herb_All.html**

Micozzi M. *Fundamentals of Complementary and Integrative Medicine* (3rd ed.). St. Louis: Saunders, 2006.

Moynihan R, Cassels A. *Selling Sickness: How the World's Biggest Pharmaceutical Companies Are Turning Us All into Patients.* New York: Nation Books, 2005.

National Center for Complementary and Alternative Medicine. **http://nccam.nih.gov**

Office of Dietary Supplements. **http://ods.od.nih.gov**

Rakel DP. *Integrative Medicine* (2nd ed.). Philadelphia: Saunders, 2007.

Snyderman R, Weil A. Integrative medicine: Bringing medicine back to its roots. *Archives of Internal Medicine* 162: 395–397, 2002. **www.bravewell.org/content/pdf/14_Snyderman_Weil_Article .pdf**

U.S. Department of Labor, Bureau of Labor Statistics. Occupational Outlook Handbook. **www.bls.gov/search/ooh.asp?ct=OOH**

A hospital should also have a recovery room adjoining the cashier's office.

— Francis O. Walsh

# Chapter 13

## HEALTH CARE DECISION MAKING

In Chapter 12, we described the structure of the U.S. health care system and types of medical care available. This leads us to the question, How can we effectively use such information to navigate the system? In this chapter, we address this question by reviewing recommendations on medical self-care, the patient-doctor relationship, and health insurance. We end this last chapter by revisiting two recurrent themes central to optimal health: health literacy and preventive health care.

## Caring for Yourself

SIGNS AND SYMPTOMS

DIAGNOSING COMMON MEDICAL PROBLEMS

HANDLING MEDICAL EMERGENCIES

PRESCRIPTION AND OTC MEDICINES

BODY ART

## Developing a Patient–Doctor Partnership

FINDING THE RIGHT DOCTOR

COMMUNICATING WITH YOUR DOCTOR

MEDICAL TESTS AND PROCEDURES

KEEPING MEDICAL RECORDS

## Understanding Health Insurance

HEALTH INSURANCE TERMINOLOGY

PRIVATE HEALTH INSURANCE: FEE FOR SERVICE AND MANAGED CARE

PUBLIC HEALTH INSURANCE: MEDICARE AND MEDICAID

CHOOSING AN APPROPRIATE PLAN

HEALTH CARE REFORM

## Striving for Optimal Health

STAYING INFORMED

PRACTICING PREVENTION

**CHOICES** we make can put us at risk of illness and injury, and significant medical expenses can result. Consider the case of Dave, a college freshman. He attended a party and over a 6-hour period consumed about 4 beers and 12 shots of whiskey. Toward the end of the evening, Dave passed out. His friends were scared when they noticed his very shallow breathing and a swollen area on his head where he had fallen and hit the floor. They took him to the emergency room at the local hospital.

Dave was semiconscious, slurring his words, and having difficulty answering questions. His friends told the emergency room doctors what happened. In order to ascertain the extent of Dave's intoxication and possible injury, the medical team performed a physical evaluation, gave him intravenous saline solution, ran blood tests, and performed a CT scan to determine if there was a serious head injury from the fall. The CT scan was normal, and it was determined that Dave would recover from his excessive drinking after his body processed the alcohol. The ER team observed him for several hours, and then he was released.

Article 13.1

Dave was lucky that his friends realized he might be in serious trouble and got him help after he passed out. He was also fortunate not to have a permanent injury. But his luck ends there, for the cost of his "bad night out" is much more than a bruise, embarrassment, and a hangover. Medical care in the United States is very expensive. Dave's treatment cost $500 for the emergency room visit, $350 for physician services, $150 for IV saline solution, $250 for blood tests, $1,500 for the CT scan, and $250 for the radiologist to evaluate the CT scan—$3,000 total. Dave was on his parent's health insurance so some of the costs get covered. However, because of the nature of the emergency room visit, and with co-payments and deductibles, Dave's parents are still responsible for $1,000 of the bill. In this instance, Dave was semiconscious when he was injured, so he had no input regarding the care he received. The emergency room was morally and legally obligated to help him. However, it was also very costly and preventable.

We do not always have a choice in the type of health issues we face in life. However, everyone faces many choices and decisions regarding health care. How much can we do on our own? How do we determine when we need to use the health care system? How do we go about finding the right doctor?

Then there are the financial reality questions about cost and health insurance. What are the health insurance options, and what particular type of plan is the right one for us? This chapter will help answer these questions. Key information and resources for making informed choices about self-care, medical care, and health insurance are provided to help you navigate the health care and insurance systems.

# ➤ Caring for Yourself

**Medical self-care** is the steps and actions you take to optimize your health and to self-treat common illnesses and injuries. When motivated consumers have access to clear, simple health information, many health problems can be prevented or treated effectively and inexpensively without a visit to the doctor's office. Consequently, in this section we'll focus on medical self-care as it relates to self-recognition of emergent signs and symptoms, and making decisions about self-treatment or seeing a health care professional. There are two key aspects of self-care: First, we must be sensitive to signs and symptoms, and second, we need to know how to acquire the relevant information.

## SIGNS AND SYMPTOMS

The terms *sign* and *symptom* are similar but not synonymous. A **sign** can be measured objectively, usually by a health care provider during a physical exam. For example, heart rate, respiratory rate, body temperature, and blood pressure are standard vital signs. Elevated blood pressure is a sign of possible heart disease. On the other hand, a **symptom** is a person's subjective perception, such as nausea or knee pain. Signs and symptoms are used together in recognizing and diagnosing medical conditions.

Being sensitive to signs and symptoms means listening to your body. Being attuned to changes in your body is central to medical self-care because you are the best judge of what is normal and routine for you and what is not. It's important to pay attention to your intuition or premonitions that something is not right—as mentioned in Chapter 11, *prodrome* is a medical term for patients' feelings or early symptoms indicating the onset of an illness. For example, most of us have a sense that we are coming down with a cold a day or two before the signs and symptoms are clearly recognizable. The true story of Carolyn Benivegna in "Breaking It Down" demonstrates the importance of knowing and listening to your body and following your intuition.

**Medical self-care** is decisions and actions that an individual can take to cope with a health problem—in particular, informed steps that one can take without seeing a health care practitioner.

A **sign** is a result of injury or illness and can be measured objectively by a health care provider.

A **symptom** is a result of injury or illness that is subjectively perceived by the patient.

Carolyn, an extremely healthy and health-conscious middle-aged woman, became alarmed when her abdomen suddenly enlarged, and she began experiencing bouts of constipation and bloated abdomen. She soon discovered that getting the correct diagnosis is not always a straightforward process. It can take a combination of luck and perseverance.

She first went to her primary care doctor. Because her symptoms seemed to be intestinal, Carolyn was referred to a specialist of the digestive system—a gastroenterologist. He ran tests to determine whether there was a bacterial infection. After ruling that out, he diagnosed her with irritable bowel syndrome. Irritable bowel syndrome (IBS) consists of several symptoms at the same time; for example, abdominal pain, constipation, and abdominal swelling often occur together. Yet, this didn't seem right to Carolyn: "I guess I would have accepted this diagnosis had it not been for my enlarged abdomen. I swear to you, it looked like I was four to five months pregnant! I therefore insisted on more tests." The doctor ordered X-rays, which also found nothing. Carolyn was again assured she had irritable bowel syndrome and was encouraged to go on her scheduled month-long trip to Europe. But she remained worried: "I couldn't wear any of my slacks or shorts because I couldn't get them buttoned. I *knew* something was radically wrong. I *insisted* on more tests."

Carolyn's doctor reluctantly scheduled a CAT scan (computerized axial tomography). This test showed an abnormal buildup of fluid in her abdomen. This finding suggested that Carolyn was indeed correct—she did *not* have IBS. Finally, a special blood test gave her a diagnosis: She had primary peritoneal cancer, a cancer involving the membrane that surrounds the organs in the abdomen and pelvis. In this case, the correct diagnosis was elusive because peritoneal cancer is closely related to ovarian cancer, yet Carolyn no longer had her ovaries (previously removed during a complete hysterectomy). Therefore, her doctors initially overlooked this type of cancer as a possible cause of her bloating and intestinal problems.

Carolyn's message is clear and direct: "I have learned that each of us must take *total* responsibility for our own health care." She knew her body well enough to realize that something serious might be wrong, and she pushed for more tests when she felt the doctor was missing something. The correct diagnosis was a direct result of her perseverance. Her actions led to getting life-saving treatment sooner

*(Continued)*

rather than later. Carolyn's story is not typical, but it's not rare, either. The main point is not that the doctor misdiagnosed her illness, but rather that Carolyn and her doctor worked *together* to solve the mystery of her illness.

You know yourself—or should know yourself—better than anyone else. Pay attention to physical and mental changes and communicate with your doctor.

Source: Adapted from Johns Hopkins Pathology, Personal Stories: Carolyn Benivegna.

### DIAGNOSING COMMON MEDICAL PROBLEMS

To adequately address the topic of common medical problems requires the power of the Internet. Several excellent online resources are available to help us identify appropriate next steps when interpreting signs and symptoms. Two resources that are highly reputable, time-tested, and designed for the layperson are the American Academy of Family Physicians website **(www.familydoctor.org)** and the *Merck Manual* online medical library **(www.merck.com/mmhe/index .html)**. Both websites are comprehensive, regularly updated, and known for their ease of use.

The familydoctor.org website has a page that is organized alphabetically by symptoms—over 40 of the most common—from abdominal pain to urination problems **(http://familydoctor.org/online/ famdocen/home/tools/symptom.html)**. Clicking on any symptom generates a decision chart that provides guidance on a course of action. Decision charts are easy to follow and logically step through the decision-making process. For example, a decision chart for headaches is presented in Figure 13.1. Following the first column under the heading of symptoms, one can scan down and follow the Yes or No branches to a probable diagnosis (second column) and then to a self-care action (third column), such as "Use an over-the-counter medicine," "Call your doctor," or "Go to the emergency room." Embedded in the website's decision chart are links to descriptions of the possible conditions that may be causing your symptoms.

The Merck website provides the online version of the *Merck Manual of Medical Information,* 2nd Home Edition. The *Merck Manual* has been a standard reference guide for physicians and pharmacists for over a century. The home edition is a plain-language version of the classic medical reference text for people with an interest in health care but no medical training. It is organized alphabetically into over 20 sections, including accidents and injuries, digestive disorders, ear-nose-throat disorders, infections, men's health issues, mental health disorders, and women's health issues. Nearly all sections have illustrated subsections

(*Continued*)

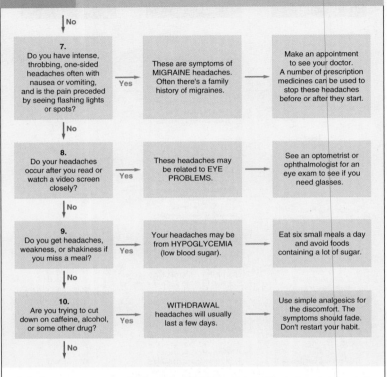

**FIGURE 13.1    A DECISION CHART FOR HEADACHES (*continued*)**

No

**7.**
Do you have intense, throbbing, one-sided headaches often with nausea or vomiting, and is the pain preceded by seeing flashing lights or spots? — Yes → These are symptoms of MIGRAINE headaches. Often there's a family history of migraines. → Make an appointment to see your doctor. A number of prescription medicines can be used to stop these headaches before or after they start.

No

**8.**
Do your headaches occur after you read or watch a video screen closely? — Yes → These headaches may be related to EYE PROBLEMS. → See an optometrist or ophthalmologist for an eye exam to see if you need glasses.

No

**9.**
Do you get headaches, weakness, or shakiness if you miss a meal? — Yes → Your headaches may be from HYPOGLYCEMIA (low blood sugar). → Eat six small meals a day and avoid foods containing a lot of sugar.

No

**10.**
Are you trying to cut down on caffeine, alcohol, or some other drug? — Yes → WITHDRAWAL headaches will usually last a few days. → Use simple analgesics for the discomfort. The symptoms should fade. Don't restart your habit.

No

Pain in one area or multiple areas of the head sometimes is accompanied by other symptoms. There are many causes for headaches.

For more information, consult your doctor. If you think the problem is serious, call your doctor right away. This tool is for general educational purposes only. It is not a substitute for medical advice. Always consult your family doctor with questions about your individual condition and circumstances.

Source: **FamilyDoctor.org.** Reprinted with permission from American Academy of Family Physicians.

on the biology of the particular topic along with specific descriptions of related illnesses and conditions including symptoms, diagnosis, and treatment.

Last, we would be remiss if we did not recommend *Take Care of Yourself: The Complete Illustrated Guide to Medical Self-Care* by James Fries, M.D., and Donald Vickery, M.D. This is arguably the finest concise book on medical self-care for the consumer. These physician-authors pioneered the use of decision charts in medical self-care. As was illustrated by Figure 13.1, a decision chart (or flow chart) is a graphical representation of a process that shows a start point, end points, and the logical steps and possible branches in between. Decision charts originated in the fields of business (quality control) and computer science (programming). As applied to medical self-care, decision charts help us make informed decisions about treatment based on interpretation of signs and symptoms.

Drs. Fries and Vickery are nationally recognized for their leadership in educating and empowering everyday folks about their own health care. *Take Care of Yourself* is one of the few books whose impact has been systematically evaluated in randomized studies. Use of this book in community and worksite studies improved health status and reduced doctor visits and medical expenditures. For readers who are parents, see the similarly acclaimed *Taking Care of Your Child* by pediatrician Robert Pantell along with Drs. Fries and Vickery.

## HANDLING MEDICAL EMERGENCIES

A final point on coping with medical problems is to consider what you would do in case of an emergency such as a heart attack, a serious fall, or a poisoning. Does the 9-1-1 system operate in your location? Where is the closest emergency room? Is your doctor's phone number readily accessible or programmed into your phone? Do you know CPR (cardiopulmonary resuscitation)? Emergencies require prompt action, so knowing what steps to take is crucial.

If you do not know CPR, or if it has been a few years since you learned it, we strongly recommend that you take a course. A basic course includes information and practice on how to assist an unconscious or choking person—an infant, child, or adult—and how to use an automated external defibrillator (AED). Even better, take a first aid course that, in addition to CPR, teaches basic skills to treat wounds and bleeding, injuries to bones and joints, extremes of hot and cold, and poisoning, bites, and stings.

In any serious accident, assume the victim is in shock to some degree. Shock is a condition of general weakness caused by physical trauma such as loss of blood (internal or external bleeding) or extreme pain or fear. People in shock may feel faint, giddy, anxious, or restless. They may feel sick, may vomit, and may lose consciousness. To assist a person in shock, take the following steps:

- Lay the person down and raise the feet above the level of the head.
- Treat obvious wounds and loosen tight clothing.
- Minimize any movement if serious neck or spine injuries are suspected.

- Cover the person with a blanket or coat and keep him or her as comfortable as possible.
- Check pulse and breathing every few minutes.
- Stay with a person in shock, because constant reassurance is extremely important.

Remember, emergencies will occur. How well we deal with them depends largely on knowing what actions to take. For further information, refer to the Mayo Clinic First Aid Guide or go to the *Merck Manual* website and click on the "Accidents and Injuries" section. (The URLs are in Website Resources at the end of this chapter.)

## PRESCRIPTION AND OTC MEDICINES

Determining which **drugs** are distributed by prescription and which are over the counter (OTC) relates to the FDA drug approval process and the pharmaceutical company's application regarding how to make a drug available to the public. Generally speaking, most **prescription (Rx) drugs** have a potential for harm that is higher than nonprescription **over-the–counter (OTC) drugs.** Therefore, use of prescription medication must be prescribed by a licensed medical professional, and the drug itself must be dispensed by a pharmacist. Some prescription drugs contain controlled substances, such as codeine, and have the potential for dependence. Others may have a very narrow safety margin between the effective dose and a lethal dose, so they require careful physician and pharmacist oversight. Over-the-counter drugs need no physician or pharmacist oversight, and when taken as directed by consumers are safe and effective.

Many prescription drugs are produced in lesser strength and are available as OTC drugs. For example, the pain reliever Motrin (also known as ibuprofen) has a prescription-strength pill that is 600 mg per tablet. But it can also be purchased over the counter in a pill that has 200 mg per tablet. The decision to make available what was once a prescription drug in an over-the-counter form also has to do with brand name marketing, market share, and profits. Sometimes it may be less expensive to purchase the prescription form of the drug than the over-the-counter strength.

Within the context of health care, a **drug** is a substance used in the diagnosis, treatment, or prevention of an illness or disease; a drug is also known as a *medicine* or *medication*. A **prescription (Rx) drug** can be sold only by a pharmacist when authorized by a written prescription from a medical practitioner, whereas an **over-the-counter (OTC) drug** can be purchased without a doctor's prescription.

One last point regarding prescription and OTC medicines has to do with the concept of generics. Every drug has a generic or chemical name. It is usually long, convoluted, and hard to pronounce; that is why a simple, easy-to-remember brand name is developed—for example, cetirizine hydrochloride is marketed and sold as Zyrtec. Generic and brand name drugs are equivalent in terms of effect and are available in both prescription and OTC forms. But a generic version is usually significantly less expensive than the brand name version of the drug.

The top prescription drugs in the United States for over a decade have been cardiovascular medicines to reduce high cholesterol (statins), to treat hypertension (antihypertensives), and to thin blood (anticoagulants). These drugs reduce the risk of stroke and heart attack. The best-selling prescription drug every year since 2000 has been Lipitor, a cholesterol reducer. Other top-selling prescription drugs include antibiotics, antidepressants, anti-ulcer drugs (for heartburn), and analgesics (for pain). In 2010, total prescription drug expenditures in the United States exceeded $307 billion, which was close to $1,000 per American.

Article 13.2

### Finding the Right OTC Medicines

Unlike a medicine prescribed by a doctor, an OTC medicine is generally selected by the individual. The top three types of OTC medications are for colds and coughs, pain, and heartburn. The number of choices is surprisingly high and can be intimidating. Thankfully, all OTC medicines have standardized drug facts labels that use simple language and an easy-to-read format. This is required by the FDA so that consumers can more easily compare products and follow dosage instructions. An example of a drug label is presented in Figure 13.2.

Article 13.3

A few precautions should be mentioned. If taking more than one OTC medicine, compare the active ingredients. You don't want to be taking multiple doses of the same medication in different products. Also, many common brands have multiple products—often different combinations of active ingredients. The brand packaging may be similar so it's wise to double check the label each time you purchase a product. Don't misuse OTC medicines by taking them longer or in higher doses than recommended. Don't hesitate to discuss your needs with a pharmacist. Pharmacists are trained and willing to assist you in finding the right medicine for your particular condition. If symptoms persist, see your doctor.

Everyone should keep a few basic medications and medical supplies on hand to deal with minor illnesses and accidents. A basic home pharmacy should include common OTC drugs such as pain and fever medications, cold and allergy medications, cough medications, and upset stomach medications. Each of these is briefly discussed below.

**FIGURE 13.2     EXAMPLE OF OTC DRUG FACTS LABEL**

### Drug Facts

| Active ingredient (in each tablet) | Purpose |
|---|---|
| Chlorpheniramine maleate 2 mg...................................................................Antihistamine | |

**Uses** temporarily relieves these symptoms due to hay fever or other upper respiratory allergies;
■ sneezing    ■ runny nose    ■ itchy, watery eyes    ■ itchy throat

**Warnings**
**Ask a doctor before use if you have**
■ glaucoma  ■ a breathing problem such as emphysema or chronic bronchitis
■ trouble urinating due to an enlarged prostrate gland

**Ask a doctor or pharmacist before use if you are** taking tranquilizers or sedatives

**When using this product**
■ you may get drowsy          ■ avoid alcoholic drinks
■ alcohol, sedatives, and tranquilizers may increase drowsiness
■ be careful when driving a motor vehicle or operating machinery
■ excitability may occur, especially in children

**If pregnant or breast-feeding,** ask a health professional before use.
**Keep out of reach of children.** In case of overdose, get medical help or contact a Poison Control Center right away.

**Directions**

| adults and children 12 years and over | take 2 tablets every 4 to 6 hours; not more than 12 tablets in 24 hours |
|---|---|
| children 6 years to under 12 years | take 1 tablet every 4 to 6 hours; not more than 6 tablets in 24 hours |
| children under 6 years | ask a doctor |

**Other information** store at 20-25° C (68-77° F)    ■ protect from excessive moisture

**Inactive ingredients** D&C yellow no. 10, lactose, magnesium stearate, microcrystalline cellulose, pregelatinized starch

Source: FDA **(www.fda.gov).**

In addition, your medicine kit should contain an antiseptic such as hydrogen peroxide to clean minor cuts, bandages and adhesive tape to protect such wounds, and a thermometer to check body temperature.

## Pain and Fever Medications

Inflammation (redness and swelling) and headache pain are the two most common types of pain. Medications that help to relieve pain are called *analgesics.* Common analgesics include non-steroidal anti-inflammatory drugs (NSAIDS) and acetaminophen. NSAIDs include four drugs: aspirin (common brand names are Bayer and St. Joseph), ibuprofen (Advil, Motrin), naproxen (Aleve), and ketoprofen (Orudis). NSAIDs, as the name indicates, also reduce inflammation (redness and swelling) if taken in substantial dosage. The common brand name for acetaminophen is Tylenol. Some products contain both aspirin and acetaminophen (Excedrin Extra Strength, Excedrin Migraine, Vanquish).

Side effects from OTC pain relievers aren't common for healthy adults who use these medications only occasionally. However, side effects can be a concern with long-term use. For example, NSAIDs can cause gastrointestinal problems, from upset stomach to bleeding in the digestive tract. In general, acetaminophen should be the first choice for pain and fever relief in children and adults because of its greater safety. Children with fever should not be given aspirin or products containing aspirin due to the risk of developing a potentially fatal condition called Reye's syndrome. If you use pain relievers often, talk to your doctor about which drug will be most effective for you.

### Cold and Allergy Medications

Common OTC cold medications such as Actifed and Contac are generally combinations of three kinds of drugs: a pain and fever reducer (acetaminophen, aspirin, ibuprofen), a decongestant such as pseudoephedrine to shrink swollen nasal passages and reduce congestion, and an antihistamine such as chlorpheniramine to dry the nasal passages and block allergies. Decongestants may cause insomnia and antihistamines drowsiness, although individual responses vary widely.

For treating colds and flu, the most important drug is the pain and fever reducer, along with standard treatment such as drinking plenty of fluids (water, fruit juices, clear soups) and getting additional rest. To treat allergy symptoms, the primary drugs are the decongestants and antihistamines. Because the cold-flu-allergy illnesses often overlap, people sometimes inadvertently overdose on these drugs by taking several products without realizing that they contain some of the same ingredients. Be sure to read the labels and know the active drugs in each medication. To be more selective in treating symptoms, you may wish to use single drugs instead of the combination medications.

### Cough Medications

There are three types of coughs: congested and productive, congested and nonproductive, and dry and nonproductive. Congested and productive means that the lungs have excess mucus, and coughing allows the person to spit up or expectorate the phlegm. Congested and nonproductive means that while extra mucus is present, coughing does nothing to remove it from the lungs. Finally, in dry and nonproductive coughs there is no congestion—hence, no expectorating.

OTC cough medications contain expectorants such as guaifenesin and/or antitussives such as dextromethorphan. Expectorants stimulate the flow of fluid in the lungs and aid in breaking up and removing the phlegm through coughing. Antitussives suppress the cough center in the brain so the urge to cough is reduced.

Knowing the type of cough you have can indicate the type of cough medication you should use. With a dry and nonproductive cough, the main objective is to stop the cough, so a medication with an antitussive should help. A congested and productive cough might not need any treatment, since your body is already expectorating the phlegm on its own. Congested and nonproductive coughs might require an expectorant to make them productive. When in doubt ask the pharmacist, and you will be directed to the correct medication. Finally, if a cough lasts more than 10 days be sure to see a physician.

### Upset Stomach and Constipation Medications

Dyspepsia, or upset stomach, is a common medical condition that can be treated using OTC antacids or acid reducers. When the stomach becomes too acidic, gas—both painful and unpleasant—is the result. Antacids are very effective at neutralizing the stomach acid, and the effects are felt almost immediately. Common antacids include calcium carbonate (Tums, Rolaids), sodium bicarbonate (Alka-Seltzer), bismuth subsalicylate (Pepto-Bismol), and magnesium (Maalox).

Antacids are designed to treat occasional dyspepsia. If a person has frequent dyspepsia or other common problems like heartburn or gastroesophageal reflux disease (GERD), reducing the amount of acid being secreted might be a better treatment option. These medications cause the acid-secreting cells in the stomach to decrease the amount they release. Common OTC acid reducers are Tagamet, Pepcid, Zantac, and Prevacid.

Difficulty in having a bowel movement or passing dry, hard stools is a very unpleasant but common condition called *constipation*. Most cases of constipation can be prevented by taking in the recommended amount of fiber in the diet, drinking plenty of water, and exercising. However, there are times when a person will want to treat constipation with laxatives.

There are two main options for OTC laxatives: bulk forming and bowel stimulating. Bulk-forming laxatives (Metamucil) are fiber. Once in the bowel the additional fiber creates a bulkier stool, and that facilitates a bowel movement. Bowel-stimulating laxatives (ex-lax, Feen-a-Mint, Correctol) contain chemicals that irritate the bowel wall and cause excessive fluid to be absorbed into the bowel. The combination of irritation and fluid results in cramping and the immediate need for a bowel movement (usually multiple bowel movements). Bulk-forming laxatives are generally safe whereas too-frequent use of bowel-stimulating laxatives can result in weakening of the bowel wall and physical dependence on the laxative.

### Reducing Prescription and OTC Medication Mistakes

Americans take more drugs per capita than people in any other nation. Based on personal experience, we know that most of us, our family members, and those we live with take one or more OTC or prescription medications on a regular or occasional basis. According to a recent estimate by the Institute of Medicine, in any given week 3 out of 10 U.S.

adults take five or more different medications. These medications can be found in many different places—a counter, a table, or a drawer in bathrooms, bedrooms, or the kitchen. With so many drugs being taken by so many people, medication errors are not uncommon. To prevent mistakes, consider applying these tips on safe storage and use of medications.

- Keep medications in their original containers.
- Store as indicated regarding temperature, light, and humidity.
- Keep your medications separate from those of others in the household as well as from pets' medications and household chemicals.
- Turn on the light when you take your medication.
- Store medicines where children can't see or reach them.
- Periodically check expiration dates and discard and replace as appropriate.
- Don't take someone else's prescription medication.

These simple steps can reduce errors, minimize confusion, and lessen the likelihood of drug misuse.

### Accessing Information on Prescription and OTC Medicines

The number of medicines available today is vast, numbering in the thousands. An Internet source that provides consumer information on both prescription and OTC medicines is the PDR Health website (**www.pdrhealth.com/drug_info**) sponsored by the publisher of the *Physicians' Desk Reference (PDR)* series. Updated annually, the *Physicians' Desk Reference* is the authoritative source for prescription drug information used by physicians and other health care professionals. The 2010 edition is over 3,000 pages! A companion volume is the *PDR for Nonprescription Drugs*. The PDR Health website translates information from these two PDR texts into nontechnical explanations about OTC and prescription drugs, including possible side effects and drug interactions. A second online source is the National Institutes of Health's MedlinePlus Drugs, Supplements, and Herbal Information web page, provided in cooperation with several pharmacy organizations (**www.nlm.nih.gov/medlineplus/druginformation.html**).

### BODY ART

The decision to get a tattoo or body piercing is a personal one. From a health perspective, it's prudent to carefully balance the pros and cons and not rush a decision. Laws and regulating authorities for tattooing vary widely among and within states. Consequently, additional precautions should be taken. Risks associated with tattoos and piercings include bloodborne diseases, skin infections, skin disorders such as scarring, and allergic reactions. Also, a number of the dyes used in

Laws regulating safe practices for body piercing and tattooing vary greatly from state to state.

tattooing have not been studied, and little is known about their toxicity. Risks are reduced if you go to a reputable and licensed tattoo or piercing studio with trained employees who follow recommended procedures such as washing their hands, wearing gloves, using only sterile disposable needles and FDA-approved dyes, and autoclaving nondisposable instruments. Under these conditions and with proper follow-up care, medical complications appear to be low.

It is not uncommon for people to grow dissatisfied with their tattoos. Several removal techniques are available—laser surgery, dermabrasion, surgical removal—but these require multiple visits, significant expense, and typically leave some scarring or skin imperfections. In short, investigate the risks and benefits, including advice from medical specialists in cosmetic surgery. If you proceed with some form of body art, be sure that the procedure will be done under the best of conditions and by an experienced professional.

✓ **NEED TO KNOW**

Medical self-care empowers people to make informed decisions and take actions to heal themselves, particularly with respect to common short-term illnesses. Knowing how to use the Internet for information on signs and symptoms, decision charts, coping with emergencies, and using medicines is key to effectively caring for yourself. Be especially vigilant if you are considering a tattoo or body piercing because state and local oversight vary widely.

## ➤ Developing a Patient–Doctor Partnership

Part of medical self-care includes knowing where to draw the line between dealing with an illness on your own and needing to see a doctor. When it comes to choosing your primary care physician, just any doctor won't do. In this section, we share strategies on finding the right doctor and developing a trusting patient–doctor partnership.

Over time, your end of this partnership will encompass more than just showing up at your doctor's office with a list of symptoms. As an active participant in your health care, you may need to inform yourself about various medical tests and treatments and perhaps at some point prepare for a hospital stay. Moreover, it's certainly wise for you to maintain a complete personal medical record. We'll provide some guidelines on each of these points in the following paragraphs.

## FINDING THE RIGHT DOCTOR

Regardless of how many times you may move or switch health plans, you can always use the same approach to finding a primary care doctor. Typically your insurance plan includes a directory of primary care doctors from which to choose. The size of the pool of potential physicians depends on the size of the student health center or the type of health plan, but you will generally have some latitude in selecting a doctor. As discussed in Chapter 12, selecting a board-certified physician is wise. In the practice of modern medicine, having only an M.D. (doctor of medicine) or D.O. (doctor of osteopathy) degree without the additional training required for board certification is just not good enough, so it's best to check your potential doctor's credentials before you start seeing him or her. Also remember that a primary care physician is typically a family practitioner or internist, though women may have the additional option of choosing a gynecologist to be their primary care doctor.

Self Assessment 13.1

Ask your family, friends, and coworkers for recommendations. Let them know that in addition to making sure the doctor is board certified, your aim is to find a doctor who shares your perspective about the patient–doctor relationship—that it is a partnership rather than a one-way relationship in which the doctor dispenses medical care to the patient. Another possible selection criterion is the gender of the doctor. It is natural for most people to want a doctor of the same gender. You may feel more comfortable and be better able to communicate frankly and openly with a doctor of the same gender.

In your initial office visit, you'll want to assess the manner or presence of the doctor and your comfort level with him or her. This is less tangible and involves impressions but is an important consideration. If you are not comfortable with a particular doctor, it doesn't mean he or she is not a good physician; rather the doctor may simply not be a good match for you. It may take several sessions with a doctor before you are able to decide whether he or she is the right doctor for you. To help with this process, ask yourself the following questions:

- Is this doctor a good listener?
- Does this doctor answer my questions completely and in terms I understand?

- Does this doctor ask for my input when options are available?
- Does this doctor use medicines conservatively?
- Does this doctor appear interested in me as a person and in my overall health?
- Does this doctor seem to give me quality patient time?
- Am I comfortable talking with this doctor, or am I intimidated or anxious?
- Do I have a high degree of trust and confidence in this doctor?

Answers to these questions will highlight how compatible you would be with the doctor. The more compatible you are, the more likely a meaningful patient–doctor partnership will be developed.

## COMMUNICATING WITH YOUR DOCTOR

Both you and your doctor have responsibilities when it comes to making the most of an office visit and developing a solid partnership. Always remember that communicating with your doctor goes both ways. For an effective patient–doctor interaction to occur, we need to appreciate the larger health care delivery context in which doctors work. They are often overworked, behind schedule, and pressured to spend only a few minutes with each patient. Patients—in addition to being sick or having a medical concern—are often frustrated with traffic, parking, and paperwork and tired of waiting and being shuffled from one room to another. Is it so surprising that the doctor wants to immediately focus on your chief complaint, and you are less than articulate in describing the problem?

Many factors can hamper the patient–doctor visit. Intimidation, fear, and embarrassment are three common barriers to effective communication between patients and doctors. Doctors are esteemed for their intelligence and compassion. This high regard can be intimidating to some patients, particularly those with little knowledge about medical matters. Patients' fear of the unknown and the possible dire consequences of a troubling symptom or health condition can also interfere with logical thinking and clear communication. Other patients may be embarrassed to talk about highly personal or disconcerting issues that make them feel self-conscious or ill at ease. Your doctor is aware of these communication obstacles and will work to allay them. You too must be aware of them and strive to minimize such concerns and doubts by being forthright and trusting with your doctor.

As Drs. Fries and Vickery succinctly state in *Take Care of Yourself,* "You and your doctor need to be able to listen, explain, ask questions, understand each other, and choose options wisely." As a patient, you

# Health & the Media Communicating with Your Doctor

It is understandable that patients can feel uneasy communicating with the doctor, yet the quality of this communication is critical to the success of the doctor–patient relationship. Most patients do not have mastery over medical language, diagnosis and treatment but that really isn't necessary. What is most important is to communicate effectively during the limited amount of time spent with the doctor. To get the most out of a visit to the doctor, educate yourself, be up-front, ask questions and take a friend.

need to prepare for the office visit by being ready to describe your symptoms, their timeline, and any self-care measures you have taken, including the use of OTC medications. Ahead of time, you may want to make notes listing symptoms and key questions for reference during your visit. You should be ready to name all prescription drugs and dietary supplements that you take and all allergies and chronic medical conditions that you have. Also, it's a good idea to take a writing pad to make notes during the visit. Even a few hours later, let alone a few days later, many people have difficulty recalling the details of what their doctor said.

Depending on the severity of the illness or the complexity of the health problem, you may want to have a family member or friend take you to the doctor—not only to drive or physically assist you if needed but also to facilitate communication with the doctor. Ask someone who can ably serve as your advocate—that is, a person who can ensure that your symptoms are clearly explained and that the doctor's course of treatment is understood. Two sets of ears are always better than one.

A final point concerns advance directives. Advance directives are documents (e.g., living will, power of attorney) that specify the type of medical care you want if you are too sick to express your wishes. Although people who are terminally or seriously ill are more likely to have advance directives, those in good health may also want to consider them in case of a catastrophic accident or sudden serious illness. Advance directives deal with a variety of issues—for example, whether to resuscitate or not, use of breathing machines and feeding tubes, and organ donation. Discuss the options for medical care under these special circumstances with your doctor. Once you establish advance directives, be sure to share them with your doctor as well as your family. Knowing your wishes ahead of time will avoid confusion later.

## MEDICAL TESTS AND PROCEDURES

Your physician may want to conduct tests to help make a diagnosis. Many standard tests are done on blood and urine. For example, a CBC (complete blood count) is a routine test that provides information about white blood cells, red blood cells, and platelets. Abnormal variations in the number, type, size, and shape of cells may indicate an infection, anemia, or a host of other conditions. The basic urine test, or urinalysis, screens for urinary tract infections, metabolic disease, and kidney disorders by examining the urine physically, chemically, and microscopically. The results of such tests may lead your doctor to order more specialized tests to help in making a diagnosis. Dozens of clinical lab tests are available; a comprehensive listing and descriptions are available at Lab Tests Online (**www.labtestsonline.org**).

Your doctor may order a medical imaging test, too. From routine X-rays and ultrasound imaging to more complex CT (computed tomography) and PET (positron emission tomography) scans, these tests—which fall within the specialty of radiology—can provide important clues to abnormalities that exist or may be developing within the internal tissues and organs of the body. For example, MRI (magnetic resonance imaging) uses radiofrequency waves in a strong magnetic field to generate detailed pictures of soft-tissue structures around bones. Especially useful in diagnosing sports injuries, MRI can show even small tears in ligaments and muscles around the

A magnetic resonance imaging (MRI) scan.

spine and major joints (knee, shoulder, hip, elbow). RadiologyInfo (**www.radiologyinfo.org**), developed by the American College of Radiology, is an excellent website to answer consumer questions about medical imaging and radiation therapies.

The more complex your illness or disease, the more likely your doctor will refer you to a specialist for an expert opinion. This in turn may lead to further testing or medical procedures requiring specialized hospital equipment and facilities. As described in Chapter 12, this sequence reflects the widening circle of medical care from primary care to secondary and tertiary care. Ideally, your primary care physician will receive copies of the results of all tests and procedures and continue to coordinate overall medical care. For example, you can discuss a specialist's diagnosis and treatment options with your primary care doctor. If you feel uneasy or uncertain regarding a recommendation for a major surgical or medical treatment, you should not hesitate to get a second opinion. Good doctors will understand your concern and not take offense. An excellent consumer resource that provides interactive health tutorials on common diagnostic, surgical, and treatment procedures is available at MedlinePlus (**www.nlm.nih.gov/medlineplus/ tutorial.html**).

There will be times when you, a family member, or a close friend must be admitted to a hospital. Many illnesses and injuries are successfully treated in hospitals. Indeed, many lives are saved. Yet, hospitals are also dangerous places; far too many errors occur resulting in unnecessary death and disability. Consequently, it's important to feel confident about the hospital of choice and to take reasonable precautions. Discuss this issue with your physician and ask questions about the hospital's experience in performing the particular treatment or procedure. Is it routinely done, and what is their safety record?

Once you are admitted to the hospital, consider the following tips to reduce the risk of medical errors:

- Carefully read and fully understand any consent form before signing.
- Find out why tests or treatments are being performed.
- Discuss the results of tests with your doctor.
- Know the purpose and side effects of all medications, whether given by mouth, injection, or intravenous (IV) administration.
- Be sure that all health care workers wash their hands before they have physical contact with you.
- Understand the follow-up treatment plan when you are discharged.

Remember you have the right to be fully informed of all procedures, so never hesitate to ask questions or express concerns. If necessary, be persistent: Ask to speak to the supervisory nurse or discuss concerns with your doctor. If you will be incapacitated for a prolonged period, try to arrange to have a capable advocate oversee your care and ask questions on your behalf.

## KEEPING MEDICAL RECORDS

Your current primary care doctor should have a complete medical file on you. However, if you are like most people, you probably have your health information scattered across multiple providers and facilities. For this reason alone, it's important to keep your own complete, updated, and easily accessible personal health record. Based on a national survey by the Harris Poll, only two in five adults keep personal or family health records, yet almost all of those who don't keep health records think it would be a good idea to do so. Simply put, it's an important task to take on, and you are in the best position to do it. In fact, it's necessary if you are to be a full partner in your health care.

A personal health record is a collection of key information about your health (or the health of someone you're caring for, such as a parent or a child) that you actively maintain and update. It can contain any information that affects your health, including information that your doctor may not have, such as your exercise routines, dietary habits, and over-the-counter drugs you routinely take. Keeping a personal health record can reduce or eliminate duplicate procedures or processes, which saves health care costs, your time, and the provider's time.

A straightforward approach to a personal health record is to organize paperwork into categories such as the following:

1. *General information:* Include medical exam results, blood profiles, and other measures such as height, weight, waist circumference, and blood pressure. Organ donor authorization or living wills should also be kept here.

2. *Specific medical conditions:* Keep a separate file for these so they can be easily updated.

3. *Prescription drugs and dosages:* Keep a record of all prescription drugs, both those you take regularly and those you have taken for specific illnesses. Be sure to note any allergies or side effects.

4. *Insurance information and medical bills:* A separate file for health insurance and medical bills is necessary. Include a description of coverage, instructions and forms for filing, a ledger of payments for bills, and a log of phone calls and written communications on bills that require follow-up or resolution.

Regardless of how smart or healthy we may be, our memory alone is not adequate for keeping a personal health record! So get your records together and start filing in an organized fashion if you haven't already developed a system. Or set up your system now and start using it with your next physician visit or medical test. Like any organizational system, it takes some time at first, but it will be well worth your while.

Electronic health records (EHR) are now commonly used by health professionals and agencies. An EHR is a single complete (electronic) record of a patient's profile, diagnoses, allergies, and lab results that can be continually updated by *all* clinicians involved in treating the patient. Connectivity would extend to labs, pharmacies, hospitals, and insurers as well as to the patient. EHR is a major information technology initiative within both the federal government (HHS Health Information Technology, **http://healthkit.hhs.gov**) and the private sector (American Health Information Management Association, **www.ahima.org**). The advantages seem clear—improved efficiency and integration of medical services should result in better patient care and significant cost savings. There is little doubt that the EHR is spreading through the health care system. The question is how long it will take for widespread adoption. In the meantime, be sure to maintain your own medical records.

✓ **NEED TO KNOW**

One must be proactive to find a compatible primary care physician and to develop an effective patient–doctor partnership. Understanding how to optimize patient–doctor communication and how to access basic information about medical tests and procedures is our responsibility as active participants in our own health care. Taking precautions to minimize medical errors in hospitals and keeping an updated personal medical record are other actions that informed consumers can take to improve their health care.

# ➤ Understanding Health Insurance

The ideal way to access the services of our health care system and to receive quality care is by having "good" health insurance. However, just because one has health insurance doesn't mean that worries about health care are over. Unfortunately, health insurance is not user-friendly. It requires knowledge both to select the right plan and then to use it. A case in point—try to get a health insurance representative on the phone and you'll typically be routed through a prolonged queuing system. When you finally make contact with a live human, that person may seem disinterested and less than helpful. By educating ourselves about health insurance options and coverage, we can do much to minimize the pitfalls and barriers that appear to be so widespread. In this section, we'll provide practical tips on selecting and navigating the health insurance system.

## HEALTH INSURANCE TERMINOLOGY

Insurance has its own language, and a common mistake consumers make is to assume they understand what a word means. Knowing the insurance language increases the likelihood of using the system more effectively and reducing health care costs. The insurance company is often called the *insurance carrier,* and the insured person is the *subscriber.* Subscribers pay **premiums,** usually on a monthly basis, to hold an insurance policy. The policy is based on the (insurance) concept of indemnity, which means "assumption of risk." In the case of health insurance, the insurance company assumes the majority of medical costs within limitations defined in the policy. Many insurance plans have **deductibles,** which is the amount of money a subscriber must pay for medical services (e.g., treatments, tests, doctor's visits) before the insurance company pays.

Exclusions are those services not covered by the insurance policy. Since insurance companies are for-profit businesses, health insurance policies often control costs by excluding coverage of certain treatments, drugs, or office visits. One important type of exclusion is known as *preexisting conditions.* These are specific diseases or conditions (e.g., heart disease, cancer, diabetes) that are known to exist when you sign up for your insurance. If you have preexisting conditions, your policy may not pay for related treatments for either a specific time or ever.

A **premium** is the amount of money the subscriber pays to maintain the health insurance policy. A **deductible** is the additional cost the subscriber pays per medical service before the insurance company pays.

It is critical to carefully read and compare differences in coverage of available policies before enrolling in a specific plan.

Generally, health insurance in the United States is either private or public. Private health insurance is the most common with about 60 percent of Americans receiving coverage through employer-sponsored plans and 9 percent through individually purchased plans. Public health insurance, which includes government-supported Medicare and Medicaid, provides coverage to a smaller proportion of Americans. Both types of health insurance—private and public—will be reviewed in the following sections.

## PRIVATE HEALTH INSURANCE: FEE FOR SERVICE AND MANAGED CARE

There are two basic types of plans under the private health insurance umbrella: fee for service and managed care.

### Fee for Service

A **fee-for-service (FFS) plan**—also known as a *traditional indemnity plan*—was the predominant type of health insurance in the United States into the latter part of the 20th century, though it only makes up a small percentage of policies today. There are two major components to FFS: basic and major medical. Basic health insurance is primarily hospital insurance, and major medical includes just about everything else—physicians, diagnostic testing, and medications. In both basic and major medical, a deductible must be met before the insurance begins paying for a person's medical bills. FFS plans cover a percentage of the remaining amount—typically 80 percent of the total costs. The policyholder is responsible for paying the deductible and the remaining 20 percent of the cost.

FFS has advantages. The chief advantage is the freedom to select physicians and medical care services. However, this freedom of choice comes, quite literally, at a high cost—consumers pay significantly more for medical care under the typical FFS plan than they do under a managed care plan.

### Managed Care

There are two primary types of **managed care plans:** preferred provider organizations and health maintenance organizations.

---

**Fee-for-service (FFS) plans,** or traditional indemnity plans, allow subscribers the greatest choice of doctors and hospitals but at a greater cost.

**Managed care plans** such as PPOs and HMOs limit subscribers to specific networks of doctors and hospitals but provide medical care at lower costs.

**Preferred Provider Organization.** Preferred provider organizations (PPOs) are groups of health care providers and hospitals who negotiate plans with an insurance carrier. The PPO agrees to charge the insurance company's subscribers reduced fees for their services. In exchange, the PPO-affiliated facilities and personnel get a higher volume of clients and quicker payment from the insurance company. PPO insurance policyholders can opt to go "out of network" and receive care from doctors and hospitals that are not part of their PPO. However, out-of-network services are much more expensive than in-network services.

The way most PPOs work is that a client selects a primary care physician (PCP) from a list of doctors in that particular network. The PCP will be the point of contact when medical care is being sought, providing primary care as well as coordinating any referrals to secondary care or diagnostic and treatment services. Patients can see their PCP as often as they want for a predetermined office visit co-payment. A co-payment—or simply "co-pay"—is a relatively small portion of the overall cost of the actual visit. For example, if a doctor charges $80 for an office visit, the co-pay for the patient might be only $20. The remaining $60 is paid by the insurance company.

When referred by their PCP to facilities for tests or to other in-network specialists, the patient is also charged reduced fees for those providers' services. If for some reason the patient does not get a PCP referral for secondary care or opts to go out of network, then the insurance company often still reimburses the patient for some of those costs, but not nearly as much as it does for in-network providers who were visited with a PCP referral.

A PPO is a cost-effective way to receive medical care. There are fewer out-of-pocket expenses than with an FFS plan. However, there is also less choice among doctors and treatment options. PPO administrators can be reluctant to approve payment of certain services, which means that a person with this type of insurance may need to be assertive to use the system effectively. PPOs are popular, accounting for about 50 percent of the health insurance market.

**Health Maintenance Organization.** Health maintenance organizations (HMOs) are plans that allow access to primary, secondary, and tertiary care within a health network. There are many slightly varying models of the HMO, and in promotional materials an insurance company may refer to a staff model, group model, independent practice association model, or point-of-service plan. But regardless of the HMO model used, the basic approach is that the HMO, after premiums are paid, will provide all the medical care one "needs" for no additional charge or for a small co-pay.

For example, an HMO patient can be seen for a broad range of services from an office visit for a sore throat to tertiary care involving major surgery and only pay $10–$30 per visit or service beyond the normal monthly premium. These are by far the lowest-cost plans for consumers. The downside of HMOs is that in order to receive care at rock-bottom costs, the patient abdicates most decision making and control over choice in hospitals, testing clinics, doctors, and the like. HMOs are designed to save money, and they do this by rationing services. A patient may wait for a longer period of time to receive certain diagnostic tests in an HMO than in a PPO, and treatment options may be more limited than in other types of plans.

Brief explanations of the main types of HMOs follow:

- *Staff model HMOs* typically include a free-standing facility owned by the HMO where all the doctors and clinical professionals are salaried employees. It is a primary care version of one-stop shopping for doctor appointments, testing, and even filling of prescriptions.

- *Group model HMO* is a group of private practice doctors that contracts with a corporate HMO and agrees to serve HMO patients at a reduced rate. The HMO pays the group at the pre-negotiated rate, and the group pays its own doctors. The group model HMO is a contract, not a facility. Other clinical services that an HMO patient may need are also negotiated with laboratories and pharmacies.

- *Independent practice association (IPA)* is another HMO structure whereby private practice physicians contract with the HMO to see HMO patients at a prenegotiated rate. Similar to the group model HMO, the IPA includes large numbers of private practice physicians.

- *Point-of-service (POS)* is a relatively new type of HMO structure. The POS allows members more choice in selecting providers and services because they have the option of going out of the network and seeing a physician of their choice, not the choice of the HMO. However, the co-pay is higher if an out-of-network physician is used.

HMOs are approximately 45 percent of the health insurance market.

Table 13.1 provides an overview of the various types of plans including what the plans offer, methods of cost control, and the advantages and disadvantages. The structures of these plans are constantly changing, and sometimes it is difficult to distinguish between an HMO and a PPO. Regardless, it is imperative that consumers know what plan they have and what is covered. When you select a health insurance plan, you are entering into a business agreement.

**TABLE 13.1    PRIVATE HEALTH INSURANCE: COMPARISON OF COMMON TYPES**

| TYPE OF PLAN | WHAT IT OFFERS | COST CONTROL METHODS | ADVANTAGES | DISADVANTAGES |
|---|---|---|---|---|
| Fee for Service (Indemnity) | Services from any doctor or hospital | None except screening for fraudulent claims | Choice of any doctor or hospital | Claim forms to file; preventive services not covered |
| Indemnity with Utilization Review | Services from any doctor or hospital | Prior approval required for hospitalization and some outpatient procedures | Choice of any doctor and access to any hospital after prior approval | Additional paperwork to get approval for some services; preventive services not covered |
| Preferred Provider Organization (PPO) | Services from any doctor or hospital, but at lower cost to those using network providers | Discounts negotiated with doctors and hospitals; prior approval required for hospitalization and some outpatient procedures | Higher rate of reimbursement when using doctors and hospitals in the network | Higher cost for services outside network; extra paperwork to get approval of some services; preventive services are not always covered |
| HMO—Staff/ Group Model | Services from hospitals under contract with HMO or salaried doctors at HMO medical centers | Primary care doctors at HMO medical centers manage services; hospital fees are discounted | Low co-payments; preventive care covered; no claim forms | Must use the HMO medical center doctors and hospitals |
| HMO—Independent Doctors (IPA) | Services from any hospital or independent doctor affiliated with HMO | Primary care doctors manage services; hospital and physician fees are discounted | Low co-payments; preventive care covered; no claim forms | Must use approved doctors and hospitals |
| HMO—Point of Service (POS) | Services from any doctor or hospital, but at lower cost to those using network providers | Within network, primary care doctors manage utilization of services; hospital and physician fees are discounted | Within network, lower co-payments; preventive care covered; no claim forms | Higher cost for services outside network; extra paperwork to get approval of some services |

Since the 1960s, the federal government has provided health care to two vulnerable groups of Americans—the elderly and the poor. The program for elderly people (aged 65 and older) is Medicare, and it is funded completely by the federal government. There are two parts to Medicare: Part A covers hospitalizations, and Part B covers medical expenses such as laboratory tests, physical therapy, and mental health services. Medical expenses are not entirely covered by either Part A or Part B. There are small premiums and deductibles and certain limitations in coverage. This can be a problem for older people of modest means. Because Medicare doesn't cover every expense, many recipients elect to purchase supplemental policies. Finally, Medicare Part C allows for private health insurance companies to provide Medicare services, and Medicare Part D is prescription drug insurance.

Medicaid, the other type of public health insurance, is for individuals whose income is below the poverty level. Medicaid is a joint federal–state program where each pays for half the program. Potential recipients must qualify for Medicaid to receive services. Like other insurance plans, both Medicare and Medicaid negotiate discounted rates of reimbursement with physicians and hospitals. With Medicaid in particular, reimbursements for providers tend to be quite low compared to what private-sector insurance companies pay for the same services—in fact they are so low that many physicians will not accept Medicaid patients.

This reduced access to health care for Medicaid patients is problematic. It results in many poor individuals having to use the emergency room for their care, which can cost 20 times as much as a physician's visit. Furthermore, because of limited access, some people wait too long to be seen. When they finally are evaluated, they may be so sick that they require hospitalization or other costly medical service.

Both Medicare and Medicaid have undergone many changes over the decades and will undergo even greater changes in the years ahead. These public health programs are well intentioned but no longer cost effective. The graying of America, escalating health care costs, and the current tax system all contribute to the dilemma. The political debate will continue until a legislative solution is found. As voters we need to stay abreast of the issues and encourage legislators to explore options that are both cost effective and provide health care access to all.

## CHOOSING AN APPROPRIATE PLAN

An unwise choice of a health insurance plan can have a significant negative financial impact. Simply put, choosing the wrong plan can quickly lead to excessive medical bills. This in turn can add to the emotional burden that one is already facing in dealing with a medical condition.

Having the right plan for your needs can allow you to focus on getting better without the added stress of limited access or affordability.

Health insurance plans offered as an employee benefit often have fixed benefits because the insurance was prenegotiated on the part of the organization (employer). Most often, these plans are reasonably good; however, it is still important to fully understand the choices and the specific plan and its coverage.

There is no one-size-fits-all "best" insurance plan. What is best for an individual depends on a variety of factors including age, gender, personal health history, current health status, family situation, and financial means. These factors must be considered along with whether you are willing to pay more to have more control over your treatment or prefer to pay less and are willing to relinquish control. Here are some key issues to consider as you formulate questions to ask about health insurance plans.

### Choice of Doctors

Does a particular doctor you already see accept the insurance you are considering? Or are there a large number of doctors in the network?

### Facilities—Proximity and Quality

Is the insurance plan–sponsored hospital too far from your home to be convenient? The hospital or clinic might be nearby, but does it have a reputation for quality care? What is the quality of the outpatient and inpatient facilities? Will you have access to diagnostic tools like MRIs and CT scans?

### Waiting Periods

Is there a waiting period if you have a preexisting condition such as asthma, diabetes, heart disease, or cancer? If there is a waiting period, can you afford to pay for treatment out of pocket in the interim? Make sure your treatments won't be excluded indefinitely before you sign up for a plan.

### Health Screenings

How easy is it to get routine health screenings like cholesterol profiles, Pap smears, and mammograms? Does the plan let women go to a gynecologist for an annual exam without going through their primary care physician?

### Other Features/Options

If you (or your spouse) are or may become pregnant, what type of prenatal coverage is available? If a family member needs long-term care, is convalescent care provided in the plan? Are dental and vision care covered?

Once a decision has been made regarding appropriate services, then cost becomes a major factor. Be sure you understand how much the premiums, deductibles, and co-pays are. For employer-sponsored plans, talk to a benefits officer and ask a lot of what-if questions. Create possible scenarios for yourself (and family), and see if the answers are acceptable. If they are acceptable, then most likely you have appropriate coverage. If not, you may want to add additional services to your coverage or purchase a different policy.

Prices of policies purchased on the open market as an individual or family are determined by age, previous medical conditions, family history, and results of a comprehensive physical exam. It is not inexpensive, but it is necessary. Remember that not knowing what is covered or how a policy works is not an acceptable excuse for avoiding a health care bill.

## ✓ NEED TO KNOW

Private health insurance plans can be broadly categorized as fee for service or managed care. Fee-for-service plans provide maximum choice but can require significant out-of-pocket expenses. Managed care is generally offered as either a preferred provider organization (PPO) or a health maintenance organization (HMO). PPOs provide some choice in providers and facilities, yet keep out-of-pocket costs fairly low. HMOs provide comprehensive care within a specific network of doctors and facilities while minimizing out-of-pocket expenses. Medicare and Medicaid are government-funded programs that provide health care for elderly and poor people, respectively. When choosing a health care plan, take the time to carefully study the available options and select the plan that best meets your needs.

## HEALTH CARE REFORM

Over $2.5 trillion is spent on health care in the United States each year. That's approximately 16 percent of the country's gross domestic product. The United States spends the most of any country in the world on health care, yet the United States ranks 28th in life expectancy and 29th in infant mortality. The United States also currently has 40–50 million people who do not have access to care, either because they have no insurance or they are underinsured. Some countries such as Sweden, Italy, and Japan spend half of what the United States does on health care, yet they have better outcomes. To make matters worse, health care costs are the leading cause of personal bankruptcy in the United States today.

Nearly everyone—policymakers, economists, and the general public—tends to agree that the high cost of U.S. health care is unsustainable

Article
13.4

Self
Assessment
13.2

and causes a myriad of problems. Some argue that this ever-increasing cost will be the next economic bubble to burst. Recognizing the problems that come from steadily increasing health care costs is not new. Presidents Nixon, Carter, and Clinton all wanted some degree of health care reform during their administrations but were unsuccessful in drafting legislation that was passed. Health care in America had its first major change in decades when, in 2010, President Barack Obama was successful in getting the Patient Protection and Affordable Care Act (PPACA) passed.

PPACA primarily is a series of reforms that will increase the number of Americans who have health insurance. Provisions of the law phase in over a 10-year period, so that by 2019 almost all Americans will be covered by some form of health insurance. As well, the law mandates some key health care items that now must be covered by health insurance policies.

Some of PPACA has already phased in. For example, before the legislation passed, companies could deny insurance coverage to individuals with preexisting medical conditions. That meant a person with asthma or a past history of cancer treatments might be able to purchase an insurance policy, but the insurance company would often refuse to pay for any tests, medication, or treatments for the very thing that needed the most monitoring in those individuals. The reason insurance companies operated in this manner was that most are for-profit companies in the United States. From a business perspective, insurance firms want to keep the pool of policyholders as healthy (and as unlikely to incur big medical bills) as possible to keep profits up. But what makes sense for businesses doesn't necessarily result in a good outcome for the general public. Not only were people with preexisting conditions at risk for great financial hardship due to being underinsured or uninsured, but their predicament also ultimately led to poor quality care.

Now because of PPACA, adults who had been denied coverage because of preexisting medical conditions can get insurance from a high-risk insurance pool. Likewise, insurance companies can no longer revoke existing policies if people get ill, as the new law bans lifetime limits on policyholder coverage. Preventative services such as vaccinations and mammograms now must be fully covered, and small businesses will also be eligible for tax credits if they offer insurance to employees.

One PPACA change that directly impacts college students came into effect in 2011. Parents may now keep children on the family health insurance through age 26. Previously, insurance companies could remove children from parents' policies as early as age 19. This added to the problem of so many uninsured Americans, as most young adults either attend school or work at lower-paying jobs that often do not offer insurance.

**TABLE 13.2    KEY PPACA CHANGES TO THE U.S. HEALTH INSURANCE SYSTEM**

| RULE | PROBLEM IT ADDRESSES | PHASED IN |
|------|----------------------|-----------|
| Parents may insure children through age 26. | Many young adults went without insurance during college and/or early in their careers. | 2011 |
| Preexisting condition exclusions and lifetime policy expense caps are banned. | Those needing treatment often could not obtain it or went into bankruptcy paying for it without insurance. | 2011 |
| Preventative care must be included in policies. | Many of the least expensive old-style policies didn't cover basics such as mammograms or vaccinations. | 2011 |
| Health insurance exchanges are created. | Previously difficult to compare the cost and type of coverage among different insurance companies. | 2014 |
| There are penalties for not having health insurance. | The trade-off of increasing health insurance coverage is that everyone is required to get a policy. | 2019 |

The most sweeping change of PPACA is that it mandates that all Americans must have insurance by the end of the phase-in period or pay a penalty. The idea is that if insurance companies are being forced to cover more treatments with less exclusions, then everyone should take part in the system and buy policies. To aid in increasing the number of policies, in 2014 each state will establish health insurance exchanges so that it is easier for individuals to shop around. There will also be tax credits for people who make too much money to be eligible for Medicaid but are still low income. Table 13.2 displays the key changes of PPACA.

### PPACA Controversies and Criticisms

PPACA attempts to correct some of the structural problems and inequities in our health care delivery system. If the Congressional Budget Office (CBO) is correct, implementing the law will result in two things: Americans will have better access to the health care delivery system, and there may be overall cost savings.

The issue of the cost of the law has been hotly contested, with estimates of federal savings varying by billions of dollars depending

Understanding Health Insurance

**FIGURE 13.3** **HOW PEOPLE GET HEALTH COVERAGE UNDER THE AFFORDABLE CARE ACT BEGINNING IN 2014**

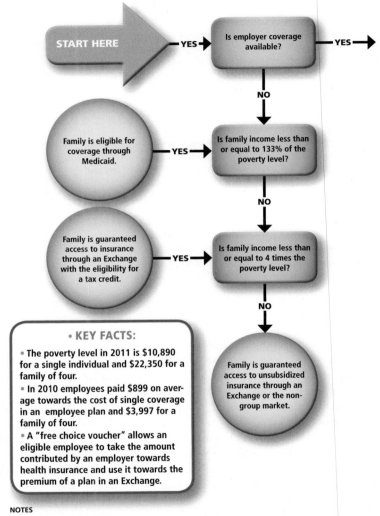

**START HERE** —YES→ Is employer coverage available? —YES→

NO ↓

Family is eligible for coverage through Medicaid. ←YES— Is family income less than or equal to 133% of the poverty level?

NO ↓

Family is guaranteed access to insurance through an Exchange with the eligibility for a tax credit. ←YES— Is family income less than or equal to 4 times the poverty level?

NO ↓

Family is guaranteed access to unsubsidized insurance through an Exchange or the non-group market.

**• KEY FACTS:**

• The poverty level in 2011 is $10,890 for a single individual and $22,350 for a family of four.

• In 2010 employees paid $899 on average towards the cost of single coverage in an employee plan and $3,997 for a family of four.

• A "free choice voucher" allows an eligible employee to take the amount contributed by an employer towards health insurance and use it towards the premium of a plan in an Exchange.

**NOTES**

• Some states may have higher income eligibility levels for Medicaid.

• In some cases, children may be eligible for public coverage through Medicaid or CHIP while their parents are covered through an employer or an Exchange.

• Undocumented immigrants are ineligible for Medicaid and may not purchase coverage in an Exchange or receive a tax credit.

• In general, people are required to obtain coverage or pay a penalty, but those whose health insurance premiums exceed 8% of family income (after tax credits or employer contributions are taken into account ) will not be penalized if they choose not to purchase coverage.

Source: Reprinted with permission from the Henry J. Kaiser Family Foundation, Menlo Park, California.

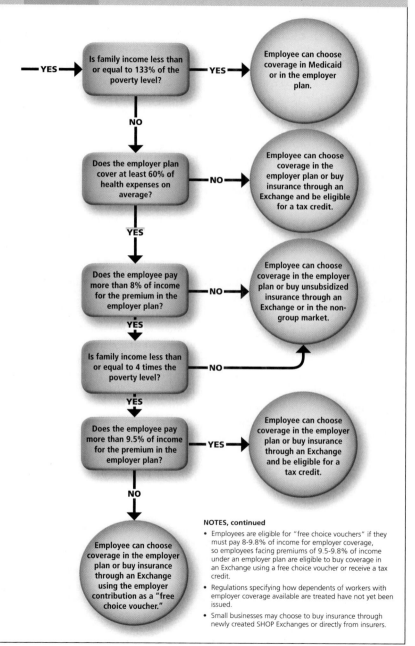

→YES→ Is family income less than or equal to 133% of the poverty level? →YES→ Employee can choose coverage in Medicaid or in the employer plan.

NO

Does the employer plan cover at least 60% of health expenses on average? —NO— Employee can choose coverage in the employer plan or buy insurance through an Exchange and be eligible for a tax credit.

YES

Does the employee pay more than 8% of income for the premium in the employer plan? —NO— Employee can choose coverage in the employer plan or buy unsubsidized insurance through an Exchange or in the non-group market.

YES

Is family income less than or equal to 4 times the poverty level? —NO—

YES

Does the employee pay more than 9.5% of income for the premium in the employer plan? —YES— Employee can choose coverage in the employer plan or buy insurance through an Exchange and be eligible for a tax credit.

NO

Employee can choose coverage in the employer plan or buy insurance through an Exchange using the employer contribution as a "free choice voucher."

**NOTES, continued**

- Employees are eligible for "free choice vouchers" if they must pay 8-9.8% of income for employer coverage, so employees facing premiums of 9.5-9.8% of income under an employer plan are eligible to buy coverage in an Exchange using a free choice voucher or receive a tax credit.

- Regulations specifying how dependents of workers with employer coverage available are treated have not yet been issued.

- Small businesses may choose to buy insurance through newly created SHOP Exchanges or directly from insurers.

upon which variables and time periods are examined. It is also possible that not every group will see the same savings across the board. For example, the government and low-income citizens could see overall health care expenditures decrease, while costs for the average, middle-income American might actually go up.

One criticism of PPACA says that the act was passed too quickly. There is some merit to this complaint, for while the problem of increasing costs and restricted access grew larger for decades, the final law came together very quickly under a brief window where the U.S. House, Senate, and presidency were all held by a majority of Democrats. Many people felt the law was rushed through at a time when the country had other problems to address, such as the war on terrorism and a bad economy. Still others wonder if the cost-saving estimates will ultimately hold true.

The complaint that PPACA is socialized medicine is false. The majority of Americans have loudly stated they do not want socialized medicine—although it is less clear if the public understands what socialized medicine actually is. For example, the elderly are quite happy with their Medicare. If one examines the structure of Medicare, it is very close to being a type of socialized medicine. Medicare covers all citizens over age 65, and the government sets the reimbursement rates for services and providers.

Many Americans like their interactions with our "old" health care system, warts and all. If you have insurance and can afford the premiums, you have a wide variety of choices, an array of services, and easy access to care. Those who get the best of care may not realize or be concerned that the system is unfair or problematic for others. But like it or not, the ever-increasing costs of the traditional system are considered unsustainable, which is what ultimately led to the passage of PPACA. Figure 13.3 lays out the steps to obtaining health insurance with PPACA.

### ✓ NEED TO KNOW

The Patient Protection and Affordable Care Act (PPACA) is the most significant attempt at health care reform since Medicare and Medicaid in the mid-1960s. PPACA will in some way affect every American, including young adults. For example, young adults can stay on their parent's health insurance until age 26. When PPACA is fully implemented most Americans should have access to medical care. It is expected that there will be some changes to PPACA. To that end, it is important that citizens access valid and reliable information sources to understand how PPACA will affect them and to keep informed of the implementation of PPACA.

# ➤ Striving for Optimal Health

In Chapter 1, we set up a personal health roadmap directing you to selected destinations on fundamental health behaviors, medical conditions, and health care topics. Our aim has been to provide you with the knowledge, confidence, and motivation to explore a variety of paths in pursuit of a healthier life. As we come to the end of the last chapter, we're completing our journey by returning to the starting point. As seen in Figure 13.4, let's remember that our health is determined by a combination of interacting factors including genetics, behaviors, environments, policies and interventions, and access to health care. All factors can contribute to varying degrees based on an individual's circumstances and surroundings. However, for most Americans, health is largely determined by lifestyle choices and behaviors. The fact that each of us has the potential to significantly affect our own health may seem obvious to us today. In actuality, the necessary knowledge and resources to support this statement have been realized only within the last few generations.

We trust that you view the concept of health much differently now. At this point, defining health as simply the absence of disease and illness seems shortsighted and self-limiting. We hope you have gained an appreciation for health as a multidimensional concept directly related to your quality of life. And this includes your quality of life *right now and in the weeks and months ahead.* Striving for optimal health is not just about reducing chronic disease and disability in

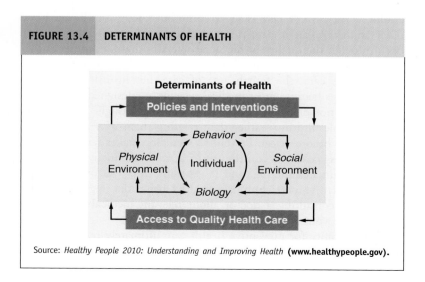

**FIGURE 13.4    DETERMINANTS OF HEALTH**

Source: *Healthy People 2010: Understanding and Improving Health* (**www.healthypeople.gov**).

middle age and beyond; it's also about feeling good and functioning at a high level today. To this end, staying informed and practicing prevention go hand in hand with living a full and healthy life.

## STAYING INFORMED

Staying informed is all about health literacy. As discussed in Chapter 1, *health literacy* means having the knowledge and skills to successfully access, analyze, and interpret relevant information to answer personal health questions. Common questions relate to seeking guidance on dealing with a health condition or changing a health behavior. Health literacy also encompasses a working knowledge of the health care system, which has been the focus of this and the previous chapter.

Self-directed learning, effective communication, and critical thinking— three threads of health literacy—have been emphasized throughout *iHealth*. It's important to continue to develop your skills in these areas beyond this course. Health literacy also assumes a mindfulness and a curiosity that motivates continual learning. Hopefully, this mind-set is present or will develop with time. Recommended Internet sites on general health information for the consumer are listed at the end of the chapter.

## PRACTICING PREVENTION

As shown in Figure 13.5, health care encompasses four areas: acute care, chronic care, palliative care, and preventive care. The majority of all health care involves treatment of acute illnesses and injuries and control of chronic diseases. Acute care is predominant among younger adults, while chronic care is more common among middle-aged and older adults. Palliative care is an emerging area of care that focuses on improving the quality of life of people who have a serious or life-threatening disease by controlling pain and providing comfort.

Preventive care, the fourth area of care, has historically received little emphasis because most medical systems are designed to treat and cure illness, not prevent it. The tide is turning though. The value of *keeping* people healthy—rather than treating them *after* they develop disease—has become clear. Preventive medicine makes sense in several ways—it's less costly, it contributes to a more productive workforce, it reduces human suffering, and it generally improves overall quality of life. Preventive care comprises healthy behaviors, regular wellness exams, and consulting a doctor about relevant medical and lifestyle strategies for your individual situation.

Responsibility for preventive health care ultimately rests with each individual. Selecting a prevention-minded doctor and a health insurance

**FIGURE 13.5    HEALTH CARE EMPHASIS AREAS**

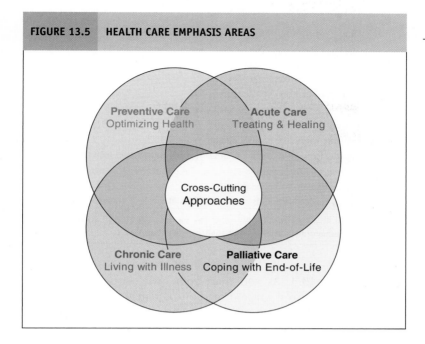

plan that encompasses prevention are important choices. Following through by undergoing age- and gender-appropriate screening tests according to evidence-based guidelines is an important habit to establish. These tests are listed under "Adult Health Resources" on the website of the Agency for Healthcare Research and Quality **(www.ahrq .gov/ppip/adguide).** Yet, as discussed throughout this book, perhaps the most important steps are those we take every day—our personal actions, especially those related to eating, exercising, sexual behavior, drug use, and managing stress.

Many of you now have a better appreciation for the challenges involved with changing a health behavior. It's generally much more complex than people realize, particularly today when social conditioning and environmental design often favor health-compromising behaviors. Developing healthy behaviors requires planning and strategies. Conceptual frameworks and examples have been provided to help you implement positive lifestyle changes.

Always remember that health is more than just physical health—it's a multidimensional concept encompassing physical, emotional, intellectual, social, and spiritual elements. Striving for optimal health is an active, ongoing process. Fundamental health-promoting actions are

**TABLE 13.3    TEN ACTION STEPS TO BEING HEALTHY**

1. Focus your efforts on things that matter; inform yourself about risks and benefits.
2. Don't smoke or use tobacco products.
3. Eat a balanced diet and handle foods safely.
4. If you drink alcoholic beverages, keep your intake moderate.
5. Exercise regularly.
6. Achieve and maintain a healthy weight.
7. Protect yourself against AIDS and other sexually transmitted infections.
8. See your doctors for scheduled screening and preventive maintenance.
9. Always separate drinking and driving.
10. Use safety devices—such as seat belts, helmets, safety glasses—every time.

Source: Adapted from *Make 2008 the Healthiest Year Yet,* American Council on Science and Health **(www.acsh.org/publications/pubID.1648/pub_detail.asp).**

listed in Table 13.3. As you chart your own course toward better health, tailor your own list and map out a plan. Implement positive actions, maintain other healthy behaviors, and resolve to stay on track. Good health habits provide a strong foundation for a full life. Making informed decisions about health care and practicing prevention further strengthen this foundation.

## ✓ NEED TO KNOW

Our health is determined by a combination of factors from the realms of heredity, lifestyle, environment, and health care policy and access. All factors can contribute to varying degrees based on a person's circumstances and surroundings. However, for most Americans, our health is largely determined by our own lifestyle choices and behaviors. We each chart a course that either strengthens or weakens our health. Staying informed and practicing prevention are two key elements in striving for optimal health.

## ARTICLES

13.1 "Health Disparities: A Case for Closing the Gap." *Healthreform .gov.* A government report highlights the problems that led to health care reform.

13.2 "Are You Ready for a World Without Antibiotics?" *The Guardian.* Resistant bacteria are becoming such an important issue that the era of antibiotics might just be coming to a close.

13.3 "Abuse of Prescription and Over the Counter Medications." *Journal of the American Board of Family Medicine.* Abuse of both prescription and over-the-counter medications are becoming a major problem in the United States.

13.4 "America, the Doctor Will See You Now." *Time.* The Patient Protection and Affordable Care Act (PPACA) is one of the most significant pieces of legislation ever passed. PPACA has many moving parts so the implementation will be challenging. This article highlights those challenges.

## SELF-ASSESSMENTS

13.1 Finding the Right Doctor
13.2 Health Reform Quiz

## Website Resources

### GENERAL

Agency for Healthcare Research and Quality **www.ahrq.gov**
Food and Drug Administration **www.fda.gov**
Joint Commission on Accreditation of Healthcare Organizations
    **www.jointcommission.org/GeneralPublic**
Kaiser Family Foundation **www.kff.org**

### COMMON MEDICAL PROBLEMS

American Academy of Family Physicians (Search by Symptom)
    **http://familydoctor.org/online/famdocen/home/tools/ symptom.html**
*Merck Manual of Medical Information,* 2nd Home Edition
    **www.mercksource.com/pp/us/cns/cns_merckmanualhome.jsp**

## HANDLING MEDICAL EMERGENCIES

CPR and First Aid courses (Contact Your Local Chapter)
- American Heart Association **www.americanheart.org**
- American Red Cross **www.redcross.org**
- National Safety Council **www.nsc.org**

Mayo Clinic First Aid Guide
**www.mayoclinic.com/health/FirstAidIndex/FirstAidIndex**

## PRESCRIPTION AND OTC MEDICINES

MedlinePlus Drug Information
**www.nlm.nih.gov/medlineplus/druginformation.html**
National Council on Patient Information and Education
**www.talkaboutrx.org**
PDRhealth (Physicians' Desk Reference)
**www.pdrhealth.com/drugs/drugs-index.aspx**

## FINDING THE RIGHT DOCTOR

American Board of Medical Specialties
**www.abms.org/Who_We_Help/Consumers**
Specialty Boards, American Osteopathic Association
**www.do-online.osteotech.org/index.cfm?PageID=crt_**
**memboards**

## MEDICAL TESTS AND PROCEDURES

Lab Tests Online **www.labtestsonline.org**
MedlinePlus Health Tutorials
**www.nlm.nih.gov/medlineplus/tutorial.html**
RadiologyInfo **www.radiologyinfo.org**

## UNDERSTANDING HEALTH INSURANCE

Agency for Healthcare Research and Quality (Choosing a Health Plan)
**www.ahrq.gov/consumer/qnt/qnthplan.htm**
America's Health Insurance Plans (AHIP)
**www.ahip.org/content/default.aspx?bc=41**
Patient Protection and Affordable Care Act (PPACA)
**www.healthreform.gov**

## STAYING INFORMED

Centers for Disease Control and Prevention (CDC)
**www.cdc.gov**

Columbia University's Health Q & A
**www.goaskalice.columbia.edu**
healthfinder® **www.healthfinder.gov**
Healthline **www.healthline.com**
Mayo Clinic **www.mayoclinic.com**
MedlinePlus **http://medlineplus.gov**

**PRACTICING PREVENTION**

Adult Health Resources **www.ahrq.gov/ppip/adguide**

## Knowing the Language

deductible, 476
drug, 462
fee-for-service (FFS) plans, 477
managed care plans, 477
medical self-care, 456

over-the-counter (OTC) drug, 462
premium, 476
prescription (Rx) drug, 462
sign, 456
symptom, 456

## Understanding the Content

1. What are signs, symptoms, and decision charts?
2. What are three common types of OTC medications that should be available in every home?
3. What characteristics would you like to see in a primary care physician?
4. What is a personal health record? What information should it include?
5. What are the two main types of private health insurance? Contrast and compare.

## Exploring Ideas

1. A key to effective medical self-care is knowing how much to do on your own and knowing when to contact your doctor. Think of two instances in which you were sick and sought medical care. Apply the signs and symptoms in each instance to the self-care resources (familydoctor.org, mercksource.com) and see what steps are recommended. Are the steps similar to or different from how you proceeded when you were sick?
2. Our current health care system offers several levels of care to diagnose and treat a vast array of illnesses and injuries from the

simplest to the most complex. As a patient, how can one efficiently access and utilize medical care? What health care suggestions about finding a doctor or using a hospital would you give to a friend who is moving to the United States from another country?

3. Typically, young adults can choose from many different health plans. Assume a 25-year-old had two major medical costs in a year: $1,700 for an emergency room visit to check on a possible concussion and $450 incurred from a visit to his primary care physician to treat an infection (including blood tests and Rx drug). To what degree would these charges be covered by your health plan versus different plans of two friends? Compare bottom-line costs by incorporating insurance premiums and deductibles.

## Selected References

Agency for Healthcare Research and Quality. Choosing a Health Plan (AHRQ). **www.ahrq.gov/consumer/qnt/qnthplan.htm**

AHRQ. Healthcare Cost and Utilization Project. **www.ahrq.gov/data/hcup**

AHRQ. Medical Expenditure Panel Survey. **www.ahrq.gov/data/mepsix.htm**

AHRQ. 20 Tips to Help Prevent Medical Errors. **www.ahrq.gov/consumer/20tips.htm**

America's Health Insurance Plans (AHIP). Questions and Answers about Health Insurance: A Consumer Guide. August 2007. **www.ahip.org/content/default.aspx?bc=41|329|20888**

Aspden P, Wolcott J, Bootman J, Cronenwett L (eds.). *Preventing Medication Errors.* Washington, DC: Institute of Medicine, National Academies Press, 2007.

Center on Budget and Policy Priorities. More Americans, including more children, now lack health insurance. August 31, 2007. **www.cbpp.org/8-28-07health.htm**

Consumer Healthcare Products Association. OTC Sales by Category, 2005–2009. **www.chpa-info.org/pressroom/sales_category.aspx**

Drug Topics. Pharmacy Facts and Figures. **http://drugtopics.modernmedicine.com/Pharmacy+Facts+ &+Figures**

Fries JF, Vickery DM. *Take Care of Yourself: The Complete Illustrated Guide to Medical Self-Care* (9th ed.). Cambridge, MA: Da Capo Press, 2009.

Harris Interactive. Two in Five Adults Keep Personal or Family Health Records and Almost Everybody Thinks This Is a Good Idea. August 10, 2004. **www.harrisinteractive.com/news/allnewsbydate.asp?NewsID=832**

Johns Hopkins Pathology. Personal Stories: Carolyn Benivegna. **www.ovariancancer.jhmi.edu/stories2.cfm?personID=15**

Kaiser Family Foundation. *Health Care and the Middle Class: More Costs and Less Coverage.* July 24, 2009. **www.kff.org/healthreform/7951.cfm**

Koh HK, Sebelius KG. Promoting prevention through the Affordable Care Act. *New England Journal of Medicine,* September 13, 2010.

Kokoska M, Eisenberg L, Stack B, Trimmer J, Taylor M. Health care for all? A single or multiple payer system. *Otolaryngology—Head and Neck Surgery* 143: 16, 2010.

MayoClinic.com. Tattoos: Risks and precautions to know first. February 16, 2008. **www.mayoclinic.com/health/tattoos-and-piercings/MC00020**

National Coalition on Health Care. Health Insurance Cost. 2009. **www.nchc.org/facts/cost.shtml**

Ornish D. *The Spectrum: A Scientifically Proven Program to Feel Better, Live Longer, Lose Weight, and Gain Health.* New York: Ballantine, 2007.

Ornish D. Yes, prevention is cheaper than treatment. *Newsweek,* April 24, 2008. **www.newsweek.com/id/133751/**

Pantell RH, Fries JF, Vickery DM. *Taking Care of Your Child: A Parent's Illustrated Guide to Complete Medical Care* (8th ed.). Cambridge, MA: Da Capo Press, 2009.

United Health Foundation. Communicate with Your Health Care Team. **www.unitedhealthfoundation.org/comm.html**

U.S. Department of Health and Human Services. Medicare. **www.medicare.gov**

*U.S. News & World Report.* America's Best Health Plans 2009. **http://health.usnews.com/sections/health/health-plans/index.html**

The online articles complement the main topics presented in the *iHealth* text. Collectively, they provide a library of readings representing the breadth, depth, and complexity of personal health issues. A variety of cross-cutting themes are found within the articles: aging/death; behavior change; consumerism; diversity/social justice; environment; health communication; health policy/regulation; mind, body, and spirit; preventive medicine; relationships; safety; science/technology; and society/culture. The following table lists each article by its affiliated *iHealth* chapter and secondary themes.

| Article | TITLE | SOURCE | SECONDARY THEMES |
|---------|-------|--------|------------------|
| 1.1 | Aging Well: Toward a Way of Life for All People | *Preventing Chronic Disease* | • Aging/Death<br>• Diversity/Social Justice<br>• Mind, Body, and Spirit<br>• Preventive Medicine<br>• Society/Culture |
| 1.2 | No Truth to the Fountain of Youth | *Scientific American* | • Aging/Death<br>• Consumerism<br>• Science/Technology<br>• Society/Culture |
| 1.3 | Simple Tools for Understanding Risks: From Innumeracy to Insight | *British Medical Journal* | • Consumerism<br>• Health Communication<br>• Health Policy/Regulation<br>• Safety |
| 1.4 | Global Warming: No Big Deal? | *The Atlantic* | • Consumerism<br>• Environment<br>• Health Communication<br>• Safety |
| 1.5 | Getting Serious about the Prevention of Chronic Diseases | *Preventing Chronic Disease* | • Consumerism<br>• Environment<br>• Health Policy/Regulation<br>• Preventive Medicine<br>• Safety |
| 2.1 | You Are Also What You Drink | *New York Times* | • Behavior Change<br>• Consumerism<br>• Preventive Medicine<br>• Society/Culture |
| 2.2 | How I Learned to Love Breakfast (Or at Least What to Eat for It) | *New York Magazine* | • Behavior Change<br>• Consumerism<br>• Preventive Medicine<br>• Science/Technology |
| 2.3 | Ancel Keys, PhD, Acclaimed Researcher and Promoter of Mediterranean Diet | Author Phillip B. Sparling | • Behavior Change<br>• Health Communication<br>• Preventive Medicine<br>• Society/Culture |
| 2.4 | Six Rules for Eating Wisely | *Time* | • Behavior Change<br>• Consumerism<br>• Environment<br>• Preventive Medicine<br>• Society/Culture |
| 3.1 | The Play of the Year | *Sports Illustrated* | • Diversity/Social Justice<br>• Mind, Body, and Spirit<br>• Society/Culture |
| 3.2 | Should Athletes Stretch Before Exercise? | Gatorade Sports Science Institute | • Health Communication<br>• Preventive Medicine<br>• Science/Technology |

*(Continued)*

| Article | TITLE | SOURCE | SECONDARY THEMES |
|---------|-------|--------|------------------|
| 3.3 | Body Image: Are You Imagining the Wrong Image? | *ACSM's Health and Fitness Journal* | • Behavior Change<br>• Mind, Body, and Spirit<br>• Relationships<br>• Society/Culture |
| 3.4 | The Courage to Start: A Guide to Running for Your Life | Excerpt from book by same name | • Behavior Change<br>• Mind, Body, and Spirit<br>• Society/Culture |
| 4.1 | How We Get Addicted | *Time* | • Behavior Change<br>• Mind, Body, and Spirit<br>• Preventive Medicine<br>• Society/Culture |
| 4.2 | America's Most Dangerous Drug | *Newsweek* | • Health Policy/Regulation<br>• Society/Culture |
| 4.3 | A Host of Trouble | *U.S. News & World Report* | • Relationships<br>• Society/Culture |
| 4.4 | Screening and Brief Intervention for Underage Drinkers | *Mayo Clinic Proceedings* | • Behavior Change<br>• Preventive Medicine<br>• Society/Culture |
| 5.1 | Hooking Up and Hanging Out: Casual Sexual Behavior Among Adolescents | University of Florida—IFAS Extension | • Health Communication<br>• Mind, Body, and Spirit<br>• Society/Culture |
| 5.2 | I Got Your Back: Friends' Understandings Regarding College Student Spring Break Behavior | *Journal of Youth Adolescence* | • Health Communication<br>• Relationships<br>• Society/Culture |
| 5.3 | Speed Dating | *Current Directions in Psychological Science* | • Health Communication<br>• Relationships<br>• Society/Culture |
| 5.4 | A Longitudinal Perspective on Dating Violence Among Adolescent and College Age Women | *American Journal of Public Health* | • Relationships<br>• Safety<br>• Society/Culture |
| 6.1 | Poll Shows Stress Pains Many in College | *USA Today* | • Mind, Body, and Spirit<br>• Relationships<br>• Society/Culture |
| 6.2 | Strong Medicine Speaks: Recollections from the Matriarch of a Once Hidden Tribe | *Smithsonian.com* | • Diversity/Social Justice<br>• Mind, Body, and Spirit<br>• Society/Culture |
| 6.3 | Professors' Guide: Top Ten Secrets to College Success | *U.S. News & World Report* | • Behavior Change<br>• Consumerism<br>• Society/Culture |

| 6.4 | Change in Lifestyle Is the Best Kind of Cure | Milwaukee-Wisconsin Journal Sentinel | • Behavior Change<br>• Mind, Body, and Spirit<br>• Preventive Medicine |
|---|---|---|---|
| 6.5 | Unraveling Beliefs | Edge.org | • Behavior Change<br>• Diversity/Social Justice<br>• Mind, Body, and Spirit<br>• Society/Culture |
| 7.1 | A Nation of Wimps | Psychology Today | • Health Communication<br>• Relationships<br>• Society/Culture |
| 7.2 | Mental Health Service Utilization Among College Students in the United States | Journal of Nervous and Mental Disease | • Consumerism<br>• Health Policy/Regulation<br>• Mind, Body, and Spirit |
| 7.3 | Conceptualizing the Engaging Bystander Approach to Sexual Violence Prevention on College Campuses | Journal of College Student Development | • Relationships<br>• Safety |
| 7.4 | Sleep Debt and Depression in Female College Students | Psychiatry Research | • Behavior Change Mind, Body, and Spirit |
| 8.1 | Paul Dudley White, MD, Preventive Cardiologist and Exercise Advocate | Author Phillip B. Sparling | • Behavior Change<br>• Health Communication<br>• Preventive Medicine<br>• Science/Technology |
| 8.2 | Lowering LDL Cholesterol Without Drugs | U.S. News & World Report | • Behavior Change<br>• Consumerism<br>• Health Communication<br>• Preventive Medicine |
| 8.3 | Sedentary Behavior: Emerging Evidence for a New Health Risk | Mayo Clinic Proceedings | • Behavior Change<br>• Health Communication<br>• Preventive Medicine<br>• Society/Culture |
| 8.4 | Americans Confused about Effects of Wine, Sea Salt on Health | Medical News Today | • Consumerism<br>• Health Communication<br>• Preventive Medicine |
| 9.1 | The Deadliest Cancer | Newsweek | • Consumerism<br>• Health Policy/Regulation<br>• Science /Technology |
| 9.2 | Getting to the Root of Testicular Cancer | ED Insider | • Consumerism<br>• Science/Technology |

(*Continued*)

| Article | TITLE | SOURCE | SECONDARY THEMES |
|---|---|---|---|
| 9.3 | The Sunscreen Myth: How Sunscreen Products Actually Promote Cancer | *Natural News.com* | • Consumerism<br>• Health Communication<br>• Science/Technology |
| 9.4 | Conquering Cancer in the 21st Century: Leading a Movement to Save More Lives Worldwide | *Health Education and Behavior* | • Health Policy/Regulation<br>• Science/Technology<br>• Society/Culture |
| 10.1 | How and Where Fat Is Stored Predicts Disease Risk Better Than Weight | University of Texas Southwestern Medical Center | • Health Communication<br>• Preventive Medicine<br>• Science/Technology |
| 10.2 | Type 2 Diabetes Surges in People Younger Than 20 | *Washington Post* | • Behavior Change<br>• Health Communication<br>• Society/Culture |
| 10.3 | Creating a Family Culture of Healthy Eating One Step at a Time | *Diabetes Health* | • Behavior Change<br>• Health Communication<br>• Relationships<br>• Society/Culture |
| 11.1 | Adolescents at Risk: The Case for Meningococcal Vaccine | *Journal of Adolescent Health* | • Behavior Change<br>• Health Communication<br>• Health Policy/Regulation |
| 11.2 | Genital Herpes: A Hidden Epidemic | *FDA Consumer* | • Health Communication<br>• Health Policy/Regulation |
| 11.3 | Getting to Know Human Papillomavirus (HPV) and the HPV Vaccines | *Journal of the American Osteopathic Association* | • Health Communication<br>• Health Policy/Regulation |
| 11.4 | A Way Forward: The National HIV/AIDS Strategy and Reducing HIV Incidence in the United States | *Journal of Acquired Immune Deficiency Syndrome* | • Diversity/Social Justice<br>• Health Communication<br>• Health Policy/Regulation |
| 12.1 | Yes, Prevention Is Cheaper Than Treatment | *Newsweek* | • Consumerism<br>• Health Policy/Regulation<br>• Preventive Medicine<br>• Society/Culture |
| 12.2 | Improving Health Care Quality | *Permanente Journal* | • Consumerism<br>• Health Communication<br>• Health Policy/Regulation<br>• Safety |
| 12.3 | Treat the Patient, not the CT Scan | *New York Times* | • Health Communication<br>• Mind, Body, and Spirit<br>• Relationships<br>• Science/Technology |

| 12.4 | Alternative Medicine Is Mainstream | *Wall Street Journal* | • Consumerism<br>• Health Policy/Regulation<br>• Preventive Medicine<br>• Society/Culture |
|------|------|------|------|
| 13.1 | Health Disparities: A Case for Closing the Gap | *Healthreform.gov* | • Diversity/Social Justice<br>• Health Policy/Regulation<br>• Preventive Medicine<br>• Society/Culture |
| 13.2 | Are You Ready for a World Without Antibiotics? | *The Guardian* | • Consumerism<br>• Health Communication<br>• Health Policy/Regulation<br>• Society/Culture |
| 13.3 | Abuse of Prescription and Over the Counter Medications | *Journal of the American Board of Family Medicine* | • Health Policy/Regulation<br>• Society/Culture |
| 13.4 | America, the Doctor Will See You Now | *Time* | • Consumerism<br>• Health Policy/Regulation<br>• Society/Culture |

**Phillip B. Sparling** is a Professor of Applied Physiology and Health Behavior in the College of Sciences at Georgia Institute of Technology (Georgia Tech). He received his undergraduate degree from Duke University and master's and doctorate from the University of Georgia. In addition to being a teacher and researcher at Georgia Tech for three decades, he has been a Fulbright Scholar at the University of Cape Town Medical School in South Africa, a Senior Scientist at the Centers for Disease Control and Prevention (CDC) in Atlanta, and a Visiting Research Professor in the School of Population Health at the University of Queensland in Australia. He has published some 70 peer-reviewed articles in scientific and medical journals. Dr. Sparling is a Fellow of the AAHPERD Research Consortium, American College of Sports Medicine, National Academy of Kinesiology, and the Society of Behavioral Medicine. His current work focuses on real-world projects that enable individuals and communities to change lifestyle behaviors to prevent and control chronic diseases.

**Kerry J. Redican** is a Professor of Public Health and Co-Director of the Master of Public Health program in the Virginia Maryland Regional College of Veterinary Medicine at Virginia Tech. He is also a Professor in the Virginia Tech Carilion School of Medicine. His education includes a bachelor's degree from California State University at Long Beach, M.S.P.H. from the UCLA School of Public Health, Ph.D. from the University of Illinois at Champaign-Urbana, and M.P.H. in health administration from the University of North Carolina at Chapel Hill. As a faculty member at Virginia Tech for over three decades, he has been actively involved in development, implementation, and evaluation of health education programs in schools and communities. He is a co-author of four textbooks and has over 60 publications in health journals. Dr. Redican is a Fellow of the American School Health Association and has served on the Board of Directors of the American Association for Health Education and as President of the Virginia Association for Health, Physical Education, Recreation, and Dance.

# PHOTO CREDITS

# INDEX

Page numbers in boldface indicate key term definition. Page numbers followed by *t* indicate material in table, *f* indicate material in a figure or an illustration. Numbers followed by *a* indicate material covered in an online *iHealth* article; the number indicates the chapter number and sequence in which the online article can be found.

# Stress: The Constant Challenge

## LOOKING AHEAD...

**After reading this chapter, you should be able to**

- Explain what stress is and how people react to it—physically, emotionally, and behaviorally
- Describe the relationship between stress and disease
- List common sources of stress
- Describe techniques for preventing and managing stress
- Put together a plan for successfully managing the stress in your life

## TEST YOUR KNOWLEDGE

1. **Which of the following events can cause stress?**
   a. taking out a loan
   b. failing a test
   c. graduating from college

2. **Exercise stimulates which of the following?**
   a. analgesia (pain relief)
   b. birth of new brain cells
   c. relaxation

3. **High levels of stress can impair memory and cause physical changes in the brain.**
   True or false?

4. **Which of the following can result from chronic stress?**
   a. violence
   b. heart attack
   c. stroke

5. **Because eating induces relaxation, it is an excellent means of coping with stress.**
   True or false?

## ANSWERS

1. **ALL THREE.** Stress-producing factors can be pleasant or unpleasant and can include physical challenges, goal achievement, and events that are perceived as negative.

2. **ALL THREE.** Regular exercise is linked to improvements in many dimensions of wellness.

3. **TRUE.** Low levels of stress may improve memory, but high stress levels impair learning and memory.

4. **ALL THREE.** Chronic—or ongoing—stress can last for years. People who suffer from long-term stress may ultimately become violent toward themselves or others. They also run a greater-than-normal risk for certain ailments, especially cardiovascular disease.

5. **FALSE.** Eating to cope with stress may lead to weight gain and to binge eating, a behavior associated with eating disorders.

L ike the term *wellness*, *stress* is a word many people use without really understanding its precise meaning. Stress is popularly viewed as an uncomfortable response to a negative event, which probably describes *nervous tension* more than the cluster of physical and psychological responses that actually constitute stress. In fact, stress is not limited to negative situations; it is also a response to pleasurable physical challenges and the achievement of personal goals.

Whether stress is experienced as pleasant or unpleasant depends largely on the situation and the individual. Because learning effective responses to stress can enhance psychological health and help prevent a number of serious diseases, stress management can be an important part of daily life.

As a college student, you may be in one of the most stressful times of your life (see the box "The Perceived Stress Scale"). This chapter explains the physiological and psychological reactions that make up the stress response and describes how these reactions can be risks to good health. The chapter also presents methods of managing stress.

## WHAT IS STRESS?

In common usage, the term *stress* refers to two different things: situations that trigger physical and emotional reactions, *and* the reactions themselves. This text uses the more precise term **stressor** for a situation that triggers

**stressor** Any physical or psychological event or condition that produces physical and emotional reactions.

**stress response** The physical and emotional reactions to a stressor.

**stress** The general physical and emotional state that accompanies the stress response.

**autonomic nervous system** The branch of the nervous system that controls basic body processes; consists of the sympathetic and parasympathetic divisions.

**parasympathetic division** A division of the autonomic nervous system that moderates the excitatory effect of the sympathetic division, slowing metabolism and restoring energy supplies.

**sympathetic division** A division of the autonomic nervous system that reacts to danger or other challenges by almost instantly accelerating body processes.

**norepinephrine** A neurotransmitter released by the sympathetic nervous system onto specific tissues to increase their function in the face of increased activity; when released by the brain, causes arousal (increased attention, awareness, and alertness); also called *noradrenaline*.

**endocrine system** The system of glands, tissues, and cells that secrete hormones into the bloodstream to influence metabolism and other body processes.

physical and emotional reactions and the term **stress response** for those reactions. A first date and a final exam are examples of stressors; sweaty palms and a pounding heart are symptoms of the stress response. We'll use the term **stress** to describe the general physical and emotional state that accompanies the stress response. So, a person taking a final exam experiences stress.

Each individual's experience of stress depends on many factors, including the nature of the stressor and how it is perceived. Stressors take many different forms. Some occur suddenly and don't last long or repeat, like a fire in the building you live in. Others, like air pollution or quarreling parents, can continue for a long time. The memory of a stressful occurrence can itself be a stressor years after the event, such as the memory of the loss of a loved one. Responses to stressors can include a wide variety of physical, emotional, and behavioral changes. A short-term response might be an upset stomach or insomnia, whereas a long-term response might be a change in your personality or social relations.

## Physical Responses to Stressors

Imagine a near miss: As you step off the curb, a car careens toward you. With just a fraction of a second to spare, you leap safely out of harm's way. In that split second of danger and in the moments following it, you experience a predictable series of physical reactions. Your body goes from a relaxed state to one prepared for physical action to cope with a threat to your life.

Two systems in your body are responsible for your physical response to stressors: the nervous system and the endocrine system. Through rapid chemical reactions affecting almost every part of your body, you are primed to act quickly and appropriately in time of danger.

**Actions of the Nervous System** The nervous system consists of the brain, spinal cord, and nerves. Part of the nervous system is under voluntary control, as when you tell your arm to reach for a chocolate. The part that is not under conscious supervision—for example, the part that controls the digestion of the chocolate—is the **autonomic nervous system**. In addition to digestion, it controls your heart rate, breathing, blood pressure, and hundreds of other involuntary functions.

The autonomic nervous system consists of two divisions:

- The **parasympathetic division** is in control when you are relaxed; it aids in digesting food, storing energy, and promoting growth.

- The **sympathetic division** is activated during times of arousal, including exercise, and when there is an emergency, such as severe pain, anger, or fear.

Sympathetic nerves use the neurotransmitter **norepinephrine** to exert their actions on nearly every organ, sweat gland, blood vessel, and muscle to enable your

## The Perceived Stress Scale

Many symptoms of excess stress are easy to notice. The following test can help you determine how much stress you have experienced in the past week.

Answer each question with a number: Never = 0; Almost never = 1; Sometimes = 2; Fairly often = 3; Very often = 4.

In the past week, how often have you . . .

1. Been upset because of something that happened unexpectedly?
2. Felt that you were unable to control the important things in your life?
3. Felt nervous and "stressed"?
4. *Felt confident about your ability to handle your personal problems?
5. *Felt that things were going your way?
6. Found that you could not cope with all the things you had to do?
7. *Been able to control irritations in your life?
8. *Felt that you were on top of things?
9. Been angered because things happened that were outside of your control?
10. Felt difficulties were piling up so high that you could not overcome them?

To calculate your score, add your answers to questions 1, 2, 3, 6, 9, and 10, and subtract your answers to questions 4, 5, 7, and 8 (the questions with the asterisks). The result is your total score. Add your answers to find your score.

If your total score is above 14, you should take time to develop effective stress-management techniques. This chapter describes many coping strategies that can aid you in dealing with college stressors. Your school's counseling center also can provide valuable support.

**SOURCE:** Cohen, S., and G. Williamson. 1988. Perceived stress in a probability sample of the United States. In *The Social Psychology of Health:* Claremont Symposium on Applied Social Psychology, ed. S. Spacapan and S. Oskamp. Newbury Park, CA: Sage.

---

body to handle an emergency. In general, the sympathetic division commands your body to stop storing energy and to use it in response to a crisis.

**Actions of the Endocrine System**   During stress, the sympathetic nervous system triggers the **endocrine system.** This system of glands, tissues, and cells helps control body functions by releasing **hormones** and other chemical messengers into the bloodstream to influence metabolism and other body processes. These chemicals act on a variety of targets throughout the body. Along with the nervous system, the endocrine system prepares the body to respond to a stressor.

**The Two Systems Together**   How do both systems work together in an emergency? Let's go back to your near collision with a car. Both reflexes and higher cognitive areas in your brain quickly make the decision that you are facing a threat, and your body prepares to meet the danger. Chemical messages and the actions of sympathetic nerves cause the release of key hormones, including **cortisol** and **epinephrine.** These hormones trigger the physiological changes shown in Figure 2.1, including these:

- Heart and respiration rates accelerate to speed oxygen through the body.
- Hearing and vision become more acute.
- The liver releases extra sugar into the bloodstream to boost energy.
- Perspiration increases to cool the skin.
- The brain releases **endorphins**—chemicals that can inhibit or block sensations of pain—in case you are injured.

Taken together, these almost-instantaneous physical changes are called the **fight-or-flight reaction.** They give you the heightened reflexes and strength you need to dodge the car or deal with other stressors. Although these physical changes may vary in intensity, the same basic set of physical reactions occurs in response to any type of stressor—positive or negative, physical or psychological.

**The Return to Homeostasis**   Once a stressful situation ends, the parasympathetic division of your autonomic nervous system takes command and halts the stress response. It restores **homeostasis,** a state in which blood pressure, heart rate, hormone levels, and other vital functions are maintained within a narrow range of normal. Your parasympathetic nervous system calms your body down, slowing a rapid heartbeat, drying sweaty palms, and returning breathing to normal. Gradually, your body resumes its normal "housekeeping" functions, such as digestion and temperature regulation. Damage that may have been sustained during the fight-or-flight reaction is

**TERMS**

**hormone**   A chemical messenger produced in the body and transported in the bloodstream to target cells or organs for specific regulation of their activities.

**cortisol**   A steroid hormone secreted by the cortex (outer layer) of the adrenal gland; also called *hydrocortisone.*

**epinephrine**   A hormone secreted by the medulla (inner core) of the adrenal gland that affects the functioning of organs involved in responding to a stressor; also called *adrenaline.*

**endorphins**   Brain secretions that have pain-inhibiting effects.

**fight-or-flight reaction**   A defense reaction that prepares a person for conflict or escape by triggering hormonal, cardiovascular, metabolic, and other changes.

**homeostasis**   A state of stability and consistency in an individual's physiological functioning.

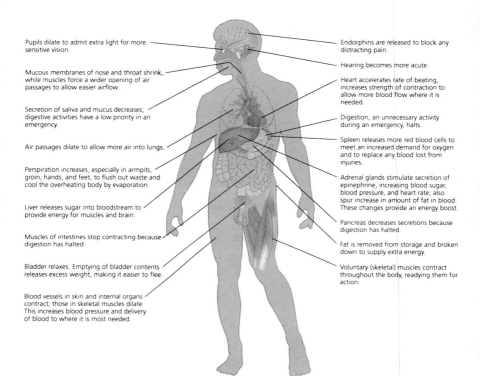

Pupils dilate to admit extra light for more sensitive vision.

Mucous membranes of nose and throat shrink, while muscles force a wider opening of air passages to allow easier airflow.

Secretion of saliva and mucus decreases; digestive activities have a low priority in an emergency.

Air passages dilate to allow more air into lungs.

Perspiration increases, especially in armpits, groin, hands, and feet, to flush out waste and cool the overheating body by evaporation.

Liver releases sugar into bloodstream to provide energy for muscles and brain.

Muscles of intestines stop contracting because digestion has halted.

Bladder relaxes. Emptying of bladder contents releases excess weight, making it easier to flee.

Blood vessels in skin and internal organs contract; those in skeletal muscles dilate. This increases blood pressure and delivery of blood to where it is most needed.

Endorphins are released to block any distracting pain.

Hearing becomes more acute.

Heart accelerates rate of beating, increases strength of contraction to allow more blood flow where it is needed.

Digestion, an unnecessary activity during an emergency, halts.

Spleen releases more red blood cells to meet an increased demand for oxygen and to replace any blood lost from injuries.

Adrenal glands stimulate secretion of epinephrine, increasing blood sugar, blood pressure, and heart rate; also spur increase in amount of fat in blood. These changes provide an energy boost.

Pancreas decreases secretions because digestion has halted.

Fat is removed from storage and broken down to supply extra energy.

Voluntary (skeletal) muscles contract throughout the body, readying them for action.

**FIGURE 2.1   The fight-or-flight reaction.** In response to a stressor, the autonomic nervous system and the endocrine system prepare the body to deal with an emergency.

repaired. The day after you narrowly dodge the car, you wake up feeling fine. In this way, your body can grow, repair itself, and acquire new reserves of energy. When the next crisis comes, you'll be ready to respond again, instantly.

**The Fight-or-Flight Reaction in Modern Life**  The fight-or-flight reaction is a part of our biological heritage, and it's a survival mechanism that has served humans well. In modern life, however, it is often absurdly inappropriate. Many of the stressors we face in everyday life do not require a physical response—for example, an exam, a mess left by a roommate, or a stoplight. The fight-or-flight reaction prepares the body for physical action regardless of whether such action is a necessary or appropriate response to a particular stressor.

## Emotional and Behavioral Responses to Stressors

We all experience a similar set of physical responses to stressors, which make up the fight-or-flight reaction. These responses, however, vary from person to person and from one situation to another. People's perceptions of potential stressors—and of their reactions to such stressors—also vary greatly. For example, you may feel confident about taking exams but be nervous about talking to people you don't know, while your roommate may love challenging social situations but may be nervous about taking tests. Many factors, some external and some internal, help explain these differences.

Your cognitive (mental) appraisal of a potential stressor strongly influences how you view it. Two factors that can

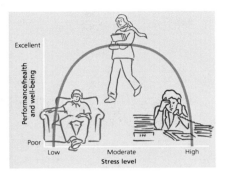

**FIGURE 2.2 Stress level, performance, and well-being.**
A moderate level of stress challenges individuals in a way that promotes optimal performance and well-being. Too little stress, and people are not challenged enough to improve; too much stress, and the challenges become stressors that can impair physical and emotional health.

reduce the magnitude of the stress response are successful prediction and the perception of control. For instance, receiving course syllabi at the beginning of the term allows you to predict the timing of major deadlines and exams. Having this predictive knowledge also allows you to exert some control over your study plans and can thus help reduce the stress caused by exams.

Cognitive appraisal is highly individual and strongly related to emotions. The facts of a situation—Who? What? Where? When?—typically are evaluated fairly consistently from person to person. But evaluation with respect to personal outcome varies: What does this mean for me? Can I do anything about it? Will it improve or worsen? If a person perceives a situation as exceeding her or his ability to cope, the result can be negative emotions and an inappropriate stress response. If, on the other hand, a person perceives a situation as a challenge that is within her or his ability to manage, more positive and appropriate responses are likely. A certain amount of stress, if coped with appropriately, can help promote optimal performance (Figure 2.2).

**Effective and Ineffective Responses** Common emotional responses to stressors include anxiety, depression, and fear. Although emotional responses are determined in part by inborn personality or temperament, we often can moderate or learn to control them. Coping techniques are discussed later in the chapter.

Behavioral responses to stressors—controlled by the **somatic nervous system,** which manages our conscious actions—are entirely under our control. Effective behavioral responses such as talking, laughing, exercising, meditating, learning time-management skills, and becoming more

assertive can promote wellness and enable us to function at our best. Ineffective behavioral responses to stressors include overeating, expressing hostility, and using tobacco, alcohol, or other drugs.

**Personality and Stress** Some people seem to be nervous, irritable, and easily upset

by minor annoyances. Others are calm and composed even in difficult situations. Scientists remain unsure just why this is or how the brain's complex emotional mechanisms work. But **personality**—the sum of cognitive, behavioral, and emotional tendencies—clearly affects how people perceive and react to stressors. To investigate the links among personality, stress, and wellness, researchers examine different clusters of characteristics, or "personality types."

- **Type A.** People with Type A personality are described as ultracompetitive, controlling, impatient, aggressive, and even hostile. Type A people have a higher perceived stress level and more problems coping with stress. They react explosively to stressors and are upset by events that others would consider only annoyances. Studies indicate that certain characteristics of the Type A pattern—anger, cynicism, and hostility—increase the risk of heart disease.
- **Type B.** The Type B personality is relaxed and contemplative. Type B people are less frustrated by daily events and more tolerant of the behavior of others.
- **Type C.** The Type C personality is characterized by anger suppression, difficulty expressing emotions, feelings of hopelessness and despair, and an exaggerated response to minor stressors. This heightened response may impair immune functions.

Studies of Type A and C personalities suggest that expressing emotions is beneficial but habitually expressing exaggerated stress responses or hostility is unhealthy.

Researchers have also looked for personality traits that enable people to deal more successfully with stress. One such trait is *hardiness*, a particular form of optimism. People with a hardy personality view potential stressors as

**somatic nervous system** The branch of the peripheral nervous system that governs motor functions and sensory information, largely under conscious control.

**personality** The sum of behavioral, cognitive, and emotional tendencies.

TERMS

challenges and opportunities for growth and learning, rather than as burdens. They see fewer situations as stressful, and react less intensely to stress than nonhardy persons might. Hardy people are committed to their activities, have a sense of inner purpose and an inner locus of control, and feel at least partly in control of their lives.

The term *resilience* refers to personality traits associated with social and academic success in at-risk populations, such as people from low-income families and those with mental or physical disabilities. Resilient people tend to set goals and face adversity through individual effort. There are three basic types of resilience, and each one determines how a person responds to stress:

*Effective behavioral responses can lessen stress; ineffective ones only worsen it.*

- **Nonreactive resilience,** in which a person does not react to a stressor
- **Homeostatic resilience,** in which a person may react strongly but returns to baseline functioning quickly
- **Positive growth resilience,** in which a person learns and grows from the stress experience

Resilience is associated with emotional intelligence and violence prevention.

You probably can't change your basic personality, but you can change your typical behaviors and patterns of thinking. You can also use positive stress-management techniques like those described later in the chapter.

**Cultural Background**  Young adults from around the world come to America for a higher education; most students finish college with a greater appreciation for other cultures and worldviews. The clashing of cultures, however, can be a big source of stress for many students—especially when it leads to disrespectful treatment, harassment, or violence. It is important to remember that everyone's reaction to stress is influenced by his or her family and cultural background. Learning to accept and appreciate the cultural backgrounds of other people is both a mind-opening experience and a way to avoid stress over cultural differences.

**Gender**  Our gender role—the activities, abilities, and behaviors our culture expects of us based on our sex—can affect our experience of stress. Some behavioral responses to stressors, such as crying or openly expressing anger, may be deemed more appropriate for one gender than the other.

A person's emotional and behavioral responses to stressors depend on many different factors, including personality, gender, and cultural background. Research suggests that women are more likely than men to respond to stressors by seeking social support, a pattern referred to as tend-and-befriend.

Strict adherence to gender roles, however, can limit one's response to stress and can itself become a source of stress. Gender roles can also affect one's perception of a stressor. If a man derives most of his self-worth from his work, for example, retirement may be more stressful for him than for a woman whose self-image is based on several different roles.

See the box "Women, Men, and Stress" for more on gender and stress.

**Experience**  Past experiences can profoundly influence the evaluation of a potential stressor. Consider someone who has had a bad experience giving a speech in the past. He or she is much more likely to perceive an upcoming speech as stressful than someone who has had positive public speaking experiences.

## The Stress Experience as a Whole

As Table 2.1 shows, the physical, emotional, and behavioral symptoms of excess negative stress are distinct. But

| Table 2.1 | Symptoms of Excess Stress | | |
| --- | --- | --- | --- |
| **PHYSICAL SYMPTOMS** | **EMOTIONAL SYMPTOMS** | **BEHAVIORAL SYMPTOMS** | |
| Dry mouth | Anxiety | Crying | |
| Excessive perspiration | Depression | Disrupted eating habits | |
| Frequent illnesses | Edginess | Disrupted sleeping habits | |
| Gastrointestinal problems | Fatigue | Harsh treatment of others | |
| Grinding of teeth | Hypervigilance | Problems communicating | |
| Headaches | Impulsiveness | Sexual problems | |
| High blood pressure | Inability to concentrate | Social isolation | |
| Pounding heart | Irritability | Increased use of tobacco, alcohol, or other drugs | |
| Stiff neck or aching lower back | Trouble remembering things | | |

they are also intimately interrelated. The more intense the emotional response, the stronger the physical response. Effective behavioral responses can lessen stress; ineffective ones only worsen it. Sometimes people have such intense responses to stressors or such ineffective coping techniques that they need professional help to overcome the stress in their lives. More often, however, people can learn to handle stressors on their own.

## STRESS AND HEALTH

According to the American Psychological Association, 43% of adult Americans suffer from stress-related health problems. The role of stress in health is complex, but evidence suggests that stress can increase vulnerability to many ailments. Several theories have been proposed to explain the relationship between stress and disease.

### The General Adaptation Syndrome

Biologist Hans Selye was one of the first scientists to develop a comprehensive theory of stress and disease. Based on his work in the 1930s and 1940s, Selye coined the term **general adaptation syndrome (GAS)** to describe what he believed to be a universal and predictable response pattern to all stressors. As mentioned earlier, some stressors (such as attending a party) are pleasant, and others (such as getting a bad grade) are unpleasant. In the GAS theory, the stress triggered by a pleasant stressor is called **eustress**; stress brought on by an unpleasant stressor is called **distress**. The sequence of physical responses associated with GAS is the same for eustress and distress and occurs in three stages (Figure 2.3):

- *Alarm.* The alarm stage includes the complex sequence of events brought on by the fight-or-flight reaction. At this stage, the body is more susceptible to disease or injury because it is geared up to deal with a crisis. Someone in this stage may experience headaches, indigestion, anxiety, and disrupted eating or sleep patterns.
- *Resistance.* With continued stress, the body develops a new level of homeostasis in which it is more resistant

**FIGURE 2.3 The general adaptation syndrome.** During the alarm phase, a lower resistance to injury is evident. With continued stress, resistance to injury is actually enhanced. With prolonged exposure to repeated stressors, exhaustion sets in, with a return of low resistance levels seen during acute stress.

to disease and injury than usual. In this stage, a person can cope with normal life and added stress.
- *Exhaustion.* The first two stages of GAS require a great deal of energy. If a stressor persists, or if several stressors occur in succession, general exhaustion sets in. This is not the sort of exhaustion you feel after a long, busy day. Rather, it's a life-threatening type of physiological exhaustion.

### Ask yourself

QUESTIONS FOR CRITICAL THINKING AND REFLECTION
Think of the last time you faced a significant stressor. How did you respond? List the physical, emotional, and behavioral reactions you experienced. Did these responses help you deal with the stress, or did they interfere with your efforts to handle it?

**general adaptation syndrome (GAS)** A pattern of stress responses consisting of three stages: alarm, resistance, and exhaustion.

**eustress** Stress resulting from a pleasant stressor.

**distress** Stress resulting from an unpleasant stressor.

# Women, Men, and Stress

Men and women alike experience stress, but they experience it differently.

## Women and Stress

Women are more likely than men to find themselves balancing multiple roles, such as those of student, spouse, and parent. Women who work outside the home still do most of the housework—although today's husbands are helping in greater numbers than previous generations did—and housework isn't limited to cleaning or doing laundry. For example, more than 60% of women make all decisions about their family's health care, including decisions about elderly parents. The combined pressures of home, workplace, and school can create very high stress levels.

## Men and Stress

Men who fit a traditional male gender role may feel compelled to be in charge at all times. This may create tension in interpersonal situations and limit men's ability to build a support network. Such men may keenly feel the responsibility to support a family, which can compound existing pressures at home and work.

## Perceptions of Stress

In late 2009, the American Psychological Association released the results of its annual "Stress in America" survey. The survey shows the different views American men and women have of their personal stress. Respondents said stress affects them in the following ways:

|  | Women | Men |
|---|---|---|
| Irritability or anger | 51% | 39% |
| Fatigue | 49% | 37% |
| Urge to cry | 46% | 16% |
| Lack of interest, motivation, energy | 45% | 35% |
| Headache | 43% | 24% |
| Feeling depressed or sad | 42% | 26% |

The survey also shows that women are more likely than men to cope with stress through behaviors such as overeating or taking prescription medications.

## Physiological Differences

Levels of testosterone (the primary male hormone, responsible for many masculine traits) increase from puberty onward, so men tend to have higher blood pressure than women of the same age. This factor contributes to greater wear on the male circulatory system, sometimes increasing a man's risk for cardiovascular disease. A part of the brain that regulates emotions, the amygdala, is sensitive to testosterone. This may be one reason that men are more likely than women to find certain situations (such as social interactions) to be stressful.

Conversely, women have higher levels of oxytocin (a hormone involved in social interaction and mood regulation) and are more likely to respond to stressors by seeking social support. This coping response may give women a longevity advantage over men by decreasing the risk of some stress-related disorders. It does not, however, free women from stress-related ailments, and women are more likely than men to suffer stress-related hypertension, depression, and obesity.

connect
ACTIVITY

---

## Allostatic Load

Although the GAS model is still viewed as a key conceptual contribution to the understanding of stress, some aspects of it are considered outdated. For example, increased susceptibility to disease after repeated or prolonged stress is now thought to be due to the effects of the stress response itself rather than to a depletion of resources (exhaustion state). In particular, long-term overexposure to stress hormones such as cortisol has been linked with health problems. Further, although physical stress reactions promote homeostasis (resistance stage), they also have negative effects on the body.

The long-term wear and tear of the stress response is called the **allostatic load**. A person's allostatic load depends on many factors, including genetics, life experiences, and emotional and behavioral responses to stressors. A high allostatic load may be due to frequent stressors, poor adaptation to common stressors, an inability to shut down the stress response, or imbalances in the stress response of different body systems. High allostatic load is linked to heart disease, hypertension, obesity, and reduced brain and immune functioning. In other words, when your allostatic load exceeds your ability to cope, you are more likely to get sick.

## Psychoneuroimmunology

One of the most fruitful areas of current research into the relationship between stress and disease is **psychoneuroimmunology (PNI)**. PNI is the study of the interactions among the nervous system, the endocrine system, and the immune system. The underlying premise of PNI is that stress, through the actions of the nervous and endocrine systems, impairs the immune system and thereby affects health.

A complex network of nerve and chemical connections exists between the nervous, endocrine, and immune systems. In general, increased levels of cortisol are linked to a decreased number of immune system cells, or *lymphocytes* (see Chapter 17 for more on the immune system). Epinephrine appears to promote the release of lymphocytes but at the same time reduces their efficiency. Scientists have identified hormone-like substances called *neuropeptides* that appear to translate stressful emotions into biochemical events, some of which impact the immune system, providing a physical link between emotions and immune function.

Different types of stress may affect immunity in different ways. For instance, during **acute stress** (typically lasting between 5 and 100 minutes), white blood cells move into the skin, where they enhance the immune response. During a stressful event sequence, such as a personal trauma and the events that follow, however, there are typically no overall significant immune changes. Chronic (ongoing) stressors such as unemployment have negative effects on almost all functional measures of immunity. **Chronic stress** may cause prolonged secretion of cortisol and may accelerate the course of diseases that involve inflammation, including multiple sclerosis, heart disease, and type 2 diabetes.

Mood, personality, behavior, and immune functioning are intertwined. For example, people who are generally pessimistic may neglect the basics of health care, become passive when ill, and fail to engage in health-promoting behaviors. People who are depressed may reduce physical activity and social interaction, which may in turn affect the immune system and the cognitive appraisal of a stressor. Optimism, successful coping, and positive problem solving, on the other hand, may positively influence immunity.

## Links Between Stress and Specific Conditions

Although much remains to be learned, it is clear that people who have unresolved chronic stress in their lives or who handle stressors poorly are at risk for a wide range of health problems. In the short term, the problem might be just a cold, a stiff neck, or a stomachache. Over the long term, the problems can be more severe—cardiovascular disease (CVD), high blood pressure, impaired immune function, or a host of other problems.

> **66%** of American adults have been diagnosed with one or more chronic conditions.
>
> —American Psychological Association, 2009

**Cardiovascular Disease** During the stress response, heart rate increases and blood vessels constrict, causing blood pressure to rise. Chronic high blood pressure is a major cause of *atherosclerosis*, a disease in which blood vessels become damaged and caked with fatty deposits. These deposits can block arteries, causing heart attacks and strokes. The stress response can precipitate a heart attack in someone with atherosclerosis. The stress response can also cause stress cardiomyopathy ("broken heart syndrome"), a condition that mimics a heart attack but doesn't damage the heart.

Certain emotional responses may increase a person's risk of CVD. As described earlier, people who tend to react to situations with anger and hostility are more likely to have heart attacks than are people with less explosive, more trusting personalities.

Stress has also been linked to other risk factors for CVD, including elevated cholesterol. For example, inflammation is a key component of the damage to blood vessels that leads to heart attacks. Stress increases inflammation throughout the body. Stress-induced increases in inflammatory messenger molecules are also linked to elevated levels of homocysteine and c-reactive protein (CRP), two compounds that appear to be markers for CVD risk. Stress-related depression and anger are associated with elevated homocysteine levels, and job-related exhaustion is linked to high CRP levels in some people. Elevated CRP

## Ask yourself

QUESTIONS FOR CRITICAL THINKING AND REFLECTION

Have you ever been so stressed that you felt ill in some way? If so, what were your symptoms? How did you handle them? Did the experience affect the way you reacted to other stressful events?

**psychoneuroimmunology (PNI)** The study of the interactions among the nervous, endocrine, and immune systems.

**acute stress** Stress immediately following a stressor; may last only minutes or may turn into chronic stress.

**chronic stress** Stress that continues for days, weeks, or longer.

Ongoing stress has been shown to make people more vulnerable to everyday ailments, such as colds and allergies.

psychological problems such as depression, panic attacks, anxiety, eating disorders, and post-traumatic stress disorder (PTSD). PTSD, which afflicts war veterans, rape and child abuse survivors, and others who have suffered or witnessed severe trauma, is characterized by nightmares, flashbacks, and a diminished capacity to experience or express emotion. (For information on psychological health, see Chapter 3.)

**Altered Immune Function**    PNI research helps explain how stress affects the immune system. Some of the health problems linked to stress-related changes in immune function include vulnerability to colds and other infections, asthma and allergy attacks, susceptibility to cancer, and flare-ups of chronic diseases such as genital herpes and HIV infection.

**Other Health Problems**    Many other health problems may be caused or worsened by excessive stress, including the following:

- Digestive problems such as stomachaches, diarrhea, constipation, irritable bowel syndrome, and ulcers
- Tension headaches and migraines (see the box "Headaches: A Common Symptom of Stress")
- Insomnia and fatigue
- Injuries, including on-the-job injuries caused by repetitive strain
- Menstrual irregularities, impotence, and pregnancy complications

levels have also been implicated in insulin resistance and the development of diabetes, which is in turn a risk factor for CVD. Clearly, stress reduction can improve cardiovascular health. See Chapter 15 for more on CVD.

**Psychological Problems**    The hormones and other chemicals released during the stress response cause emotional as well as physical changes. Stress also activates the enzyme PKC, which influences the brain's prefrontal cortex. Excess PKC can negatively affect focus, judgment, and the ability to think clearly. Moreover, many stressors are inherently anxiety-producing, depressing, or both. Stress has been found to contribute to

## COMMON SOURCES OF STRESS

Recognizing potential sources of stress is an important step in successfully managing the stress in your life.

### Major Life Changes

Any major change in your life that requires adjustment and accommodation can be a source of stress. Early adulthood and the college years are associated with many significant changes, such as moving out of the family home. Even changes typically thought of as positive—graduation, job promotion, marriage—can be stressful.

Clusters of life changes, particularly those that are perceived negatively, may be linked to health problems in some people. Personality and coping skills, however, are important moderating influences. People with a strong support network and a stress-resistant personality are less likely to become ill in response to life changes than people with fewer resources.

**Headaches: A Common Symptom of Stress**

More than 45 million Americans suffer from chronic, recurrent headaches. Headaches come in various types but are often grouped into three major categories: tension headaches, migraines, and cluster headaches. Other types of headaches have underlying organic causes, such as sinus congestion or infection.

### Tension Headaches

Approximately 90% of all headaches are *tension headaches*, characterized by a dull, steady pain, usually on both sides of the head. It may feel as though a band of pressure is tightening around the head, and the pain may extend to the neck and shoulders. Acute tension headaches may last from hours to days, while chronic tension headaches may occur almost every day for months or even years.

Psychological stress, poor posture, and immobility are the leading causes of tension headaches. There is no cure, but the pain can sometimes be relieved with over-the-counter painkillers and with therapies such as massage, acupuncture, relaxation, hot or cold showers, and rest.

If your headaches are frequent, keep a diary with details about the events surrounding each one. If you can identify the stressors that are consistently associated with your headaches, you can begin to gain more control over the situation. If you suffer persistent tension headaches, you should consult your physician.

### Migraines

*Migraines* typically progress through a series of stages lasting from several minutes to several days. They may produce a variety of symptoms including throbbing pain that starts on one side of the head and may spread, heightened sensitivity to light, visual disturbances such as flashing lights, nausea, and fatigue. About 70% of migraine sufferers are women, and migraine headaches may have a genetic component.

Research suggests that people who get migraines may have abnormally excitable nerve cells in their brains. When triggered, these nerve cells send a wave of electrical activity throughout the brain, which in turn causes migraine symptoms. Potential triggers include menstruation, stress, fatigue, atmospheric changes, specific sounds or odors, and certain foods. The frequency of attacks varies from a few in a lifetime to several per week.

Keeping a headache journal can help a migraine sufferer identify headache triggers—the first step to avoiding them. In addition, many new treatments can help reduce the frequency, severity, and duration of migraines.

### Cluster Headaches

*Cluster headaches* are extremely severe headaches that cause intense pain in and around one eye. They usually occur in clusters of one to three headaches each day over a period of weeks or

months, alternating with periods of remission in which no headaches occur. About 90% of people with cluster headaches are male.

There is no known cause or cure for cluster headaches, but a number of treatments are available. During cluster periods, it is important to refrain from smoking cigarettes and drinking alcohol, because these activities can trigger attacks.

For more information on treating headaches and when a headache may signal a serious illness, see Appendix B.

## Daily Hassles

Although major life changes are stressful, they seldom occur regularly. Researchers have proposed that minor problems—life's daily hassles, such as losing your keys or wallet—can be an even greater source of stress because they occur much more often.

People who perceive hassles negatively are likely to experience a moderate stress response every time they are faced with one. Over time, this can take a significant toll on health. Studies indicate that for some people, daily hassles contribute to a general decrease in overall wellness.

## College Stressors

College is a time of major changes and minor hassles. For many students, college means being away from home and

family for the first time. Nearly all students share stresses like the following:

- *Academic stress.* Exams, grades, and an endless workload await every college student but can be especially troublesome for students just out of high school.
- *Interpersonal stress.* Most students are more than just students; they are also friends, children, employees, spouses, parents, and so on. Managing relationships while juggling the rigors of college life can be daunting, especially if some friends or family members are less than supportive.
- *Time pressures.* Class schedules, assignments, and deadlines are an inescapable part of college life. But these time pressures can be drastically compounded for students who also have a job and/or family responsibilities.

- *Financial concerns.* The majority of college students need financial aid not just to cover the cost of tuition but also to survive from day to day while in school. For many, college life isn't possible without a job, and the pressure to stay afloat financially competes with academic and other stressors.
- *Worries about the future.* As college life comes to an end, students face life after college. This means thinking about a career, choosing a place to live, and leaving the friends and routines of school behind.

As mentioned earlier, test anxiety is a source of stress for many students. To learn some proven techniques for overcoming test anxiety, see the Behavior Change Strategy at the end of this chapter.

## Job-Related Stressors

Americans rate their jobs as a key source of stress in their lives. According the 2009 Stress in America survey, about 41% of working Americans say they typically feel tense or stressed out while at work. Tight schedules and overtime leave less time to exercise, socialize, and engage in other stress-proofing activities. While daily work activities can be stressful enough on their own, stress can be even worse for people who are left out of important decisions relating to their jobs. When workers are given the opportunity to shape how their jobs are performed, job satisfaction goes up and stress levels go down.

If job-related (or college-related) stress is severe or chronic, the result can be **burnout,** a state of physical, mental, and emotional exhaustion. Burnout occurs most often in highly motivated and driven individuals who come to feel that their work is not recognized or that they are not accomplishing their goals. People in the helping professions—teachers, social workers, caregivers, police officers, and so on—are also prone to burnout. For some people who suffer from burnout, a vacation or leave of absence may be appropriate. For others, a reduced work schedule, better communication with superiors, or a change in job goals may be necessary. Improving time-management skills can also help.

## Social Stressors

Social networks can be real or virtual. Both types can help improve your ability to deal with stress, but any social network can also become a stressor in itself.

**burnout** A state of physical, mental, and emotional exhaustion.

**Real Social Networks**   Although social support is a key buffer against stress, your interactions with others can themselves be a source of stress. The college years, in particular, can be a time of great change in interpersonal relationships. The larger community where you live can also act as a stressor.

Social stressors include prejudice and discrimination. You may feel stress as you try to relate to people of other ethnic or socioeconomic groups. If you are a member of a minority ethnic group, you may feel pressure to assimilate into mainstream society, or to spend as much time as possible with others who share your ethnicity or background. If English is not your first language, you may face the added burden of conducting daily activities in a language with which you are not comfortable. All these pressures can become significant sources of stress. (See the box "Diverse Populations, Discrimination, and Stress.")

**Virtual Social Networks**   Technology can help you save time, but it can also increase stress. Being electronically connected to work, family, and friends all the time can impinge on your personal space, waste time, and distract you from your current real situation. If you are "always on"—that is, always available by voice or text messaging—some friends or colleagues may think it's all right to contact you anytime, even if you're in class or trying to work, and they may expect an immediate reponse. The convenience of staying electronically connected comes at a price.

## Environmental Stressors

Have you tried to eat at a restaurant where the food was great, but the atmosphere was so noisy that it put you on edge? This is an example of an environmental stressor—a condition or event in the physical environment that causes stress. Examples of typical environmental stressors include the following:

- Natural disasters
- Acts of violence
- Industrial accidents
- Intrusive noises or smells

Like the noisy atmosphere of some restaurants, many environmental stressors are mere inconveniences that are easy to avoid. Others, such as pollen or construction noise, may be unavoidable daily sources of stress. For those who live in poor or violent neighborhoods or in a war-torn country, environmental stressors can be major stressors (see the box "Coping After Violence on Campus").

## Internal Stressors

Some stressors are found not in our environment but within ourselves. We pressure ourselves to reach goals and

## Diverse Populations, Discrimination, and Stress

Stress is universal, but in diverse multi-ethnic and multicultural nations such as the United States, some groups face special stressors and have higher-than-average rates of stress-related physical and emotional problems. These groups include ethnic minorities, the poor, those with physical or mental disabilities, and those with atypical sexual orientations.

Discrimination occurs when people speak or act according to their prejudices—biased, negative beliefs or attitudes toward some group. Blatant examples are painting a swastika on a Jewish studies house or defacing a sculpture depicting a same-sex couple holding hands. More subtle examples are when an African American student notices that white shopkeepers in a mostly white college town tend to keep a close eye on him, a male-to-female transgender individual is treated with less respect by her professors and peers, a student using a wheelchair finds no accessible bathrooms, or an obese woman overhears remarks about eating and self-control.

Recent immigrants to the United States have to learn to live in a new society. This requires a balance between assimilating and changing to be like the majority, and maintaining a connection to their own culture, language, and religion. The process of acculturation is generally stressful, especially when the person's background is radically different from that of the people he or she is now living among. Parental expectations generate stress if they are too high or too low. If too high, the child may work too hard in an attempt to succeed at everything; if too low, the child may not work hard enough to succeed at anything.

Both immigrants and minorities that have lived for generations in the United States can face job- and school-related stressors because of stereotypes and discrimination. They may make less money in comparable jobs with comparable levels of education and may find it more difficult to achieve leadership positions.

However, on a positive note, many who experience hardship, disability,

or prejudice develop effective, goal-directed coping skills and are successful at overcoming obstacles and managing the stress they face.

---

continually evaluate our progress and performance. Striving to reach goals can enhance self-esteem if the goals are reasonable. Unrealistic expectations, however, can be a significant source of stress and can damage self-esteem. Other internal stressors are physical and emotional states such as illness and exhaustion; these can be both a cause and an effect of unmanaged stress.

> *Some stressors are found within ourselves.*

## MANAGING STRESS

You can control the stress in your life by taking the following steps:

- Shore up your support system
- Improve your communication skills
- Develop healthy exercise, eating, and sleeping habits
- Learn to identify and moderate individual stressors

The effort required is well worth the time. People who manage stress effectively not only are healthier but have more time to enjoy life and accomplish goals.

### Social Support

Having the support of friends and family members seems to contribute to the well-being of body and mind. Research supports this conclusion, as the following examples demonstrate:

- Among college students living in overcrowded apartments, a study revealed that those students with a strong social support system were less distressed by their cramped quarters than were the loners who navigated life's challenges on their own.
- Young adults who have strong relationships with their parents tend to cope with stress better than peers with poor parental relationships.
- Many studies show that married people live longer than single people (including those who are divorced, widowed, or never married) and have lower death rates from practically all causes.

## Coping After Violence on Campus

Stories of violence on American campuses have become all too familiar:

• In May 2010, a University of Virginia student was beaten to death. Shortly afterwards, her boyfriend was arrested and charged with her murder.

• In December 2009, a disgruntled student opened fire in class at Northern Virginia Community College, apparently trying to shoot the teacher. No one was injured in the shooting.

• In March 2008, an Auburn University student died from gunshot wounds sustained during a robbery. A day later, a University of North Carolina student was killed while being robbed.

• On February 14, 2008, a former Northern Illinois University student walked into one of the school's lecture halls and fatally shot five students before killing himself. Gunfire injured at least 16 other people.

• On April 16, 2007, a student killed 28 students and 5 teachers and injured 29 others during two attacks at Virginia Polytechnic Institute and State University (Virginia Tech). The attacker was acting out fantasies of revenge in a drama that held the nation's attention for weeks.

School shootings are not uniquely American events. They also occur at schools in other countries, including countries where access to guns is much more tightly controlled than in the United States.

People react to news of school violence in different ways, depending on

their proximity to the event and its recency. In the case of school massacres, people far from the site may suffer emotional reactions simply from watching endless coverage on television.

Responses to violence include disbelief, shock, fear, anger, resentment, anxiety, mood swings, irritability, sadness, depression, panic, guilt, apathy, feelings of isolation or powerlessness, and many of the symptoms of excess stress. Some people affected by such violence develop post-traumatic stress disorder (PTSD), a more serious condition.

In the case of the Virginia Tech shootings, the school and community mobi-

lized quickly to respond to the expected surge in behavioral health needs generated by the attack. Hotline calls and emergency room visits increased dramatically, especially during the second and third weeks following the shootings. Information sources and support groups were established for people grieving the loss of friends, family, neighbors, or colleagues. Volunteers contacted each family that was directly affected by the shootings to offer help in making arrangements and other services.

If you are affected by a disastrous event such as a school shooting or terrorist attack, take these steps:

• Be sure that you have the best information about what happened, whether a continuing risk is present, and what you can do to avoid it. That information may be posted on Web sites or on local radio or TV stations.

• Don't expose yourself to so much media coverage that it overwhelms you.

• Take care of yourself. Use the stress-relief techniques discussed in this chapter.

• Share your feelings and concerns with others. Be a supportive listener.

• If you feel able, help others in any way you can, such as by volunteering to work with victims.

• If you feel emotionally distressed days or weeks after the event, consider asking for professional help.

---

Social support can provide a critical counterbalance to the stress in our lives. Give yourself time to develop and maintain a network of people you can count on for emotional support, feedback, and nurturing. If you believe you don't have enough social support, consider becoming a volunteer to help build your network of friends and to enhance your spiritual wellness (see the box "Altruism: Is Doing Good Good for Your Health?").

## Communication

Communicating in an assertive way that respects the rights of others—while protecting your own rights—can prevent stressful situations from getting out of control.

Some people have trouble either telling others what they need or saying no to the needs of others. They may suppress their feelings of anger, frustration, and resentment, and they may end up feeling taken advantage of or suffering in unhealthy relationships. At the other extreme are people who express anger openly and directly by being verbally or physically aggressive or indirectly by making critical, hurtful comments to others. Their abusive behavior pushes other people away, so they also have problems with relationships.

Better communication skills can help everyone form and maintain healthy relationships. Chapter 3 includes a detailed discussion of anger and its impact on health and relationships. Chapter 4 discusses strategies for building healthy relationships, including positive communication techniques.

## Altruism: Is Doing Good Good for Your Health?

Ethics and religion have long told us that it is more blessed to give than to receive. Now scientists from many disciplines are finding empirical support for the notion that altruism—unselfish love and giving—benefits the giver at least as much as the receiver. These benefits come in the form of better psychological health, better physical health, and longer life.

One study of more than 7000 older adults over the age of 70 found that volunteering was associated with delayed mortality—that is, the more frequently people volunteered, the longer they lived compared with people who didn't volunteer. Another study found that longer life was associated with more years of volunteering, suggesting that people who start giving early in life reap benefits over their lifetime. In surveys, people who volunteer report fewer colds and headaches, improved sleeping and eating patterns, and some relief from the discomfort of chronic diseases such as asthma and arthritis.

What is the chain of events leading from altruism to health benefits, from volunteering to improved well-being, better health, and longer life? Scientists have proposed several mechanisms:

- Better immune system functioning. Altruistic love may block or reduce the stress response, which is known to suppress the immune system. A healthier immune system is more effective at fighting off infection and illness.

- Better cardiovascular health. The stress response also affects the cardiovascular system, increasing heart rate and raising blood pressure. Altruistic love may protect the heart and blood vessels from the damaging effects of stress.

- Activation of the relaxation response. Altruistic love may activate the relaxation response, the opposite of the stress response, inducing feelings of warmth, calm, and happiness. This response may be mediated by the release of hormones and neurotransmitters.

- Pain relief. Altruistic love may reduce sensations of pain by inducing the release of endorphins, brain chemicals that block pain and produce feelings of euphoria. Endorphins may account for the experience known as "helper's high," similar to "runner's high," which makes people feel happier, stronger, and more energetic.

- Increase in the frequency and depth of positive emotions, such as happiness and calmness. Positive emotions may reduce the burden of psychological and physiological stress and thereby provide benefits for health-related physiological processes.

- Increased self-esteem and positive beliefs about self-efficacy and self-worth.

- Better overall mental health. The combination of positive feelings and increased self-esteem are conducive to

improved mental health. Part of the effect may come from reducing self-absorption, taking an outward focus, and shifting attention away from the individual's perceived problems.

- Better social integration, more social support. Volunteering provides people with meaningful social roles and a sense of purpose, as well as opportunities for social contact. For older adults, volunteering can enhance a shift toward developmentally appropriate goals, such as giving back and being generative, in contrast to an earlier focus on career.

- Improved spiritual health. Altruism provides an avenue for putting deeply felt values into practice.

Studies show that not all giving is the same—for example, donating money does not have the same beneficial health effects as volunteering that involves personal contact. A few simple guidelines can help you get the most out of giving:

- Choose a volunteer activity that puts you in contact with people.

- Make helping voluntary. Obligatory helping can actually increase stress levels.

- Volunteer with a group. Sharing your interests with other volunteers increases social support. Volunteering seems to have the most benefits for people who also have other close relationships and social interests.

- Know your limits. Helping that goes beyond what you can handle depletes your own resources and is detrimental to your health.

If you want to incorporate more giving and helping into your life, look for opportunities to volunteer on your campus or in your community. Many colleges have lists of volunteer opportunities, ranging from tutoring to assisting in community gardens. If your schedule doesn't allow volunteering at this time, you can still help others with small acts of kindness, empathy, and compassion, such as listening to a friend's problems or writing a note to an aging relative. Getting in the habit of helping now can set you on a lifetime course of health-promoting altruistic actions.

SOURCES: Harris, A. H. S., and C. E. Thoresen. 2005. Volunteering is associated with delayed mortality in older people: Analysis of the Longitudinal Study of Aging. *Journal of Health Psychology* 10(6), 739–752; Sternberg, E. M. 2001. Approaches to defining mechanisms by which altruistic love affects health. Research Topic White Paper #3, Institute for Research on Unlimited Love, Altruism, Compassion, Service (http://www.altruists.org/f72; retrieved October 20, 2010); Pembroke, G. 2007. Compassion Rx: The many health benefits of altruism (http://epages.wordpress.com/2007/10/26/compassion-rx-the-many-health-benefits-of-altruism; retrieved October 20, 2010).

## Ask yourself

**QUESTIONS FOR CRITICAL THINKING AND REFLECTION**

What are the top two or three stressors in your life right now? Are they new to your life—as part of your college experience—or are they stressors you've experienced in the past? Do they include both positive and negative experiences (eustress and distress)?

## Exercise

Exercise helps maintain a healthy body and mind and even stimulates the birth of new brain cells. Regular physical activity can also reduce many of the negative effects of stress. Consider the following examples:

- Taking a long walk can help decrease anxiety and blood pressure.
- A brisk 10-minute walk can leave you feeling more relaxed and energetic for up to 2 hours.
- People who exercise regularly react with milder physical stress responses before, during, and after exposure to stressors.
- In a study, people who took three brisk 45-minute walks each week for 3 months reported fewer daily hassles and an increased sense of wellness.

These findings should not be surprising, because the stress response mobilizes energy resources and readies the body for physical emergencies. If you experience stress and do not physically exert yourself, you are not completing the energy cycle. You may not be able to exercise while your daily stressors occur—during class, for example, or while sitting in a traffic jam—but you can be active at other times of the day. Physical activity allows you to expend the nervous energy you have built up and trains your body to more readily achieve homeostasis following stressful situations.

It isn't hard to incorporate light to moderate exercise into your day. The important thing is to find an activity that you enjoy, so it can become a habit and a regular stress reducer.

For some people, however, exercise can become just one more stressor in a highly stressed life. People who exercise compulsively risk overtraining, a condition characterized by fatigue, irritability, depression, and diminished athletic performance. An overly strenuous exercise program can even make you sick by compromising your immune function. (For details on creating a safe and effective exercise program, see Chapter 13.)

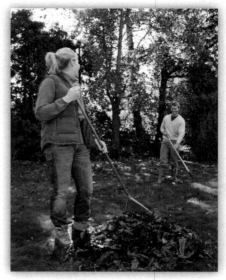

Exercise—even light activity—can be an effective antidote to stress.

## Nutrition

A healthy diet gives you an energy bank to draw from whenever you experience stress. Eating wisely also can enhance your feelings of self-control and self-esteem. Learning the principles of sound nutrition is easy, and sensible eating habits rapidly become second nature when practiced regularly. (For information on nutrition and healthy eating habits, see Chapter 12.)

For the purposes of managing stress, you may find it especially helpful to limit or avoid caffeine. Although one or two cups of coffee a day probably won't hurt you, caffeine is a mildly addictive stimulant that leaves some people jittery, irritable, and unable to sleep. Consuming caffeine during stressful situations can raise blood pressure and increase levels of cortisol.

While your diet has an effect on the way your body handles stress, the reverse is also true. Excess stress can negatively affect the way you eat. Many people, for example, respond to stress by overeating; other people skip meals or stop eating altogether during stressful periods. Both responses are not only ineffective (they don't address the causes of stress), but potentially unhealthy.

## Sleep

Most adults need 7–9 hours of sleep every night to stay healthy and perform their best. Getting enough sleep isn't just good for you physically. Adequate sleep also improves mood, fosters feelings of competence and self-worth, enhances mental functioning, and supports emotional functioning.

**How Sleep Works** Sleep occurs in two phases: **rapid eye movement (REM) sleep** and **non–rapid eye movement (NREM) sleep.** A sleeper goes through several cycles of non-REM and REM sleep each night.

NREM sleep actually includes four stages of successively deeper sleep. As you move through these stages of sleep, a variety of physiological changes occur, including the following:

- Blood pressure drops.
- Respiration and heart rates slow.
- Body temperature declines.
- Growth hormone is released.
- Brain wave patterns become slow and even.

During REM sleep, dreams occur. REM sleep is characterized by the rapid movement of the eyes under closed eyelids. Heart rate, blood pressure, and breathing rate rise, and brain activity increases to levels equal to or greater than those during waking hours. Muscles in the limbs relax completely, resulting in a temporary paralysis. (This total relaxation may prevent you from acting out your dreams while you're asleep.)

**Sleep and Stress** Stress hormone levels in the bloodstream vary throughout the day and are related to sleep patterns. Peak concentrations occur in the early morning, followed by a slow decline during the day and evening. Concentrations return to peak levels during the final stages of sleep and in the early morning hours. Stress hormone levels are low during non-REM sleep and increase during REM sleep. With each successive sleep cycle during the night, REM sleep lasts a little longer. This increase in REM sleep duration with each sleep cycle may underlie the progressive increase in circulating stress hormones during the final stages of sleep.

Even though stress hormones are released during sleep, it is the *lack* of sleep that has the greatest impact on

> *Most adults need 7–9 hours of sleep every night to stay healthy and perform their best.*

stress. In someone who is suffering from **sleep deprivation** (not getting enough sleep over time), mental and physical processes steadily deteriorate. A sleep-deprived person experiences headaches, feels irritable, is unable to concentrate, and is more prone to forgetfulness. Poor-quality sleep has long been associated with stress and depression. A small 2008 study of female college students further associated sleep deprivation with an increased risk of suicide.

Acute sleep deprivation slows the daytime decline in stress hormones, so evening levels are higher than normal. A decrease in total sleep time also causes an increase in the level of stress hormones. Together, these changes may cause an increase in stress hormone levels throughout the day and may contribute to physical and mental exhaustion. Extreme sleep deprivation can lead to hallucinations and other psychotic symptoms, as well as to a significant increase in heart attack risk.

**Sleep Problems** According to the National Sleep Foundation's 2009 Sleep in America Poll, 20% of American adults sleep an average of less than 6 hours per night. (Compare this to the recommended 7–9 hours per night.) Although many of us can attribute the lack of sleep to long work days and family responsibilities, as many as 70 million Americans suffer from chronic sleep disorders—medical conditions that prevent them from sleeping well.

According to National Sleep Foundation polls, more than 50% of adults report having trouble falling asleep or staying asleep—a condition called **insomnia.** The most common causes of insomnia are lifestyle factors, such as high caffeine or alcohol intake before bedtime; medical problems, such as a breathing disorder; and stress. About 75% of people who suffer from chronic insomnia report some stressful life event at the onset of their sleeping problems. (For more information, see the box "Overcoming Insomnia.")

TERMS

**rapid eye movement (REM) sleep**   The portion of the sleep cycle during which dreaming occurs.

**non-rapid eye movement (non-REM) sleep**   The portion of the sleep cycle that involves deep sleep; non-REM sleep includes four states of successively deeper sleep.

**sleep deprivation**   A lack of sleep over a period of time.

**insomnia**   A sleep problem involving the inability to fall or stay asleep.

# Overcoming Insomnia

Most people can overcome insomnia by discovering the cause of poor sleep and taking steps to remedy it. If your insomnia lasts more than 6 months and interferes with daytime functioning, you should probably talk to a sleep specialist in a medical center. Sleeping pills are not recommended for chronic insomnia because they can be habit-forming; they also lose their effectiveness over time.

If you're bothered by insomnia, try the following:

• Determine how much sleep you need to feel refreshed the next day, and don't sleep longer than that.

• Go to bed at the same time every night and, more important, get up at the same time every morning, 7 days a week, regardless of how much sleep you got. Don't nap during the day if you can help it. If you fall asleep in the afternoon, make the nap short—less than 30 minutes.

• Exercise every day, but not too close to bedtime. Your metabolism takes up to 6 hours to slow down after exercise.

• Avoid caffeine late in the day, and alcohol before bedtime (it causes disturbed, fragmented sleep). If you take any medications (prescription or not), ask your doctor or pharmacist if they are known to interfere with sleep.

• Do what you can to make your sleeping environment quiet, dark, and a comfortable temperature. Overhearing music or talking can make it hard to sleep.

• Have a light snack before bedtime; you'll sleep better if you're not hungry.

• Use your bed only for sleep. Don't eat, read, study, or watch television in bed.

• Relax before bedtime with a bath, a book, music, or relaxation exercises.

• If you don't fall asleep in 15–20 minutes, or if you wake up and can't fall asleep again, get out of bed, leave the room if possible, and do something monotonous until you feel sleepy. Try distracting yourself with imagery; imagine yourself on a pleasant vacation or enjoying some beautiful scenery. Don't turn on bright lights or watch TV.

• If sleep problems persist, ask your physician for a referral to a sleep specialist in your area. You may be a candidate for a sleep study—an overnight evaluation of your sleep pattern that can uncover many sleep-related disorders.

---

Another type of chronic sleep problem, called **sleep apnea**, occurs when a person stops breathing while asleep. Apnea can be caused by a number of factors, but it typically results when the soft tissue at the back of the mouth (such as the tongue or soft palate) "collapses" during sleep, blocking the airway (Figure 2.4). When breathing is interrupted, so is sleep, as the sleeper awakens repeatedly throughout the night to begin breathing again. In most cases, this occurs without the sleeper's even being aware of it. However, the disruption to sleep can be significant, and over time acute sleep deprivation can result from apnea. There are several treatments for apnea, including the use of medications, a special apparatus that helps keep the airway open during sleep, and surgery.

## Time Management

Learning to manage your time can be crucial to coping with everyday stressors. Overcommitment, procrastination, and even boredom are significant stressors for many people. Along with gaining control of nutrition and exercise to maintain a healthy energy balance, time management is an important element in a wellness

program. Try these strategies for improving your time-management skills:

• *Set priorities.* Divide your tasks into three groups: essential, important, and trivial. Focus on the first two, and ignore the third.

• *Schedule tasks for peak efficiency.* You've undoubtedly noticed you're most productive at certain times of the day (or night). Schedule as many of your tasks for those hours as you can, and stick to your schedule.

• *Set realistic goals and write them down.* Attainable goals spur you on. Impossible goals, by definition, cause frustration and failure. Fully commit yourself to achieving your goals by putting them in writing.

• *Budget enough time.* For each project you undertake, calculate how long it will take to complete. Then tack on another 10–15%, or even 25%, as a buffer.

• *Break up long-term goals into short-term ones.* Instead of waiting for large blocks of time, use short amounts of time to start a project or keep it moving.

• *Visualize the achievement of your goals.* By mentally rehearsing your performance of a task, you will be able to reach your goal more smoothly.

• *Keep track of the tasks you put off.* Analyze the reasons you procrastinate. If the task is difficult or unpleasant, look for ways to make it easier or more fun.

• *Consider doing your least-favorite tasks first.* Once you have the most unpleasant ones out of the way, you can work on the tasks you enjoy more.

• *Consolidate tasks when possible.* For example, try walking to the store so that you run your errands and exercise in the same block of time.

**sleep apnea**   The interruption of normal breathing during sleep.

Tongue — Soft palate
Uvula

Blocked airway

**FIGURE 2.4 Sleep apnea.** Sleep apnea occurs when soft tissues surrounding the airway relax, "collapsing" the airway and restricting airflow.

• *Identify quick transitional tasks.* Keep a list of 5- to 10-minute tasks you can do while waiting or between other tasks, such as watering your plants, doing the dishes, or checking a homework assignment.

• *Delegate responsibility.* Asking for help when you have too much to do is no cop-out; it's good time management. Just don't delegate the jobs you know you should do yourself.

• *Say no when necessary.* If the demands made on you don't seem reasonable, say no—tactfully, but without guilt or apology.

• *Give yourself a break.* Allow time for play—free, unstructured time when you can ignore the clock. Don't consider this a waste of time. Play renews you and enables you to work more efficiently.

• *Avoid your personal "time sinks."* You can probably identify your own time sinks—activities, like watching television, surfing the Internet, or talking on the phone, that consistently use up more time than you anticipate and put you behind schedule. Some days, it may be best to avoid problematic activities altogether; for example, if you have a big paper due, don't sit down for a 5-minute TV break if it is likely to turn into a 2-hour break. Try a 5-minute walk if you need to clear your head.

• *Stop thinking or talking about what you're going to do, and just do it!* Sometimes the best solution for procrastination is to stop waiting for the right moment and just get started. You will probably find that things are not as bad as you feared, and your momentum will keep you going.

## Striving for Spiritual Wellness

Spiritual wellness is associated with greater coping skills and higher levels of overall wellness. It is a very personal wellness component, and there are many ways to develop it (see the box "Paths to Spiritual Wellness"). Researchers have linked spiritual wellness to longer life expectancy, reduced risk of disease, faster recovery, and improved emotional health. Although spirituality is difficult to study, and researchers aren't sure how or why spirituality seems to improve health, several explanations have been offered.

• *Social support.* Attending religious services or participating in volunteer organizations helps people feel that they are part of a community with similar values and promotes social connectedness and caring.

• *Healthy habits.* Some of the paths to spiritual wellness may encourage healthy behaviors, such as eating a vegetarian diet or consuming less meat and alcohol, and may discourage harmful habits like smoking.

• *Positive attitude.* Spirituality can give a person a sense of meaning and purpose in life, and these qualities create a more positive attitude in the person, which in turn helps her or him cope with life's challenges.

• *Moments of relaxation.* Spiritual practices such as prayer, meditation, and immersion in artistic activities can reduce stress by eliciting the relaxation response.

Spirituality provides an ethical path to personal fulfillment that includes connectedness with self, others, and a higher power or larger reality. Spiritual wellness can make you more aware of your personal values and can help clarify them. Without an awareness of personal values, you might be driven by immediate desires and the passing demands of others. Living according to values means considering your options carefully before making a choice, choosing between options without succumbing

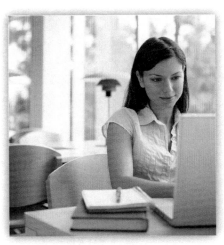

Managing the many commitments of adult life—including work, school, and parenthood—can sometimes feel overwhelming and produce a great deal of stress. Time-management and problem-solving skills, including careful scheduling with a date book or handheld computer, can help people cope with busy days.

## Paths to Spiritual Wellness

Spiritual wellness means different things to different people. For many, it involves developing a set of guiding beliefs, principles, or values that give purpose and meaning to life. It helps people achieve a sense of wholeness within themselves and in their relationships with others. Spiritual wellness influences people on an individual level, as well as on a community level, where it can bond people together through compassion, love, forgiveness, and self-sacrifice.

There are many paths to spiritual wellness. One of the most common is organized religion. The major religions provide paths for transforming the self in ways that can lead to greater happiness and serenity and reduce feelings of anxiety and hopelessness. For example, in Christianity, salvation means turning away from the selfish ego and to God's sovereignty and grace, where a joy is found that frees the believer from anxious self-concern and despair. *Islam* is the word for a kind of self-surrender leading to peace with God. Buddhism teaches how to detach oneself from selfish desire, leading to compassion for the suffering of others and freedom from fear-engendering illusions. Judaism emphasizes the social and ethical redemption the Jewish community can experience if it follows the laws of God.

Religions teach specific techniques for achieving these transformations of the self: prayer, both in groups and in private;

meditation; the performance of rituals and ceremonies symbolizing religious truths; and good works and service to others. Religious organizations also usually offer social and material support to members who might otherwise be isolated.

Spiritual wellness does not require participation in organized religion. Many people find meaning and purpose in other ways. By spending time in nature or working on environmental issues, people can experience continuity with the natural world. Spiritual wellness can come through helping others in one's community or by promoting human rights, peace and harmony among people, and opportunities for human development on a global level. Other people develop spiritual wellness through art or through their personal relationships.

How would you define spiritual wellness and its role in your life? What beliefs and practices do you associate with your sense of spiritual wellness? To achieve overall well-being, it is important to take time out to consider what you can do to help your spiritual side flourish.

---

to outside pressures that oppose your values, and making a choice and acting on it rather than doing nothing.

## Confiding in Yourself Through Writing

Keeping a diary is analogous to confiding in others, except that you are confiding in yourself. This form of coping with severe stress may be especially helpful for those who are shy or introverted and find it difficult to open up to others. Although writing about traumatic and stressful events may have a short-term negative effect on mood, over the long term, stress is reduced and positive changes in health occur. A key to promoting health and well-being through journaling is to write about your emotional responses to stressful events. Set aside a special time each day or week to write down your feelings about stressful events in your life.

## Cognitive Techniques

Some stressors arise in our own minds. Ideas, beliefs, perceptions, and patterns of thinking can add to our stress level. Each of the following techniques can help you change unhealthy thought patterns to ones that will help you cope with stress. As with any skill, mastering these techniques takes practice and patience.

**Think and Act Constructively** Think back to the worries you had last week. How many of them were needless? Think about things you *can* control. Try to stand aside from the problem, consider the positive steps you can take

to solve it, and then carry them out. Remember, if you can successfully predict that a stressor will occur, you can better control your response to it. In the evening, try to predict stressful events you might encounter the following day. Then decide how to handle them constructively. This may mean dealing positively with an unpleasant person or figuring out how to stay focused during a boring class. By taking a constructive approach, you can prevent stressors from becoming negative events and perhaps even turn them into positive experiences.

**Take Control** A situation often feels more stressful if you feel you're not in control of it. Time may seem to be slipping away before a big exam, for example. Unexpected obstacles may appear in your path, throwing you off course. When you feel your environment is controlling you instead of the other way around, take charge! Concentrate on what is possible to control, and set realistic goals. Be confident of your ability to succeed.

**Problem-Solve** Students with greater problem-solving abilities report easier adjustment to university life, higher motivation levels, lower stress levels, and higher grades. When you find yourself stewing over a problem, sit down with a piece of paper and do some problem solving. Try this approach:

1. Define the problem in one or two sentences.
2. Identify the causes of the problem.

3. Consider alternative solutions; don't just stop with the most obvious one.
4. Weigh positive and negative consequences for each alternative.
5. Make a decision—choose a solution.
6. Make a list of tasks you must perform to act on your decision.
7. Begin to carry out your list; if you're unable to do that, temporarily turn to other things.
8. Evaluate the outcome and revise your approach if necessary.

**Modify Your Expectations**   Expectations are exhausting and restricting. The fewer expectations you have, the more you can live spontaneously and joyfully. The more you expect from others, the more often you will feel let down. And trying to meet the expectations others have of you is often futile.

**Stay Positive**   If you beat up on yourself—"Late for class again! You can't even cope with college! How do you expect to ever hold down a professional job?"—change your inner dialogue. Talk to yourself as you would to a child you love: "You're a smart, capable person. You've solved other problems; you'll handle this one. Tomorrow you'll simply schedule things so you get to class with a few minutes to spare." (Chapter 3 has more information on self-talk.)

*Problem-solving skills can improve your motivation, stress level, and grades.*

**Practice Affirmations**   One way of cultivating the positive is to systematically repeat positive thoughts, or *affirmations*, to yourself. For example, if you react to stress with low self-esteem, you might repeat sentences such as "I approve and accept myself completely" and "It doesn't matter what others say, but what I believe." Saying affirmations to yourself every day may make them automatic and help you change the way you react.

**Cultivate Your Sense of Humor**   When it comes to stress, laughter may be the best medicine. Even a fleeting smile produces changes in your autonomic nervous system that can lift your spirits. And a few minutes of belly laughing can be as invigorating as brisk exercise. Hearty laughter elevates your heart rate, aids digestion, eases pain, and triggers the release of endorphins and other pleasurable and stimulating chemicals in the brain. After a good laugh, your muscles go slack; your pulse and blood pressure dip below normal. You are relaxed. Cultivate the ability to laugh at yourself, and you'll have a handy and instantly effective stress reliever.

**Focus on What's Important**   A major source of stress is trying to store too much data. Forget unimportant details (they will usually be self-evident) and organize important information. One technique you can try is to "chunk" the important material into categories. If your next exam covers three chapters from your textbook, consider each chapter a chunk of information. Then break down each chunk into its three or four most important features. Create a mental outline that allows you to trace your way from the most general category down to the most specific details. This technique can be applied to managing daily responsibilities as well.

## Relaxation Techniques

The **relaxation response** is a physiological state characterized by a feeling of warmth and quiet mental alertness. This is the opposite of the fight-or-flight reaction. When the relaxation response is triggered by a relaxation technique, heart rate, breathing, and metabolism slow down. Blood pressure and oxygen consumption decrease. At the same time, blood flow to the brain and skin increases, and brain waves shift from an alert beta rhythm to a relaxed alpha rhythm. Practiced regularly, relaxation techniques can counteract the debilitating effects of stress.

If you decide to try a relaxation technique, practice it daily until it becomes natural to you, and then use it whenever you feel the need. You may feel calmer and more refreshed after each session. You'll know you've mastered a deep relaxation technique when you start to see subtle changes in other areas of your life: You may notice you've been encountering fewer hassles, working more efficiently, or enjoying more free time. None of the techniques takes long to do.

**Progressive Relaxation**   Unlike most of the other methods of relaxation, progressive relaxation requires no imagination, willpower, or self-suggestion. You simply tense and relax the muscles in your body, group by group. The technique, also known as deep muscle relaxation, helps you become aware of the muscle tension that occurs when you're under stress. When you consciously relax those muscles, other systems of the body get the message and ease up on the stress response.

Start, for example, with your right fist. Inhale as you tense it. Exhale as you relax it. Repeat. Next, contract and relax your right upper arm. Repeat. Do the same with your left arm. Then, beginning at your forehead and ending at your feet, contract and relax your other muscle groups. Repeat each contraction at least once, breathing in as you tense, breathing out as you relax. To speed up

> **relaxation response**   A physiological state characterized by a feeling of warmth and quiet mental alertness.

# Meditation and the Relaxation Response

Here is a simple technique for eliciting the relaxation response.

## The Basic Technique

1. Pick a word, phrase, or object to focus on. If you like, you can choose a word or phrase that has a deep meaning for you, but any word or phrase will work. Some meditators prefer to focus on their breathing.

2. Take a comfortable position in a quiet environment, and close your eyes if you aren't focusing on an object.

3. Relax your muscles.

4. Breathe slowly and naturally. If you're using a focus word or phrase, silently repeat it each time you exhale. If you're using an object, focus on it as you breathe.

5. Keep a passive attitude. Disregard thoughts that drift in.

6. Continue for 10–20 minutes, once or twice a day.

7. When you're finished, sit quietly for a few minutes with your eyes first closed and then open. Then stand up.

## Suggestions

- Allow relaxation to occur at its own pace; don't try to force it. Don't be surprised if you can't quiet your mind for more than a few seconds at a time; it's not a reason for anger or frustration. The more you ignore the intrusions, the easier doing so will become.

- If you want to time your session, peek at a watch or clock occasionally, but don't set a jarring alarm.

- The technique works best on an empty stomach, before a meal or about 2 hours after eating. Avoid times of day when you're tired—unless you want to fall asleep.

- Although you'll feel refreshed even after the first session, it may take a month or more to get noticeable results. Be patient. Eventually the relaxation response will become so natural that it will occur spontaneously, or on demand, when you sit quietly for a few moments.

---

the process, tense and relax more muscles at one time—both arms simultaneously, for instance. With practice, you'll be able to relax very quickly and effectively by clenching and releasing only your fists.

**Visualization** Also known as *imagery,* **visualization** lets you daydream without guilt. Athletes find that the technique enhances sports performance, and visualization is even part of the curriculum at U.S. Olympic training camps. You can use visualization to help you relax, change your habits, or perform well—whether on an exam, a stage, or a playing field.

Next time you feel stressed, close your eyes. Imagine yourself floating on a cloud, sitting on a mountaintop, or lying in a meadow. Involve all your senses; imagine the sounds, the smells, and the other sensations that would be part of the scene. Your body will respond as if the imagery were real. An alternative: Close your eyes and imagine a deep purple light filling your body. Now change the color into a soothing gold. As the color lightens, so should your distress.

Visualization can also be used to rehearse for an upcoming event and enhance performance. By experiencing an event ahead of time in your mind, you can practice coping with any difficulties that may arise. Think positively, and you can "psych yourself up" for a successful experience.

**Meditation** The need to periodically stop our incessant mental chatter is so great that, from ancient times, hundreds of forms of **meditation** have developed in cultures all over the world. Meditation is a way of telling the mind to be quiet for a while. Because meditation has been at the core of many Eastern religions and philosophies, it has acquired an "Eastern" mystique that has caused some people to shy away from it. Yet meditation requires no special knowledge or background. Whatever philosophical, religious, or emotional reasons may be given for meditation, it is potentially useful for reducing stress. According to a 2008 study, college students who learned how to use meditation for stress management were able to significantly reduce their daily stress levels. Further, those students found it easier to forgive others for perceived wrongdoings and spent less time focusing on negative thoughts.

Meditation helps you tune out the world temporarily, removing you from both internal and external sources of stress. The "thinker" takes time out to become the "observer"—calmly attentive, without analyzing, judging, comparing, or rationalizing. Regular practice of this quiet awareness will subtly carry over into your daily life, encouraging physical and emotional balance no matter what confronts you. For a step-by-step description of a basic meditation technique, see the box "Meditation and the Relaxation Response."

Another form of meditation, known as *mindfulness meditation,* involves paying attention to physical sensations, perceptions, thoughts, and imagery. Instead of focusing on a word or object to quiet the mind, you observe thoughts that occur without evaluating or judging them. Development of this ability requires regular practice but may eventually result in a more objective view of one's perceptions. It is believed that a greater understanding of one's moment-to-moment thought processes (mindful awareness) provides a richer and more vital sense of life and improves coping. Studies also suggest that people who rate high in mindfulness are less anxious and better able to deal with stress; among people with specific health problems, mindfulness can provide substantial benefits.

**Deep Breathing**  Your breathing pattern is closely tied to your stress level. Deep, slow breathing is associated with relaxation. Rapid, shallow, often irregular breathing occurs during the stress response. With practice, you can learn to slow and quiet your breathing pattern, thereby also quieting your mind and relaxing your body. Breathing techniques can be used for on-the-spot tension relief as well as for long-term stress reduction.

The primary goal of many breathing exercises is to change your breathing pattern from chest breathing to diaphragmatic ("belly") breathing. (The diaphragm is a sheet of muscle and connective tissue that divides the chest and abdominal cavities.) Except when sleeping, most adults breathe by expanding their chest and raising their shoulders rather than by expanding their abdomen. Diaphragmatic breathing is slower and deeper than chest breathing. To practice diaphragmatic breathing, lie on your back and place one hand on your chest and one hand on your abdomen to monitor your breathing. Take a slow, deep breath through your nose and into your belly. Your abdomen should rise significantly and your chest only slightly. Think of filling your belly with air. Exhale gently through your mouth. Once you become familiar with belly breathing, you can use it anywhere, any time, to dispel tension and stress.

**Yoga**  Hatha yoga, the most common yoga style practiced in the United States, emphasizes physical balance and breath control. It integrates components of flexibility, muscular strength and endurance, and muscle relaxation; it also sometimes serves as a preliminary to meditation. A session of yoga typically involves a series of postures, each held for a few seconds to several minutes, which involve stretching and balance and coordinated breathing. Yoga can induce the relaxation response and promote body awareness and flexibility. If you are interested in trying yoga, it's best to take a class from an experienced instructor.

**Tai chi**  This martial art (in Chinese, *taijiquan*) is a system of self-defense that incorporates philosophical concepts from Taoism and Confucianism. In addition to self-defense, tai chi aims to bring the body into balance and harmony to promote health and spiritual growth. It teaches practitioners to remain calm and centered, to conserve and concentrate

Listening to soothing music leads to reduced levels of the stress hormone cortisol.

energy, and to manipulate force by becoming part of it—by "going with the flow." Tai chi is considered the gentlest of the martial arts. Instead of quick and powerful movements, tai chi consists of a series of slow, fluid, elegant movements, which reinforce the idea of moving *with* rather than *against* the stressors of everyday life. As with yoga, it's best to start tai chi with a class led by an experienced instructor.

**Listening to Music**  Listening to music is another method of inducing relaxation. It can influence pulse, blood pressure, and the electrical activity of muscles. Studies of newborns and hospitalized stroke patients have shown that listening to soothing, lyrical music can lessen depression, anxiety, and stress levels. Researchers have found that exposure to soothing music leads to reduced levels of the stress hormone cortisol and causes changes in the electrical activity in the brain.

To experience the stress-management benefits of music yourself, set aside a time to listen. Choose music that you enjoy and that makes you feel relaxed.

**Biofeedback**  Biofeedback helps people reduce the stress response by enabling them to become more

**biofeedback**  A technique in which monitoring devices help a person become conscious of unconscious body processes, such as body temperature or blood pressure, in order to exert some control over them.

**TERMS**

## The Green Way to Manage Stress

Need a way to beat your stress? Look no further than your own back yard, local park, or nearby hiking trail. Mounting evidence shows that people who get outdoors—or just get to look out a window once in a while—experience an almost instant, if short-term, reduction in stress. Scientists are investigating "natural stress reduction" as an easy and inexpensive booster to cognitive and behavioral approaches to stress management. High-tech replications of nature won't do, though—it has to be the real thing.

In a 2008 study at the University of Washington, participants were set up in two similar office environments with one difference. Some of the offices were equipped with plasma TV screens that displayed videos of a relaxing outdoor setting. The other offices were equipped with windows overlooking an actual outdoor setting. The volunteers were asked to perform a series of stress-inducing work tasks, and then their heart rates were measured. The volunteers with window views recovered from their stress significantly more quickly than the volunteers who viewed a natural scene on TV. The study not only supported the idea that exposure to nature can reduce stress but also demonstrated that facsimiles of nature have little or no effect on stress.

Other studies have yielded similar results. For example, one study looked at hospital patients who were recovering from recent surgery. Patients whose rooms offered a window view of the outdoors needed fewer pain relievers than similar patients with no outdoor view. Recent research on children with attention deficit hyperactivity disorder (ADHD) revealed that spending time in green play settings improved the children's ability to focus and concentrate, at least temporarily (see Chapter 3 for more on this topic).

Why do we benefit so much from communing with nature or even just seeing it through a window? Perhaps it's because we're born nature lovers. The term *biophilia* was coined to describe the innate affinity humans have for nature and living things. In his book *Biophilia*, biologist Edward O. Wilson proposed that people feel a deep connection with the natural world and that this bond is rooted in our biology, perhaps because our species evolved in the context of living systems. According to this theory, we are attracted to plants and animals—we seek them out, surround ourselves with them, and get positive feelings from them—because they have always helped sustain life, including the life of our species.

**connect** ACTIVITY

Whether this hypothesis is true or not, many people are attracted to nature and experience relief from stress just being in natural settings. The next time you're struggling with a term paper or feeling frazzled by your electronic devices, try stepping outside and spending some time under the trees. You may find yourself feeling surprisingly soothed, relaxed, and refreshed.

For a detailed discussion of environmental health—how the environment affects you and how you affect the environment—see Chapter 19.

**SOURCES:** Grind, B., and G. G. Patil. 2009. Biophilia: Does visual contact with nature impact on health and well-being? *International Journal of Environmental Research and Public Health* 6(9): 2332–2343; Kahn, P. H., et al. 2008. A plasma display window? The shifting baseline problem in a technologically mediated natural world. *Journal of Environmental Psychology* 28(2008) 192–199; Faber Taylor, A., and Sullivan, W. C. 2001. Coping with ADD: The surprising connection to green play settings. *Environment and Behavior* 33(1): 54–77.

---

aware of their level of physiological arousal. It involves electrical monitoring of some measure of the physiological stress response, such as perspiration, heart rate, skin temperature, or muscle tension. The subject receives feedback about his or her condition through the use of sound (a tone or music), light, or a meter or dial. For example, as heart rate increases, the tone becomes louder; as it decreases, the tone becomes softer. In this way, people can learn to reduce their physiological stress response through conscious control even without biofeedback.

The point of biofeedback training is to learn how relaxation feels, how to induce relaxation, and how to transfer this skill to daily life (without the use of electronic equipment). In addition to monitoring equipment, biofeedback usually also requires the initial help of a therapist, stress counselor, or technician.

Other relaxation techniques include massage, hypnosis and self-hypnosis, and autogenic training. To learn more about these and other techniques for inducing the relaxation response, refer to For More Information at the end of the chapter. In addition, many people are familiar

with the relaxing effects of nature; for more on this topic, see the box "The Green Way to Manage Stess."

## Counterproductive Coping Strategies

College is a time when you'll learn to adapt to new and challenging situations and gain skills that will last a lifetime. It is also a time when many people develop counterproductive and unhealthy habits in response to stress. Such habits can last well beyond graduation.

**Tobacco Use**  Many young adults who never smoked in high school smoke their first cigarette in college, usually at a party or bar or in a dorm with friends. Many smokers report that smoking helps them to cope with stress by providing a feeling of relaxation, giving them something to do with their hands in social situations, or breaking up monotony and routine.

Cigarettes and other tobacco products contain *nicotine*, a chemical that enhances the actions of neurotransmitters. Nicotine can make you feel relaxed and even increase your ability to concentrate, but it is highly addictive.

ON THE ENVIRONMENT

In fact, nicotine dependence itself is considered a psychological disorder. Cigarette smoke also contains substances that cause heart disease, stroke, lung cancer, and emphysema. These negative consequences far outweigh any beneficial effects, and tobacco use should be avoided. The easiest thing to do is to not start.

See Chapter 11 for more on the health effects of tobacco use and for tips on how to quit.

**Use of Alcohol and Other Drugs**   No college experience is complete without a party or two. Letting loose, dancing, laughing, and interacting with others—all are part of college parties and all can be very effective short-term coping strategies. However, partying in college is usually associated with drinking alcohol. Keg parties and drinking games can be fun, but they contribute to binge drinking and other forms of alcohol abuse. Like nicotine, alcohol is addictive, and many alcoholics find it hard to relax without a drink. Having a few drinks might make you feel temporarily at ease, and drinking until you're intoxicated may help you forget your current stressors. However, using alcohol to deal with stress places you at risk for all the short- and long-term problems associated with alcohol abuse. It also does nothing to address the actual causes of stress in your life. Although moderate alcohol consumption may have potential health benefits for some people, many college students have patterns of drinking that detract from wellness. For more on the responsible use of alcohol, refer to Chapter 10.

Using other psychoactive drugs to cope with stress is also usually counterproductive:

• Caffeine raises cortisol levels and blood pressure and can make you feel more stressed; caffeine also disrupts sleep. Other stimulants, such as amphetamines, can activate the stress response. They also affect the same areas of the brain that are involved in regulating the stress response.

• Marijuana use is relatively common among college students, who report that they smoke marijuana in an effort to induce relaxation and for "mind expansion." Use of marijuana causes a brief period of euphoria and decreased short-term memory and attentional abilities. Physiological effects clearly show that marijuana use doesn't cause relaxation; in fact, some neurochemicals in marijuana act to enhance the stress response, and getting high on a regular basis can elicit panic attacks. To compound this, withdrawal from marijuana may also be associated with an increase in circulating stress hormones.

• Opioids such as morphine and heroin can mimic the effects of your body's natural painkillers and act to reduce anxiety. However, tolerance to opioids develops quickly, and many users become dependent.

For more information on the use of psychoactive drugs, see Chapter 9.

**Unhealthy Eating Habits**   The nutrients in the food you eat provide energy and the substances needed to

Eating candy and other sugary foods is not a healthy way to cope with stress. Eating junk food can lead to weight gain and other long-term health problems.

maintain your body. Eating is also psychologically rewarding. The feelings of satiation and sedation that follow eating produce a relaxed state. However, regular use of eating as a means of coping with stress may lead to unhealthy eating habits. In fact, a survey by the American Psychological Association revealed that about 25% of Americans use food as a means of coping with stress or anxiety. These "comfort eaters" are twice as likely to be obese as average Americans.

Certain foods and supplements are sometimes thought to fight stress. Carbohydrates may reduce the stress response by promoting activity of the parasympathetic nervous system; however, a high-carbohydrate diet can lead to excessive weight gain in sedentary people and is not recommended as a strategy for coping with stressors. In addition, some evidence suggests that greater ingestion of carbohydrates, simple sugars, and fatty foods may actually be a predisposing factor for psychological distress. Many dietary supplements are marketed for stress reduction, but supplements are not required to meet the same standards as medications in terms of safety, effectiveness, and manufacturing (see Chapters 12 and 20).

## CREATING A PERSONAL PLAN FOR MANAGING STRESS

What are the most important sources of stress in your life? Are you coping successfully with these stressors? No single strategy or program for managing stress will work for everyone, but you can use the principles of behavior management described in Chapter 1 to tailor a plan specifically to your needs. The most important starting point for a successful stress-management plan is to learn to listen to your body. When you learn to recognize the stress response and the emotions and thoughts that accompany it, you'll be in a position to take charge of that crucial moment and handle it in a healthy way.

### Identifying Stressors

Before you can learn to manage the stressors in your life, you have to identify them. Many experts recommend keeping a stress journal for a week or two (see Figure 2.5). Each time you feel or express a stress response, record the time and the circumstances in your journal. Note what you were doing at the time, what you were thinking or feeling, and the outcome of your response.

After keeping your journal for a few weeks, you should be able to identify your key stressors and spot patterns in how you respond to them. Take note of the people, places, events, and patterns of thought and behavior that cause you the most stress. You may notice, for example, that mornings are usually the most stressful part of your day.

| STRESS JOURNAL | | DATE 9-18-11 |
|---|---|---|
| TIME | STRESSOR | REACTION/COPING STRATEGY |
| 7:45 AM | Tara wouldn't get out of the shower | Yelled at her, started an argument |
| 8:35 AM | Late for class | Slouched in back of room; chewed my nails |
| 11:55 AM | Dad called to discuss credit card debt | Cried, skipped lunch and went out to smoke with Greg |
| 5:30 PM | Power outage at dorm, couldn't study | Took a walk with Tara, made up for arguing this morning, then went to library to study |
| 7:45 PM | Ed called, asked to borrow money | Stayed calm, put down phone and counted to 10, then explained that he already owes me $50. |
| 8:30 PM | Ed called, angry, said he wanted to break up | Argued on phone, then went out with Tara for a drink |

**FIGURE 2.5 A sample stress journal.** Tracking stressful events and reactions can help you understand how you normally cope with stress.

Or you may discover that when you're angry at your roommate, you're apt to respond with behaviors that only make matters worse. Keeping a journal allows you to be analytical about what produces the most stress in your life and fills in where your conscious memory fails you.

### Designing Your Plan

Once you've identified the key stressors in your life, choose the stress reduction techniques that will work best for you and create an action plan for change. Finding a buddy to work with you can make the process more fun and increase your chances of success. Some experts recommend drawing up a formal contract with yourself.

> The most important starting point for a successful stress-management plan is to *learn* to listen to *your body.*

Whether or not you complete a contract, it's important to design rewards into your plan. You might treat yourself to a special breakfast in a favorite restaurant on the weekend (as long as you eat a nutritious breakfast every weekday morning). It's also important to evaluate your plan regularly and redesign it as your needs change. Under times of increased stress, for example, you might want to focus on good eating, exercise, and relaxation habits. Over time, your new stress-management skills will become almost automatic. You'll feel better, accomplish more, and reduce your risk of disease.

### Getting Help

If the techniques discussed so far don't provide you with enough relief from the stress in your life, you might want to learn more about specific areas to work on. Excellent self-help guides can be found in bookstores or the library. Additional resources are listed in the For More Information section at the end of the chapter.

Your student health center or student affairs office can tell you whether your campus has a peer counseling program. Such programs are usually staffed by volunteer students with special training that emphasizes maintaining confidentiality. Peer counselors can guide you to other campus or community resources or can simply provide understanding.

Support groups are typically organized around a particular issue or problem. In your area, you might find a support group for first-year students; for reentering students; for single parents; for students of your ethnicity, religion, or national origin; for people with eating disorders; or for rape survivors. The number of such groups has increased in recent years as more and more people discover how therapeutic it can be to talk with others who share the same situation.

Short-term psychotherapy can also be tremendously helpful in dealing with stress-related problems. Your student health center may offer psychotherapy on a sliding-fee scale; the county mental health center in your area may do the same. If you belong to any type of religious organization, check to see whether pastoral counseling is available. Your physician can refer you to psychotherapists in your community. Not all therapists are right for all people, so be prepared to have initial sessions with several. Choose the one you feel most comfortable with.

## Connect to your Choices

Have you ever thought about why you handle stress the way you do? Many factors can influence the choices we make about stress management, some not as obvious as others. Do you try to do too much and then take your frustration out on other people because that's how stress was handled in your family? Do you blow off steam with alcohol on weekends because that's what your friends are doing? Do you dismiss relaxation techniques like yoga, meditation, or deep breathing because you think they're only for a certain type of person?

**What are the external factors that influence your choices about stress management? What are your inner motivations and core values, and how do they affect your choices? Based on what you learned in this chapter, will you make some different choices in the future? If so, what will they be?**

Go online to Connect to complete this activity.
www.mcgraw-hillconnect.com

## TIPS FOR TODAY AND THE FUTURE

For the stress you can't avoid, develop a range of stress-management techniques and strategies.

### RIGHT NOW YOU CAN
- Practice deep breathing for 5–10 minutes.
- Visualize a relaxing, peaceful place and imagine yourself experiencing it as vividly as possible. Stay there as long as you can.
- Do some stretching exercises.
- Get out your datebook and schedule what you'll be doing the rest of today and tomorrow. Pencil in a short walk and a conversation with a friend.

### IN THE FUTURE YOU CAN
- Take a class or workshop that can help you overcome a source of stress, such as one in assertiveness training or time management.
- Find a way to build relaxing time into every day. Just 15 minutes of meditation, stretching, or massage can induce the relaxation response.

## SUMMARY

- When confronted with a stressor, the body undergoes a set of physical changes known as the fight-or-flight reaction. The sympathetic nervous system and endocrine system act on many targets in the body to prepare it for action.

- Emotional and behavioral responses to stressors vary among individuals. Ineffective responses increase stress but can be moderated or changed.

- Factors that influence emotional and behavioral responses to stressors include personality, cultural background, gender, and past experiences.

- The general adaptation syndrome (GAS) has three stages: alarm, resistance, and exhaustion.

- A high allostatic load characterized by prolonged or repeated exposure to stress hormones can increase a person's risk of health problems.

- Psychoneuroimmunology (PNI) looks at how the physiological changes of the stress response affect the immune system and thereby increase the risk of illness.

- Health problems linked to stress include CVD, colds and other infections, asthma and allergies, cancer, flare-ups of chronic diseases, psychological problems, digestive problems, headaches, insomnia, and injuries.

- A cluster of major life events that require adjustment and accommodation can lead to increased stress and an increased risk of health problems. Minor daily hassles increase stress if they are perceived negatively.

- Sources of stress associated with college may be academic, interpersonal, time-related, or financial pressures.

- Job-related stress is common, particularly for employees who have little control over decisions relating to their jobs. If stress is severe or prolonged, burnout may occur.

- New and changing relationships, prejudice, and discrimination are examples of interpersonal and social stressors.

- Social support systems help buffer people against the effects of stress and make illness less likely. Good communication skills foster healthy relationships.

- Exercise, nutrition, sleep, and time management are wellness behaviors that reduce stress and increase energy.

- Cognitive techniques for managing stress involve developing new and healthy patterns of thinking, such as practicing problem solving, monitoring self-talk, and cultivating a sense of humor.

- The relaxation response is the opposite of the fight-or-flight reaction. Techniques that trigger it, including progressive relaxation, imagery, meditation, and deep breathing, counteract the effects of chronic stress. Counterproductive coping strategies include smoking, drinking, and unhealthy eating.

- A successful individualized plan for coping with stress begins with the use of a stress journal or log to identify and study stressors and inappropriate behavioral responses. Completing a contract and recruiting a buddy can help your stress-management plan succeed.

- Additional help in dealing with stress is available from self-help books, peer counseling, support groups, and psychotherapy.

## FOR MORE INFORMATION

### BOOKS

Greenberg, J. 2010. *Comprehensive Stress Management.* 12th ed. New York: McGraw-Hill. *Provides a clear explanation of the physical, psychological, sociological, and spiritual aspects of stress and offers numerous stress-management techniques.*

Kabat-Zinn, J. 2006. *Coming to Our Senses: Healing Ourselves and the World Through Mindfulness.* New York: Hyperion. *Explores the connections among mindfulness, health, and physical and spiritual well-being.*

Pennebaker, J. W. 2004. *Writing to Heal: A Guided Journal for Recovering from Trauma and Emotional Upheaval.* Oakland, Calif.: New Harbinger Press. *Provides information about using journaling to cope with stress.*

Seaward, B. L. 2009. *Managing Stress: Principles and Strategies for Health and Well-Being.* 6th ed. Boston: Jones and Bartlett. *A comprehensive textbook for college students.*

### ORGANIZATIONS AND WEB SITES

*American Headache Society.* Provides information for consumers and clinicians about different types of headaches, their causes, and their treatment.
http://www.americanheadachesociety.org/
*American Psychiatric Association: Healthy Minds, Healthy Lives.* Provides information on mental wellness developed especially for college students.
http://www.healthyminds.org
*American Psychological Association.* Provides information on stress management and psychological disorders.
http://www.apa.org
http://www.apa.org/helpcenter
*Association for Applied Psychophysiology and Biofeedback.* Provides information about biofeedback and referrals to certified biofeedback practitioners.
http://www.aapb.org
*Benson-Henry Institute for Mind Body Medicine.* Provides information about stress-management and relaxation techniques.
http://www.massgeneral.org/bhi/
*National Institute of Mental Health (NIMH).* Publishes informative brochures about stress and stress management as well as other aspects of mental health.
http://www.nimh.nih.gov
*National Sleep Foundation.* Provides information about sleep and how to overcome sleep problems such as insomnia and jet lag.
http://www.sleepfoundation.org
*The American Institute of Stress.* A resource of in-depth information on stress, its causes, and its treatments.
http://www.stress.org

## SELECTED BIBLIOGRAPHY

American College Health Association. 2009. *American College Health Association–National College Health Assessment II Reference Group Executive Summary, Fall 2009.* Linthicum, Md.: American College Health Association.

American Psychological Association. 2009. *Stress in America 2009.* Washington, D.C.: American Psychological Association.

American Psychological Association. 2010. *How Does Stress Affect Us?* (http://www.apa.org/helpcenter/stress-effects.aspx; retrieved October 20, 2010).

American Psychological Association. 2010. *Learning to Deal with Stress* (http://www.apa.org/helpcenter/stress-learning.aspx; retrieved October 20, 2010).

American Psychological Association. 2010. *Mind/Body Health: Stress* (http://www.apa.org/helpcenter/stress.aspx; retrieved October 20, 2010).

Caldwell, K., et al. 2010. Developing mindfulness in college students through movement-based courses: Effects on self-regulatory self-efficacy, mood, stress, and sleep quality. *Journal of American College Health* 58(5): 433–442.

Centers for Disease Control. 2010. *Coping with a Disaster or Traumatic Event: Information for Individuals and Families* (http://emergency.cdc.gov/mentalhealth/general.asp; retrieved October 20, 2010).

Hefner, J., and D. Eisenberg. 2009. Social support and mental health among college students. *American Journal of Orthopsychiatry* 79(4): 491–499.

Flugel Colle, K. F., et al. 2010. Measurement of quality of life and participant experience with the mindfulness-based stress reduction program. *Complementary Therapies in Clinical Practice* 16(1): 36–40.

Freedman, N. 2010. Treatment of obstructive sleep apnea syndrome. *Clinics in Chest Medicine* 31(2): 187–201.

Frequent headaches, hidden dangers. 2006. *Consumer Reports on Health,* June.

Headaches. 2006. *Journal of the American Medical Association* 295(19): 2320.

Hook, J. N., et al. 2010. Empirically supported religious and spiritual therapies. *Journal of Clinical Psychology* 66(1): 46–72.

Institute of Medicine Committee on Sleep Medicine and Research. 2006. *Sleep Disorders and Sleep Deprivation: An Unmet Public Health Problem,* ed. H. R. Colton and B. M. Altevogt. Washington, D.C.: National Academies Press.

Mayo Foundation for Medical Education and Research. 2008. *Stress: Win control over the stress in your life* (http://www.mayoclinic.com/health/stress/SR00001; retrieved October 20, 2010).

National Sleep Foundation. 2010. *2010 Sleep in America Poll.* Washington, D.C.: National Sleep Foundation.

Nordboe, D. J., et al. 2007. Immediate Behavioral Health Response to the Virginia Tech Shootings. *Disaster Medicine and Public Health Preparedness* 1(Suppl. 1.): S31–S32.

Roddenberry, A., and K. Renk. 2010. Locus of control and self-efficacy: Potential mediators of stress, illness, and utilization of health services in college students. *Child Psychiatry and Human Development* 41(4): 353–370.

Telles, S., et al. 2009. Effect of a yoga practice session and a yoga theory session on state anxiety. *Perceptual and Motor Skills* 109(3): 924–930.

The New York Times. 2010 Update. *Times Topics: School Shootings* (http://topics.nytimes.com/top/reference/timestopics/subjects/s/school_shootings/index.html; retrieved October 20, 2010).

Torpy, J. M. 2008. Chronic stress and the heart. *Journal of the American Medical Association* 298(14): 1722.

U.S. Department of Health and Human Services, National Institutes of Health. 2009. *Stress* (http://www.nlm.nih.gov/medlineplus/stress.html; retrieved October 20, 2010).

# Dealing with Test Anxiety

Do you perform as well as you should on tests? Does anxiety interfere with your ability to study effectively before a test and to think clearly in the test situation? If so, you may be experiencing test anxiety. Two effective methods can help you deal with test anxiety: systematic desensitization and success rehearsal.

## Systematic Desensitization

Systematic desensitization is based on the premise that you can't feel anxiety and be relaxed at the same time.

**Phase I: Constructing an Anxiety Hierarchy** Begin the first phase by thinking of ten or more situations related to your fear, such as hearing the announcement of the test date in class, studying for the test, sitting in the classroom waiting for the test to begin, reading the test questions, and so on. Write each situation on an index card, using a brief phrase to describe it on one side of the card. On the other side, list several realistic details or prompts that will help you vividly imagine yourself actually experiencing the situation. For example, if the situation is "hearing that 50% of the final grade will be based on the two exams," the prompts might include details such as "sitting in the big lecture auditorium in Baily Hall," "taking notes in my blue notebook," and "listening to Professor Smith's voice."

Next, arrange your cards in order, from least-tense to most-tense situation. Rate each situation to reflect the amount of anxiety you feel when you encounter it in real life, to confirm your anxiety hierarchy. Assign ratings on a scale of 0–100, and make sure the distances between items are fairly small and about equal. When you're sure your anxiety hierarchy is a true reflection of your feelings, number the cards.

**Phase II: Learning and Practicing Muscle Relaxation** The second phase of the program involves learning to relax your muscles and to recognize when they are relaxed (see the description of progressive relaxation in this chapter). As you become proficient at this technique, you'll be able to go into a deeply relaxed state within just a few minutes. When you can do this, go on to the next phase of the program.

**Phase III: Implementing the Desensitization Program** Use the quiet place where you practiced your relaxation exercises. Sit comfortably and place your stack of numbered cards within reach. Take several minutes to relax completely, and then look at the first card, reading both the brief phrase and the descriptive prompts. Close your eyes and imagine yourself in that situation for about 10 seconds. Then put the card down and relax completely for about 30 seconds. Look at the card again, imagine the situation for 10 seconds, and relax again for 30 seconds.

At this point, evaluate your current level of anxiety about the situation on the card in terms of the rating scale you devised earlier. If your anxiety level is 10 or below, relax for 2 minutes and go on to the second card. If it's higher than 10, repeat the routine with the same card until the anxiety decreases.

If you have difficulty with a particular item, go back to the previous item and try it again. If you still can't visualize it without anxiety, try to construct three new items with smaller steps between them and insert them before the troublesome item. You should be able to move through one to four items per session.

Sessions can be conducted from twice a day to twice a week and should last no longer than 20 minutes. It's helpful to graph your progress in a way that has meaning for you.

After you have successfully completed your program, you should be desensitized to the real-life situations that previously caused anxiety. If you find that you experience some anxiety in the real situations, take 30 seconds or a minute to relax completely, just as you did when you were practicing.

## Success Rehearsal

To practice this variation on systematic desensitization, take your hierarchy of anxiety-producing situations and vividly imagine yourself successfully dealing with each one. Create a detailed scenario for each situation, and use your imagination to experience genuine feelings of confidence. Recognize your negative thoughts ("I'll be so nervous I won't be able to think straight") and replace them with positive ones ("Anxiety will keep me alert so I can do a good job").

Proceed one step at a time, thinking as you go of strategies for success that you can later implement. These might include the following:

- Before the test, find out everything you can about it—its format, the material to be covered, the grading criteria. Ask the instructor for practice materials. Study in advance; don't just cram the night before. Avoid all-nighters.

- Devise a study plan. This might include forming a study group with one or more classmates or outlining what you will study, when, where, and for how long. Generate your own questions and answer them.

- In the actual test situation, sit away from possible distractions, listen carefully to instructions, and ask for clarification if you don't understand a direction.

- During the test, answer the easiest questions first. If you don't know an answer and there is no penalty for incorrect answers, guess. If there are several questions you have difficulty answering, review the ones you have already handled. Figure out approximately how much time you have to cover each question.

- For math problems, try to estimate the answer before doing the precise calculations.

- For true-false questions, look for qualifiers such as *always* and *never*. Such questions are likely to be false.

- For essay questions, look for key words in the question that indicate what the instructor is looking for in the answer. Develop a brief outline of your answer, sketching out what you will cover. Stick to your outline, and keep track of the time you're spending on your answer. Don't get caught with unanswered questions when time is up.

- Remain calm and focused throughout the test. Don't let negative thoughts rattle you. Avoid worrying about past performance, how others are doing, or the negative consequences of a poor test grade. If you start to become nervous, take some deep breaths and relax your muscles completely for a minute or so.

The best way to counter test anxiety is with successful test-taking experiences. The more times you succeed, the more your test anxiety will recede. If you find that these methods aren't sufficient to get your anxiety under control, you may want to seek professional help.

# CHAPTER 9

# The Use and Abuse of Psychoactive Drugs

## LOOKING AHEAD...

After reading this chapter, you should be able to

- Define and discuss the concepts of addictive behavior, substance abuse, and substance dependence
- Explain factors contributing to drug use and dependence
- List the major categories of psychoactive drugs and describe their effects, methods of use, and potential for abuse and dependence
- Discuss social issues related to psychoactive drug use and its prevention and treatment
- Evaluate the role of drugs and other addictive behaviors in your life and identify your risk factors for abuse or dependence

## TEST YOUR KNOWLEDGE

1. Addictions always involve drugs that cause physical withdrawal symptoms when the person stops taking them.
   True or false?

2. Which of the following is the most widely used illegal drug among college-age Americans?
   a. cocaine
   b. hallucinogens
   c. marijuana

3. Caffeine use can produce physical dependence.
   True or false?

4. Which of the following drugs is most addictive?
   a. marijuana
   b. nicotine
   c. LSD

5. About what percentage of street drugs contain the promised primary ingredient?
   a. 50%
   b. 75%
   c. 90%

## ANSWERS

1. **FALSE.** Both assertions in this statement are wrong. Addiction does not always involve a drug, but even when it does, withdrawing from that drug may not result in physical symptoms.

2. **C.** Marijuana ranks first, followed (in order) by hallucinogens and cocaine. Alcohol remains by far the most popular drug among college-age Americans.

3. **TRUE.** Regular users of caffeine develop physical tolerance, needing more caffeine to produce the same level of alertness. Many experience withdrawal symptoms when they reduce their caffeine intake.

4. **B.** Nicotine is believed to be the most highly addictive psychoactive drug.

5. **A.** This figure is even lower for drugs that are difficult to obtain or manufacture. Street drugs may be sold in unsafe dosages and are often mixed with cheaper, more hazardous substances.

The use of **drugs** for both medical and social purposes is widespread in America (Table 9.1). Many people believe that every problem has or should have a chemical solution. For fatigue, many turn to caffeine; for insomnia, sleeping pills; for anxiety or boredom, alcohol or other recreational drugs. Advertisements, social pressures, and the human desire for quick solutions to life's difficult problems all contribute to the prevailing attitude that drugs can ease all pain. But benefits often come with consequences, and drug use can—and, in many cases, does—pose serious or even life-threatening ones.

The most serious consequences are abuse and addiction. The drugs most often associated with abuse are **psychoactive drugs**—those that alter a person's experiences or consciousness. In the short term, psychoactive drugs can cause **intoxication**, a state in which sometimes unpredictable physical and emotional changes occur. A person who is intoxicated may experience potentially serious changes in physical functioning. His or her emotions and judgment may be affected in ways that lead to uncharacteristic and unsafe behavior. In the long term, recurrent drug use can have profound physical, emotional, and social effects.

This chapter introduces the concept of addictive behavior, then focuses on the major classes of psychoactive drugs, their effects, their potential for abuse and addiction, and other issues related to their use. Alcohol and nicotine—two of the most widely used and most harmful psychoactive drugs—are discussed in Chapters 10 and 11.

## ADDICTIVE BEHAVIOR

Although addiction is most often associated with drug use, many experts now extend the concept of addiction to other behaviors. **Addictive behaviors** are habits that have gotten out of control, with resulting negative effects on a person's health. Looking at the nature of addiction

TERMS

VITAL STATISTICS

| Table 9.1 | Nonmedical Drug Use Among Americans, 2008 |
| --- | --- |

| | PERCENTAGE USING SUBSTANCE IN THE PAST 30 DAYS | | |
| --- | --- | --- | --- |
| | COLLEGE-AGE AMERICANS | | ALL AMERICANS |
| | AGE 18–20 | AGE 21–25 | AGE 12 AND OLDER |
| ILLICIT DRUGS | 21.5 | 18.4 | 8.0 |
| Marijuana and Hashish | 18.7 | 15.0 | 6.1 |
| Cocaine | 1.6 | 1.5 | 0.7 |
| Crack | 0.2 | 0.2 | 0.1 |
| Heroin | 0.2 | 0.2 | 0.1 |
| Methamphetamine | 0.1 | 0.3 | 0.1 |
| Hallucinogens | 2.3 | 1.3 | 0.4 |
| LSD | 0.3 | 0.3 | 0.1 |
| PCP | 0.0 | 0.0 | 0.0 |
| Ecstasy | 1.3 | 0.6 | 0.2 |
| Inhalants | 0.5 | 0.2 | 0.3 |
| Nonmedical Use of Psychotherapeutics | 6.0 | 5.8 | 2.5 |
| Pain Relievers | 4.8 | 4.4 | 1.9 |
| OxyContin | 0.4 | 0.4 | 0.2 |
| Tranquilizers | 1.7 | 1.7 | 0.7 |
| Stimulants | 1.0 | 1.1 | 0.4 |
| Sedatives | 0.1 | 0.3 | 0.1 |
| TOBACCO (ALL FORMS) | 39.6 | 42.6 | 28.4 |
| Cigarettes | 33.5 | 37.1 | 23.9 |
| Smokeless tobacco | 5.8 | 5.1 | 3.5 |
| Cigars | 13.4 | 9.9 | 5.3 |
| Pipe tobacco | 1.9 | 1.0 | 0.8 |
| ALCOHOL | 48.7 | 69.5 | 51.6 |
| Binge alcohol use | 33.7 | 46.0 | 23.3 |

**SOURCE:** Substance Abuse and Mental Health Services Administration. 2009. *Results from the 2008 National Survey on Drug Use and Health: National Findings.* Rockville, Md.: Office of Applied Studies, NSDUH Series H-36, HHS Publication No. SMA 09-4434.

and a range of addictive behaviors can help us understand similar behaviors when they involve drugs.

### What Is Addiction?

Today, scientists view **addiction** as a psychological or physical dependence on a substance or behavior. This type of dependence is defined by four key characteristics:

- A compulsive desire for a drug
- The need to increase the dosage associated with physical or psychological dependence
- Harmful effects to the addict
- Harm to society

Historically, the term *addiction* was applied only when the habitual use of a drug produced chemical changes in the user's body. One such change is physical **tolerance**, in which the body adapts to a drug so that the initial dose no longer produces the original emotional or psychological effects. This process, caused by chemical changes, means the user has to take larger and larger doses of the drug to achieve the same high. (Tolerance is discussed in greater detail later in the chapter.) The concept of addiction as a disease process, one based in brain chemistry rather than a moral failing, has led to many advances in the understanding and treatment of drug addiction.

Some scientists think that other behaviors may share some of the chemistry of drug addiction. They suggest that activities like gambling, eating, exercising, and sex release brain chemicals that cause a pleasurable rush in much the same way that psychoactive drugs do. The brain's own chemicals thus become the "drug" that can cause addiction. These theorists suggest that all addictions—whether to drugs or to pleasurable activities—have a common mechanism in the brain. In this view, addiction is partly the result of our own natural wiring.

The view that addiction is based in our brain chemistry does *not* imply that people are not responsible for their addictive behavior. Many experts believe that it is inaccurate and counterproductive to think of all bad habits and excessive behaviors as diseases. They point to other factors, especially lifestyle and personality traits, that play key roles in the development of addictive behaviors.

## Characteristics of Addictive Behavior

Experts have identified some general characteristics typically associated with addictive behaviors:

- *Reinforcement.* Addictive behaviors reinforce themselves. The behavior either produces pleasurable physical and/or emotional states, or relieves negative ones.

- *Compulsion or craving.* The addict feels a strong compulsion—a compelling need—to engage in the behavior, often accompanied by obsessive planning for the next opportunity to perform it.

- *Loss of control.* The addict loses control over the behavior and cannot block the impulse to do it.

- *Escalation.* Addiction often involves a pattern of escalation: More and more of the substance or activity is required to produce its desired effects.

- *Negative consequences.* The behavior continues despite serious negative consequences, such as problems with academic or job performance, personal relationships, and health; legal or financial troubles are also typical.

## The Development of Addiction

We all engage in activities that are potentially addictive. Some of these activities can be good for you if they are done appropriately and in moderation. But if a behavior starts to be excessive, it may become an addiction.

An addiction often starts when a person does something to bring pleasure or avoid pain. The activity may be drinking a beer, using the Internet, playing the lottery, or going shopping. If it works, the person is likely to repeat it. He or she becomes increasingly dependent on the behavior, and tolerance may develop; that is, the person needs more of the behavior to feel the same effect. Eventually, the behavior becomes a central focus of the person's life, and there is a deterioration in other areas, such as school performance or relationships. The behavior no longer brings pleasure, but it is necessary to avoid the pain of going without it. What started as a seemingly innocent way of feeling good becomes a prison.

*When taken to a compulsive level, even healty activities can turn into addictive behaviors.*

Although many common behaviors are potentially addictive, most people who engage in them do not develop problems. The reason lies in the combination of factors that are involved in the development of addiction, including personality, lifestyle, heredity, the social and physical environment, and the nature of the substance or behavior in question. For a behavior to become an addiction, these diverse factors must come together in a certain way. For example, nicotine (the psychoactive drug in tobacco) has a very high potential for physical addiction, but you must submit to the temptation to start using tobacco—whether prompted by peer pressure, stress, or personality traits—in order to develop an addiction to it.

## Characteristics of People with Addictions

The causes and course of an addiction are extremely varied, but people with addictions (commonly referred to as *addicts*) seem to share some characteristics. Many use a substance or activity as a substitute for healthier coping strategies. People vary in their ability to manage their lives, and those who have the most trouble dealing with stress and painful emotions may be more susceptible to addiction.

Some people may have a genetic predisposition to addiction to a particular substance; such predispositions may involve variations in brain chemistry. People with addictive disorders usually have a distinct preference for a particular addictive behavior. They also often have problems with impulse control and self-regulation, and tend to be risk-takers.

## Examples of Addictive Behaviors

Some behaviors that are not related to drugs can become addictive for some people. Such behaviors can include eating, watching TV, and playing video games. Any substance or activity that becomes the focus of a person's life at the expense of other needs and interests can be damaging to health.

**Compulsive Gambling**   Compulsive gamblers cannot control the urge to gamble, even in the face of ruin. The consequences of compulsive gambling are not just financial; the suicide rate of compulsive gamblers is 20 times higher than that of the general population. About 1% of adult Americans are compulsive (pathological) gamblers, and another 2% are "problem gamblers." Some 42% of college students gamble at least once in a year, and about 3% gamble at least once a week.

**QUICK STATS**

**48** states and the District of Columbia allow some form of legalized gambling.

—National Council on Problem Gambling, 2010

The American Psychiatric Association (APA) recognizes pathological gambling as a mental disorder associated with 10 characteristic behaviors, including preoccupation with gambling, unsuccessful efforts to quit, using gambling to escape problems, and lying to family members to conceal the extent of gambling. Many compulsive gamblers also have drug and alcohol abuse problems.

**Compulsive Exercising**   When taken to a compulsive level, even healthy activities can turn into harmful addictions. For example, compulsive exercising is now recognized as a serious departure from normal behavior. Compulsive exercising is often accompanied by more severe psychiatric disorders such as anorexia nervosa and bulimia (Chapter 14). Traits often associated with compulsive exercising include an excessive preoccupation and dissatisfaction with body image, use of laxatives or vomiting to lose weight, and development of other obsessive-compulsive symptoms.

**Work Addiction**   People who are excessively preoccupied with work are often called *workaholics*. Work addiction, however, is actually based on a set of specific symptoms, including the following:

- An intense work schedule
- The inability to limit one's own work schedule
- The inability to relax, even when away from work
- Failed attempts at curtailing the intensity of work (in some cases)

Work addicts are likely to neglect other aspects of life. For example, work addicts may exercise less, spend less time with family and friends, and avoid social activities.

Work addiction typically coincides with a well-known risk factor for cardiovascular disease—the Type A personal-

Many college students have gotten caught up in the poker craze.

ity (Chapter 15). Traits associated with Type A personality include competitiveness, ambition, drive, time urgency, restlessness, hyperalertness, and hostility.

**Sex and Love Addiction**   More controversial is the notion of addiction to sex or love. Behaviors associated with sex addiction include an extreme preoccupation with sex, a compulsion to have sex repeatedly in a given period of time, spending a great deal of time and energy looking for partners or having sex, using sex as a means of relieving painful feelings, and suffering negative emotional, personal, and professional consequences as a result of sexual activities.

Some experts are reluctant to call compulsive sexual activity a true addiction. However, even therapists who challenge the concept of sex addiction recognize that some people become overly preoccupied with sex, cannot seem to control their sex drive, and act in potentially harmful ways in order to stay satisfied. This pattern of sexual behavior seems to meet the criteria for addictive behaviors discussed earlier.

**Compulsive Buying or Shopping**   A compulsive buyer repeatedly gives in to the impulse to buy more than he or she needs or can afford. Compulsive spenders usually buy luxury items rather than daily necessities, even though they are usually distressed by their

## Is Internet Use a Problem for You?

To assess the extent to which your Internet use is creating problems in your life, answer the following questions using this point scale:

| | |
|---|---|
| Rarely | 1 point |
| Occasionally | 2 points |
| Frequently | 3 points |
| Often | 4 points |
| Always | 5 points |

_____ 1. How often do you find that you stay online longer than you intended?

_____ 2. How often do you neglect household chores to spend more time online?

_____ 3. How often do you prefer the excitement of the Internet to intimacy with your partner?

_____ 4. How often do you form new relationships with fellow online users?

_____ 5. How often do others in your life complain about the amount of time you spend online?

_____ 6. How often do your grades or schoolwork suffer because of the amount of time you spend online?

_____ 7. How often do you check your email before something else that you need to do?

_____ 8. How often does your job performance or productivity suffer because of the Internet?

_____ 9. How often do you become defensive or secretive when someone asks you what you do online?

_____ 10. How often do you block out disturbing thoughts about your life with soothing thoughts about the Internet?

_____ 11. How often do you find yourself anticipating when you will go online again?

_____ 12. How often do you fear that life without the Internet would be boring, empty, and joyless?

_____ 13. How often do you snap, yell, or act annoyed if someone bothers you while you are online?

_____ 14. How often do you lose sleep due to late-night log-ins?

_____ 15. How often do you feel preoccupied with the Internet when offline or fantasize about being online?

_____ 16. How often do you find yourself saying "just a few more minutes" when online?

_____ 17. How often do you try to cut down on the amount of time you spend online and fail?

_____ 18. How often do you try to hide how long you've been online?

_____ 19. How often do you choose to spend more time online over going out with others?

_____ 20. How often do you feel depressed, moody, or nervous when you are offline, which goes away once you are back online?

Add the points associated with your responses to get your final score. The higher your score, the more problems your Internet usage is causing you. Here's a general scale to help you evaluate your score:

**20–49 points:** You are an average online user. You may surf the Web a bit too long at times, but you have control over your usage.

**50–79 points:** You are experiencing occasional or frequent problems because of the Internet. You should consider their full impact on your life.

**80–100 points:** Your Internet usage is causing significant problems in your life. You should evaluate the impact of the Internet on your life and start thinking about how to address the problems.

**SOURCE:** Netaddiction.com. *Internet Addiction Test* (http://www.netaddiction.com/index.php?option=com_bfquiz&view=onepage&catid=46&Itemid=106; retrieved November 3, 2010).

behavior and its social, personal, and financial consequences. Some experts link compulsive shopping with neglect or abuse during childhood; it also seems to be associated with eating disorders, depression, and bipolar disorder.

**Internet Addiction** In the 15 years since the Internet became widely available, millions of Americans have become compulsive Internet users—as much as 10% of the U.S. population, by some estimates. To spend more time online, Internet addicts skip other important activities. Compulsive Internet users often spend their work time online, a fact that has led many employers to adopt strict Internet usage policies. Despite negative financial, social, or academic consequences, compulsive Internet users don't feel able to stop. As with other addictive behaviors, online addicts may be using their behavior to alleviate stress or avoid painful emotions (see the box "Is Internet Use a Problem for You?").

## DRUG USE, ABUSE, AND DEPENDENCE

The substances most commonly associated with addiction are psychoactive drugs. Drugs are chemicals other than food that are intended to affect the structure or function of the body. They include prescription medicines such as antibiotics and antidepressants; nonprescription or over-the-counter (OTC) substances such as alcohol, tobacco, and caffeine products; and illegal substances such as LSD and heroin.

### The Drug Tradition

Using drugs to alter consciousness is an ancient and universal pursuit. People have used alcohol for celebration and intoxication for thousands of years. People in all parts of the world have exploited the psychoactive properties of plants, such as the coca plant in South America and the opium poppy in the Far East.

In the nineteenth century, chemists began extracting the active chemicals from medicinal plants, such as morphine from the opium poppy and cocaine from the coca leaf. This was the beginning of modern **pharmacy,** the art of compounding drugs, and of **pharmacology,** the science and study of drugs. It was also the start of the era of man-made psychoactive drugs, from codeine to methamphetamine, which continues to the present.

Drug addiction among Americans was more common by 1900 than at any time before or since. In the early 1900s, concerns about drug addiction and the need to regulate drug sales and manufacture led to new federal drug laws in the United States. Middle-class use of regulated drugs dropped, and drug use became restricted to, and increasingly identified with, criminal subcultures.

Nonmedical (recreational) drug use expanded in America during the 1960s and 1970s, reaching a peak in 1979. Drug use rates then declined until the early to mid-

**Ask Yourself**

QUESTIONS FOR CRITICAL THINKING AND REFLECTION
Have you ever repeatedly or compulsively engaged in a behavior that had negative consequences? What was the behavior, and why did you continue? Did you ever worry that you were losing control? Were you able to bring the behavior under control?

1990s, when drug use rates began to rise in certain age groups. Between 2002 and 2007, however, use of illicit drugs, including marijuana and methamphetamine, declined among youths aged 12–17, as did use of alcohol and tobacco. In young adults aged 18–25, overall drug use remained stable during the same period, although there was a significant increase in the nonmedical use of narcotic pain relievers.

### Drug Abuse and Dependence

The APA's *Diagnostic and Statistical Manual of Mental Disorders* is the authoritative reference for defining all sorts of behavioral disorders, including those related to drugs. The APA has chosen not to use the term *addiction,* in part because it is so broad and has so many connotations. Instead, the APA refers to two forms of substance (drug) disorders: substance abuse and substance dependence. Both are maladaptive patterns of substance use that lead to significant impairment or distress. Although the APA's definitions are more precise and more directly related to drug use, they clearly encompass the general characteristics of addictive behavior described in the preceding section.

**Abuse** As defined by the APA, **substance abuse** involves one or more of the following characteristics:

- Recurrent drug use, resulting in a failure to fulfill major responsibilities at work, school, or home
- Recurrent drug use in situations in which it is physically hazardous, such as before or while driving
- Recurrent drug-related legal problems
- Continued drug use despite persistent social or interpersonal problems caused or worsened by the effects of the drug

The pattern of use may be constant or intermittent, and **physical dependence** may or may not be present. For example, a person who smokes marijuana once a week and cuts classes because he or she is high is abusing marijuana, even though he or she is not physically dependent.

**Dependence** Substance dependence is a more complex disorder and is what many people associate with the

> *Drug dependence can occur without a physical component (tolerance or withdrawal), based solely on compulsive use.*

idea of addiction. The seven specific criteria the APA uses to diagnose substance dependence are listed below. The first two are associated with physical dependence; the final five are associated with compulsive use. To be considered dependent, one must experience a cluster of three or more of these symptoms during a 12-month period.

1. *Developing tolerance to the substance.* When a person requires increased amounts of a substance to achieve the desired effect or notices a markedly diminished effect with continued use of the same amount, he or she has developed tolerance to the substance.

2. *Experiencing withdrawal.* In someone who has maintained prolonged, heavy use of a substance, a drop in its concentration within the body can result in unpleasant physical and cognitive **withdrawal** symptoms. Withdrawal symptoms are different for different drugs. For example, nausea, vomiting, and tremors are common for alcohol, opioids, and sedatives. Some drugs have no significant withdrawal symptoms; in some cases, withdrawal symptoms can be life-threatening.

3. *Taking the substance in larger amounts or over a longer period than was originally intended.*

4. *Expressing a persistent desire to cut down or regulate substance use.*

5. *Spending a great deal of time getting the substance, using it, or recovering from its effects.*

6. *Giving up or reducing important social, school, work, or recreational activities because of substance use.*

7. *Continuing to use the substance despite the knowledge that it is contributing to a psychological or physical problem.*

If a drug-dependent person experiences either tolerance or withdrawal, he or she is considered physically dependent. However, not everyone who experiences tolerance or withdrawal is drug dependent. For example, a hospital patient who is prescribed therapeutic doses of morphine to relieve pain may develop a tolerance to the drug and experience withdrawal symptoms when the prescription is discontinued. But without showing any signs of compulsive use, this individual would not be considered dependent.

Conversely, dependence can occur without a physical component, based solely on compulsive use. For example, people with at least three symptoms of compulsive use of marijuana who show no signs of tolerance or withdrawal

| Table 9.2 | Psychoactive Drugs and Their Potential for Producing Dependence | |
|---|---|---|
| | **POTENTIAL FOR DEPENDENCE** | |
| **DRUG** | **PHYSICAL** | **PSYCHOLOGICAL** |
| Heroin | High | High |
| Morphine | High | High |
| Hydrocodone | High | High |
| Oxycodone | High | High |
| Codeine | Moderate | Moderate |
| Gamma Hydroxybutric Acid | Moderate | Moderate |
| Benzodiazepines | Moderate | Moderate |
| Cocaine | Possible | High |
| Amphetamine/Methamphetamine | Possible | High |
| Methylphenidate | Possible | High |
| MDMA (Ecstasy) | None | Moderate |
| LSD | None | Unknown |
| PCP | Possible | High |
| Marijuana | Unknown | Moderate |
| Hashish | Unknown | Moderate |
| Alcohol | High | High |

**SOURCES:** U.S. Department of Justice, Drug Enforcement Administration. 2005. *Drugs of Abuse.* Washington, D.C.: U.S. Department of Justice.

are suffering from substance dependence. In general, dependence problems that involve physical dependence carry a greater risk of immediate general medical problems and higher relapse rates.

## Who Uses Drugs?

Drug use and abuse occur at all income and education levels, among all ethnic groups, and across all age groups (see the box "Drug Use Among College Students"). Society is concerned with the casual or recreational use of illegal drugs because it is not really possible to know when it will lead to abuse or dependence. Some casual users develop substance-related problems; others do not. Some drugs are more likely than others to lead to dependence (Table 9.2), but even some heroin or cocaine users do not meet the APA's criteria for substance dependence.

It isn't possible to accurately predict which drug users will become abusers, but young people at a high risk of *trying* drugs share certain characteristics:

- *Being young.* People who start using drugs when they're very young have a greater risk of dependence and health consequences.

**withdrawal** Physical and psychological symptoms that follow the interrupted use of a drug on which a user is physically dependent; symptoms may be mild or life-threatening.

## Drug Use Among College Students

Drug use in college has long been recognized as a significant health problem that affects many students. By some measures of substance abuse, double-digit prevalence is still the defining characteristic of drug use on college campuses for certain drugs.

According to the most recent survey data from the Substance Abuse and Mental Health Services Administration (SAMHSA), 21.5% of young adults ages 18–20 reported using an illicit drug in the past 30 days (see Table 9.1). This number represents a slight decline from 2007. The same survey shows that past-month tobacco use increased slightly and binge drinking decreased significantly in this age group, while marijuana and cocaine use remained steady.

Other surveys show that recreational drug use is fairly common among college students. According to the 2009 American College Health Association–National College Health Assessment, more than 12% of college students reported using marijuana at least once in the past 30 days. Another 13% said they had used some other drug at least once in the past 30 days.

Drug use on college campuses has been examined extensively, and many experts believe that no single factor can explain the widespread impact of this phenomenon. Family history, peer pressure, depression, anxiety, low self-esteem, and the dynamics of college

life (for example, the drive to compete and distorted perception of drug use among peers) have been suggested as potential explanations for college-age drug use.

Excessive alcohol use often accompanies illicit drug use. A 2009 SAMHSA report found that 13.5% of young adults age 18–25 had used drugs and alcohol together, and that the risk of combining drugs and alcohol increased with the number of drinks a young adult consumed during a single session. Binge drinkers were more likely than non-binge drinkers to abuse illegal drugs while drinking. In fact, the term *AOD* (Alcohol and Other Drug) has been coined to refer to this type of substance use among college students. Further, AOD use and depression and/or anxiety are generally recognized as coexisting conditions that require a comprehensive approach to prevention and treatment. Despite the growing awareness among college counselors and other health pro-

fessionals who work with college students, it is not entirely clear whether anxiety and depression precede the onset of alcohol and drug use or whether early precollege exposure to alcohol and drug use exacerbates more serious psychiatric disorders by the time a student enters college. A third line of research suggests that AOD use, depression, and anxiety share common causes such as genetic predisposition and/or family history.

However, one aspect of drug use among college students remains clear: AOD use has dramatic consequences for the educational, family, and community life of students. Poor academic performance has been linked with AOD use. Further, driving while intoxicated remains one of the most dangerous outcomes associated with AOD use affecting families and communities.

Several AOD prevention programs are now underway at college campuses. Several federal laws have been enacted to provide resources and a legislative framework for addressing AOD use at schools. The 1989 Drug-free School and Communities Act and the 1998 Higher Education Amendment are examples of concerted federal legislative efforts to encourage the development of educational policies for preventing alcohol and other drug use and providing assistance to college students at risk for these harmful behaviors.

- *Being male.* Males are twice as likely as females to abuse illicit drugs (see the box "Gender Differences in Drug Use").

- *Being a troubled adolescent.* Teens are more likely to try drugs if they have poor self-image or self-control, use tobacco, or suffer from certain mental or emotional problems.

- *Being a thrill-seeker.* A sense of invincibility is a factor in drug experimentation.

- *Being in a dysfunctional family.* A chaotic home life or parental abuse increases the risk of drug use. The same is true for children from a single-parent home or whose parents didn't complete high school.

- *Being in a peer group that accepts drug use.* Young people who are uninterested in school and earn poor grades are more likely to try drugs.

- *Being poor.* Young people who live in disadvantaged areas are more likely to be around drugs at a young age.

- *Dating young.* Adolescent girls who date boys two or more years older than themselves are more likely to use drugs.

What about people who *don't* use drugs? As a group, nonusers also share some characteristics. Not surprisingly, people who perceive drug use as risky and who disapprove of it are less likely to use drugs than those who believe otherwise. Drug use is also less common among people who have positive self-esteem and self-concept and who are assertive, independent thinkers who are not controlled by peer pressure. Self-control, social competence, optimism, academic achievement, and regular church attendance are also linked to

**Gender Differences in Drug Use**

Men are more likely than women to use, abuse, and be dependent on illicit drugs. Rates of use are similar in males and females ages 12–17, but among those 18 and older, more men than women use drugs and have problems associated with drug use (see table). Men account for about 80% of arrests for drug abuse violations, 70% of admissions for treatment, and 65% of drug-related deaths.

There are also gender differences in why and how young people use drugs. Young males tend to use alcohol or drugs for sensation seeking or to enhance their social status, factors tied to culturally based gender roles. Young women tend to use drugs to improve mood, increase confidence, and reduce inhibitions. Boys are likelier to receive offers to use drugs in public settings, whereas girls are likelier to receive offers in a private place such as a friend's residence.

Despite overall lower rates of drug use, females may have unique biological vulnerabilities to certain drugs, and they may move more quickly from use to abuse. Major life transitions, including

the physical and emotional changes associated with puberty, increase the risk of drug use and abuse for girls more than for boys. Certain other drug abuse risk factors are also more common in female adolescents, including depression, low self-esteem, eating disorders, and a history of physical or sexual abuse.

Adolescent boys and girls share some protective factors relating to drug abuse, including positive family relationships and extracurricular activities; religious involvement is protective for

both boys and girls but may be more protective for girls.

Among older men and women, marriage, children, and employment are associated with lower rates of drug abuse and dependence. Rates of drug abuse and dependence among married adults are less than half of those among unmarried adults. Similar patterns are seen when comparing adults who live with children versus those who do not live with children and adults who are employed versus those who are unemployed.

NATIONAL SURVEY RESULTS:
PERCENT REPORTING IN PAST YEAR

| | MALES | FEMALES |
|---|---|---|
| Illicit drug use* | 16.4 | 12.2 |
| Age 12–17 | 19.0 | 18.9 |
| Age 18–25 | 36.9 | 29.9 |
| Age 26 and older | 12.3 | 8.5 |
| Drove under the influence of an illicit drug | 5.5 | 2.6 |
| Illicit drug or alcohol abuse or dependence | 11.5 | 6.4 |
| Treatment for drug or alcohol dependence | 2.2 | 1.0 |

*Illicit drugs include marijuana/hashish, cocaine, heroin, hallucinogens, inhalants, and prescription-type psychotherapeutics used nonmedically.
**SOURCE:** Substance Abuse and Mental Health Services Administration. 2009. Results from the 2008 National Survey on Drug Use and Health: National Findings. Rockville, Md.: Office of Applied Studies, NSDUH Series H-36, HHS Publication No. SMA 09-4434.

lower rates of drug use (see the box "Spirituality and Drug Abuse").

Home environments are also influential: Coming from a strong family, one that has a clear policy on drug use, is another characteristic of people who don't use drugs. Young people who communicate openly with and feel supported by their parents are also less likely to use drugs.

## Why Do People Use Drugs?

Young people, especially those from middle-class backgrounds, are frequently drawn to drugs by the allure of the exciting and illegal. They may be curious, rebellious, or vulnerable to peer pressure. Young people may want to imitate adult models in their lives or in the movies. Most people who take illicit drugs do so experimentally, typically trying the drug one or more times but not continuing. The main factors in the initial choice of a drug are whether it is available and whether peers are using it.

Although some people use drugs because they have a desire to alter their mood or are seeking a spiritual experience, others are motivated by a desire to escape boredom, anxiety, depression, feelings of worthlessness, or other distressing symptoms of psychological problems. They use drugs as a way to cope with the difficulties they expe-

rience in life. The common practice in our society of seeking a drug solution to every problem is a factor in the widespread reliance on both illicit and prescription drugs.

For people living in poverty in the inner cities, many of these reasons for using drugs are magnified. The problems are more devastating, the need for escape more compelling. Further, the buying and selling of drugs provide access to an unofficial, alternative economy that may seem like an opportunity for success.

## Risk Factors for Dependence

Why do some people use psychoactive drugs without becoming dependent, whereas others aren't so lucky? The answer seems to be a combination of physical, psychological, and social factors. Research indicates that some people may be born with a brain chemistry or metabolism that makes them more vulnerable to drug dependence. Other research suggests that people who were exposed to drugs in the womb may have an increased risk of abusing drugs themselves later in life.

Psychological risk factors for drug dependence include difficulty in controlling impulses and a strong need for excitement, stimulation, and immediate gratification. Feelings of rejection, hostility, aggression, anxiety, or depression are

## Spirituality and Drug Abuse

Although there are diverse religious viewpoints on drug use, many religions infer some link between psychoactive drugs and spirituality. Some religions use drugs in the quest for spiritual transcendence: American Indian, Polynesian, African, and other indigenous religions have used psychoactive drugs such as peyote, khat, alcohol, and hashish for expanding consciousness and developing personal spirituality. Other religions view psychoactive drugs as a threat to spirituality. In Islam, for example, the consumption of alcohol and certain other drugs is strictly forbidden.

In studies of American teens and adults, spiritual or religious involvement is generally associated with a lower risk of trying psychoactive drugs and, for those who do use drugs, a lower risk of heavy use and dependence. The mechanism for this protective effect is unclear; possibilities include the adoption of a strict code of behavior or set of principles that forbids drug use, the presence of a social support system for abstinence or moderation, and the promotion of values that include avoidance of drug use.

The relationship between religious faith and avoidance of drug use appears to be even stronger in teens than in adults. One study found that teens who felt they had a personal relationship with the divine and/or who belonged to a more fundamentalist religious denomination were less likely to engage in substance use and abuse than other teens. Teens who attend 25 or more religious services per year are about half as likely to use illicit drugs as teens who attend services less frequently. Overall, people who spend time regularly engaging in spiritual practices such as prayer and transcendental meditation have lower rates of drug abuse.

People with current substance-abuse problems tend to have lower rates of religious affiliation and involvement and lower levels of spiritual wellness, characterized by a lack of a sense of meaning in life. One of the hallmarks of drug dependence is spending increasing amounts of time and energy getting and using drugs. Such a pattern of behavior inevitably reduces the resources one can devote to developing physical, emotional, and spiritual wellness.

Among people in treatment for substance abuse, higher levels of religious faith and spirituality may contribute to the recovery process. A study of people recovering from alcohol or other drug abuse found that spirituality and religiousness were associated with increased coping skills, greater optimism about life, greater resilience to stress, and greater perceived social support.

More research is needed to clarify the relationships among spirituality, religion, drug use, and recovery. One of the difficulties in conducting research in this area is the difficulty in defining and measuring spirituality and religious involvement. Spirituality is a complex part of human nature, involving behavior, belief, and experience. And although behaviors such as the spiritual practices of prayer or meditation can be measured, it is more difficult to determine what such practices mean to an individual and her or his overall sense of self.

**SOURCES:** Brown, A. E., et al. 2006. Alcohol recovery and spirituality: Strangers, friends, or partners? *Southern Medical Journal* 99(6): 654–657; Substance Abuse and Mental Health Network. 2004. Religious beliefs and substance use among youths. *NSDUH Report*, January; Dunn, M. S. 2005. The relationship between religiosity, employment, and political beliefs on substance use among high school seniors. *Journal of Alcohol and Drug Education* 49(1): 73.

also associated with drug dependence. People may turn to drugs to blot out their emotional pain.

People with mental illnesses have a very high risk of substance dependence. Research shows that about one-third of people with psychological disorders also have a substance-dependence problem; about one-third of those have mental disorder. People with two or more coexisting mental disorders are referred to as having *dual (co-occurring) disorders*. Diagnosing psychological problems among people with substance dependence can be difficult because drug intoxication and withdrawal can mimic the symptoms of a mental illness.

Social factors can influence drug dependence. These factors include growing up with a family member who abuses drugs, belonging to a peer group that emphasizes or encourages drug use, and living in poverty. Because they have easy access to drugs, health care professionals are also at a higher risk.

## Other Risks of Drug Use

Dependence is not the only serious potential consequence of drug use. In 2007, nearly 1.9 million emergency department visits were related to drug misuse or abuse (Table 9.3).

**Intoxication** People who are under the influence of drugs—intoxicated—may act in uncharacteristic and unsafe ways because both their physical and mental functioning are impaired. They are more likely to be injured from a variety of causes, to have unsafe sex, and to be involved in incidents of aggression and violence.

| Table 9.3 | Emergency Department (ED) Visits Involving Drug Use/Abuse: 2007* | |
|---|---|---|
| REASON FOR ED VISIT | ESTIMATED VISITS | PERCENTAGE OF VISITS |
| Pharmaceuticals only | 582,187 | 30.9 |
| Illicit drugs | 522,650 | 27.8 |
| Illicit drugs and alcohol | 237,936 | 12.6 |
| Alcohol and pharmaceuticals | 189,444 | 10.1 |
| Illicit drugs and pharmaceuticals | 143,783 | 7.6 |
| Alcohol only in patients younger than 21 | 137,369 | 7.3 |
| Illicit drugs with pharmaceuticals and alcohol | 69,903 | 3.7 |
| Total | 1,883,272 | 100% |

*U.S. hospitals received 116 million ED visits in 2007. About 1.6% of those visits involved drug use or abuse by the patient. (Note: percentages shown here may not equal 100 due to rounding.)

SOURCE: Substance Abuse and Mental Health Services Administration, Office of Applied Studies. 2010. *Drug Abuse Warning Network, 2007: National Estimates of Drug-Related Emergency Department Visits.* Rockville, Md.: Substance Abuse and Mental Health Services Administration.

**Ask Yourself**

QUESTIONS FOR CRITICAL THINKING AND REFLECTION
Have you ever tried a psychoactive drug for fun? What were your reasons for trying it? Who were you with, and what were the circumstances? What was your experience like? What would you tell someone else who was thinking about trying a drug?

**Unexpected Side Effects** Psychoactive drugs have many physical and psychological effects beyond the alteration of consciousness. These effects range from nausea and constipation to paranoia, depression, and heart failure. Some drugs also carry the risk of fatal overdose.

**Unknown Drug Constituents** There is no quality control in the illegal drug market, so the composition, dosage, and toxicity of street drugs are highly variable. Studies indicate that half of all street drugs don't contain their promised primary ingredient. In some cases, a drug may be present in unsafe dosages or mixed with other drugs to boost its effects. Makers of street drugs aren't held to any safety standards, so illicit drugs can be contaminated or even poisonous.

**Risks Associated with Injection Drug Use** Heroin is the most commonly injected drug, but users can also inject cocaine, amphetamines, and other drugs. Many injection drug users (IDUs) share or reuse needles, syringes, and other injection supplies, which can easily become contaminated with the user's blood. Small amounts of blood can carry enough human immunodeficiency virus (HIV) and hepatitis C virus (HCV) to be infectious. In 2008, injection drug use accounted for more than 10% of all new HIV/AIDS cases; many more were attributed to sexual contact with IDUs. Injection drug use also accounts for nearly half of new HCV infections.

**48% of confirmed new HCV infections occurred among injection drug users.**
—CDC, 2009

Unsterile injection practices can cause skin and soft tissue infections, which can progress to gangrene (tissue death) and be fatal if untreated. Other risks include endocarditis (infection of the heart valves), tuberculosis, and tetanus.

The surest way to prevent diseases related to injection drug use is never to inject drugs. IDUs should use a new needle and syringe with each injection and should use sterile water and supplies to prepare drugs. Bleach or boiling water may kill some viruses and bacteria, but are not foolproof sterilization methods. Many viruses can survive in a syringe for a month or more.

Syringe exchange programs (SEPs)—where IDUs can trade a used syringe for a new one—have been advocated to help slow the spread of HIV and reduce the rates and cost of other health problems associated with injection drug use. Opponents of SEPs argue that supplying addicts with syringes gives them the message that illegal drug use is acceptable and worsens the nation's drug problem. However, studies have shown that well-implemented SEPs do not increase the use of drugs, and most offer AIDS counseling and provide referrals to drug treatment programs. Getting people off drugs is clearly the best solution, but there are far more IDUs than treatment facilities can currently handle.

**Legal Consequences** Many psychoactive drugs are illegal, so possessing them can result in large fines and/or imprisonment. According to the Federal Bureau of Investigation (FBI), law enforcement officials made 1.7 million arrests for drug abuse violations (12% of all arrests) in 2008—more arrests than for any other offense that year.

## HOW DRUGS AFFECT THE BODY

The drugs discussed in this chapter have complex and variable effects, many of which can be traced to changes in brain chemistry. However, the same drug may affect different people differently or the same person in different ways under different circumstances. Beyond a fairly predictable general change in brain chemistry, the effects of a drug may vary depending on drug factors, user factors, and social factors.

## Changes in Brain Chemistry

Psychoactive drugs produce most of their key effects by acting on brain chemistry in a characteristic fashion. Before any changes in brain chemistry can occur, however, molecules of the drug have to be carried to the brain through the bloodstream via a particular route of administration. A drug that is taken by mouth has to dissolve in the stomach, be absorbed into the bloodstream through the lining of the small intestine, and then pass through the liver, heart, and lungs before returning to the heart to be carried via arteries to the brain. A drug that is already dissolved and is injected directly into the bloodstream will reach the brain in much less time, and drugs that are inhaled and absorbed by the lungs travel to the brain even more rapidly. The more quickly a drug reaches the brain, the more likely the user is to become dependent.

> *Psychoactive drugs work by **affecting** one or more neurotransmitters in the brain.*

Once a psychoactive drug reaches the brain, it acts on one or more **neurotransmitters,** either increasing or decreasing their concentration and actions. Cocaine, for example, affects dopamine, a neurotransmitter thought to play a key role in the process of reinforcement—the brain's way of telling itself "That's good; do the same thing again." When a neurotransmitter is released by one neuron to signal another neuron, its level or concentration is controlled in part by the re-uptake or resorption of the neurotransmitter by the releasing neuron. Cocaine inhibits the resorption of dopamine, thereby increasing the concentration of dopamine in the synapse and lengthening the time of its action (Figure 9.1). The euphoria produced by cocaine is thought to be a result of its effect on

dopamine. Heroin, nicotine, alcohol, and amphetamines also affect dopamine levels.

The duration of a drug's effect depends on many factors and may range from 5 minutes (crack cocaine) to 12 or more hours (LSD). As drugs circulate through the body, they are metabolized by the liver and eventually excreted by the kidneys in urine. Small amounts may also be eliminated in other ways, including in sweat, in breast milk, and via the lungs.

## Drug Factors

When different drugs or dosages produce different effects, the differences are usually caused by one or more of five different drug factors:

1. The **pharmacological properties** of a drug are its effects on a person's body chemistry, behavior, and psychology. Pharmacological properties also include the amount of a drug required to exert various effects, the time course of the effects, and other characteristics, such as a drug's chemical composition.

2. The **dose-response function** is the relationship between the amount of drug taken and the type and intensity of its effects. Many psychological effects of drugs reach a plateau in the dose-response function, so that increasing the dose does not increase the effect any further. With LSD, for example, the maximum changes in perception occur at a certain dose, and no further changes in perception take place if higher doses are taken. However, all drugs have more than one effect, and the dose-response functions usually are different for different effects. This means that increasing the dose of any drug may begin to result in additional effects, which are likely to be more unpleasant or dangerous at high doses.

3. The **time-action function** is the relationship between the time elapsed since a drug was taken and the intensity of its effect. A drug's effects are greatest when its concentrations in body tissues are changing fastest, especially if they are increasing.

4. The person's *drug use history* may influence the effects of a drug. A given amount of alcohol, for example, will generally affect a habitual drinker less than an occasional drinker. Tolerance to some drugs, such as LSD, builds rapidly. To experience the same effect, a user has to abstain from the drug for a period of time before that dosage will again exert its original effects.

5. The *method of use* (or *route of administration*) has a direct effect on how strong a response a drug produces. Methods of use include ingestion, inhalation, injection, and absorption through the skin or tissue linings. Drugs are usually injected in one of three ways: intravenously (IV, or mainlining), intramuscularly (IM), or subcutaneously (SC, or skin popping).

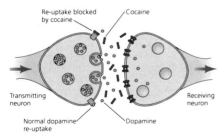

**FIGURE 9.1  Effect of cocaine on brain chemistry.** Under normal circumstances, the amount of dopamine at a synapse is controlled in part by the re-uptake of dopamine by the transmitting neuron. Cocaine blocks the removal of dopamine from a synapse; the resulting buildup of dopamine causes continuous stimulation of the receiving neurons.

## User Factors

Certain physical and psychological characteristics help determine how a person will respond to a drug. Body mass is one variable. The effects of a certain dose of a drug on a 100-pound person will be twice as great as on a 200-pound person. Other variables include general health and genetic factors. For example, some people have an inherited ability to rapidly metabolize a cough suppressant called dextromethorphan, which also has psychoactive properties. These people must take a higher-than-normal dose to get a given cough-suppressant effect.

If a person's biochemical state is already altered by another drug, this too can make a difference. Some drugs intensify the effects of other drugs, as is the case with alcohol and sedatives. Some drugs block the effects of other drugs, such as when a tranquilizer is used to relieve anxiety caused by cocaine. Interactions between drugs, including many prescription and OTC medications, can be unpredictable and dangerous.

One physical condition that requires special precautions is pregnancy. It can be risky for a woman to use any drugs at all during pregnancy, including alcohol and common OTC products like cough medicine. The risks are greatest during the first trimester, when the fetus's body is rapidly forming and even small biochemical alterations in the mother can have a devastating effect on fetal development. Even later, the fetus is more susceptible than the mother to the adverse effects of any drugs she takes. The fetus may even become physically dependent on a drug being taken by the mother and suffer withdrawal symptoms after birth.

Sometimes a person's response to a drug is strongly influenced by the user's expectations about how he or she will react (the psychological *set*). With large doses, the drug's chemical properties seem to have the strongest effect on the user's response. But with small doses, psychological (and social) factors are often more important. When people strongly believe that a given drug will affect them a certain way, they are likely to experience those effects regardless of the drug's pharmacological properties. In one study, regular users of marijuana reported a moderate level of intoxication (high) after using a cigarette that smelled and tasted like marijuana but contained no THC, the active ingredient in marijuana. This is an example of the placebo effect—when a person receives an inert substance yet responds as if it were an active drug. In other studies, subjects who smoked low doses of real marijuana that they believed to be a placebo experienced no effects from the drug. Clearly, the user's expectations had a greater effect on the smokers than the drug itself.

## Social Factors

The *setting* is the physical and social environment surrounding the drug use. If a person uses marijuana at home with trusted friends and pleasant music, the effects are likely to be different from the effects if the same dose

is taken in an austere experimental laboratory with an impassive research technician. Similarly, the dose of alcohol that produces mild euphoria and stimulation at a noisy, active cocktail party might induce sleepiness and slight depression when taken at home while alone.

## REPRESENTATIVE PSYCHOACTIVE DRUGS

The following sections and Figure 9.2 introduce six representative groups of psychoactive drugs: opioids, central nervous system (CNS) depressants, central nervous system stimulants, marijuana and other cannabis products, hallucinogens, and inhalants. Some of these drugs are classified according to how they affect the body. Others— the opioids and the cannabis products—are classified according to their chemical makeup.

### Opioids

Also called *narcotics,* opioids are natural or synthetic (laboratory-made) drugs, such as opium, morphine, heroin, methadone, codeine, hydrocodone, oxycodone, meperidine, and fentanyl. Opioids relieve pain, cause drowsiness, and induce euphoria. Especially in small doses,

**TERMS**

**neurotransmitter** A brain chemical that transmits nerve impulses.

**pharmacological properties** The overall effects of a drug on a person's behavior, psychology, and chemistry.

**dose-response function** The relationship between the amount of a drug taken and the intensity and type of the resulting effect.

**time-action function** The relationship between the time elapsed since a drug was taken and the intensity of its effect.

**high** The subjectively pleasing effects of a drug, usually felt quite soon after the drug is taken.

**placebo effect** A response to an inert or innocuous substance given in place of an active drug.

**opioid** Any of several natural or synthetic drugs that relieve pain and cause drowsiness and/or euphoria; examples are opium, morphine, and heroin; also called a *narcotic.*

**euphoria** An exaggerated feeling of well-being.

| Category | Representative drugs | Street names | Appearance | Methods of use | Short-term effects |
|---|---|---|---|---|---|
| **Opioids** | Heroin | Dope, H, junk, brown sugar, smack | White/dark brown powder; dark tar or coal-like substance | Injected, smoked, snorted | Relief of anxiety and pain; euphoria; lethargy, apathy, drowsiness, confusion, inability to concentrate; nausea, constipation, respiratory depression |
| | Opium | Big O, black stuff, hop | Dark brown or black chunks | Swallowed, smoked | |
| | Morphine | M, Miss Emma, monkey, white stuff | White crystals, liquid solution | Injected, swallowed, smoked | |
| | Oxycodone, codeine, hydrocodone | Oxy, O.C., killer, Captain Cody, schoolboy, vike | Tablets, powder made from crushing tablets | Swallowed, injected, snorted | |
| **Central nervous system depressants** | Barbiturates | Barbs, reds, red birds, yellows, yellow jackets | Colored capsules | Swallowed, injected | Reduced anxiety, mood changes, lowered inhibitions, impaired muscle coordination, reduced pulse rate, drowsiness, loss of consciousness, respiratory depression |
| | Benzodiazepines (e.g., Valium, Xanax, Rohypnol) | Candy, downers, tranks, roofies, forget-me pill | Tablets | Swallowed, injected | |
| | Methaqualone | Ludes, quad, quay | Tablets | Injected, swallowed | |
| | Gamma hydroxy butyrate (GHB) | G, Georgia home boy, grievous bodily harm | Clear liquid, white powder | Swallowed | |
| **Central nervous system stimulants** | Amphetamine, methamphetamine | Bennies, speed, black beauties, uppers, chalk, crank, crystal, ice, meth | Tablets, capsules, white powder, white crystals | Injected, swallowed, smoked, snorted | Increased heart rate, blood pressure, metabolism; increased mental alertness and energy; nervousness, insomnia, impulsive behavior; reduced appetite |
| | Cocaine, crack cocaine | Blow, C, candy, coke, flake, rock, toot | White powder, beige pellets or rocks | Injected, smoked, snorted | |
| | Ritalin | JIF, MPH, R-ball, Skippy | Tablets | Injected, swallowed, snorted | |
| **Marijuana and other cannabis products** | Marijuana | Dope, grass, joints, Mary Jane, reefer, skunk, weed | Dried leaves and stems | Smoked, swallowed | Euphoria, slowed thinking and reaction time, confusion, anxiety, impaired balance and coordination, increased heart rate |
| | Hashish | Hash, hemp, boom, gangster | Dark, resin-like compound formed into rocks or blocks | Smoked, swallowed | |
| **Hallucinogens** | LSD | Acid, boomers, blotter, yellow sunshines | Blotter paper, liquid, gelatin tabs, pills | Swallowed, absorbed through mouth tissues | Altered states of perception and feeling; nausea; increased heart rate, blood pressure; delirium; impaired motor function; numbness, weakness |
| | Mescaline (peyote) | Buttons, cactus, mesc | Brown buttons, liquid | Swallowed, smoked | |
| | Psilocybin | Shrooms, magic mushrooms | Dried mushrooms | Swallowed | |
| | Ketamine | K, special K, cat valium, vitamin K | Clear liquid, white or beige powder | Injected, snorted, smoked | |
| | PCP | Angel dust, hog, love boat, peace pill | White to brown powder, tablets | Injected, swallowed, smoked, snorted | |
| | MDMA (ecstasy) | X, peace, clarity, Adam | Tablets | Swallowed | |
| **Inhalants** | Solvents, aerosols, nitrites, anesthetics | Laughing gas, poppers, snappers, whippets | Household products, sprays, glues, paint thinner, petroleum products | Inhaled through nose or mouth | Stimulation, loss of inhibition, slurred speech, loss of motor coordination, loss of consciousness |

**FIGURE 9.2  Commonly abused drugs and their effects.**

SOURCES: The Partnership for a Drug-Free America. 2010. *Drug Guide by Name* (http://www.drugfree.org/portal/drug_guide; retrieved November 3, 2010); U.S. Drug Enforcement Agency. 2006. *Photo Library* (http://www.usdoj.gov/dea/photo_library.html; retrieved November 3, 2010); U.S. Drug Enforcement Agency. 2010. *Drug Information* (http://www.justice.gov/dea/concern/concern.htm; retrieved November 3, 2010); National Institute on Drug Abuse. 2010. *Commonly Abused Drugs* (http://www.drugabuse.gov/DrugPages/DrugsofAbuse.html; retrieved November 3, 2010).

opioids have beneficial medical uses, including pain relief and cough suppression. Opioids tend to reduce anxiety and produce lethargy, apathy, and an inability to concentrate. Opioid users become less active and less responsive to frustration, hunger, and sexual stimulation. These effects are more pronounced in novice users; with repeated use, many effects diminish.

Opioids are typically injected. They can also be absorbed into the body through the stomach, intestines, nasal membranes (from snorting or sniffing), or lungs (from smoking). Effects depend on the method of administration. If brain levels of the drug change rapidly, more immediate effects result. Although the euphoria associated with opioids is an important factor in their abuse, many people experience a feeling of uneasiness when they first use these drugs. Users also often feel nauseated and vomit, and they may have other unpleasant sensations. Even so, the abuse of opioids often results in dependence. Tolerance can develop rapidly and be pronounced. Withdrawal symptoms include cramps, chills, sweating, nausea, tremors, irritability, and feelings of panic.

Rates of heroin use have always been low, but there are periodic episodes of increased use among some groups. Use among college students remains below 1%, but between 1991 and 2000 heroin use among high school seniors more than doubled, mostly due to increased rates of sniffing or smoking the drug. Although these users avoid the special disease risks of injection drug use, including HIV infection, dependence can readily result from sniffing and smoking heroin. In addition, the potentially high but variable purity of street heroin poses a risk of unintentional overdose. Symptoms of overdose include respiratory depression, coma, and constriction of the pupils; death can result.

Nonmedical use of prescription pain relievers that contain oxycodone and hydrocodone, including Oxycontin and Vicodin, has increased in recent years (see the box "Prescription Drug Abuse Among American Teenagers"). When taken as prescribed in tablet form, these drugs treat moderate to severe chronic pain and do not typically lead to abuse. However, as is the case with other opioids, use of prescription painkillers can lead to abuse and dependence. Oxycodone and hydrocodone can be abused orally; the long-acting form of oxycodone is also sometimes crushed and snorted or dissolved and injected, providing a powerful heroin-like high. When taken in large doses or combined with other drugs, oxycodone and hydrocodone can cause fatal respiratory depression.

## Central Nervous System Depressants

Central nervous system **depressants**, also known as **sedative-hypnotics**, slow down the overall activity of the **central nervous system (CNS)**. The result can range from mild **sedation** to death, depending on the factors involved—which drug is used, how it's taken, how tolerant the user is, and so on. CNS depressants include alcohol (Chapter 10), barbiturates, and other sedatives.

**Types** The various types of barbiturates are similar in chemical composition and action, but they differ in how quickly and how long they act. Drug users call barbiturates "downers" or "downs" and refer to specific brands by names that describe the color and design of the capsules. People usually take barbiturates in capsules, but may also inject them.

Antianxiety agents, also called sedatives or **tranquilizers**, include the benzodiazepines such as Xanax, Valium, Librium, clonazepam (Klonopin), and flunitrazepam (Rohypnol, also called roofies). Other CNS depressants include methaqualone (Quaalude), etchchlorvynol (Placidyl), chloral hydrate ("mickey"), and gamma hydroxybutyrate (GHB, or "liquid ecstasy").

**Effects** CNS depressants reduce anxiety and cause mood changes, impaired muscular coordination, slurring of speech, and drowsiness or sleep. Mental functioning is also affected, but the degree varies from person to person and also depends on the kind of task the person is trying to do. Most people become drowsy with small doses, although a few become more active.

**Medical Uses** Barbiturates, antianxiety agents, and other sedative-hypnotics are widely used to treat insomnia and anxiety disorders and to control seizures. Some CNS depressants are used for their calming properties in combination with **anesthetics** before operations and other medical or dental procedures.

**From Use to Abuse** People are usually introduced to CNS depressants either through a medical prescription or through drug-using peers. The use of Rohypnol and GHB

---

**depressant, or sedative-hypnotic** A drug that decreases nervous or muscular activity, causing drowsiness or sleep.

**central nervous system (CNS)** The brain and spinal cord.

**sedation** The induction of a calm, relaxed, often sleepy state.

**tranquilizer** A CNS depressant that reduces tension and anxiety.

**anesthetic** A drug that produces a loss of sensation with or without a loss of consciousness.

TERMS

## Prescription Drug Abuse Among American Teenagers

According to the 2008 National Survey on Drug Use and Health (NSDUH), nearly 21% of Americans over age 11 have used prescription-type psychotherapeutic drugs for nonmedical reasons at least once in their life, and more than 6 million Americans have done so in the past 30 days. Prescription-type drugs include pain relievers, tranquilizers, stimulants, and sedatives that are legally available only by prescription, as well as similar over-the-counter (OTC) drugs.

Although Americans have been abusing prescription drugs like Valium for decades, the rapidly growing trend of abuse among teenagers is a major source of concern. Over the last decade, the number of middle- and high school students who misuse prescription and OTC medications has increased dramatically. The 2008 NSDUH shows that well over a million Americans ages 12–20 abused a prescription drug in the past 30 days.

According to another survey, the CDC's Youth Risk Behavior Surveillance for 2009, 20.2% of American high school students have taken prescription drugs at least once without a doctor's prescription. The rate of abuse increases steadily through the grade levels, with 15.1% of freshman and 25.8% of seniors misusing prescription medications. The CDC's study also found that more white students (23.0%) abuse prescription drugs than do Hispanic (17.2%) or black (11.8%) students. Males and females abuse prescription drugs at about the same rate.

Aside from marijuana, prescription-type drugs are the most abused drugs

among teenagers. The most commonly abused are painkillers (OxyContin, Vicodin), depressants (sleeping pills, anti-anxiety medications), and stimulants (Ritalin, Adderall). The most commonly abused OTC drugs are cough and cold remedies containing the cough suppressant dextromethorphan, an ingredient in Robitussin and Nyquil. According to the Substance Abuse and Mental Health Services Administration (SAMSHA), 1 million Americans ages 12–25 used OTC cough and cold medicines recreationally in 2006.

The primary reason for the increase in abuse of prescription-type drugs is their availabiltiy. Teens report getting

drugs from relatives and buying them without a prescription over the Internet. They also commonly get them from one another, at school or at parties where drugs are openly exchanged.

In addition, teens apparently choose prescription-type drugs because they believe they are safer than illicit drugs, but this is not the case. Just like their illegal counterparts, these medications carry the risk of dependency, addiction, and lethal overdose, particularly when combined with alcohol. Between 2004 and 2008, emergency department visits due to prescription painkiller abuse increased by more than 110%, and more than 71,000 children are taken to the ED each year for overdoses of OTC medications. In response to the challenge of prescription drug abuse, the government has launched public health campaigns and public service announcements aimed at educating both parents and teens about the dangers of these seemingly innocuous substances.

SOURCE: Centers for Disease Control and Prevention. 2010. Emergency Department Visits Involving Nonmedical Use of Selected Prescription Drugs—United States, 2004–2008. Morbidity and Mortality Weekly Report 59(23): 705–709; Centers for Disease Control and Prevention. 2010. Youth Risk Behavior Surveillance—United States, 2009. Morbidity and Mortality Weekly Report Surveillance Summaries 59(SS-5): 1–142; Substance Abuse and Mental Health Services Administration. 2009. Results from the 2008 National Survey on Drug Use and Health: National Findings. Rockville, Md.: Office of Applied Studies, NSDUH Series H-36, HHS Publication No. SMA 09-4434.

---

is often associated with dance clubs and raves (see the box "Club Drugs"). The abuse of CNS depressants by a medical patient may begin with repeated use for insomnia and progress to dependence through increasingly larger doses at night, coupled with doses during stressful times during the day.

Most CNS depressants, including alcohol, can lead to physical dependence. Tolerance, sometimes for up to 15 times the usual dose, can develop with repeated use. Tranquilizers have been shown to produce physical dependence even at ordinary prescribed doses. Withdrawal symptoms can be more severe than those accompanying opioid dependence and are similar to the DTs of alcoholism (see Chapter 10). They may begin as anxiety, shaking,

and weakness but may turn into convulsions and possibly cardiovascular collapse and death.

While intoxicated, people on depressants cannot function well. They are confused and are frequently obstinate, irritable, and abusive. Even prescription use of benzodiazepines has been associated with an increased risk of automobile crashes. After long-term use, depressants like alcohol can lead to poor health and brain damage, with impaired ability to reason and make judgments.

**Overdosing with CNS Depressants** Too much depression of the central nervous system slows respiration and may stop it entirely. CNS depressants are particularly dangerous in combination with another depressant,

# Club Drugs

Some people refer to club drugs as soft drugs because they see them as recreational—for the casual, weekend user—rather than as addictive. But club drugs have many potential negative effects and are particularly potent and unpredictable when mixed with alcohol. Substitute drugs are often sold in place of club drugs, putting users at risk for taking dangerous combinations of unknown drugs.

**MDMA** *(ecstasy, E, X, XTC, Adam, hug drug, lover's speed):* Taken in pill form, MDMA (methylenedioxymethamphetamine) is a stimulant with mildly hallucinogenic and amphetamine-like effects. Users may experience euphoria, increased energy, and a heightened sense of belonging. In club settings, using MDMA can produce dangerously high body temperature and potentially fatal dehydration; some users experience confusion, depression, anxiety, paranoia, muscle tension, involuntary teeth clenching, blurred vision, nausea, and seizures. Even low doses can affect concentration, judg-

ment, and driving ability. Tolerance can develop, leading users to take the drug more frequently, to use higher doses, or to combine MDMA with other drugs to enhance the drug's effects.

In addition to MDMA, many ecstasy tablets include other drugs such as methamphetamine, ephedrine, or cocaine. At high doses or mixed with other drugs, MDMA is extremely dangerous; most deaths linked to MDMA have occurred as a result of multidrug toxicity or traumatic injuries.

MDMA increases the activity of three neurotransmitters: serotonin, dopamine, and norepinephrine. Increases in serotonin are likely the cause of the drug's mood-elevating effects, but use of MDMA can deplete the brain of serotonin and may cause an emotional let-down (sadness, irritability, etc.) in the days following use.

MDMA users perform worse than nonusers on complex cognitive tasks of memory, attention, and general intelligence. Long-term effects may include physical symptoms and psychological problems such as confusion or paranoia. Research suggests that pregnant women who use MDMA are at increased risk for having a baby with congenital malformations and long-term impairment in memory and other cognitive functions.

**LSD** *(acid, boomers, yellow sunshines, red dragon):* A potent hallucinogen, LSD (lysergic acid diethylamide) is sold in tablets or capsules, in liquid form, or on small squares of paper called blotters. LSD increases heart rate and body temperature and may cause nausea, tremors, sweating, numbness, and weakness.

**Ketamine** *(special K, vitamin K, K, cat valium, jet):* A veterinary anesthetic that can be taken in powdered or liquid form, ketamine may cause hallucinations and impaired attention and memory. At higher doses, ketamine can cause delirium, amnesia, high blood pressure, and

potentially fatal respiratory problems. Tolerance to ketamine develops rapidly.

**GHB** *(Georgia home boy, G, grievous bodily harm, liquid ecstasy):* GHB (gamma hydroxybutyrate) can be produced in clear liquid, white powder, tablet, and capsule form. GHB is a CNS depressant that in large doses or when taken in combination with alcohol or other depressants can cause sedation, loss of consciousness, respiratory arrest, and death. GHB may cause prolonged and potentially life-threatening withdrawal symptoms.

Some products sold as dietary supplements for bodybuilding, weight loss, or insomnia contain the chemically similar compounds GBL (gamma butyrolactone) or BD (butanediol). It is illegal to sell products containing GHB, GBL, or BD for human consumption. The FDA has issued several warnings to prevent such items from being sold to the public.

**Rohypnol** *(roofies, roche, forget-me pill):* Taken in tablet form, Rohypnol (flunitrazepam) is a sedative that is ten times more potent than Valium. Its effects, which are magnified by alcohol, include reduced blood pressure, dizziness, confusion, gastrointestinal disturbances, and loss of consciousness. Users of Rohypnol may develop physical and psychological dependence on the drug.

Several club drugs are used as "date rape drugs." Because they can be added to beverages surreptitiously, these drugs may be unknowingly consumed by intended rape victims. In addition to depressant effects, some drugs also cause *anterograde amnesia,* the loss of memory of things occurring while under the influence of the drug. Because of concern about such drugs, Congress passed the "Drug-Induced Rape Prevention and Punishment Act," which increased federal penalties for use of any controlled substance to aid in sexual assault (see Chapter 21).

such as alcohol. People who combine depressants with alcohol account for thousands of emergency department visits and hundreds of overdose deaths each year. Rohypnol is ten times more potent than Valium and can be fatal if combined with alcohol. GHB is often produced clandestinely, resulting in widely varying degrees of purity; it has been responsible for many poisonings and deaths.

# Central Nervous System Stimulants

CNS **stimulants** speed up the activity of the nervous or muscular system. Under their influence, the heart rate accelerates, blood pressure rises, blood vessels constrict, the pupils and bronchial tubes dilate, and gastric and adrenal secretions increase. There is greater muscular tension and sometimes an increase in motor activity. Small doses usually make people feel more awake and alert, less fatigued and bored. The most common CNS stimulants are cocaine, amphetamines, nicotine (Chapter 11), ephedrine, and caffeine.

**Cocaine** Usually derived from the leaves of coca shrubs that grow high in the Andes in South America, cocaine is a potent CNS stimulant. For centuries, natives of the Andes have chewed coca leaves both for pleasure and to increase their endurance. For a short time during the nineteenth century, some physicians were enthusiastic about the use of cocaine to cure alcoholism and addiction to the painkiller morphine. Enthusiasm waned after the drug's adverse side effects became apparent.

Cocaine—also known as coke or snow—quickly produces a feeling of euphoria, which makes it a popular recreational drug. Cocaine use surged in popularity during the early 1980s, when the drug's high price made it a status drug. The introduction of crack cocaine during the 1980s made the drug available in smaller quantities and at lower prices to more people. The typical recreational user shifted rapidly from wealthy professionals snorting powdered cocaine to poor inner-city smokers of crack cocaine. Cocaine use peaked in 1985 with an estimated 3% of adult Americans reporting use.

**METHODS OF USE** Cocaine is usually snorted and absorbed through the nasal mucosa or injected intravenously, providing rapid increases of the drug's concentration in the blood and therefore fast, intense effects. Another method of use involves processing cocaine with baking soda and water, yielding the ready-to-smoke form of cocaine known as crack. Crack is typically available as small beads or pellets smokable in glass pipes. The tiny but potent beads can be handled more easily than cocaine powder and marketed in smaller, less expensive doses.

**EFFECTS** The effects of cocaine are usually intense but short-lived. The euphoria lasts from 5 to 20 minutes and ends abruptly, to be replaced by irritability, anxiety, or slight depression. When cocaine is absorbed via the lungs, by either smoking or inhalation, it reaches the brain in about 10 seconds, and the effects are particularly intense. This is part of the appeal of smoking crack. The effects from IV injections occur almost as quickly—in about 20 seconds. Since the mucous membranes in the nose briefly slow absorption, the onset of effects from snorting takes 2–3 minutes. Heavy users may inject cocaine intravenously every 10–20 minutes to maintain the effects.

The larger the cocaine dose and the more rapidly it is absorbed into the bloodstream, the greater the immediate—and sometimes lethal—effects. Sudden death from cocaine is most commonly the result of excessive CNS stimulation that causes convulsions and respiratory collapse, irregular heartbeat, extremely high blood pressure, blood clots, and possibly heart attack or stroke. Although rare, fatalities can occur in healthy young people; among people aged 18–59, cocaine users are seven times more likely than nonusers to have a heart attack. Chronic cocaine use produces inflammation of the nasal mucosa, which can lead to persistent bleeding and ulceration of the septum between the nostrils. The use of cocaine may also cause paranoia and/or aggressiveness.

Although the use of cocaine decreased in the general U.S. population after 1985, cocaine is responsible for more deaths and emergency room visits than any other illicit drug. This presumably reflects the fact that smoking crack is more toxic than snorting powdered cocaine. Most deaths result from people using cocaine in combination with another substance, such as alcohol or heroin.

**ABUSE AND DEPENDENCE** When steady cocaine users stop taking the drug, they experience a sudden "crash" characterized by depression, agitation, and fatigue, followed by a period of withdrawal. Their depression can be temporarily relieved by taking more cocaine, reinforcing its continued use. A binge cocaine user may go for weeks or months without using any cocaine and then take large amounts repeatedly. Although not physically dependent, a binge cocaine user who misses work or school and risks serious health consequences is clearly abusing the drug.

**COCAINE USE DURING PREGNANCY** Cocaine rapidly passes from the mother's bloodstream into the placenta and can have serious effects on the fetus. A woman who uses cocaine during pregnancy is at higher risk for miscarriage, premature labor, and stillbirth. She is more likely to deliver a low-birth-weight baby who has a small head circumference. Her infant may be at increased risk for defects of the genitourinary tract, cardiovascular system, central nervous system, and extremities. It is difficult to pinpoint the effects of cocaine because many women who use cocaine also use tobacco and/or alcohol.

---

**TERMS**

**stimulant** A drug that increases nervous or muscular activity.

**state dependence** A situation in which information learned in a drug-induced state is difficult to recall when the effect of the drug wears off.

**psychosis** A severe mental disorder characterized by a distortion of reality; symptoms might include delusions or hallucinations.

Infants whose mothers use cocaine may also be born intoxicated. They are typically irritable and jittery and do not eat or sleep normally. These characteristics may affect their early social and emotional development because it may be more difficult for adults to interact with them. Cocaine also passes into breast milk and can intoxicate a breastfeeding infant.

**Amphetamines**  Amphetamines (uppers) are a group of synthetic chemicals that are potent CNS stimulants. Some common drugs in this family are amphetamine (Benzedrine), dextroamphetamine (Dexedrine), and methamphetamine (Methedrine). Crystal methamphetamine (also called ice) is a smokable, high-potency form of methamphetamine, or meth. Crystal meth is easy to manufacture and cheaper than crack cocaine, and it produces a similar but longer-lasting euphoria. The use of crystal meth can quickly lead to dependence.

**EFFECTS**  Small doses of amphetamines usually make people feel more alert. Amphetamines generally increase motor activity but do not measurably alter a normal, rested person's ability to perform tasks calling for challenging motor skills or complex thinking. When amphetamines improve performance, it is primarily by counteracting fatigue and boredom. In small doses, amphetamines increase heart rate and blood pressure and change sleep patterns.

Amphetamines are sometimes used to curb appetite, but after a few weeks the user develops tolerance and higher doses are necessary. When people stop taking the drug, their appetite usually returns, and they gain back the weight they lost unless they have made permanent changes in eating behavior.

**FROM USE TO ABUSE**  Much amphetamine abuse begins as an attempt to cope with a temporary situation. A student cramming for an exam or an exhausted long-haul truck driver can go a little longer by taking amphetamines, but the results can be disastrous. The likelihood of making bad judgments significantly increases. The stimulating effects may also wear off suddenly, and the user may precipitously feel exhausted or fall asleep ("crash").

Another problem is **state dependence,** the phenomenon whereby information learned in a certain drug-induced state is difficult to recall when the person is not in that same physiological state. Test performance may deteriorate when students use drugs to study and then take tests in their normal, nondrug state. (Users of antihistamines may also experience state dependence.)

**DEPENDENCE**  Repeated use of amphetamines, even in moderate doses, often leads to tolerance and the need for increasingly larger doses. The result can be severe disturbances in behavior, including a temporary state of paranoid **psychosis,** with delusions of persecution and episodes of unprovoked violence. If injected in large doses, amphetamines produce a feeling of intense pleasure, followed by

sensations of vigor and euphoria that last for several hours. As these feelings wear off, they are replaced by feelings of irritability and vague uneasiness. Long-term use of amphetamines at high doses can cause paranoia, hallucinations, delusions, and incoherence.

Methamphetamine is more addictive and dangerous than most forms of amphetamine because it is more toxic and its effects last longer (see the box "Meth and the Environment: A Toxic Impact"). In the short term, meth can cause rapid breathing, increased body temperature, insomnia, tremors, anxiety, and convulsions. Meth use has been linked to high-risk sexual behavior and increased rates of STDs, including HIV infection. In the long term, the effects of meth can include weight loss, severe acne, hallucinations, paranoia, violence, and psychosis. Meth use causes extensive tooth decay and tooth loss, a condition referred to as "meth mouth." Meth takes a toll on the user's heart and can cause heart attack and stroke. Methamphetamine users have signs of brain damage similar to those seen in Parkinson's disease patients that appear to persist even after drug use ceases, causing impaired memory and motor coordination. Withdrawal from meth causes symptoms that may include muscle aches and tremors, profound fatigue, deep depression, despair, and apathy. Chronic high-dose use is often associated with pronounced psychological cravings and obsessive drug-seeking behavior.

Women who use amphetamines during pregnancy risk premature birth, stillbirth, low birth weight, and early infant death. Babies born to amphetamine-using mothers have a higher incidence of cleft palate, cleft lip, and deformed limbs. They may also experience symptoms of withdrawal from amphetamines.

**Ritalin**  A stimulant with amphetamine-like effects, Ritalin (methylphenidate) is used to treat attention-deficit/hyperactivity disorder (ADHD). When taken orally at prescribed levels, it has little potential for abuse. When injected or snorted, however, dependence and tolerance can rapidly result.

**Ephedrine**  Although somewhat less potent than amphetamine, ephedrine produces stimulant effects. Ephedrine has been linked to heart arrhythmia, stroke, psychotic reactions, seizures, and some deaths, and it may be particularly dangerous at high doses or when combined with another stimulant such as caffeine. The FDA has banned the sale of ephedrine (see Chapter 14).

**Caffeine**  Caffeine is probably the most popular psychoactive drug and also one of the most ancient. It is found in coffee, tea, cocoa, soft drinks, headache remedies, and OTC preparations like NōDōz.

*In addition to being one of the most popular psychoactive drugs, caffeine is one of the most ancient.*

# Meth and the Environment: A Toxic Impact

Most people know about the toxic effects of methamphetamine on users' health. Fewer people are aware of the toxic effects meth has on the environment.

Although most meth sold in the United States comes from large-scale drug trafficking organizations, the do-it-yourself appeal of meth production has led to the proliferation of small-scale clandestine labs across the country. Users and dealers set up meth labs in kitchens, bathrooms, garages, and abandoned buildings and cook up the drug using commonly available household and automotive chemicals. Although meth labs are found in urban and suburban areas, they are particularly prevalent in rural areas, where it is easier to escape detection.

One meth ingredient, pseudoephedrine, a drug found in cold and allergy medications, is now restricted to behind-the-counter sale in pharmacies, as part of a national attempt to stem the "meth epidemic." Other, more toxic ingredients include engine starter fluid (ether), paint thinner, acetone, freon, anhydrous ammonia, iodine, red phosphorus (used in matches and road flares), brake cleaner (toluene), drain cleaner (sodium hydroxide/lye), battery acid (sulfuric acid), hydrochloric acid, reactive chemicals (sodium or lithium), and gasoline additives (methanol, alcohol). Because many of these ingredients are volatile and flammable, explosions and fires are common occurrences in meth labs.

For every pound of meth produced in a meth lab, about 5 pounds of toxic waste are created. This toxic waste is usually dumped down the drain, in yards or fields, or by back roads,

creating toxic waste sites. Poisonous fumes from the waste are released into the air, and toxic chemicals contaminate streams and leach into water supplies. Livestock have been killed by these poisons, as have trees and vegetation. People have stumbled on meth dump sites, which can be recognized by strong chemical odors or the presence of items like empty containers of antifreeze or lye or equipment like rubber tubing or gas cans.

When a waste dump or clandestine lab is discovered, a cleanup has to be undertaken, following EPA regulations. Private contractors with specialized training and equipment provide hazardous waste removal and disposal services to local and state law enforcement agencies and the U.S. Drug Enforcement Administration. The cost of a cleanup ranges from the hundreds to the thousands of dollars, paid by taxpayers. Additional costs come from property damage, lowered property values, medical care for innocent bystanders (including children), and criminal justice expenses. Houses and other structures used as meth labs are often so toxic they have to be destroyed.

Meth isn't the only drug with a negative effect on the environment. An estimated 60% of outdoor marijuana cultivation in the United States takes place on public land, especially the remote parts of national parks and forests. Growers use fertilizers and pesticides to grow the plants and poisons to kill deer and bear who wander too close to the crops. For every acre of forest used to grow marijuana, 10 acres are damaged by toxic chemicals.

In Central and South America, millions of acres of rainforest have been burned and cleared for the production of coca plants, contributing to soil erosion, air and water pollution, flooding, and global warming. Poisonous chemicals are used to produce cocaine in jungle labs, endangering hundreds of species of mammals, birds, and fish. For every 2 pounds of coca paste produced, 1300 pounds of trash are generated and 200 gallons of water contaminated.

What can be done to reduce the impact of drug production on the environment? One answer lies in reducing the demand for drugs. In 2010, Mexican president Felipe Calderon blamed the United States for the drug wars in his country, saying Mexico is located next to the country with the highest levels of drug consumption in the world and likening the United States to "the biggest drug addict in the world." Even if the Mexican president was being dramatic, reducing the American addiction to illicit drugs would go a long way toward improving the welfare of the global environment.

**SOURCES:** U.S. DEA. 2010. *Environmental Impacts of Methamphetamine* (http://www.justice.gov/dea/concern/meth_environment.html; retrieved November 3, 2010); U.S. DEA. 2009. *Demand Reduction, Costs to Society* (http://www.justthinktwice.com/costs/DamagetoEnvironment.cfm; retrieved November 3, 2010); U.S. DEA. 2005. *Comprehensively Combating Methamphetamine: Impact on Health and the Environment* (http://www.justice.gov/dea/speeches/s102005.html; retrieved November 3, 2010); Booth, W. 2010. *Mexico's deadly drug violence claims hundreds of lives in past 5 days*. June 6 (http://www.washingtonpost.com; retrieved November 3, 2010).

(Table 9.4 lists typical levels of caffeine in several popular beverages.) In ordinary doses, caffeine produces greater alertness and a sense of well-being. It also decreases feelings of fatigue or boredom; using caffeine may enable a person to keep at physically tiring or repetitive tasks longer. Such use is usually followed, however, by a sudden letdown. Caffeine does not noticeably influence a person's ability to perform complex mental tasks unless fatigue, boredom, or other factors have already affected normal performance.

| Table 9.4 | Caffeine Content of Popular Beverages | |
|---|---|---|
| | SERVING SIZE | TYPICAL CAFFEINE LEVEL (MG)* |
| **COFFEE** | | |
| Regular coffee, brewed | 8 oz. | 95 |
| Regular coffee, instant | 8 oz. | 93 |
| Espresso | 1 oz. | 64 |
| Decaffeinated coffee, brewed | 8 oz. | 5 |
| Decaffeinated coffee, instant | 8 oz. | 2 |
| **TEA** | | |
| Regular tea, brewed | 8 oz. | 47 |
| Decaffeinated tea, brewed | 8 oz. | 2 |
| Green tea, brewed | 8 oz. | Varies |
| **SODA** | | |
| Code Red Mountain Dew | 12 oz. | 54 |
| Mello Yello | 12 oz. | 53 |
| Diet Coke | 12 oz. | 47 |
| Dr. Pepper, Diet Dr. Pepper | 12 oz. | 41 |
| Sunkist Orange Soda | 12 oz. | 41 |
| Pepsi | 12 oz. | 38 |
| Coca-Cola Classic, Diet Pepsi | 12 oz. | 35 |
| **ENERGY DRINKS** | | |
| No Name | 8.4 oz. | 280 |
| SoBe No Fear | 16 oz. | 174 |
| Monster Energy, Rockstar | 16 oz. | 160 |
| SoBe Adrenaline Rush | 16 oz. | 152 |
| Full Throttle, Full Throttle Fury | 16 oz. | 144 |
| AMP Energy Drink | 16 oz. | 143 |
| Red Bull | 8.3 oz. | 76 |
| Vault | 8 oz. | 47 |

*Caffeine levels vary greatly by brand of product, manner of preparation, and amount consumed. The amounts shown here are averages based on tests conducted by a variety of organizations. The U.S. Food and Drug Administration limits the amount of caffeine in cola and pepper soft drinks to 71 milligrams per 12-ounce serving. To find the exact amount of caffeine in any product, check that product's label.

SOURCES: Center for Science in the Public Interest. 2007. *Caffeine Content of Food & Drugs* (http://www.cspinet.org/new/cafchart.htm; retrieved November 3, 2010); Mayo Clinic. 2008. *Caffeine Content in Tea, Soda, and More* (http://www.mayoclinic.com/health/caffeine/AN01211; retrieved November 3, 2010); U.S. Department of Agriculture, Agricultural Research Service. 2009. *USDA National Nutrient Database for Standard Reference, Release 22* (http://www.ars.usda.gov/ba/bhnrc/ndl; retrieved November 3, 2010).

Caffeine mildly stimulates the heart and respiratory system, increases muscular tremor, and enhances gastric secretion. Higher doses may cause nervousness, anxiety, irritability, headache, disturbed sleep, and gastric irritation or peptic ulcers. In people with high blood pressure, caffeine can cause blood pressure to rise even further above normal; in people with type 2 diabetes, caffeine may cause glucose and insulin levels to rise after meals.

Some people, especially children, are quite vulnerable to the adverse effects of caffeine. They become wired: hyperactive and overly sensitive to any stimulation in their environment. In rare instances, the disturbance is so severe that there is misperception of their surroundings—a toxic psychosis.

Drinks containing caffeine are rarely harmful for most people, but some tolerance develops, and withdrawal symptoms of irritability, headaches, and even mild depression do occur. Thus, although we don't usually think of caffeine as a dependence-producing drug, for some people it is. People can usually avoid problems by simply decreasing their daily intake of caffeine; if intake is decreased gradually, withdrawal symptoms can be reduced or avoided. About 80–90% of American adults consume caffeine regularly; the average daily intake is about 280 mg.

## Marijuana and Other Cannabis Products

Marijuana is the most widely used illegal drug in the United States (cocaine is second). About 47% of Americans have tried marijuana at least once. In 2008, nearly 19% of 18–20-year-old and 15% of 21–25-year-old Americans reported using marijuana at least once within the past month.

Marijuana is a crude preparation of various parts of the Indian hemp plant *Cannabis sativa*, which grows in most parts of the world. THC (tetrahydrocannabinol) is the main active ingredient in marijuana. Based on THC content, the potency of marijuana preparations varies widely. Marijuana plants that grow wild often have less than 1% THC in their leaves. When selected strains are cultivated by separation of male and female plants (*sinsemilla*), the bud leaves from the flowering tops may contain 7–8% THC. Hashish, a potent preparation made from the thick resin that exudes from the marijuana leaves, may contain up to 14% THC.

These various preparations have all been known and used for centuries, so the frequently heard claim that today's marijuana is more potent than the marijuana of the 1970s is not strictly true. However, a greater proportion of the marijuana sold today is the higher-potency (and more expensive) sinsemilla; hence, the average potency of street marijuana has increased.

Marijuana is usually smoked, but it can also be ingested. The classification of marijuana is a matter of some debate. For this reason, it is treated separately here.

**Short-Term Effects and Uses**   As is true with most psychoactive drugs, the effects of a low dose of marijuana are strongly influenced both by the user's expectations and by past experiences. At low doses, marijuana users typically experience euphoria, a heightening of subjective sensory experiences, a slowing down of the perception of passing time, and a relaxed, laid-back attitude. These pleasant effects are the reason this drug is so widely used. With moderate doses, marijuana's effects become stronger, and the user can also expect to have impaired memory function, disturbed thought patterns, lapses of attention, and feelings of **depersonalization**, in which the mind seems to be separated from the body.

At higher doses, marijuana's effects are determined mostly by the drug itself rather than by the user's expectations and setting. Very high doses produce feelings of depersonalization, as well as marked sensory distortion and changes in body image (such as a feeling that the body is very light). Inexperienced users sometimes think these sensations mean they are going crazy and become anxious or even panicky. Unexpected reactions are the leading reason for emergency department visits by users of marijuana or hashish.

Physiologically, marijuana increases heart rate and dilates certain blood vessels in the eyes, which creates the characteristic bloodshot eyes. The user may also feel less inclined toward physical exertion and may feel particularly hungry or thirsty. THC affects parts of the brain controlling balance, coordination, and reaction time; thus marijuana use impairs driving performance. The combination of alcohol and marijuana is even more dangerous: Even a low dose of marijuana, when combined with alcohol, significantly impairs driving performance and increases crash risk.

In 1999, the Institute of Medicine determined that some compounds in marijuana may have legitimate medical use. For example, marijuana has been shown to ease pain, reduce nausea, and increase appetite. These benefits led several states to approve the use of "medical marijuana" by extremely ill patients, with physician monitoring. However, because growing, selling, or possessing marijuana is a federal crime, the Supreme Court has held that state laws permitting medical marijuana use cannot supersede federal law. This means anyone who uses marijuana for medical reasons—even in a state that approves such use—can still be prosecuted under federal drug laws, although the Obama administration made it known that it would not pursue such prosecutions. Currently, more than 30 states have medical marijuana laws on their books.

**Long-Term Effects**   The most probable long-term effect of smoking marijuana is respiratory damage, including impaired lung function and chronic bronchial irritation. Although there is no evidence linking marijuana use to lung cancer, it may cause changes in lung tissue that promote cancer growth. Marijuana users may be at increased risk for emphysema and cancer of the head and neck; among people with chronic conditions like cancer and AIDS, marijuana use is associated with increased risk of fatal lung infections. (These are key reasons the Institute of Medicine has recommended the development of alternative methods of delivering the potentially beneficial compounds in marijuana.) Heavy users may experience learning problems, as well as subtle impairments of attention and memory that may or may not be reversible following long-term abstinence. Long-term use may also decrease testosterone levels and sperm counts and increase sperm abnormalities.

Heavy marijuana use during pregnancy may cause impaired fetal growth and development, low birth weight, and increased risk of ectopic pregnancy. Marijuana may act synergistically with alcohol to increase the damaging effects of alcohol on the fetus. THC rapidly enters breast milk and may impair an infant's early motor development.

**Dependence**   Regular users of marijuana can develop tolerance; some develop dependence, and researchers estimate that 1.5% of Americans meet the APA criteria for marijuana dependence. Withdrawal symptoms may occur in the majority of dependent or heavy users; common symptoms include anger or aggression, irritability,

Marijuana is the most widely used illegal drug in the United States.

nervousness or restlessness, sleep difficulties, and decreased appetite or weight loss.

## Hallucinogens

**Hallucinogens** are a group of drugs whose predominant pharmacological effect is to alter the user's perceptions, feelings, and thoughts. Hallucinogens include the following:

- LSD (lysergic acid diethylamide)
- Mescaline
- Psilocybin
- STP (4-methyl-2,5-dimethoxyamphetamine)
- DMT (dimethyltryptamine)
- MDMA (3,4-methylene-dioxymethamphetamine)
- Ketamine
- PCP (phencyclidine)

These drugs are most commonly ingested or smoked.

**LSD**  LSD is one of the most powerful psychoactive drugs. Tiny doses will produce noticeable effects in most people, such as an altered sense of time, visual disturbances, an improved sense of hearing, mood changes, and distortions in how people perceive their bodies. Dilation of the pupils and slight dizziness, weakness, and nausea may also occur. With larger doses, users may experience a phenomenon known as **synesthesia**, feelings of depersonalization, and other alterations in the perceived relationship between the self and external reality.

Many hallucinogens induce tolerance so quickly that after only one or two doses their effects decrease substantially. The user must then stop taking the drug for several days before his or her system can be receptive to it again. These drugs cause little drug-seeking behavior and no physical dependence or withdrawal symptoms.

The immediate effects of low doses of hallucinogens are largely determined by expectations and setting. Many effects are hard to describe because they involve subjective and unusual dimensions of awareness—the **altered states of consciousness** for which these drugs are famous. For this reason, hallucinogens have acquired a certain aura not associated with other drugs. People have taken LSD in search of a religious or mystical experience or in the hope of exploring new worlds. During the 1960s, some psychiatrists gave LSD to their patients to help them talk about their repressed feelings.

A severe panic reaction, which can be terrifying in the extreme, can result from taking any dose of LSD. It is impossible to predict when a panic reaction will occur. Some LSD users report having had hundreds of pleasurable and ecstatic experiences before having a bad trip, or bummer. If the user is already in a serene mood and feels no anger or hostility and if he or she is in secure surroundings with trusted companions, a bad trip may be less likely, but a tranquil experience is not guaranteed.

Even after the drug's chemical effects have worn off, spontaneous flashbacks and other psychological disturbances can occur. **Flashbacks** are perceptual distortions and bizarre thoughts that occur after the drug has been entirely eliminated from the body. Although they are relatively rare phenomena, flashbacks can be extremely distressing. They are often triggered by specific psychological cues associated with the drug-taking experience, such as certain mood states or even types of music.

**Other Hallucinogens**  Most other hallucinogens have the same general effects as LSD, but there are some variations. For example, a DMT or ketamine high does not last as long as an LSD high; an STP high lasts longer. MDMA has both hallucinogenic and amphetamine-like properties. Tolerance to MDMA develops quickly, and high doses can cause anxiety, delusions, and paranoia. (See the box "Club Drugs" for more on MDMA.)

PCP reduces and distorts sensory input, especially proprioception, the sensation of body position and movement; it creates a state of sensory deprivation. PCP was initially used as an anesthetic but was unsatisfactory because it caused agitation, confusion, and delirium (loss of contact with reality). Because it can be easily made, PCP is often available illegally and is sometimes used as an inexpensive replacement for other psychoactive drugs.

The effects of ketamine are similar to those of PCP—confusion, agitation, aggression, and lack of coordination—but they tend to be less predictable. Tolerance to either drug can develop rapidly.

Mescaline, derived from the peyote cactus, is the ceremonial drug of the Native American Church. It causes effects similar to LSD, including altered perception and feeling; increased body temperature, heart rate, and blood pressure; weakness and trembling; and sleeplessness. Mescaline is expensive, so most street mescaline is diluted LSD or a mixture of other drugs. Hallucinogenic effects can be obtained from certain mushrooms (*Psilocybe mexicana*, or "magic mushrooms"), certain morning glory seeds, nutmeg, jimsonweed, and other botanical products, but unpleasant side effects, such as dizziness, have limited the popularity of these products.

---

**depersonalization**  A state in which a person loses the sense of his or her reality or perceives his or her body as unreal.

**hallucinogen**  Any of several drugs that alter perception, feelings, or thoughts; examples are LSD, mescaline, and PCP.

**synesthesia**  A condition in which a stimulus evokes not only the sensation appropriate to it but also another sensation of a different character, such as when a color evokes a specific smell.

**altered states of consciousness**  Profound changes in mood, thinking, and perception.

**flashback**  A perceptual distortion or bizarre thought that recurs after the chemical effects of a drug have worn off.

## Inhalants

Inhaling certain chemicals can produce effects ranging from heightened pleasure to delirium and death. Inhalants fall into several major groups:

- Volatile solvents, which are found in products such as paint thinner, glue, and gasoline
- Aerosols, which are sprays that contain propellants and solvents
- Nitrites, such as butyl nitrite and amyl nitrite
- Anesthetics, which include nitrous oxide, or laughing gas

Inhalant use tends to be highest among younger adolescents and declines with age; in 2008, 3.9% of teens ages 12–17 had used inhalants during the past year, as had 1.6% of young adults ages 18–25.

Inhalant use is difficult to control because inhalants are easy to obtain. They are present in a variety of seemingly harmless products, from dessert-topping sprays to underarm deodorants, that are both inexpensive and legal. Using the drugs also requires no illegal or suspicious paraphernalia. Inhalant users get high by sniffing, snorting, "bagging" (inhaling fumes from a plastic bag), or "huffing" (placing an inhalant-soaked rag in the mouth).

Although different in makeup, nearly all inhalants produce effects similar to those of anesthetics, which slow down body functions. Low doses may cause users to feel slightly stimulated; at higher doses, users may feel less inhibited and less in control. Sniffing high concentrations of the chemicals in solvents or aerosol sprays can cause a loss of consciousness, heart failure, and death. High concentrations of any inhalant can also cause death from suffocation by displacing oxygen in the lungs and central nervous system. Deliberately inhaling from a bag or in a closed area greatly increases the chances of suffocation. Other possible effects of the excessive or long-term use of inhalants include damage to the nervous system; hearing loss; increased risk of cancer; and damage to the liver, kidneys, and bone marrow.

**Ask Yourself**

Do you know any young teens who may be at risk for using inhalants? If so, would you try to intervene in some way? What would you tell a youngster to convince him or her to stop inhaling chemicals?

**67%** of inhalant users were under the age of 18 when they first tried it.

—SAMHSA, 2009

QUICK STATS

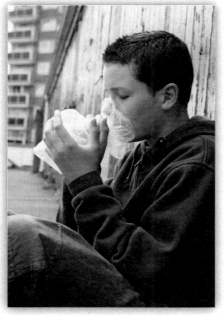

Inhalant use is difficult to monitor and control because inhalants are found in many inexpensive and legal products.

## DRUG USE: THE DECADES AHEAD

Drug research will undoubtedly provide new information, new treatments, and new chemical combinations in the decades ahead. New psychoactive drugs may present unexpected possibilities for therapy, social use, and abuse. Making honest and unbiased information about drugs available to everyone, however, may cut down on their abuse.

Although the use of some drugs, both legal and illegal, has declined dramatically since the 1970s, the use of others has held steady or increased. Mounting public concern has led to great debate and a wide range of opinions about what should be done. Efforts to combat the problem include workplace drug testing, tougher law enforcement and prosecution, and treatment and education. With drugs entering the country on a massive scale from South America, Southeast Asia, and elsewhere, and being distributed through tightly controlled drug-smuggling organizations and street gangs, the success of any program is uncertain.

## Drugs, Society, and Families

The economic cost of drug abuse is staggering. According to the National Institute on Drug Abuse, the cost to society of illicit drug abuse alone is $181 billion annually. That figure exceeds $500 billion when combined with the costs of alcohol and tobacco use, including health care, criminal justice, and lost productivity. But the costs are more than just financial; they are also paid in human pain and suffering.

The relationship between drugs and crime is complex. The criminal justice system is inundated with people accused of crimes related to drug possession, sale, or use. The FBI reports that more than 1.7 million arrests are made annually for drug violations; at any given time, more than 100,000 people are in jail for violating drug laws. Many assaults and murders are committed when people try to acquire or protect drug territories, settle disputes about drugs, or steal from dealers. Violence and gun use are common in neighborhoods where drug trafficking is prevalent. Addicts commit more robberies and burglaries than criminals not on drugs. People under the influence of drugs, especially alcohol, are more likely to commit violent crimes like rape and murder than people who do not use drugs. Although often associated with poor inner-city areas and ethnic minorities, drug-related problems affect all groups and every area of the country (see the box "Drug Use and Ethnicity").

Drug use is also a health care issue for society. In the United States, illegal drug use leads to more than 800,000 emergency department admissions and nearly 20,000 deaths annually. Although it is in the best interest of society to treat addicts who want help, there is not nearly enough space in treatment facilities to help the millions of Americans who need immediate treatment. Drug addicts who want to quit, especially those among the urban poor, often have to wait a year or more for acceptance into a residential care or other treatment program.

Drug abuse also takes a toll on individuals and families. Children born to women who use drugs such as alcohol, tobacco, or cocaine may have long-term health problems. Drug use in families can become a vicious cycle. Observing adults around them using drugs, children assume it is an acceptable way to deal with problems. Abuse, neglect, lack of opportunity, and unemployment become contributing factors to drug use and serve to perpetuate the cycle.

## Legalizing Drugs

Pointing out that many of the social problems associated with drugs are related to prohibition rather than to the effects of the drugs themselves, some people have argued for various forms of drug legalization or decriminalization. Proposals range from making drugs such as marijuana and heroin available by prescription to allowing licensed dealers to sell some of these drugs to adults. Proponents argue that legalizing some currently illicit drugs—but putting controls on them similar to those used for alcohol, tobacco, and prescription drugs—could eliminate many of the problems. A measure to legalize recreational marijuana use and allow it to be sold and taxed was placed on the ballot in California in November 2010. Voters defeated that proposal by a significant margin.

Opponents of drug legalization argue that allowing easier access to drugs would expose many more people to possible abuse and dependence. Drugs would be cheaper and easier to obtain, and drug use would be more socially acceptable. Legalizing drugs could cause an increase in drug use among children and teenagers. Opponents point out that alcohol and tobacco are major causes of disease and death in our society and that they should not be used as models for other practices.

## Drug Testing

The workplace is another segment of our society where drug use is common. According to data from recent surveys, the majority of substance users hold full-time jobs and constitute a significant public health problem in the workplace. Drug use in the workplace not only creates health problems for individual users, but it has a *Many American businesses **require workers to take drug tests;** a substantial number of employers offer counseling and treatment support for workers who test positive.* negative effect on productivity and on safety of coworkers. People who use drugs at work face higher rates of absenteeism, poor health, and a greater likelihood of harming themselves or others in the workplace.

Statistics from the federal government show that 8.4% of full-time workers were illicit drug users in 2007. In absolute numbers, approximately 13.1 million current illicit drug users and 13 million heavy alcohol users were full-time workers in 2007. Illicit drug use is highest among workers in the food industry and construction sectors, while heavy alcohol use is greatest among construction, mining, and repair workers. Premature death, illness, and disability—factors associated with the economic and health burden of lost productivity—are estimated to run as high as $114 billion for drug use and $179 billion for heavy alcohol use.

The extent of the problem has given rise to the development of workplace policies to help workers regain their health and well-being. Workplace policies developed to address the problem often include drug testing and referral services. Despite controversial aspects of drug testing in the workplace, a growing number of U.S. workers recognize the need for such screening.

**DIMENSIONS OF DIVERSITY**

## Drug Use and Ethnicity

Surveys of the U.S. population find a variety of trends in drug use and abuse among ethnic groups (see table). In addition to these general trends, there are also trends relating to specific drugs. For example, cocaine use is more prevalent among whites than among other groups, and hallucinogen use is more prevalent among American Indians and Alaska Natives.

However, as is true for many areas of health, ethnic trends are influenced by a complex interplay of other factors:

- *Educational status:* Adults with four or more years of college are more likely to have *tried* illicit drugs than are people of the same age who never finished high school. *Current* drug use, however, is lower among college graduates than among people with less education. Among teens, poor school performance is associated with a higher risk of drug use.

- *Employment status:* Most adult drug users are employed, but rates of current drug use are much higher among people who are unemployed or who work part-time compared with those who are employed full-time.

| NATIONAL SURVEY RESULTS, 2008 | | |
|---|---|---|
| | LIFETIME DRUG USE (PERCENT) | PAST YEAR DRUG USE (PERCENT) |
| White | 50.7 | 14.4 |
| Black or African American | 46.1 | 16.9 |
| Hispanic or Latino | 36.4 | 12.3 |
| Asian American | 21.2 | 7.4 |
| American Indian and Alaska Native | 57.6 | 19.5 |
| Native Hawaiian and Pacific Islander American | N/A | N/A |
| Two or more races | 56.1 | 22.2 |

Note: Results shown in percentages of each population group.
N/A = Data not available.

- *Parental education and socioeconomic status:* Students from poor families have higher rates of *early* drug use compared with students from wealthier families. By the twelfth grade, the differences disappear. Socioeconomic status and parental education are closely linked.

- *Geographic area:* Current drug use in the United States is highest in the West and Midwest; drug use is also higher in metropolitan and urban areas compared with more rural areas. People living in communities with high rates of poverty, crime, and unemployment have higher-than-average rates of drug use and abuse. Specific drugs may also be more available—and their abuse more prevalent—in certain regions or communities.

Strong cultural identity is associated with reduced risk of drug use and abuse among all groups. The following factors may contribute to lower rates of drug use among such groups:

- *Parental and community disapproval of drug and alcohol use:* Parents of Asian American children tend to have more restrictive drug and alcohol use norms than African American and white parents. Black parents tend to monitor their children's activities and friendships more closely than white parents.

Parental disapproval of drug use is often tied to greater perceived risk of drug use—and lower rates of drug use—among teens.

- *Close family ties:* Asian American teens are the likeliest to come from intact homes. Respect for authority and family loyalty are strongly valued among many Asian American populations. Black teens, although least likely to come from intact homes, often come from single-parent households with close extended family ties. Teens from cohesive and stable families are less likely to use drugs.

- *Focus on schooling and education:* Teens from families who value education and where parents help with homework and limit weeknight time with friends have lower rates of drug use. Asian Americans have twice the rate of college graduation compared with other groups.

**SOURCES:** Johnston, L. D., et al. 2009. *Monitoring the Future: National Results on Adolescent Drug Use—Overview of Key Findings, 2008.* Bethesda, Md.: National Institute on Drug Abuse, NIH Publication No. 09-7401; Substance Abuse and Mental Health Services Administration, Office of Applied Studies. 2009. *Results from the 2008 National Survey on Drug Use and Health: National Findings.* Rockville, Md.: Office of Applied Studies, NSDUH Series H-36, HHS Publication No. SMA 09-4434.

Many companies test current and prospective employees for drug use.

Most drug testing involves a urine test; a test for alcohol involves a blood test or a breath test. The accuracy of these tests has improved in recent years, so there are fewer opportunities for people to cheat or for the tests to yield inaccurate results. If a person tests positive for drugs, the employer may provide drug counseling or treatment, suspend the employee until he or she tests negative, or fire the individual.

The FDA has approved several over-the-counter home drug testing kits designed to allow parents to check their children for drug use. Urine samples are collected at home; preliminary results may be available immediately, but final results require that the sample be sent to a laboratory for analysis. Many experts, including the American Academy of Pediatrics, advise against the use of home tests in cases of suspected drug use; instead, they recommend a comprehensive evaluation by a qualified health care professional.

## Treatment for Drug Dependence

Treatment for drug dependence is sometimes characterized by discrete episodes of short-term abstinence and relapse. Regardless of the therapeutic approach used for drug dependence, many individuals undergoing treatment will often slide back into their drug habits. Often, this backsliding results in worsening of the original substance-abuse problem. For some substances, the period from abstinence to relapse occurs within one year after treatment.

Preventing relapse and maintaining long-term cessation of drug use is an exceedingly complex medical goal. Medical interventions based on pharmaceutical aids to enhance the individual's long-term commitment to change and stay drug-free remains a distant and elusive goal. Relapse prevention research is instead increasingly focusing on the need to expand the behavioral repertoire of skills needed to decrease the risk of recidivism among individuals receiving drug-treatment services.

**Medication-Assisted Treatment**   Medications are increasingly being used in addiction treatment—to reduce the craving for the abused drug or to block or oppose its effects. Perhaps the best-known medication for drug abuse is methadone, a synthetic drug used as a substitute for heroin. Use of methadone prevents withdrawal reactions and reduces the craving for heroin; it enables dependent people to function normally in social and vocational activities, although they remain dependent on methadone. The narcotic buprenorphine, approved for treatment of opioid addiction, also reduces cravings. Many other medications are under study; drugs used specifically in the treatment of nicotine and alcohol dependence are discussed in Chapters 10 and 11.

**2.1 million** Americans received treatment for illicit drug abuse in 2008.

—SAMHSA, 2009

QUICK STATS

Medication therapy is relatively simple and inexpensive and is therefore popular among patients, health care providers, and insurance companies. However, the relapse rate is high. Combining drug therapy with psychological and social services improves success rates, underscoring the importance of psychological factors in drug dependence.

**Treatment Centers**   Treatment centers offer a variety of short-term and long-term services, including hospitalization, detoxification, counseling, and other mental health services. The therapeutic community is a specific type of center, a residential program run in a completely drug-free atmosphere. Administered by ex-addicts, these programs use confrontation, strict discipline, and unrelenting peer pressure to attempt to resocialize the addict with a different set of values. Halfway houses, transitional settings between a 24-hour-a-day program and independent living, are an important phase of

## Choosing a Drug-Treatment Program

When evaluating different facilities or programs for drug treatment, consider the following issues:

• *What type of treatment or facility is most appropriate?* Intensive outpatient treatment is available through many community mental health centers, as well as through specialized drug-treatment facilities. Such programs typically require several sessions per week, combining individual therapy, group counseling, and attendance at 12-step meetings. Residential, or inpatient, facilities may be associated with a medical facility such as a hospital, or they may be freestanding programs that focus solely on substance-abuse treatment. Some residential treatment programs last longer or cost more per week than many health insurance plans will cover.

• *How will treatment be paid for?* Many health insurance plans limit residential treatment to a maximum of 3 weeks or less. They may also require that you first attempt a less expensive form of treatment before they will approve coverage for a residential facility.

• *Is there likely to be a need for medical support?* Chronic alcoholics or abusers of other CNS depressants may experience life-threatening seizures or other withdrawal symptoms during the first few days of detoxification. Malnutrition is common among substance abusers, and injection drug users may suffer from local infections and bloodborne diseases such as hepatitis or HIV infection. Medical problems such as these are best handled in an inpatient program with good medical support.

• *What is the level of professional training of the staff?* Is there a medical doctor on-site or making frequent visits? Are there trained nurses? Licensed psychologists or social workers? Many successful programs are staffed primarily by recovering alcoholics or drug users. Those staff members should have training and certification as addiction specialists.

• *Does the program provide related services, such as family and job counseling and post-treatment follow-up?* These types of services are extremely important for the long-term success of drug-abuse treatment.

• *Can you visit the facility and speak with the staff and clients?* A prospective client and his or her family should be allowed to visit any treatment center or program.

---

treatment for some people. Strategies for evaluating programs are given in the box "Choosing a Drug-Treatment Program."

**Groups and Peer Counseling** Groups such as Alcoholics Anonymous (AA) and Narcotics Anonymous (NA) have helped many people. People treated in drug substitution programs or substance-abuse treatment centers are often urged or required to join a self-help group as part of their recovery. These groups follow a 12-step program. Group members' first step is to acknowledge that they have a problem over which they have no control. Peer support is a critical ingredient of these programs, and members usually meet at least once a week. Each member is paired with a sponsor to call on for advice and support if the temptation to relapse becomes overwhelming. With such support, thousands of substance-dependent people have been able to recover, remain abstinent, and reclaim their lives. Chapters of AA and NA meet on some college campuses; community-based chapters are listed in the phone book and in local newspapers.

Many colleges also have peer counseling programs, in which students are trained to help other students who have drug problems. A peer counselor's role may be as limited as referring a student to a professional with expertise in substance dependence for an evaluation or as involved as helping arrange a leave of absence from school for participation in a drug-treatment program. Most peer counseling programs are founded on

principles of strict confidentiality. Peer counselors may also be able to help students who are concerned about a classmate or loved one with an apparent drug problem (see the box "If Someone You Know Has a Drug Problem . . ."). Information about peer counseling programs is usually available from the student health center.

**Harm Reduction Strategies** Recognizing that many attempts at treatment are at first unsuccessful and that a drug-free society may be an unobtainable goal, some experts advocate the use of harm reduction strategies. The goal of harm reduction is to minimize the negative effects of drug use and abuse; a common example is the use of designated drivers to reduce alcohol-related motor vehicle crashes. In terms of illicit drugs, drug substitution programs such as methadone maintenance are one form of harm reduction; although participants remain drug dependent, the negative individual and social consequences of their drug use are reduced. Syringe exchange programs, designed to reduce transmission of HIV and hepatitis C, are another harm reduction approach. Some experts have also suggested free testing of street drugs for purity and potency to help users avoid unintentional toxicity or overdose.

**Codependency** Many treatment programs also offer counseling for those who are close to drug abusers. Drug abuse takes a toll on friends and family members, and counseling can help people work through painful

## If Someone You Know Has a Drug Problem . . .

Changes in behavior and mood in someone you know may signal a growing dependence on drugs. Signs that a person's life is beginning to focus on drugs include the following:

- Sudden withdrawal or emotional distance
- Rebellious or unusually irritable behavior
- A loss of interest in usual activities or hobbies
- A decline in school performance
- A sudden change in the chosen group of friends
- Changes in sleeping or eating habits
- Frequent borrowing of money or stealing
- Secretive behavior about personal possessions, such as a backpack or the contents of a drawer
- Deterioration of physical appearance

If you believe a family member or friend has a drug problem, locate information about drug treatment resources available on campus or in your community. Communicate your concern, provide him or her with information about treatment options, and offer your support during treatment. If the person continues to deny having a problem, talk with an experienced counselor about setting up an intervention—a formal, structured confrontation designed to end denial by having family, friends, and other caring people present their concerns to the drug user. Participants in an intervention would indicate the ways in which the individual is hurting others as well as himself or herself. If your friend or family member agrees to treatment, encourage him or her to attend a support group such as Narcotics Anonymous or Alcoholics Anonymous.

And finally, examine your relationship with the abuser for signs of codependency. If necessary, get help for yourself; friends and family of drug users can often benefit from counseling.

feelings of guilt and powerlessness. **Codependency,** in which a person close to the drug abuser is controlled by the abuser's behavior, sometimes develops. Codependent people may come to believe that love, approval, and security are contingent on their taking care of the abuser. People can become codependent naturally because they want to help when someone they love becomes dependent on a drug. They may assume that their good intentions will persuade the drug user to stop.

Codependent people often engage in behaviors that remove or soften the effects of drug use on the user—so-called *enabling* behaviors. However, the habit of enabling can inhibit a drug abuser's recovery because the person never has to experience the consequences of his or her behavior. Often, the enabler is dependent, too—on the patterns of interaction in the relationship. People who need to take care of others often marry people who need to be taken care of. Children in these families often develop the same behavior pattern as one of their parents, by either becoming helpless or becoming a caregiver. For this reason, many treatment programs involve the whole family.

Have you ever been an enabler in a relationship? You may have, if you've ever done any of the following:

- Given someone one more chance to stop abusing drugs, then another, and another . . .
- Made excuses or lied for someone to his or her friends, teachers, or employer
- Joined someone in drug use and blamed others for your behavior
- Lent money to someone to continue drug use
- Stayed up late waiting for or gone out searching for someone who uses drugs

- Felt embarrassed or angry about the actions of someone who uses drugs
- Ignored the drug use because the person got defensive when you brought it up
- Not confronted a friend or relative who was obviously intoxicated or high on a drug

If you come from a codependent family or see yourself developing codependency relationships or engaging in enabling behaviors, consider acting now to make changes in your patterns of interaction. Remember, you cannot cause or cure drug dependence in another person.

### Preventing Drug Abuse

Obviously, the best solution to drug abuse is prevention. Government attempts at controlling the drug problem have historically focused on stopping the production, importation, and distribution of illegal drugs. A new national drug policy announced in 2010, however, redirects federal funding and efforts into stopping the demand for drugs. Developing persuasive antidrug educational programs offers the best hope for solving the drug problem in the future. Indirect approaches to prevention involve building young people's self-esteem, improving their academic skills, and increasing their recreational opportunities. Direct approaches involve providing information

---

**codependency** A relationship in which a non–substance-abusing partner or family member is controlled by the abuser's behavior; codependent people frequently engage in enabling behaviors.

TERMS

## Ask yourself

Do you know someone who may have a drug problem? What steps, if any, have you taken to help that person? If you were using drugs and felt that things had gone out of control, what would you want your friends to do for you?

about the adverse effects of drugs and teaching tactics that help students resist peer pressure to use drugs in various situations. Developing strategies for resisting peer pressure is one of the more effective techniques.

Prevention efforts need to focus on the different motivations individuals have for using and abusing specific drugs at different ages. For example, grade-school children seem receptive to programs that involve their parents or well-known adults such as professional athletes. Adolescents in junior or senior high school are often more responsive to peer counselors. Many young adults tend to be influenced by efforts that focus on health education. For all ages, it is important to provide nondrug alternatives—such as recreational facilities, counseling, greater opportunities for leisure activities, and places to socialize—that speak to the individual's or group's specific reasons for using drugs. Reminding young people that most people, no matter what age, are *not* users of illegal drugs, do *not* smoke cigarettes, and do *not* get drunk frequently is a critical part of preventing substance abuse.

## Connect to your Choices

Have you ever thought about why you make the choices you do about drugs? Many factors can influence the drug-related choices we make, some not as obvious as others. If you use drugs—or if you don't—have you been influenced by attitudes toward drug use in your family or peer group? Do you take drugs when they're offered at parties because it's easier than saying no? Are you influenced by the lyrics of songs that make drug use sound glamorous?

**What are the external factors that influence your drug-related choices? What are your inner motivations and core values, and how do they affect your choices? Based on what you learned in this chapter, will you make some different choices in the future? If so, what will they be?**

**Go online to Connect to complete this activity. www.mcgraw-hillconnect.com**

## TIPS FOR TODAY AND THE FUTURE

**RIGHT NOW YOU CAN**
- If you are a regular caffeine user, look for ways to cut back.
- Consider whether you or someone you know might benefit from drug counseling. Find out what types of services are available on campus or in your area.

**IN THE FUTURE YOU CAN**
- Study the drug-related attitudes of people you know. For example, talk to two older adults and two fellow students about their attitudes toward legalizing marijuana. What are the differences in their opinions, and how do they account for them?
- Analyze media portrayals of drug use. As you watch TV shows and movies, note the way they depict drug use among people of different ages and backgrounds. How realistic are the portrayals, in your view? Think about the influence they have on you and your peers.

## SUMMARY

- Addictive behaviors are self-reinforcing. Addicts experience a strong compulsion for the behavior and a loss of control over it; an escalating pattern of abuse with serious negative consequences may result.

- The sources or causes of addiction include heredity, personality, lifestyle, and environmental factors. People may use an addictive behavior as a means of alleviating stress or painful emotions.

- Many common behaviors are potentially addictive, including gambling, shopping, sexual activity, Internet use, eating, and working.

- Drug abuse is a maladaptive pattern of drug use that persists despite adverse social, psychological, or medical consequences.

- Drug dependence involves taking a drug compulsively, which includes neglecting constructive activities because of it and continuing to use it despite experiencing adverse effects resulting from its use. Tolerance and withdrawal symptoms are often present.

- Reasons for using drugs include the lure of the illicit; curiosity; rebellion; peer pressure; and the desire to alter one's mood or escape boredom, anxiety, depression, or other psychological problems.

- Psychoactive drugs affect the mind and body by altering brain chemistry. The effect of a drug depends on the properties of the drug and how it's used (drug factors), the physical and psychological characteristics of the user (user factors), and the physical and social environment surrounding the drug use (social factors).

# Changing Your Drug Habits

This behavior change strategy focuses on one of the most commonly used drugs—caffeine. If you are concerned about your use of a different drug or another type of addictive behavior, you can devise your own plan based on this one and on the steps outlined in Chapter 1.

Because caffeine supports certain behaviors that are characteristic of our culture, such as sedentary, stressful work, you may find yourself relying on coffee (or tea, chocolate, or cola) to get through a busy schedule. Such habits often begin in college. Fortunately, it's easier to break a habit before it becomes entrenched as a lifelong dependency.

When you are studying for exams, the forced physical inactivity and the need to concentrate even when fatigued may lead you to overuse caffeine. But caffeine doesn't help unless you are already sleepy. And it does not relieve any underlying condition (you are just more tired when it wears off). How can you change this pattern?

## Self-Monitoring

Keep a log of how much caffeine you eat or drink. Use a measuring cup to measure coffee or tea. Using Table 9.4, convert the amounts you drink into an estimate expressed in milligrams of caffeine. Be sure to include all forms, such as chocolate bars and OTC medications, as well as caffeine candy, colas, cocoa or hot chocolate, chocolate cake, tea, and coffee.

## Self-Assessment

At the end of the week, add up your daily totals and divide by 7 to get your daily average in milligrams. How much is too much? At more than 250 mg per day, you may well be experiencing some adverse symptoms. If you are experiencing at least five of the following symptoms, you may want to cut down.

- Restlessness
- Nervousness
- Excitement
- Insomnia
- Flushed face
- Excessive sweating
- Gastrointestinal problems
- Muscle twitching
- Rambling thoughts and speech
- Irregular heartbeat
- Periods of inexhaustibility
- Excessive pacing or movement

## Set Limits

Can you restrict your caffeine intake to a daily total, and stick to this contract? If so, set a cutoff point, such as one cup of coffee. Pegging it to a specific time of day can be helpful, because then you won't confront a decision at any other point (and possibly fail). If you find you cannot stick to your limit, you may want to cut out caffeine altogether; abstinence can be easier than moderation for some people. If you experience caffeine withdrawal symptoms (headache, fatigue), you may want to cut your intake more gradually.

## Find Other Ways to Keep Up Your Energy

If you are fatigued, it makes sense to get enough sleep or exercise more, rather than drowning the problem in coffee or tea. Different people need different amounts of sleep; you may also need more sleep at different times, such as during a personal crisis or an illness. Also, exercise raises your metabolic rate for hours afterward—a handy fact to exploit when you need to feel more awake and want to avoid an irritable caffeine jag. And if you've been compounding your fatigue by not eating properly, try filling up on complex carbohydrates such as whole-grain bread or crackers instead of candy bars.

**Tips on Cutting Out Caffeine** Here are some more ways to decrease your consumption of caffeine:

- Keep some noncaffeinated drinks on hand, such as decaffeinated coffee, herbal teas, mineral water, bouillon, or ice water.
- Alternate between hot and very cold liquids.
- Fill your coffee cup only halfway.
- Avoid the office or school lunchroom or cafeteria and the chocolate sections of the grocery store. (Often people drink coffee or tea and eat chocolate simply because they're available.)
- Read labels of over-the-counter medications to check for hidden sources of caffeine.

---

- Opioids relieve pain, cause drowsiness, and induce euphoria; they reduce anxiety and produce lethargy, apathy, and an inability to concentrate.

- CNS depressants slow down the overall activity of the nerves; they reduce anxiety and cause mood changes, impaired muscular coordination, slurring of speech, and drowsiness or sleep.

- CNS stimulants speed up the activity of the nerves, causing acceleration of the heart rate, a rise in blood pressure, dilation of the pupils and bronchial tubes, and an increase in gastric and adrenal secretions.

- Marijuana usually causes euphoria and a relaxed attitude at low doses; very high doses produce feelings of depersonalization and sensory distortion. The long-term effects may include chronic bronchitis and cancer; use during pregnancy may impair fetal growth.

- Hallucinogens alter perception, feelings, and thought and may cause an altered sense of time, visual disturbances, and mood changes.

- Inhalants are present in a variety of everyday products; they can cause delirium. Their use can lead to loss of consciousness, heart failure, suffocation, and death.

- Economic and social costs of drug abuse include the financial costs of law enforcement, treatment, and health care and the social costs of crime, violence, and family problems. Drug testing and drug legalization have been proposed to address some of the problems related to drug abuse.

- Approaches to treatment include medication, treatment centers, self-help groups, and peer counseling; many programs also offer counseling to family members.

## FOR MORE INFORMATION

### BOOKS

Aue, P. W. 2007. *Teen Drug Abuse: Opposing Viewpoints.* San Diego: Greenhaven Press. *Explores key issues relating to drug use and abuse by teenagers.*

Hanson, G. R., et al. 2008. *Drugs and Society,* 10th ed. Boston: Jones & Bartlett. *Discusses the impact of drug abuse on individuals' lives and on the broader society.*

Ksir, C., C. L. Hart, and O. S. Ray. 2010. *Drugs, Society, and Human Behavior,* 14th ed. New York: McGraw-Hill. *Examines drugs and behavior from the behavioral, pharmacological, historical, social, legal, and clinical perspectives.*

Lessa, N. R., et al. 2006. *Wiley Concise Guides to Mental Health: Substance Use Disorders.* New York: Wiley. *A clearly written introduction to the diagnosis and treatment of various kinds of substance abuse.*

Murphy, P. J. M., and M. Shlafer. 2006. *Over-the-Counter Drugs of Abuse.* New York: Chelsea House Publications. *An up-to-date discussion of nonprescription medicines and their abuse.*

Rosen Publishing. 2009. *Drug Abuse and Society Series.* New York: Rosen Publishing. *A series of short books, each exploring a different type of drugs—from prescription medicine to club drugs—and their use and abuse.*

### ORGANIZATIONS, HOTLINES, AND WEB SITES

*ClubDrugs.Gov.* Provides information on drugs commonly classified as "club drugs."
http://www.clubdrugs.gov

*Do It Now Foundation.* Provides youth-oriented information about drugs.
http://www.doitnow.org

*Drug Enforcement Administration: Drug Information.* Provides basic facts about major drugs of abuse, including penalties for drug trafficking.
http://www.dea.gov/concern/concern.htm

*Gamblers Anonymous.* Includes questions to help diagnose gambling problems and resources for getting help.
http://www.gamblersanonymous.org

*Higher Education Center for Alcohol and Other Drug Abuse and Violence Prevention.* Gives information about alcohol and drug abuse on campus and links to related sites.
http://www.higheredcenter.org

*Indiana Prevention Resource Center.* A clearinghouse of information on substance-abuse topics, including specific psychoactive drugs and issues such as drug testing and drug legalization.
http://www.drugs.indiana.edu

*Narcotics Anonymous (NA).* Similar to Alcoholics Anonymous, NA sponsors 12-step meetings and provides other support services for drug abusers.
http://www.na.org
There are also 12-step programs that focus on specific drugs:
Cocaine Anonymous
http://www.ca.org
Marijuana Anonymous
http://www.marijuana-anonymous.org

*National Center on Addiction and Substance Abuse (CASA) at Columbia University.* Provides information about the costs of substance abuse to individuals and society.
http://www.casacolumbia.org

*National Clearinghouse for Alcohol and Drug Information.* Provides statistics, information, and publications on substance abuse, including resources for people who want to help friends and family members overcome substance-abuse problems.
http://ncadi.samhsa.gov

*National Council on Problem Gambling.* Provides information and help for people with gambling problems and their families, including a searchable directory of counselors.
http://www.ncpgambling.org

*National Drug Information, Treatment, and Referral Hotlines.* Sponsored by the SAMHSA Center for Substance Abuse Treatment, these hotlines provide information on drug abuse and on HIV infection as it relates to substance abuse; referrals to support groups and treatment programs are available.
800-662-HELP
800-729-6686 (Spanish)
800-487-4889 (TDD for hearing impaired)

*National Institute on Drug Abuse.* Develops and supports research on drug-abuse prevention programs.
http://www.drugabuse.gov

*Substance Abuse and Mental Health Services Administration (SAMHSA).* Provides statistics, information, and other resources related to substance-abuse prevention and treatment.
http://www.samhsa.gov

See also the listings for Chapters 10 and 11.

## SELECTED BIBLIOGRAPHY

American Psychiatric Association. 2000. *Diagnostic and Statistical Manual of Mental Disorders,* 4th ed., text revision. *(DSM-IV-TR).* Washington, D.C.: American Psychiatric Association.

Beers, M. H., et al. 2006. *The Merck Manual of Diagnosis and Therapy,* 18th ed. New York: Wiley.

Centers for Disease Control and Prevention. 2006. Methamphetamine Use and HIV Risk Behaviors Among Heterosexual Men. *Morbidity and Mortality Weekly Report* (55)10: 273–277.

Centers for Disease Control and Prevention. 2009. Surveillance for Acute Viral Hepatitis—United States, 2007. *Morbidity and Mortality Weekly Report Surveillance Summaries* 58(SS–3): 1–30.

Centers for Disease Control and Prevention. 2010. *HIV Surveillance Report, 2008; vol. 20* (http://www.cdc.gov/hiv/topics/surveillance/resources/reports; retrieved November 3, 2010).

Colfax, G., et al. 2005. Longitudinal patterns of methamphetamine, popper (amyl nitrite), and cocaine use and high-risk sexual behavior among a cohort of San Francisco men who have sex with men. *Journal of Urban Health,* 28 February [epub].

Grant, J. E., et al. 2006. Multicenter investigation of the opioid antagonist nalmefene in the treatment of pathological gambling. *American Journal of Psychiatry* 163(2): 303–312.

Hurd, Y. L., et al. 2005. Marijuana impairs growth in mid-gestation fetuses. *Neurotoxicology and Teratology* 27(2): 221–229.

Iannone, M., et al. 2006. Electrocortical effects of MDMA are potentiated by acoustic stimulation in rats. *BMC Neuroscience* 7: 13.

Jefferson, D. J. 2005. America's most dangerous drug. *Newsweek*, 8 August, 41–48.

Kim, S. W., et al. 2006. Pathological gambling and mood disorders: Clinical associations and treatment implications. *Journal of Affective Disorders* 92(1): 109–116.

Johnston, L. D., et al. 2009. *Monitoring the Future: National results on adolescent drug use—Overview of key findings, 2008.* Bethesda, Md.: National Institute on Drug Abuse, NIH Publication No. 09-7401.

Mahowald, M. L., J. A. Singh, and P. Majeski. 2005. Opioid use by patients in an orthopedics spine clinic. *Arthritis and Rheumatology* 52(1): 312–321.

Messinis, L., et al. 2006. Neuropsychological deficits in long-term frequent cannabis users. *Neurology* 66(5): 737–739.

National Council on Problem Gambling. 2010. *What Is Problem Gambling?* (http://www.ncpgambling.org/i4a/pages/index.cfm?pageid=1; retrieved November 3, 2010).

National Institute on Drug Abuse. 2008. *Comorbidity: Addiction and Other Mental Illnesses.* Bethesda, Md.: National Institute on Drug Abuse, NIH Publication No. 08-5771.

Office of National Drug Control Policy. 2010. *2010 National Strategy* (http://www.whitehousedrugpolicy.gov/strategy/; retrieved November 3, 2010).

Parrott, A. C. 2005. Chronic tolerance to recreational MDMA (3,4-methylenedioxymethamphetamine) or ecstasy. *Journal of Psychopharmacology* 19(1): 71–83.

Ren, S., et al. 2006. Effect of long-term cocaine use on regional left ventricular function as determined by magnetic resonance imaging. *American Journal of Cardiology* 97(7): 1085–1088.

Savoca, M. R., et al. 2005. Association of ambulatory blood pressure and dietary caffeine in adolescents. *American Journal of Hypertension* 18(1): 116–120.

Substance Abuse and Mental Health Services Administration, Office of Applied Studies. 2009. *The NSDUH Report: Concurrent Illicit Drug and Alcohol Use.* Rockville, Md.: Office of Applied Studies, NSDUH 128.

Substance Abuse and Mental Health Services Administration, Office of Applied Studies. 2009. *Results from the 2008 National Survey on Drug Use and Health: National Findings.* Rockville, Md.: Office of Applied Studies, NSDUH Series H-36, HHS Publication No. SMA 09-4434.

Substance Abuse and Mental Health Services Administration, Office of Applied Studies. 2010. *Drug Abuse Warning Network, 2007: National Estimates of Drug-Related Emergency Department Visits.* Rockville, Md.: Substance Abuse and Mental Health Services Administration.

U.S. Department of Justice, Federal Bureau of Investigation. 2009. *Crime in the United States: 2008* (http://www.fbi.gov/ucr/cius2008/index.html; retrieved November 3, 2010).

Wareing, M., et al. 2005. Visuo-spatial working memory deficits in current and former users of MDMA ("ecstasy"). *Human Psychopharmacology* 20(2): 115–23.

Waska, R. 2006. Addictions and the quest to control the object. *American Journal of Psychoanalysis* 66(1): 43–62.

Zakzanis, K. K., and Z. Campbell. 2006. Memory impairment in now abstinent MDMA users and continued users: A longitudinal follow-up. *Neurology* 66(5): 740–741.